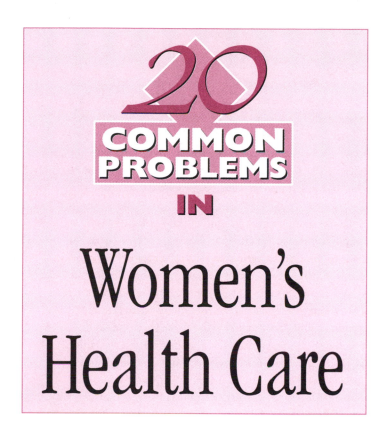

20 COMMON PROBLEMS IN

Women's Health Care

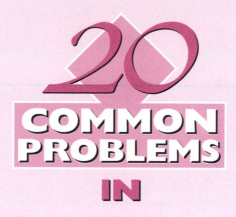

20 COMMON PROBLEMS

IN

Women's Health Care

EDITORS

MINDY A. SMITH, M.D., M.S.

Associate Professor, Department of Family Practice, College of Human Medicine,
Michigan State University, East Lansing, Michigan

LESLIE A. SHIMP, Pharm.D., M.S.

Associate Professor of Pharmacy, College of Pharmacy and Assistant Professor of Pharmacy
in Family Medicine, Medical School, University of Michigan, Ann Arbor, Michigan

SERIES EDITOR

BARRY D. WEISS, M.D.

Professor of Clinical Family and Community Medicine
University of Arizona College of Medicine, Tucson, Arizona

McGraw-Hill

Health Professions Division

New York   St. Louis   San Francisco   Auckland   Bogotá   Caracas   Lisbon   London   Madrid
Mexico City   Milan   Montreal   New Delhi   San Juan   Singapore   Sydney   Tokyo   Toronto

McGraw-Hill

A Division of The **McGraw·Hill** *Companies*

20 COMMON PROBLEMS IN WOMEN'S HEALTH CARE

1 2 3 4 5 6 7 8 9 0 DOCDOC 00

ISBN 0-07-069767-1

This book was set in Garamond by V&M Graphics, Inc.
The editors were Martin Wonsiewicz, Susan Noujaim, and Nicky Panton.
The production supervisor was Catherine Saggese.
The cover designer was Marsha Cohen/Parallelogram.
The color insert was designed by Robert Freese.
The index was prepared by Geraldine Beckford.

R. R. Donnelley and Sons Company was printer and binder.

This book is printed on acid-free paper.

Library of Congress Cataloging-in-Publication Data

20 common problems in women's health care / editors, Mindy A. Smith, Leslie
   A. Shimp.
      p.   ;   cm.
   Includes bibliographical references and index.
   ISBN 0-07-069767-1
   1. Women—Diseases. 2. Women—Health and hygiene. I. Title: Twenty com-
mon problems in women's health care. II. Smith, Mindy A. III. Shimp, Leslie A.
[DNLM: 1. Women's Health. 2. Maternal Health Services. 3. Women's Health
Services. WA 309 Z4 2000]
RC48.6.A15 2000
616′.0082—dc21   99–054486

We dedicate this book to the many wonderful women who've touched our lives.
To our nurturers in the form of grandmothers
(Fanny, Frieda, Helen G., and
Helen M.),
mothers (Dotty and Peggy),
and
daughters (Emma and Jenny),
supportive and inspirational colleagues and friends,
our students who teach and challenge us,
and our patients who invite us into their lives with
trust and who provide the impetus for continued learning
and improved understanding;
and to four special and supportive men in our lives
(Arthur, Fred, Gary, and Nick).

Contents

Contributors

ABUSE OF WOMEN (CHAPTER 7)

Valerie J. Gilchrist, M.D.
Professor and Chair
Department of Family Medicine
NEOUCOM
Rootstown, Ohio

BREAST DISORDERS (CHAPTER 16)

Mindy A. Smith, M.D., M.S.
Associate Professor
Department of Family Practice
College of Human Medicine
Michigan State University
East Lansing, Michigan

Linda Boyd, D.O.
Assistant Professor
Department of Family Medicine
New Jersey Medical School
Newark, New Jersey

Janet R. Osuch, M.D.
Professor
Department of Surgery
Michigan State University
East Lansing, Michigan

Kendra Schwartz, M.D., M.S.P.H.
Associate Professor
Department of Family Practice
Wayne State University
Detroit, Michigan

DEPRESSION AND ANXIETY
(CHAPTER 9)

Jonathan G. A. Henry, M.D.
Medical Director
Clinton-Eaton-Ingham Community Health Board
and
Clinical Assistant Professor
Department of Psychiatry
Michigan State University
College of Human Medicine
East Lansing, Michigan

FAMILY PLANNING (CHAPTER 2)

Mindy A. Smith, M.D., M.S.
Associate Professor
Department of Family Practice
College of Human Medicine
Michigan State University
East Lansing, Michigan

Leslie A. Shimp, Pharm.D., M.S.
Associate Professor of Pharmacy
College of Pharmacy
and
Assistant Professor of Pharmacy in Family Medicine,
Medical School
University of Michigan
Ann Arbor, Michigan

GALLBLADDER DISEASE
(CHAPTER 19)

Diana Curran, M.D.
Clinical Assistant Professor
Department of Family Medicine
University of North Carolina - Chapel Hill
and
Medical Director
Hendersonville Family Practice Residency Program
Hendersonville, North Carolina

GASTROINTESTINAL DISORDERS (CHAPTER 18)

Rosemary R. Berardi, Pharm.D., F.A.S.H.P.
Professor of Pharmacy
College of Pharmacy
University of Michigan
and
Clinical Pharmacist Gastroenterology
Department of Pharmacy
University of Michigan
Ann Arbor, Michigan

Juliana Chan, Pharm.D.
Research Assistant Professor of Pharmacy Practice
and Pharmacotherapist
Digestive and Liver Diseases
College of Pharmacy
University of Illinois at Chicago
Chicago, Illinois

Ellen M. Zimmermann, M.D.
Assistant Professor of Medicine
Department of Internal Medicine
Division of Gastroenterology
School of Medicine
University of Michigan
Ann Arbor, Michigan

HYPERTENSION AND ISCHEMIC HEART DISEASE (CHAPTER 17)

James P. Olson, M.D.
Assistant Director
Sparrow Hospital Family Practice Residency
Michigan State University Affiliated
Mason, Michigan

Duane Warren, Pharm.D., B.C.P.S.
Assistant Adjunct Professor
Department of Family Practice
College of Human Medicine
Michigan State University
East Lansing, Michigan
and
Director of Clinical Services
Pharmacy Group Practice Associates
Okemos, Michigan

MENSTRUAL DISORDERS (CHAPTER 13)

Louise Parent-Stevens, Pharm.D., B.C.P.S.
Clinical Assistant Professor
Department of Pharmacy Practice
College of Pharmacy
University of Illinois at Chicago
Chicago, Illinois

Elizabeth A. Burns, M.D., M.A.
Professor and Head of Department of Family Medicine
University of Illinois at Chicago
Chicago, Illinois

MENOPAUSE (CHAPTER 4)

Leslie A. Shimp, Pharm.D., M.S.
Associate Professor of Pharmacy
College of Pharmacy
and
Assistant Professor of Pharmacy in Family Medicine,
Medical School
University of Michigan
Ann Arbor, Michigan

Mindy A. Smith, M.D., M.S.
Associate Professor
Department of Family Practice
College of Human Medicine
Michigan State University
East Lansing, Michigan

MISCARRIAGE (CHAPTER 15)

Louise Acheson, M.D., M.S.
Associate Professor
Department of Family Medicine
Case Western Reserve University
Cleveland, Ohio

OBESITY AND EATING DISORDERS (CHAPTER 6)

Elizabeth A. Alexander, M.D., M.S.
Professor
Department of Family Practice
Michigan State University
College of Human Medicine
East Lansing, Michigan

Leslie A. Shimp, Pharm.D., M.S.
Associate Professor of Pharmacy
College of Pharmacy
and
Assistant Professor of Pharmacy in Family Medicine,
Medical School
University of Michigan
Ann Arbor, Michigan

Mindy A. Smith, M.D., M.S.
Associate Professor
Department of Family Practice
College of Human Medicine
Michigan State University
East Lansing, Michigan

OSTEOPOROSIS (CHAPTER 20)

Barbara Kaplan-Machlis, Pharm.D.
Associate Professor of Clinical Pharmacy and Family Medicine
West Virginia University-Charleston Division
School of Pharmacy
Charleston, West Virginia

Kathleen P. Bors, M.D.
Assistant Professor of Family Medicine
West Virginia University-Charleston Division
Family Medicine Center of Charleston
Charleston, West Virginia

PRENATAL CARE (CHAPTER 3)

Margaret R. Helton, M.D.
Clinical Assistant Professor
University of North Carolina
Department of Family Medicine
Chapel Hill, North Carolina

RELATIONAL PROBLEMS (CHAPTER 10)

Jenny Speice, Ph.D.
Senior Instructor of Psychiatry and Medicine
Primary Care Institute and Wynne Center for Family Research
University of Rochester School of Medicine and Dentistry
Rochester, New York

Audrey Farley, M.D.
Director
Brighton Women's Health Center
Brighton, Colorado

Susan McDaniel, Ph.D.
Professor of Psychiatry and Family Medicine
Primary Care Institute and Wynne Center for Family Research
University of Rochester School of Medicine
Rochester, New York

SEXUALITY (CHAPTER 5)

Linda A. Bernhard, Ph.D., R.N.
Associate Professor
Department of Adult Health and Illness Nursing and
Department of Women's Studies
The Ohio State University
Columbus, Ohio

Robert W. Birch, Ph.D., F.A.A.C.S.
Psychologist and Certified Sex Therapist
Department of Family Relations and Human Development
Family Therapy Program
The Ohio State University
Columbus, Ohio

SEXUALLY TRANSMITTED DISEASES AND PELVIC INFLAMMATORY DISEASE (CHAPTER 14)

Charles D. Ponte, PharmD., C.D.E., B.C.P.S., F.A.S.H.P., F.C.C.P., F.A.Ph.A.
Professor of Clinical Pharmacy and Family Medicine
West Virginia University
Morgantown, West Virginia

Karen M. Gross, M.D.
Assistant Professor of Family Medicine
Department of Family Medicine
West Virginia University
Morgantown, West Virginia

SUBSTANCE ABUSE (CHAPTER 8)

Bertram Stoffelmayr, Ph.D.
Professor
Department of Psychiatry
Michigan State University
East Lansing, Michigan

William C. Wadland, M.D., M.S.
Professor and Chair
Department of Family Practice
Michigan State University
East Lansing, Michigan

Sally K. Guthrie, Pharm.D.
Associate Professor
University of Michigan
College of Pharmacy
Ann Arbor, Michigan

**THE WOMEN'S HEALTH
MAINTENANCE
EXAMINATION** (CHAPTER 1)

Henry C. Barry, M.D., M.S.
Associate Professor
Department of Family Practice
Michigan State University
East Lansing, Michigan

Mark H. Ebell, M.D., M.S.
Associate Professor
Department of Family Practice
Michigan State University
East Lansing, Michigan

URINARY INCONTINENCE
(CHAPTER 12)

Leslie A. Shimp, Pharm.D., M.S.
Associate Professor of Pharmacy
College of Pharmacy
and
Assistant Professor of Pharmacy in Family Medicine,
Medical School
University of Michigan
Ann Arbor, Michigan

James F. Peggs, M.D.
Clinical Associate Professor and Associate Chair
Department of Family Medicine
School of Medicine
University of Michigan
Ann Arbor, Michigan

VULVA AND VAGINAL DISEASE
(CHAPTER 11)

Judith A. Suess, M.D., M.P.H.
Assistant Professsor
Department of Family Practice
College of Human Medicine
Michigan State University
East Lansing, Michigan

Claudia Holzman, D.V.M., M.P.H., Ph.D.
Assistant Professor
Department of Epidemiology
College of Human Medicine
Michigan State University
East Lansing, Michigan

Preface

This book is a part of the McGraw-Hill *20 Common Problems* series, a new series devoted to the common clinical problems seen daily in outpatient primary care practice. The purpose of this book is to provide comprehensive information on the common problems that women bring to their primary care health providers. The topics were chosen based on data obtained from the National Ambulatory Medical Care Survey and the National Center for Health Statistics and published papers about why women visit their health care providers and the kinds of problems they bring to these encounters. In addition, we sought advice from colleagues, friends, patients, and family members about the concerns of today's women. It was after one of these interesting and fruitful conversations that we added the final chapter to our list of 19 others. Based on the comment "the most common health care problem for women is men," the chapter on relational problems was born.

Women's Health Care

Women have unique medical problems and health care needs. Although federal health statistics demonstrate an improvement in the health status of men in the United States, the health status of women has not improved. This discrepancy raised the concern as to whether the health care system was addressing the needs of women. In particular, two issues were noted.

The first issue is that the health care needs of women transcend reproductive health concerns. Women's health care has been defined as "the screening, diagnosis, and management of conditions that are unique to women, more prevalent in women, more serious among women, have different risk factors for women, and/or require different interventions in women."[1] Women's health care needs extend beyond reproductive health concerns; the majority of health care women receive, even during their reproductive years, is not obstetric care. In 1997, the Federated Council for Internal Medicine (FCIM) developed consensus recommendations for competencies in women's health for primary care medical residents.[1] The chapters in this text cover over 90 percent of the topics included on the FCIM list. In addition, it is important for the definition of women's health to consider the sociocultural and emotional aspects of health as well as the physical aspects. These aspects influence the perception of women about the quality of care they receive and ultimately affect health care outcomes, by influencing the likelihood of health-promoting or health-threatening behaviors.

The second issue involves the lack of data from clinical trials on the management of diseases in women, which has contributed to compromises in the quality of medical care for women.[2] Clearly, women differ biologically from men in numerous ways. Factors such as body size, lean/fat ratios in body tissues, and the hormonal milieu can modify the effects of drugs, including appropriate dosage and drug metabolism. The documented inadequate diagnosis and management of heart disease in women is a powerful example of the clinical significance of ignoring gender differences. The authors of several chapters in this text, particularly the chapters on cardiovascular disease and substance abuse, have noted that the absence of research on women detracts from clinical knowledge and patient care. Fortunately, policy changes at the National Institutes of Health (NIH) and the Food and Drug Administration promote the inclusion of women in clinical trials, the study of diseases prevalent in women, and the importance of testing drugs in a broader range of patients, including women of childbearing age. In addition, a re-examination of the issue of conducting studies in pregnant women is attempting to balance the desire to protect the fetus with the need for better information on the best approaches for managing chronic illness during pregnancy and the influence of pregnancy on drug kinetics and on therapeutic and adverse effects. A recent NIH-sponsored trial on the treatment of women positive for human immunodeficiency virus with AZT (which showed decreased transmission of the disease for treated women) demonstrated the benefit to infants of studying drug therapy during pregnancy.

About this Book

One unique feature of this book is the focus on common problems. In our review of texts on women's health, we identified two dominant approaches to writing about women's health. Some books present highly detailed information about literally hundreds of potential problems encountered but no clear guidance about the diagnosis or management of the most likely problem. Conversely, other books present brief summaries of topics with outlines of steps in the work-up or treatment of a particular problem, but no depth or rationale is offered to support the approach proposed. It is often difficult in clinical practice to find a text with the right mix of clinically relevant information with enough detail to provide an understanding of the topic and yet easy access to information on the work-up and treatment options. By limiting the material presented to the most common problems seen in ambulatory care settings, we believe that this book provides just this mix of comprehensiveness with practical approaches based on evidence when possible. Each chapter has an extensive reference list, offering readers the opportunity to review the original literature and form their own opinions about the data presented.

Most chapters have multiple authors, including family physicians, primary care internists, pharmacists, and behavior medicine practitioners who offer their expertise and practical guidance from a practice-based perspective. Chapters therefore include many tables and algorithms where information on the diagnostic and treatment options are easily viewed and important aspects of drug therapy such as costs and side effects are quickly identified. The emphasis of the chapters is on empowerment of patients, providing education about options and negotiating care in the context of women's beliefs, values, and culture. Management sections of the chapters expand treatment options, including alternative/complementary choices, so that practitioners have maximal flexibility to select what appears to be optimal therapy while providing an alternative plan if the initial choice fails or is not tolerated.

The topics covered in this book are grouped into five areas. The section *Preventive Care and Health Maintenance* covers the topics of the health maintenance examination, family planning, prenatal care, and menopause. Evidence-based guidelines are emphasized and screening strategies, along with their rationales, are presented. Although recognizing that many providers who read this book do not offer pregnancy care, this chapter also provides information about symptom management and treatment options for common acute illnesses experienced by all women. In addition, these chapters provide information about how and when to discuss the issues that women face throughout their lives to optimize preventive care.

The sections *Womanhood: Choices and Challenges* and *Women in Trouble* offer the provider an in-depth understanding of the biopsychosocial and cultural aspects of women's sexuality and sexual dysfunctions, eating disorders and obesity, abuse, substance abuse, depression and anxiety, and relational problems. These often hidden problems have serious consequences for women, especially when unrecognized. The chapters offer concrete ways to identify and assist women with these problems and return them to healthy functioning. Issues about options in management and referrals assist providers in initiating treatment and offering guidance for patients without feeling overwhelmed.

A book on women's health is not complete without a review of common gynecologic concerns and this section of the book covers the topics of vaginitis, incontinence, menstrual disorders, sexually transmitted disease, miscarriage, and breast disorders. These chapters include figures to assist in the recognition of likely problems and present tables of treatment options based on their efficacy, cost, and availability (including nonprescription options). Because this section is limited to only common problems, the chapters have expanded information on the management of these problems throughout life, including safe options for pregnant and lactating mothers as well as optimal treatment for the elderly or those with special concerns or illness that may complicate treatment. In addition, information is provided on resources in the form of books or websites for patients and providers to expand the ability of providers to educate and support women.

The final section of the book presents common health problems that have a strong influence on women because of their high prevalence or unique aspects of their presentation or treatment. These problems include cardiovascular disease, gastrointestinal disorders, gallbladder disease, and osteoporosis. The chapter on cardiovascular disease offers recommendations based on the most recent published national guidelines and all chapters provide both in-depth and easy-to-access diagnostic and treatment approaches.

All chapters in this book are organized into multiple subsections making information easy to find. Diagnostic and treatment algorithms allow readers to quickly scan the information and locate the path that seems best for their particular patient.

In summary, this book is unique in that it is based on the current best evidence and provides detailed diagnostic and management options, including prescription and nonprescription drugs and alternative/complementary approaches. The concerns of women who present for care are discussed in the context of their unique biology and cultural perspectives. Finally, this book is distinctive in that it covers common issues relevant to women across the life span.

Who Should Read this Book

This text is highly relevant to all clinicians who provide primary care for women, including family physicians, internists, obstetricians/gynecologists, nurse practitioners, physician assistants, and pharmacists. In addition, medical students may find this text easy to read during their required rotations in family practice, internal medicine, and obstetrics/gynecology. There are few books that prepare students for the diagnosis and management of common problems experienced by the women students are likely to encounter in the office setting. This book offers practical and easily accessed information, in the form of algorithms, figures, and tables (that present cost as well as efficacy data) to allow for rapid and cost-effective decision-making during the medical encounter.

Finally, because of the strong focus on drug treatment presented, this book is appropriate for pharmacy students training in outpatient settings alongside medical students and residents. Clinical training for these students now includes more emphasis on advanced pharmacy services in ambulatory settings. As more women's health products move from prescription to nonprescription status, pharmacists will need greater training experience in the area of the management of common problems in women's health.

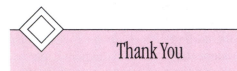

Thank You

We would like to thank our many authors whose expertise and painstaking efforts turned our sometimes sketchy outlines into comprehensive and informative chapters. The collaborative nature of our relationships with them and with the series editor, Dr. Barry Weiss, have enriched this experience for us in many ways. We know that the reader will benefit from the final product of their work.

References

1. American College of Physicians: Comprehensive women's health care: the role and commitment of internal medicine. *Am J Med* 103: 451, 1997.
2. Merkatz RB: Inclusion of women in clinical trails: a historical overview of scientific, ethical, and legal issues. *J Obstet Gynecol Neonatal Nurs* 27:78, 1998.

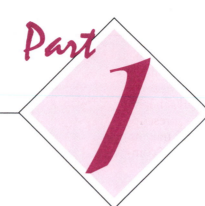

Part

1

Preventive Care/ Health Maintenance

Henry C. Barry
Mark H. Ebell

The Women's Health Maintenance Examination

Overview

The health maintenance examination (HME) is focused on providing women with clinical preventive services. These services include traditional screening tests, education about life-style choices and their consequences, and measures aimed at primary and secondary prevention of disease. Clinical preventive services are an important reason that women seek care and help explain why women are more likely to have an identified primary care physician, are more likely to see that physician during any given year, and are more likely than men to have more than one physician.[1]

A woman's choice of provider is strongly related to her economic status. Wealthier women are much more likely to have both a family physician or internist and an obstetrician/gynecologist, whereas less affluent women, those with comorbidities, and those with a worse self-perceived health status are more likely to have a family physician or internist as their sole source of care.[1] Based on a survey of seven common preventive services (complete physical examination, blood pressure, cholesterol, clinical breast examination, mammogram, pelvic examination, and Pap smear), women who see an obstetrician/gynecologist are more likely to receive these services than women seeing a family physician or internist (5.5 services versus 4.9 services, $P < .05$).[1] However, most elements of the complete physical examination (including pelvic examination) are not recommended by the United States Preventive Services Task Force for screening purposes, and clinical breast examination is optional in women who have had a mammogram.[2] It is, therefore, unclear whether women seen by obstetrician/gynecologists received better care or simply more care.

Given the greater likelihood that women seen by internists and family physicians are poor and have comorbidities, it is possible that limited access or appropriate selectivity can explain the lower number of preventive services provided. For example,

poor women are less likely to be able to afford a mammogram, and women who have had a hysterectomy (and who may therefore be less likely to see a gynecologist) do not need Pap tests and pelvic examinations. More research is needed to understand how different specialists provide clinical preventive services and whether the appropriate number of services are being ordered by each group.

In this chapter, we discuss the goals and organization of the HME. We also describe the criteria for a good screening test, so clinicians can evaluate new tests and procedures as they become available in the coming years. The recommendations for screening are largely based on the Guide to Clinical Preventive Services of the United States Preventive Services Task Force (USPSTF).[2] This book is highly recommended as a primary reference for every clinician who provides health care services to women because the recommendations for prevention are based on high-quality original research evidence.

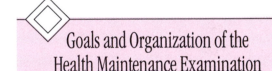

Goals and Organization of the Health Maintenance Examination

Goals of the Health Maintenance Examination

The goal of the HME is to provide appropriate clinical preventive services to the patient, based on her age, race, life-style, and other risk factors. Tailoring the HME is important because providing unnecessary services is costly and time-consuming. It can even be harmful if it leads to unnecessary invasive testing or inappropriate therapeutic recommendations. For example, the clinical breast examination in a 20-year-old woman (not recommended by the USPSTF) might lead to an unnecessary biopsy and significant emotional trauma. It may also lead that woman to label herself as high risk for breast cancer, when her risk is actually not altered by the presence or absence of benign breast diseases.

What Makes a Good Screening Test?

Medical conditions are appropriate candidates for clinical preventive services when they are common or have important health consequences. Effective and acceptable interventions must be available to treat the condition once identified. For example, it would be difficult to justify screening programs for brain malignancy or pancreatic cancer because these conditions are relatively uncommon and treatment regimens are generally not very effective. Most importantly, detection and treatment during the asymptomatic phase of the illness must provide important benefits to patients compared with treatment once symptoms are clinically apparent. Cervical cancer and breast cancer are good examples of such conditions.

In addition, the characteristics of available screening tests are important. The tests should be accurate enough to detect disease in the asymptomatic phase, while not subjecting too many patients to the discomfort, worry, and cost of "working-up" a false-positive screening test. Accuracy can be described in many ways, including sensitivity, specificity, predictive value, and likelihood ratios. Although a full discussion of these terms (defined in Table 1-1) is beyond the scope of this chapter, it is important to understand the trade-off between sensitivity and specificity. As sensitivity increases, specificity decreases, and vice versa. A lower sensitivity increases the risk of missing a woman with the disease (higher false-negative rate), whereas a lower specificity increases the risk of labeling a healthy woman as diseased (higher false-positive rate). Screening programs often will use a highly sensitive, less specific test for the initial screen (such as the enzyme-linked immunosorbent assay for HIV infection) and follow it with a highly specific test (the Western blot) to eliminate the false-positive results. Another example is mammography followed by breast biopsy.

Organization of the Health Maintenance Examination

SCREENING

Age- and risk factor–specific recommendations for screening during the history, physical examination, and laboratory evaluation phases of the HME are discussed below. They are based on

Table 1-1

Definitions of Terms

TERM	DEFINITION
Primary prevention	Prevention of disease before it is manifest (e.g., immunizations)
Secondary prevention	Prevention of complications when disease is present (e.g., early detection and treatment of breast cancer)
Sensitivity	The probability of a positive test result in affected patients
Specificity	The probability of a negative test result in unaffected patients
Positive predictive value	The probability of disease in patients with a positive test result
Negative predictive value	The probability of no disease in patients with a negative test result
Positive likelihood ratio	A ratio of the probability of a positive test result in affected individuals compared to unaffected individuals
Negative likelihood ratio	A ratio of the probability of a negative test result in affected individuals compared to unaffected individuals

recommendations from the Guide to Clinical Preventive Services, which are summarized in Tables 1-2, 1-3, and 1-4 for easy application to clinical practice.[2]

HISTORY/COUNSELING/PATIENT EDUCATION Although patients often think of screening and health maintenance in terms of the physical examination and laboratory testing, perhaps the greatest potential

Table 1-2

Clinical Preventive Services Recommended for Women Ages 11 to 24

INTERVENTION	INTERVAL
HISTORY/COUNSELING/EDUCATION	
Assess for problem drinking	Annually
Counsel regarding: seat belt use, helmet use (bike/motorcycle), smoke detector, firearm storage and use	Annually
Counsel regarding: tobacco, drug, and alcohol use	Annually
Counsel regarding: avoidance of high-risk sexual behavior and unintended pregnancy/ contraception	Annually
Counsel regarding: diet (fat, cholesterol, fruit, vegetable), adequate calcium intake, and regular exercise	Annually
Counsel regarding: dental hygiene	Annually
Multivitamin with folic acid for women planning pregnancy	Annually
PHYSICAL EXAMINATION	
Height and weight	Annually
Blood pressure	Annually
LABORATORY EVALUATION/IMMUNIZATION	
Pap test; may be discontinued if woman had a hysterectomy for nonmalignant disease. Risk factors include multiple partners, tobacco use, early onset of sexual intercourse, and low socioeconomic status. Start when sexually active or at age 18 if sexual history is unreliable.	At least every 3 y, more often in higher-risk women*
Chlamydia screen for high-risk women. Risk factors include age under 25, new or multiple partners, history of prior STD, cervical ectopy, inconsistent use of barrier contraceptives, or unmarried.	As needed based on risk factors
Rubella serology or vaccination history	Once
Tetanus-diphtheria (Td) boosters	At age 11–16 and every 10 y thereafter
Hepatitis B	One series
MMR and varicella	By age 11 or 12

*Based on recommendations from the American College of Physicians rather than the USPSTF.
†See text for additional discussion and description of interventions for certain high-risk women.[2]
ABBREVIATIONS: MMR, Measles, Mumps, Rubella; STD, sexually transmitted disease.

Table 1-3

Clinical Preventive Services Recommended for Women Ages 25 to 64

INTERVENTION	INTERVAL
HISTORY/COUNSELING/EDUCATION	
Assess for problem drinking	Annually
Counsel regarding: seat belt use, helmet use (bike/motorcycle), smoke detector, firearm storage and use	Annually
Counsel regarding: tobacco, drug, and alcohol use	Annually
Counsel regarding: avoidance of high-risk sexual behavior and unintended pregnancy/ contraception	Annually
Counsel regarding: diet (fat, cholesterol, fruit, vegetable), adequate calcium intake, and regular exercise	Annually
Counsel regarding: dental hygiene	Annually
Multivitamin with folic acid for women planning pregnancy	Annually
Discuss hormone replacement therapy if peri- or postmenopausal	As needed
PHYSICAL EXAMINATION	
Height and weight	Annually
Blood pressure	Annually
Clinical breast examination (over age 40; best evidence to support use in ages 50–69). Added benefit of clinical breast examination in addition to mammography is uncertain.	Annually
LABORATORY EVALUATION/IMMUNIZATION	
Pap test (may be discontinued if woman had a hysterectomy for nonmalignant disease)	At least every 3 y, more often in higher-risk women*
Cholesterol (over age 45)	About every 5 y
Rubella serology or vaccination history (if childbearing age)	Once
Chlamydia screen for high-risk women. Risk factors include new or multiple partners, history of prior STD, cervical ectopy, inconsistent use of barrier contraceptives, or unmarried.	As needed based on risk factors
Tetanus-diphtheria (Td) boosters	At age 11–16 and every 10 y thereafter
Hepatitis B	One series
MMR and varicella	By age 11 or 12
Fecal occult blood testing and/or sigmoidoscopy beginning at age 50	FOBT annually or sigmoidoscopy every 3–5 y
Mammogram (over age 40; best evidence to support use in ages 50–69)	Annually

*See text for additional discussion and description of interventions for certain high-risk women.[2]
ABBREVIATIONS: FOBT, fecal occult blood testing; MMR, measles, mumps, rubella; STD, sexually transmitted disease.

Table 1-4

Clinical Preventive Services Recommended for Women Ages 65 and Older

INTERVENTION	INTERVAL
HISTORY/COUNSELING/EDUCATION	
Assess for problem drinking	Annually
Assess for hearing impairment	Annually
Counsel regarding: seat belt use, helmet use (bike/motorcycle), smoke detector, firearm storage and use	Annually
Counsel regarding: tobacco, drug, and alcohol use	Annually
Counsel regarding: avoidance of high-risk sexual behavior	Annually
Counsel regarding: diet (fat, cholesterol, fruit, vegetable), adequate calcium intake, and regular exercise	Annually
Counsel regarding: fall prevention	
Counsel regarding: dental hygiene	Annually
CPR training for household members	
Discuss hormone replacement therapy	As needed
Set water heater to under 120–130°F	Once
PHYSICAL EXAMINATION	
Height and weight	Annually
Blood pressure	Annually
Clinical breast examination (over age 40; best evidence to support use in ages 50–69). Added benefit of clinical breast examination in addition to mammography is uncertain.	Annually
Vision screening	Annually
LABORATORY EVALUATION/IMMUNIZATION	
Pap test; (may be discontinued if woman had a hysterectomy for nonmalignant disease; may consider discontinuing use after age 65 in women who have had regular previous screening with consistently normal results).	At least every 3 y, more often in higher-risk women*
TSH using sensitive assay; if undetectable or > 10 mU/L, obtain free thyroxine (over age 50)*	Once, reconsider if symptomatic
Fecal occult blood testing and/or sigmoidoscopy	FOBT annually; sigmoidoscopy every 4–5 y
Mammogram (69 or under)	Every 1 to 2 years
Pneumococcal vaccine	Once; consider revaccination if > 6 y for high-risk individuals†
Influenza vaccine	Annually
Tetanus-diphtheria (Td) boosters	Every 10 y

*Based on recommendations from the American College of Physicians rather than the USPSTF.
†Nursing home resident, renal disease, immunosuppressed, chronic cardiopulmonary disease, or hemoglobinopathy.
‡See text for additional discussion and description of interventions for certain high-risk women.[2]
ABBREVIATIONS: CPR, cardiopulmonary resuscitation; FOBT, fecal occult blood testing; TSH, thyroid-stimulating hormone.

benefit derives from simply talking to patients about their lifestyles, risk factors, family history, and habits. In younger women, who are at the greatest risk for sexually transmitted diseases, it is particularly important to address risky sexual behavior and effective contraception. Women of all ages should be asked at each visit about use of tobacco, and smokers should be offered assistance in quitting. Women of all ages should also be asked about alcohol use during their HME. The most effective screening instrument for alcohol abuse among women is the TWEAK questionnaire. Although the CAGE questionnaire is more widely used, it is less sensitive for the detection of alcohol abuse in women.[3] The TWEAK questionnaire and guidelines for interpretation are summarized in Fig. 1-1.

The USPSTF advocates a relatively long list of items to discuss with women of all ages. They include injury prevention (use of lap and shoulder belts, bicycle/motorcycle helmets, smoke detectors, and storage of firearms), diet and exercise, dental health, and the issues around sexual behavior and substance use described above. Although difficult to cover in a single HME visit, they can be addressed by creative providers using a variety of approaches:

- Patient education handouts
- Wall posters
- Collaborative efforts with nurses, medical assistants, dietitians, social workers, and midlevel providers
- Group classes

Many providers will address some of these issues over time during both acute care and HME visits, tracking their educational progress on a form or a flow sheet in the chart.

SPECIAL CONSIDERATIONS FOR OLDER WOMEN Women's educational needs change as they age. Perimenopausal women should receive counseling regarding the risks and benefits of hormone replacement therapy. In general, only women at high risk for breast cancer and low risk for coronary artery disease will not benefit from hormone replacement therapy. A useful algorithm to help patients evaluate the risks and benefits can be found in Chap. 4. Elders should be counseled to reduce the risk of falls by removing throw rugs and installing assistive devices in the bath as necessary. In a nursing home setting, the following have been identified as risk factors for falls: psychotropic medication use, prior falls, wandering, use of a cane or walker, declining functional status, age over 87, unsteady gait, ability to transfer independently, and not using a wheelchair.[4] In-home exercise training can reduce the risk of falls.[5]

PHYSICAL EXAMINATION Many of the elements of the physical examination to which patients have become accustomed, such as cardiac auscultation, bimanual pelvic examination, and assessment of the patellar tendon reflex, have little if any value as screening tests. Although appropriate in symptomatic patients, and for evaluation of specific complaints, they should not be considered a necessary element of the HME.

The only elements of the physical examination that should routinely be performed are height, weight, and blood pressure. Clinical breast examination (CBE) in addition to mammography may provide some incremental value over mammography alone. The greatest sensitivity of the CBE was observed with a 5- to 10-min examination by specially trained examiners, not practical in most office settings.[6] Breast self-examination (BSE) has a very low sensitivity (12 to 25 percent) and uncertain specificity, and many are calling its routine use into question.[7] Unfortunately, no large-scale trials have randomized women to BSE or no BSE, so good evidence is not available. In summary, CBE should be carefully performed annually by a trained health care provider. Physicians might consider training nurses or midlevel providers who can take the 5 or 10 min necessary to perform a thorough and useful CBE.

The pelvic examination has long been a traditional part of the HME. However, except as a method for obtaining Pap smears or cervical cultures, the USPSTF does not recommend pelvic

Figure 1-1

Ask your patient these five questions, and add up the points for each affirmative response:

Item	Question	Points
Tolerance	How many drinks can you hold? (2 points if ≥ 6 drinks)	2
Worried	Have close friends or relatives worried or complained about your drinking in the past year?	2
Eye openers	Do you sometimes take a drink in the morning when you first get up?	1
Amnesia	Has a friend or family member ever told you about things you said or did while you were drinking that you could not remember?	1
Kut down	Do you sometimes feel the need to cut down on your drinking?	1
	Total (range 0 to 7):	

A score of 2 or more points is approximately 87% sensitive and 87% specific for a diagnosis of alcohol abuse, while a score of 3 or more points is 77% sensitive and 93% specific. To interpret these results, refer to the table below:

Your estimate of the likelihood of alcohol abuse before doing the test	Score	Probability of alcoholism with a score in this range
10%	TWEAK ≥ 2	43%
10%	TWEAK ≥ 3	55%
20%	TWEAK ≥ 2	62%
20%	TWEAK ≥ 3	73%

The TWEAK screening questionnaire for alcohol abuse.[3]

examinations as a routine screening test.[2] Although ovarian cancers can occasionally be detected using the pelvic examination, they are usually advanced and untreatable when found this way. Because women may associate the pelvic examination with a physician's thoroughness or care, it is important that the reasons for not performing this aspect of the physical examination be carefully explained.

LABORATORY EVALUATION/IMMUNIZATION

Pap Test. The Papanicolaou test is central to the health maintenance visit for most women. Although traditionally done annually, long-term follow-up of women who have had regular Pap tests and a better understanding of the biology of cervical cancer have led to a revision in these recommendations. In some countries, a screening interval of 3 to 5 years is standard practice. The USPSTF recommends that Pap smears begin with the onset of sexual activity and be repeated at least every 3 years, with more frequent examinations reserved for women at high risk (previous abnormal Pap test, multiple partners, or early onset of sexual activity).[2] This recommendation is based on high-quality evidence from cervical cancer screening programs in Canada and Europe, which found that the incidence of invasive cervical cancer was reduced 64 percent when the interval between Pap tests was 10 years, 83.6 percent at 5 years, 90.8 percent at 3 years, 92.5 percent at 2 years, and 93.5 percent at 1 year.[8] If women have been consistently screened throughout their lives, it is reasonable to stop Pap tests at age 65.[2]

Mammography. Mammography is another important screening test for women aged 40 and older. Although some groups have recommended a "baseline" mammogram between ages 35 and 40, no evidence supports this recommendation, and the practice should be abandoned. Mammography between the ages of 40 and 49 is similarly controversial. Because the premenopausal breast tissue is denser, and cancer less common, there is less benefit of screening this age group than for women aged 50 to 69. Although this explanation may be plausible and logical, some empirical evidence fuels the controversy.

In 1995, Kerlikowske[9] reported the results of a meta-analysis of the potential benefits of screening mammography in women under age 50 compared to women over age 50. Women over age 50 receiving mammograms had a 26 percent reduction (95 percent confidence interval was 17 to 34 percent) in breast cancer mortality risk. Women

aged 40 to 49 had a 7 percent reduction in breast cancer mortality risk (95 percent confidence interval showed the range of risk varied between a benefit of 24 percent to a harm of 13 percent). In other words, based on the literature, it is possible that younger women may have some benefit, but there may also be a harm to screening. This synthesis of the literature was confirmed by a cost-effectiveness analysis.[10] When compared to women not receiving mammography, screening of women aged 50 to 69 was associated with a 12-day increase in life expectancy per woman, at a cost of $704/woman and a cost-effectiveness of $21,400/year of life saved. Screening women between the ages of 40 and 49 would increase life expectancy by 2.5 days at an additional cost of $676/woman. This translates to an incremental cost-effectiveness of $105,000/year of life saved.

This controversy was underscored by the apparently conflicting recommendations of the National Cancer Institute (NCI). The 1993 NCI recommendations spoke only to screening women over the age of 50; no evidence indicated benefit to screening younger women. In 1997, a Consensus Development Panel, after reviewing the available research, issued a statement indicating that screening with mammography for women aged 40 to 49 could not be recommended and that decisions regarding mammography in this age group should be individualized. This recommendation would have placed the decision between a woman and her health care provider. Although shared decision-making is an admirable and appropriate goal, its implementation may be a problem in the absence of decision support tools. With these latter issues under consideration, combined with Congressional pressure, the National Institutes of Health issued their latest recommendation that women over age 40 should be screened. Regardless of the controversy and ongoing debate, screening this age group has become the de facto community standard in the United States.

Discontinuing Screening. Recommendations are less clear regarding when to stop screening for cervical and breast cancer. Women who have had a hysterectomy in which the cervix was removed for nonmalignant disease do not require Pap tests.[11] For cervical cancer, the risk of new invasive cancer is extremely low beyond age 65 to 70, as long as a woman has had consistent, normal screening throughout her life. However, many low-income women have not had such screening and would benefit from continued Pap smears into their seventies. Although the USPSTF[2] found no evidence for or against mammography beyond age 69, screening should be considered for women in otherwise good health until at least age 75, given the high incidence of breast cancer among women aged 69 to 75.

Blood Tests. Many patients have come to expect "blood work" as a regular part of the HME. The focus, however, should be on lifestyle choices, education, and risk factor assessment. According to the USPSTF,[2] the only blood tests indicated for otherwise healthy women as part of the HME are blood cholesterol measurements between age 45 and 69 years of age and rubella serology for women of childbearing age who have an uncertain vaccination history. Recently, the American College of Physicians recommended that women over age 50 be screened using the sensitive thyroid-stimulating hormone (TSH) test. Free thyroxine levels, using the same blood sample, should be obtained if the TSH is either nondetectable or greater than 10 mU/L, and patients in whom both tests are abnormal should be treated. If only one is abnormal, then the patient should be retested in 4 to 6 months. It is estimated that mass screening for thyroid disease would benefit 1 of 71 women over age 50 years who are screened.[12]

MANAGEMENT STRATEGIES

Delivering health maintenance care can occur at either planned or unplanned encounters. Most providers will find it easy to address the issues discussed above when "wellness" is the primary agenda. Although a recent study[13] found that family physicians perform preventive care at about one-third of acute and chronic care visits, it is difficult to prioritize preventive care at these times. In this section, we address some ways of putting prevention into practice.

COMMON PROBLEMS IN DELIVERY OF PREVENTIVE SERVICES

A recent study by Stange and colleagues[14] provides the first comprehensive look at the day-to-day practice of a group of family physicians. Commonly performed preventive care activities during visits for illness care or chronic disease follow-up include smoking cessation (42 percent) and recommendations for exercise (42 percent) and flu shots (33 percent).[13] Additional counseling included discussions of tobacco and alcohol use, hormone replacement, diet, contraception, and screening issues. In addition to these elements, the USPSTF[2] suggests that providers keep alert for several other conditions: skin cancer, thyroid disease (especially in postpartum patients), depression, family violence, and drug and alcohol abuse. Many of these can be addressed at wellness visits as well as at other visits.

Family physicians can be attuned to individual concerns when other family members are seen. When we see a patient in the office, we frequently (just under 20 percent of the time) address health concerns of other family members![15] This "surreptitious" care often serves as an opportunity to reinforce advice given at earlier encounters, to remind patients to return for periodic examinations, or to evaluate new problems. For instance, it is common for a parent accompanying at a well child visit to inquire about a mole or some other concern.

PROMOTING GOOD HEALTH BEHAVIORS

What are the main objectives of counseling and patient education? They are twofold: to change behaviors and to improve health status.[2] Health care workers can effectively help women to control their weight,[16] begin to exercise,[17] and use contraception.[18] When health care concerns are addressed, women experience improved outcomes in hypertension,[19] breast cancer,[20] and diabetes control.[21]

There are many possible issues to be discussed, perhaps more than can be covered in the typical 30 to 45 mins set aside for the HME. Several approaches may help prioritize which issues are covered. First, identify any pressing problems (e.g., chest pain, suicidal ideations, volatile domestic circumstances, etc.) that might even force postponement of elements of the HME. Next, identify the patient's goals. What issues are on her mind? What interventions have the greatest potential impact? Tables 1-5 and 1-6 list common interventions and their impact on life expectancy for the average woman and for those at higher risk, respectively. For example, in a 35-year-old woman with mild hypertension who smokes, has a cholesterol over 200 mg/dL, and has a body mass index of 50, the single intervention with the greatest impact on life expectancy is smoking cessation. This information must then be balanced with her own sense of what is achievable and

important to her. Keep in mind that most of the published literature focuses on mortality. Some might argue that though this is an important and easily measured end-point, it is not the most important one. Quality of life, maintenance of function, and prevention of morbidity are more important for many of our patients. Fortunately, for many of the preventive interventions available, the beneficial impact on mortality is also reflected in quality of life.

Some interventions, however, involve significant trade-offs that require discussion with the patient. Three studies have evaluated the use of tamoxifen in preventing breast cancer in women at high risk*.[22–24] Two of the studies[22,23] were terminated early due to a lack of benefit and an increased rate of thromboembolic events (deep vein thrombosis and pulmonary embolism). The third study[24] was a

Table 1-5

Prevention in Women at Average Risk

DISEASE AND INTERVENTION	AGE GROUP (Y)	GAIN IN LIFE EXPECTANCY (MO)
CARDIOVASCULAR DISEASE		
Smoking cessation	35	8
Hormone replacement with estrogen only	50 (with hysterectomies)	13
CANCER		
10 y of biennial mammography	50	0.8
Pap smears	20	
Every 3 y for 55 y		3.1
Annually for 55 y		3.2
Annual fecal occult blood test plus barium		
enema or colonoscopy	50	
Every 5 y for 25 y		2.2
Every 3 y for 25 y		2.5
INFECTIOUS DISEASES		
Hepatitis B virus vaccine	Adolescents	0.12
	Adults	0.03

*The National Cancer Institute has a free (your tax dollars at work) computer program to assist in determining which women are at high risk. It may be ordered via Internet at: http://207.121.187.155/NCI_CANCER_TRIALS/zones/PressInfo/Risk/NciSignUp4.html.
SOURCE: Adapted from Wright and Weinstein.[48]

Table 1-6

Prevention in Women at Elevated Risk

DISEASE AND INTERVENTION	AGE GROUP (Y)	GAIN IN LIFE EXPECTANCY (MO)
CARDIOVASCULAR DISEASE		
Reducing diastolic blood pressure to 88 mm Hg	35 with hypertension	
Diastolic BP 90–94		11
Diastolic BP > 105		68
Reducing cholesterol to 200 mg/dL (5.2 mmol/L)	35 with hypercholesterolemia	
Cholesterol 200–239 mg/dL (5.2–6.2 mmol/L)		5
Cholesterol > 300 mg/dL (7.8 mmol/L)		76
Achieving ideal weight	35	
< 30% above ideal weight		6
> 30% above ideal weight		13
Smoking cessation	35	34
HRT with estrogen and progesterone	50	
History of coronary artery disease		11–26
At high risk for coronary artery disease		7–19
At high risk for breast cancer		−6 to 10
At high risk for hip fracture		2–13
CANCER		
Dilatation and curettage for postmenopausal bleeding followed by hysterectomy if needed	50	6
Dilatation and curettage for postmenopausal bleeding followed by hysterectomy if needed	70	2.2
Prophylactic bilateral mastectomy in woman carrying the BRCA1 or BRCA2 mutation	30	35–64
Prophylactic bilateral mastectomy in woman carrying the BRCA1 or BRCA2 mutation	50	12–28
Prophylactic bilateral oophorectomy in woman carrying the BRCA1 or BRCA2 mutation	30	4–20
Prophylactic bilateral oophorectomy in woman carrying the BRCA1 or BRCA2 mutation	50	1–10
INFECTIOUS DISEASES		
Hepatitis B virus vaccine in high-risk women	12–50	0.15–0.24

ABBREVIATIONS: BP, blood pressure; HRT, hormone replacement therapy.
SOURCE: Adapted from Wright and Weinstein.[48]

larger trial that showed benefit but involved significant trade-offs between harm and benefit. If 1000 high-risk women were treated with tamoxifen for 5 years, 18 breast cancers and 2 deaths could be prevented. However, tamoxifen would also cause two strokes, two pulmonary emboli, and two deep vein thromboses. Obviously the risks incurred by the use of this therapy are not trivial.

When strategies based on a combination of the patient's preferences and the likely benefits are prioritized, the likelihood of success increases. When women play an active role in the decision-making, they have a personal stake in carrying out the plan, thereby improving compliance with it.

The USPSTF[2] also suggests the following counseling and education strategies:

1. **Frame teaching to match the patient's perceptions.** To do this requires incorporation of the patient's beliefs and concerns, which can be elicited by asking specific questions, such as "When you think of cholesterol, what do you think of?" or "What gets in the way of changing your diet?" Women should also receive educationally appropriate and culturally sensitive educational materials. This is also an opportunity to find out what the woman's goals are or to help set goals. From this discussion, health care plans consistent with achieving those goals can be negotiated.

2. **Fully inform patients of the purposes and expected effects of interventions.** Women should be told, for instance, that Pap smears are designed to screen for cancer of the cervix. Patients should know that elevated blood pressure may not cause symptoms until advanced complications occur and that the benefit of treatment is one of reducing long-term complications.

3. **Suggest small changes rather than large ones.** Nothing is more frustrating than not attaining a goal. It can also be a daunting task to think about losing 40 lb over a period of 2 years. We should help women set intermediate, attainable goals such as losing 5 lb in 3 months. When these intermediate goals are met, the patient may attempt the next set with greater confidence.

4. **Be specific.** For example, ask women about their current exercise capacity. Advise them to exercise three times a week and to increase the duration by 10 to 25 percent a week until they achieve a goal of 30 min three to four times a week.

5. **It is sometimes easier to add a new behavior than to eliminate established ones.** Habits can be difficult to break. For instance, it might be easier for an overweight patient to begin exercising regularly than to alter the diet.

6. **Link new behaviors to old ones.** For example, take oral contraceptives after brushing teeth in the morning.

7. **Use the power of the profession.** This is a sensitive area due to potential concerns about power or control. The HME, however, is an opportunity to use simple, direct, nonjudgmental advice: "I want you to stop smoking." Sometimes guilt can be a great motivator, but use it with caution! This is a time to use expertise to guide action.

8. **Get explicit commitments from the patient.** For example, if you have a patient in the contemplative or preparation phase of smoking cessation, get her to set a quit date.

9. **Use a combination of strategies.** Use audiotapes or videotapes in addition to written materials.

10. **Involve your office staff.** Office practice efficiency can be improved by prioritizing as described above. Additionally, empowering the office staff to play a role in wellness can also be useful. For instance, the office nurse may identify if a woman needs a tetanus booster and, in the absence of contraindications, administer it before the health care provider sees the patient. The office staff may also identify patients in need of flu shots or develop tracking systems to remind women when they are due for health maintenance interventions.

11. **Refer.** Take advantage of programs available through the local hospital, your local health maintenance organization, or local chapters of agencies such as the American Heart Association or American Lung Association.

12. **Monitor progress.** Follow up by telephone or mail or in the office. Monitor progress with behavior changes, intermediate parameters (e.g., cholesterol levels, blood pressure), or for complications.

These general strategies should be supplemented with the specific strategies discussed in other chapters.

THERAPEUTIC OR PREVENTIVE MEDICATIONS AND OTHER INTERVENTIONS   At various stages in the life of women, the role of medications and other supplements should be explored. For women in their childbearing years (aged 15 to 44), it is important to discuss contraceptive needs and possible future childbearing. As discussed in Chap. 2, many contraceptive options exist. The use of folic acid for women contemplating a pregnancy should be encouraged (Table 1-7).[2] A woman's need for rubella vaccination should be considered; women

who are not immune to rubella should be immunized before they become pregnant.

With the exception of folic acid, vitamin supplements have not been proven to improve health outcomes or reduce mortality. At the core of the controversy regarding the value of dietary supplements are the questions about what level of nutrient intake optimizes health and whether an adequate intake of nutrients can be obtained from the diet. In addition to recommending an adequate intake of folic acid to young women, it is appropriate to recommend a dietary supplement of vitamin D and vitamin B_{12} for many elderly patients because it is unlikely that the diet will provide the required quantity of these nutrients.[25] Although the

Table 1-7

Dietary Sources and Recommended Doses of Commonly Used Vitamins and Minerals

DIETARY SUPPLEMENT	RECOMMENDED DOSE*/RDA	DIETARY SOURCES
β-carotene	Supplements not recommended (RDA: not established) Multivitamins: 0.6–6 mg Supplements 12–15 mg†	Dark-colored vegetables and fruits: broccoli, carrots, winter squash, spinach, cantaloupe, prunes, mango
Vitamin C	120–500 mg daily (RDA: 60 mg)	Vegetables and fruits: broccoli, sweet peppers, brussel sprouts, mango, oranges, grapefruit, strawberries, cantaloupe
Vitamin E	400–800 IU daily (RDA: 30 IU)	Vegetable oils, seeds, nuts: almonds, safflower oil, sunflower seeds
Folic acid	0.4–0.8 mg daily	Meat: liver, lean beef; eggs, dark-green leafy vegetables, yeast, enriched bread and grain products
Vitamin B_{12}	Supplement to meet RDA (RDA: 2 μg daily—adults 2.2 μg daily—pregnancy, 2.6 μg daily—lactation	Produced by microorganisms—present in meats, eggs, milk and milk products
Vitamin D	400 IU; for elderly individuals not exposed to sunlight 600–800 IU (RDA: 400 IU)	Milk and milk products that are supplemented, eggs, liver, fish, beef
Calcium	adult women <50 y of age and post-menopausal women taking estrogen—1000 mg/d; women over age 65 or postmenopausal not taking estrogen—1500 mg/d	Milk and dairy products (cheese, yogurt), calcium-fortified juices, canned sardines or salmon with bones, raw oysters, broccoli, collard greens, soybeans, tofu

*Dose associated with benefit in observational trials or known to be nontoxic.
†>20 mg daily found in several studies to be associated with increased incidence of cancer in tobacco smokers.
ABBREVIATIONS: RDA, Recommended Dietary Allowance.
SOURCE: Adapted from references 26–28.

role of vitamin C in the prevention of heart disease, cancer, and cataract formation is still controversial, the dietary requirement for vitamin C is increased by about 60 mg/d in tobacco smokers and supplementation in this population is appropriate.[26]

Among the nutrients most studied for possible health benefits and most popular among consumers are the antioxidant vitamins: C, E, and β-carotene (vitamin A precursor). Epidemiologic studies and animal data suggest that these vitamins may offer some protection against heart disease and cancers when consumed in amounts greater than the Recommended Dietary Allowances (RDA).[26,27] In contrast, randomized controlled trials have not demonstrated significant health improvement and several trials found an increased risk of lung cancer among high-risk individuals taking β-carotene.[28–30] One reason that epidemiologic studies show a benefit while controlled trials do not may be the "healthy user" effect: the better outcomes observed in people who use supplements may have been due to healthier lifestyles, greater use of preventive services, or the result of some other unmeasurable reason.[31,32] Vitamin E is the most intriguing of the antioxidant vitamins. A number of cohort and case-control studies raise the possibility that intake of vitamin E may reduce the risk of heart disease,[33] cancer,[34–37] Parkinson's disease,[38] and dementia.[39] Clinical trials are under way, and their findings will help us better inform our patients.

Given the predisposition of many Americans to use dietary supplements, it is prudent for health care providers to be able to counsel on safe/nontoxic doses and intakes of vitamins and minerals that are associated with benefit in epidemiologic studies (see Table 1-7). Many young women do not consume enough calcium in their diet, and reduced calcium intake in younger women is an important risk factor for developing postmenopausal osteoporosis.[40] Although there is no evidence that adding calcium supplements for adolescent and menstruating women reduces this risk, dietary calcium and the possible need for supplementation should be discussed.

Another issue relates to the use of aspirin. Several cohort studies, including the Nurses' Health Study, suggest that aspirin has some benefit in the primary prevention of myocardial infarction (a 25 percent reduction in risk) but not for stroke. Other randomized trials that enrolled women have shown some mixed results. Thus far, no large prospective trials of aspirin for the primary prevention of myocardial infarction or stroke in women have been completed, although one, the Women's Health Study, is ongoing.[41] Data are also inconclusive with respect to the use of aspirin among women with previous stroke or heart attack. Elwood[42] conducted a randomized controlled trial of aspirin and placebo in over 1600 patients with confirmed myocardial infarction and found a small, statistically insignificant, reduction in mortality. That study only enrolled 248 women. The Aspirin Myocardial Infarction Study[43] was another trial involving patients with previous acute myocardial infarction. Although there was a small reduction in nonfatal cardiovascular events, there was an increase in mortality among aspirin users. The authors of this study could not recommend the routine use of aspirin in survivors of acute myocardial infarction. The available studies have not enrolled sufficient numbers of women to provide good data on the risks and benefits of aspirin for women.

Alternative/Complementary Approaches. Many women use alternative/complementary approaches to maintain health. Homeopathic remedies, herbal supplements, acupuncture, chiropractic manipulation, aromatherapy, imagery, various massage techniques, and naturopathy are just a few examples of complementary practices. They are used more often than most physicians realize. In one population-based survey of 3000 adults, 49 percent used at least one nonmedically prescribed alternative therapy.[44] Users were typically more well-educated working perimenopausal women of normal weight. About 20 percent used an alternative practitioner (chiropractors, naturopaths, reflexologists, etc.); these individuals were more likely to be younger, overweight women living in rural areas.

Although many practices are unproven, some alternative practices may be beneficial. For example, supplementation with vitamin E was very popular as an alternative medicine long before it was studied in clinical trials. Among perimenopausal women with frequent hot flushes and only modest improvement with estrogen, the addition of soy protein in the diet may serve as a useful adjunct.[45] Other measures, such as acupuncture, have not been subjected to placebo-controlled trials but have become incorporated into mainstream medicine as an adjunct to smoking cessation and in managing painful conditions. The danger of dismissing alternative practices glibly is that patients may become disenfranchised from traditional beneficial practices. In addition, they may be reluctant to disclose the use of alternative treatments.

Although supplements are commonly used and some appear to be beneficial, their use is not without problems. Because the Food and Drug Administration does not regulate them, issues of quality control and consistency from lot to lot (even with the same manufacturer) are potential problems. The lack of rigorous research or published research to support many claims makes it difficult to evaluate their true benefit. The final issue relates to safety. Many patients are under the impression that, because these are "natural products," they are safe. The literature contains many reviews, case reports, and case series of toxicity associated with herbal preparations.[46] Additionally, there are many documented interactions between alternative and traditional remedies (e.g., serotonin toxicity associated with patients taking St. Johns wort and fluoxetine). Finally, there have been reports of contamination with heavy metals and other potentially toxic substances and even adulteration of preparations.[47]

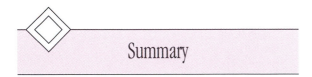

Summary

The HME is an important aspect of primary care. Not only do these visits help build rapport with patients, they help health care providers identify the health care values and goals of their patients. Knowledge of these goals and values is important in negotiating a plan of preventive care with a patient. Although these issues are often addressed at the time of a regularly scheduled checkup, it may be appropriate to address some preventive issues at illness-related visits.

References

1. Weisman CS: Women's use of health care. In: Falik MM, Collins KS (eds): *Women's Health: The Commonwealth Fund Survey.* Baltimore: The Johns Hopkins University Press; 1996;26.
2. U.S. Preventive Services Task Force: *Guide to Clinical Preventive Services*, 2nd ed. Baltimore: Williams & Wilkins; 1996.
3. Bradley KA, Boyd-Wickizer J, Powell SH, Burman ML: Alcohol screening questionnaires in women: a critical review. *JAMA* 280:166, 1998.
4. Kiely DK, Kiel DP, Burrows AB, Lipsitz LA: Identifying nursing home residents at risk for falling. *J Am Geriatr Soc* 46:551, 1998.
5. Campbell AJ, Robertson MC, Gardner MM, Norton RN, Tilyard MW, Buchner DM: Randomised controlled trial of a general practice programme of home based exercise to prevent falls in elderly women. *BMJ* 315(7115):1065, 1997.
6. Miller AB, Baines CJ, To T, Wall C: Canadian National Breast Screening Study: 2. Breast cancer detection and death rates among women aged 50 to 59 years [published erratum appears in *CMAJ* Mar 1;148(5):718, 1993]. *CMAJ* 147:1477, 1992.
7. Fletcher SW, Black W, Harris R, Rimer BK, Shapiro S: Report of the International Workshop on Screening for Breast Cancer. *J Natl Cancer Inst* 85:1644, 1993.
8. Screening for squamous cervical cancer: duration of low risk after negative results of cervical cytology and its implication for screening policies. IARC Working Group on Evaluation of Cervical Cancer Screening Programmes. *BMJ* 293(6548):659, 1986.
9. Kerlikowske K, Grady D, Rubin SM, Sandrock C, Ernster VL: Efficacy of screening mammography. A meta-analysis. *JAMA* 273:149, 1995.
10. Salzmann P, Kerlikowske K, Phillips K: Cost-effectiveness of extending screening mammography guidelines to include women 40 to 49 years of age. *Ann Intern Med* 127:955, 1997.

11. Piscitelli JT, Bastian LA, Wilkes A, Simel DL: Cytologic screening after hysterectomy for benign disease. *Am J Obstet Gynecol* 173:424, 1995.

12. Clinical guideline, part 1. Screening for thyroid disease. American College of Physicians. *Ann Intern Med* 129:141, 1998.

13. Stange KC, Flocke SA, Goodwin MA: Opportunistic preventive services delivery. Are time limitations and patient satisfaction barriers? *J Fam Pract* 46:419, 1998.

14. Stange KC, Jaen CR, Flocke SA, Miller WL, Crabtree BF, Zyzanski SJ: The value of a family physician. *J Fam Pract* 46:363, 1998.

15. Medalie JH, Zyzanski SJ, Langa D, Stange KC: The family in family practice: is it a reality? *J Fam Pract* 46:390, 1998.

16. Brownell KD, Kramer FM: Behavioral management of obesity. *Med Clin North Am* 73:185, 1989.

17. King AC, Blair SN, Bild DE, et al: Determinants of physical activity and interventions in adults. *Med Sci Sports Exerc* 24(6 suppl):S221, 1992.

18. Nathanson CA, Becker MH: The influence of client-provider relationships on teenage women's subsequent use of contraception. *Am J Public Health* 75:33, 1985.

19. Morisky DE, Levine DM, Green LW, Shapiro S, Russell RP, Smith CR: Five-year blood pressure control and mortality following health education for hypertensive patients. *Am J Public Health* 73:153, 1983.

20. Spiegel D, Bloom JR, Kraemer HC, Gottheil E: Effect of psychosocial treatment on survival of patients with metastatic breast cancer. *Lancet* 2(8668):888, 1989.

21. Padgett D, Mumford E, Hynes M, Carter R: Meta-analysis of the effects of educational and psychosocial interventions on management of diabetes mellitus. *J Clin Epidemiol* 41:1007, 1988.

22. Veronesi U, Maisonneuve P, Costa A, et al: Prevention of breast cancer with tamoxifen: preliminary findings from the Italian randomized trial among hysterectomised women. *Lancet* 352:93, 1998.

23. Powles T, Eeles R, Ashley S, et al: Interim analysis of the incidence of breast cancer in the Royal Marsden Hospital tamoxifen randomized chemoprevention trial. *Lancet* 352:98, 1998.

24. Fisher B, Costantino JP, Wickerham DL, et al: Tamoxifen for prevention of breast cancer: report of the national surgical adjuvant breast and bowel project P-1 study. *J Natl Cancer Inst* 90:1371, 1998.

25. Vitamin Supplements. *Medical Letter* 40(1032):75, 1998.

26. Weber P, Bendich AS, Schalch W: Vitamin C and human health—a review of recent data relevant to human requirements. *Int J Vit Nutr Res* 66:19, 1996.

27. Hathcock JN: Vitamins and minerals: efficacy and safety. *Am J Clin Nutr* 66:427, 1997.

28. Antioxidant vitamins. *The Rx Consultant* V(8):1, 1996.

29. The effect of vitamin E and beta carotene on the incidence of lung cancer and other cancers in male smokers. The Alpha-Tocopherol, Beta Carotene Cancer Prevention Study Group. *N Engl J Med* 330:1029, 1994.

30. Marwick C: Trials reveal no benefit, possible harm of beta carotene and vitamin A for lung cancer prevention. *JAMA* 275:422, 1996.

31. Colditz GA, Stampfer MJ, Willett WC: Diet and lung cancer. A review of the epidemiologic evidence in humans. *Arch Intern Med* 147:157, 1987.

32. Gao CM, Tajima K, Kuroishi T, Hirose K, Inoue M: Protective effects of raw vegetables and fruit against lung cancer among smokers and ex-smokers: a case-control study in the Tokai area of Japan. *Jpn J Cancer Res* 84:594, 1993.

33. Stampfer MJ, Hennekens CH, Manson JE, Colditz GA, Rosner B, Willett WC: Vitamin E consumption and the risk of coronary disease in women. *N Engl J Med* 328:1444, 1993.

34. Mezzetti M, La Vecchia C, Decarli A, Boyle P, Talamini R, Franceschi S: Population attributable risk for breast cancer: diet, nutrition, and physical exercise. *J Natl Cancer Inst* 90:389, 1998.

35. Bostick RM, Potter JD, McKenzie DR, et al: Reduced risk of colon cancer with high intake of vitamin E: the Iowa Women's Health Study. *Cancer Res* 53: 4230, 1993.

36. Slattery ML, Edwards SL, Anderson K, Caan B: Vitamin E and colon cancer: is there an association? *Nutr Cancer* 30:201, 1998.

37. Wideroff L, Potischman N, Glass AG, et al: A nested case-control study of dietary factors and the risk of incident cytological abnormalities of the cervix. *Nutr Cancer* 30:130, 1998.

38. de Rijk MC, Breteler MM, den Breeijen JH, et al: Dietary antioxidants and Parkinson disease. The Rotterdam Study. *Arch Neurol* 54:762, 1997.

39. Perrig WJ, Perrig P, Stahelin HB: The relation between antioxidants and memory performance in the old and very old. J Am Geriatr Soc 45:718, 1997.

40. Turner JG, Gilchrist NL, Ayling EM, Hassall AJ, Hooke EA, Sadler WA: Factors affecting bone min-

eral density in high school girls. *N Z Med J* 105(930):95, 1992.

41. Hennekens CH: Aspirin in the treatment and prevention of cardiovascular disease. *Annu Rev Public Health* 18:37, 1997.

42. Elwood PC, Sweetnam PM: Aspirin and secondary mortality after myocardial infarction. *Lancet* 2 (8156–8157):1313, 1979.

43. A randomized, controlled trial of aspirin in persons recovered from myocardial infarction. *JAMA* 243:661, 1980.

44. MacLennan AH, Wilson DH, Taylor AW: Prevalence and cost of alternative medicine in Australia. *Lancet* 347(9001):569, 1996.

45. Albertazzi P, Pansini F, Bonaccorsi G, Zanotti L, Forini E, De Aloysio D: The effect of dietary soy supplementation on hot flushes. *Obstet Gynecol* 91:6, 1998.

46. Bateman J, Chapman RD, Simpson D: Possible toxicity of herbal remedies. *Scott Med J* 43:7, 1998.

47. Crone CC, Wise TN: Use of herbal medicines among consultation-liaison populations. A review of current information regarding risks, interactions, and efficacy. *Psychosomatics* 39:3, 1998.

48. Wright JC, Weinstein MC: Gains in life expectancy from medical interventions—standardizing data on outcomes. *N Engl J Med* 339(6):380, 1998.

Mindy A. Smith
Leslie A. Shimp

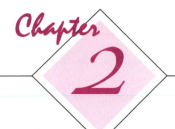

Chapter 2

Family Planning

Overview

Unplanned Pregnancy

Unplanned pregnancy is an all too common problem in primary care, and health care providers must be both attentive to patient inquiries and actively solicit information about current needs for contraception. Without the use of contraception, 85 percent of women engaging in intercourse become pregnant within 1 year. The probability of conception is 15 to 33 percent per cycle, depending on the frequency of intercourse (once a week versus every other day).[1] Viable sperm are able to remain in the genital tract for up to 5 days, but the egg, once released, is capable of being fertilized for only about 24 h. The fertile period for women, therefore, lasts about 6 days, ending within 24 h of ovulation.

According to 1995 figures from the National Survey of Family Growth,[2] 31 percent of pregnancies were unintended (65 percent for women under age 20 and 20 percent among women aged 30 to 44). The United States has the highest rate of adolescent pregnancy in the industrialized world; this is not due to higher rates of adolescent sexual activity, but to less use of effective contraception.[3] Ineffective use of contraception is likely related to a combination of limited education and poorer access to services, including lack of subsidized services and supplies. Approximately one-half of adolescent pregnancies occur within the first 6 months of sexual activity, but the average time between initiating sexual activity and seeking contraceptive advice is 1 year.[3] Psychological and social costs of early sexual activity include damaged self-esteem, involvement in exploitive relationships, unsatisfactory sexual experiences and unhealthy patterns of sexual intimacy, and decreased likelihood of completing high school and college education.[4] In addition, unprotected intercourse increases the risk of transmission of sexually transmitted diseases (STDs) and AIDS.

Problems with Current Approaches to Family Planning

Patients frequently seek advice and prescriptions for birth control. Approximately 18 percent of women's contacts with physicians focus on reproductive health, and 7 percent of visits made by women aged 15 to 44 (12.6 million) are for contraception.[5] In 1990, 59 percent of U.S. women, 15 to 44 years of age, were using contraception.[6] Unfortunately, the figures for noncontraceptive use among at-risk women aged 15 to 44 actually increased between 1988 and 1990 (from 7 to 12 percent), and among women aged 15 to 19, 22 percent were sexually active in the past month without using contraception.[6]

CONCERN ABOUT HEALTH EFFECTS

A major reason for lack of use, particularly of the most effective forms of contraception, is a concern about potential health risks and side effects of available methods. In a study of women seeking legal abortion, 93 percent claimed to have adequate knowledge of contraception, but at the time of conception only 11.5 percent used the most effective methods available (oral contraceptives [OCs] or intrauterine devices [IUDs]); concern about side effects was the most common reason for nonuse.[7]

Specific concerns about contraceptive methods were sought in a Finnish study of 3000 women aged 18 to 44.[8] Approximately half the respondents reported a concern about the risks of at least one type of contraceptive; of those, the majority of concerns (71 percent) were about OCs. Specifically, women were concerned about cardiovascular effects, cancer risk, infertility, mood changes, and weight gain. Concerns about the IUD included infection risk, effects on menstruation, and ectopic pregnancy. Interestingly, concerns about OCs were associated in multiple regression analysis with higher education, past experience, and knowledge. In reality, the health risks to women are far less with current methods of contraception than those associated with pregnancy, and some methods reduce the risks for certain health conditions (e.g., use of a combined OC reduces the risk for ovarian and endometrial cancer). Concerns about health risks and women's past experience should be addressed to assist women in making the best choices among the contraceptive options.

ACCESS AND COST

Effective contraceptive use is also determined by access to health care and financial issues. Because the most effective forms of contraception are prescription products or surgical procedures, patients with poor access to health care or limited financial means will be less likely to use contraceptive methods with greater effectiveness. The combined costs of office visits and medication can prohibit some women from obtaining the most effective contraceptives.[9] Subsidized family planning clinics, with providers located in 85 percent of U.S. counties, are an important source of contraceptive services.[10] In 1994, these clinics served almost 6.6 million women. Many of the largest sites are dependent on federal title X funding. A study from the Alan Guttmacher Institute reported that each year 24 percent of U.S. women obtain family planning services from a publicly funded clinic or a private doctor reimbursed by Medicaid; if these subsidized contraceptive services were not available, women who currently use them would have an estimated 1.3 million additional unplanned pregnancies annually.[11]

CONFIDENTIALITY

Adolescents are faced with an additional barrier to contraceptive health care—concerns about confidentiality. Many adolescents will not initiate a discussion of sexual activity and contraception with a physician if they are concerned about the conversation being shared with their parents. For adolescents in this country, lack of knowledge and difficulty obtaining contraceptives (often because of fear and embarrassment) are common.

In one study, although the majority of adolescents (66 percent) reported that they would like to discuss contraception and that they would like the physician to initiate a discussion, few (22 percent) had actually had a conversation with a health care provider.[3] Information should be readily available, both within schools and in the physician's office. A substantial body of literature demonstrates either no impact on sexual activity or a decrease with the provision of sex and contraceptive education. Health providers should initiate conversations about contraception at any available opportunity.

CULTURAL AND RELIGIOUS PERSPECTIVES

In considering optimal contraception, women's religion and cultural affiliation influence choices as well. Within the Roman Catholic church procreation is the main purpose of marriage so natural family planning and abstinence are the only condoned forms of birth control. Less restrictive positions are held by Protestant and Anglican churches where other forms of contraception are accepted.[12] In Judaism, sexual relations within marriage has two roles—procreation and fulfillment of women's sexual needs; men are duty-bound to propagate, but women are not. Therefore, prohibitions exist for the use of male contraception, including withdrawal, condom use, abstinence, and vasectomy, but other forms are acceptable.

Cultural considerations may be particularly important for immigrant groups. Although Islam, Hinduism, and Buddhism allow contraceptive use, couples may not be comfortable with certain forms of birth control for cultural reasons. For example, among Muslim, Hindu, and Sikh women, modesty may preclude the use of methods that involve self-insertion of a device into the vagina; use of a condom, OC, or IUD may be more acceptable. These aspects of women's lives must be considered before recommending a birth control method.

Contraceptive Methods

Among birth control options, sterilization is the most common method (36 percent of U.S. couples) followed by OCs (about 17 percent of U.S. women). Several surveys of U.S. women have reported condoms as the next most frequently used method of birth control (11 percent) followed by spermicide use alone and withdrawal. The diaphragm and periodic abstinence are next most common, followed in frequency of use by IUDs. Natural family planning methods are used by about 1 million ever-married women or between 2 and 3 percent of currently married couples. Progestin implants and douching are reported as the least common methods of birth control. It is estimated that 95 percent of sexually active women use contraception at some time in their lives and that each woman uses up to three different methods.

Important in the discussion of any birth control method is the reported method effectiveness. Method (theoretical failure, assuming perfect use) and user failure rates are often reported, the former determined after removing pregnancies due to imperfect use from the numerator. Unfortunately, optimal statistical methods for reporting accidental pregnancy rates have yet to be developed. The Pearl Index, used in much of the older literature, reports rates of accidental pregnancy per woman-year of use. This method, however, does not account well for the passage of time; it is unable to distinguish between a few women followed over a long period of time and a large number of women followed for a short period of time. The second method uses life table analysis to compute rates as probability of accidental pregnancy within a particular time frame. This method is now the most frequently used although it has been criticized for its lack of precision in identifying patterns of use. For example, this model assumes few drop-outs and that "exposure" to a particular method is continuous over the time period reported; this assumption is not consistent with most studies on contraception. Recently, a pilot study reported the results of a randomized trial for determining contraceptive efficacy using women who desired pregnancy but were willing to be randomized to either delay of conception (through use of the method to be tested) or no method (i.e., attempt to conceive).[13] This strategy may eliminate many of the current biases in determining user efficacy.

For the purpose of this chapter, life table analyses are used to report effectiveness and ranges of effectiveness for typical users, based on the literature. This information is presented in Table 2-1. It should be remembered that these "typical user" estimates are usually derived from study data. In practice, failure rates are likely to be higher. For example, in a report based on data from the 1995 National Survey of Family Growth, within 1 year of starting to use a reversible method of contraception, 9 percent of the respondents reported a contraceptive failure.[14] This included 7 percent of women using the OC, 9 percent using male condoms, and 19 percent using withdrawal. In addition, 31 percent had discontinued the use of the initial method selected by 6 months and 44 percent by 12 months because of method-related concerns. Although 76 percent had resumed a method within 3 months, low-income women were found to be less likely to resume any method. This speaks to a continued dissatisfaction with available methods and a need for improved counseling and follow-up.

Sterilization

Surgical sterilization is a safe, effective, and permanent form of contraception. Tubal sterilization is more frequently used by couples than vasectomy. Among U.S. women, 33 percent of those aged 30 to 35 and 50 percent of women over age 40 use this method.[6] Vasectomy is used for contraception by approximately 11 to 12 percent of U.S. couples. The number of vasectomies performed each year has been relatively stable since

1991 with about 10 vasectomies per 1000 men aged 25 to 49 years.[15] About one million sterilization procedures are performed yearly in the United States.

MECHANISM OF ACTION

Female sterilization involves occlusion of the fallopian tubes, which prevents the sperm from uniting with the egg. Tubal ligation is performed using one of five methods for tubal occlusion:

1. Partial salpingectomy (often selected in the immediate postpartum period) in which a portion of each fallopian tube is cut and tied off
2. The Pomeroy method where a small loop of each tube is tied off and the top segment of the loop excised
3. Coagulation methods—unipolar and bipolar coagulation involving electrical current, which cauterizes and blocks the tubes (the latter causing less tubal damage)
4. Silicone banding in which an occluding device is placed over the tubes
5. Use of a spring clip to occlude the tubes

The latter two methods may be more easily reversible. The majority of these procedures are performed either immediately postpartum under general or regional anesthesia or as an outpatient procedure under laparoscopic guidance.

Male sterilization, or vasectomy, involves occlusion of the vas deferens to prevent sperm from entering the ejaculate. As with tubal ligation, the methods of occlusion include ligation, cautery, clips, and combinations of these approaches, with ligation being the most commonly reported procedure. Virtually all vasectomies are performed under local anesthesia, and the majority are performed in physician's offices (urology, general surgery, and family practice). Percutaneous vasectomy, a technique more recently introduced into the United States, reduces surgery time to 10 mins and significantly decreases the incidence of complications such as infection and hematoma.

Table 2-1

Failure Rates Among Typical Users and Potential Advantages and Side Effects of Birth Control Methods

METHOD	FAILURE RATE, % IN FIRST YEAR	ANNUAL COST $*	ADVANTAGES	COMMON OR SERIOUS ADVERSE EFFECTS
Female sterilization	0.4–1.8	1200–2500†	Permanent, safe, decreased rate ovarian cancer	Ectopic pregnancy, menstrual disorders, dysmenorrhea, regret
Male sterilization	0.5–1.6	500†	Permanent, safe	Hematoma, epididymitis, orchialgia, sperm granuloma
Oral contraceptives	3.0	200–325	Fewer STDs, decreased rate of ovarian and endometrial cancer, less menstrual pain and bleeding	Cardiovascular complications, nausea, dizziness, headache, spotting, weight gain, breast tenderness, chloasma
Depo-Provera (medroxy-progesterone DMPA)	0.3	140	Less PID, decreased ovarian and endometrial cancer, easy to use	Irregular bleeding, weight gain, headaches
Norplant	0.1	170‡	Less PID, less menstrual pain and bleeding, effective for 5 y	Complications of insertion and removal, irregular bleeding
Female condom	15–21	250	Fewer STDs, nonprescription	Awkward to use
Male condom	4–12	50	Fewer STDs, reduced cervical cancer, easy, inexpensive, nonprescription, delays premature ejaculation	Discomfort, reduced sensitivity, latex allergy, reduced spontaneity
Diaphragm	3–18	155–235	Fewer STDs, decreased cervical neoplasia	Latex or spermicide allergy, bladder infection, bacterial or yeast vaginitis, toxic shock syndrome
Cervical cap	8–19	155–235	Fewer STDs, can remain in vagina longer than diaphragm	Odor, cervical erosion or laceration, other side effects same as diaphragm
Spermicide (alone)	21	85	Low cost, nonprescription, fewer STDs	Allergy, irritation
IUD (copper)	0.6–0.8	180‡	Not user-dependent, effective for 10 y	PID, perforation of uterus, increased menstrual pain and bleeding, possibly increased ectopic pregnancy
IUD (progestin)	1.5	320‡	Not user-dependent, effective for 1 y, less menstrual bleeding	Similar to copper IUD
Natural family planning		0	No chemicals or devices needed	No STD protection, unforgiving of imperfect use, requires highly motivated user
Perfect use	1–3			
Imperfect use	19–38			
Lactation	0.5–2	0	Promotes breast-feeding	Only reliable for 4–6 mo
Withdrawal	7–19	0	Readily available	No STD protection

*Cost figures from Hatcher et al.[17] †Costs for sterilization calculated as a one-time expense. ‡Assumes retention for 5 years for Norplant, 1 year for progestin IUD, and 8 years for copper IUD. ABBREVIATIONS: IUD, intrauterine device; PID, pelvic inflammatory disease; STD, sexually transmitted disease.

EFFICACY

The typical failure rate reported for tubal ligation is 0.4 percent for the first year (see Table 2-1). A recent collaborative prospective study of 10,685 women found a higher cumulative failure rate of 18.5 pregnancies per 1000 procedures over 10 years.[16] In this study, younger women (18 to 27), African American women, and those undergoing bipolar or spring clip occlusion methods had the highest failure rates. Failure rates with vasectomy are reported to be between 0.48 and 1.57 percent.

PATIENT EDUCATION

During the planning for tubal ligation, the provider should be aware of hospital or insurance policies for sterilization procedures; for example, forms may need to be completed 30 days prior to anticipated delivery for a postpartum tubal ligation if the patient is insured through Medicaid.

Following tubal ligation, women should be informed that recovery from the procedure averages about 4 days. They should plan to rest for the first 24 h and may resume activities gradually over the first week. Bathing may resume after 2 days and intercourse after 1 week. Women should be made aware that, should pregnancy occur, the risk of that pregnancy being ectopic (located outside the uterus, usually in the fallopian tube) is high (up to 50 percent). Women should know the signs and symptoms of an ectopic pregnancy such as absent menses followed by vaginal bleeding and pelvic (adnexal) pain.

Postoperative warning signs for women include fever, bleeding from the incision, and excessive pain; patients with these problems, or women who suspect a pregnancy, should seek immediate assistance. Follow-up in 1 to 2 weeks after the procedure is recommended.

BENEFITS AND SIDE EFFECTS

The major benefit of sterilization is its high efficacy resulting in freedom from worry about accidental pregnancy. Other advantages include lack of significant long-term side effects, no need for partner compliance, and no need to interrupt lovemaking. Potential short-term complications of these procedures are uncommon and include reactions to anesthesia (rare, but can be severe), bleeding (1 percent), and infection (< 1 percent). Following tubal ligation, some investigators report increases in dysmenorrhea and abnormal menstrual cycles compared to control groups of women. These findings, however, are not consistent and may be due to differences in follow-up intervals.

CONTRAINDICATIONS

It should be emphasized that sterilization is considered a permanent decision and, although reversal methods exist, success rates for a reversal resulting in a pregnancy are only 70 percent to 80 percent for tubal ligation reversal and about 50 percent for vasectomy reversal. Differences in rates appear to be based on the type of procedure (less success with electrocautery methods for women and with removal of long segments of the vas deferens for men), time since surgery (inversely related to success), and other factors such as age.

Regret about the decision and requests for reversal occur in 2 to 7 percent of individuals. Regret is higher among young patients, those who express a desire for more children, and those who suffer the loss of a child or divorce after the procedure. The issue of possible desire for future children in the case of remarriage or loss of a child should be discussed directly with women/couples seeking sterilization. For individuals or couples who express uncertainty, alternative methods should be strongly considered.

Combined Oral Contraceptives

Combined OCs contain two hormones, estrogen and progestin. The estrogen component of most OCs is ethinyl estradiol (EE). Mestranol, the other estrogen used in OCs, is a prodrug of EE and is less potent (35 μg of EE is approximately equivalent to 50 μg of mestranol). There are eight progestins contained in the current OCs marketed in the United States. They are norethindrone, norethindrone acetate, ethynodiol diacetate, norgestrel, levonorgestrel, norethynodrel, desogestrel, and norgestimate. Gestodene is awaiting approval in the United States. Comparing the different progestins is made difficult by variable progestational, androgenic, and endometrial potency. The biologic (clinical) effect of the various progestins in the current low-dose OCs, however, is similar because of adjustments in dose.

Combined OCs are available in monophasic, biphasic, and triphasic cycles, depending on the number of variations in hormone composition of active pills. Since the Food and Drug Administration (FDA) approval of a combined OC in 1960, the medication has been extensively studied and refined. There has been a continued lowering of the dose of estrogen and progestin, reducing adverse effects without compromising the contraceptive efficacy. In addition, the newer progestins (desogestrel and norgestimate) have greater selectivity (greater affinity for the progesterone versus androgen receptor) and are less androgenic, reducing androgenic side effects and adverse lipid changes. The current OCs can, therefore, be used by a broader group of women and continued by many until menopause.

MECHANISM OF ACTION

Combined OCs prevent pregnancy primarily by suppressing ovulation through inhibition of the hypothalamic-pituitary-ovarian axis. The feedback to the pituitary, created by the exogenous hormone, prevents the release of follicle-stimulating hormone (FSH) and luteinizing hormone (LH) to stimulate the ovary. Estrogenic effects include suppression of FSH, alteration of ovum transport, changes in the uterine environment (via altered uterine secretions and abnormal cellularity that hampers implantation), and acceleration of luteolysis (degeneration of the corpus luteum). Progestin effects include suppression of LH, thickening

of cervical mucus (which hampers sperm transport), inhibition of capacitation (activation of enzymes that permit the sperm to penetrate the ovum), slowed ovum transport, altered fallopian tube secretions, and endometrial changes resulting in a decidualized endometrial bed with atrophied glands that hampers implantation.

EFFICACY

The OCs are very effective; typical accidental pregnancy rates are about 3 percent. The efficacy of monophasic and multiphasic products is equivalent. Contraceptive failures are largely due to poor compliance, with the most critical error being delayed initiation of the next cycle of pills (potentially interrupting ovarian suppression). Continuance rates are approximately 71 percent at 1 year.

PRESCRIBING INFORMATION

SCREENING   The role of the provider is to screen interested women for risk factors, review side effects, and determine the most appropriate OC. Combined OCs are a good choice for women who can remember to take pills daily and want to space children. Women with acne, anovulatory or irregular periods, endometriosis, heavy or painful menses, recurrent ovarian cysts, or a family history of ovarian cancer are likely to benefit from the use of combined OCs. Conversely, women who have poor medication compliance, have previously become pregnant while using OCs, are taking long-term medications known to interfere with the effectiveness of OCs (Table 2-2), or who are over the age of 35 and smoke cigarettes are poor candidates.

PILL SELECTION   Many pill choices are available in the United States. Figure 2-1 is designed to assist clinicians in deciding which pill to prescribe.[17] The steps begin by determining whether a woman can safely use estrogen (contraindications are listed in the lower left hand side of the figure) and continue by considering the dose of estrogen, the OC cost, and a woman's needs with respect to

(text continues on page 32)

Table 2-2

Clinically Significant Drug Interactions with Oral Contraceptives (OCs)

DRUG	EFFECT	ACTION
Barbiturates (phenobarbital, primidone—Mysoline)	Loss of OC effectiveness	Use alternative contraceptive or titrate OC dose to avoid breakthrough bleeding; consider use of BUM
Caffeine	Action of caffeine may be enhanced	If caffeine-related CNS or cardiovascular effects are noted, limit or abstain from use
Carbamazepine (Tegretol, Epitol)	Loss of OC effectiveness	Use alternative contraceptive or titrate OC dose to avoid breakthrough bleeding; consider use of BUM
Corticosteroids	Increased availability of steroids	Reduction in steroid dose may be needed; enhanced effect or toxicity possible
Griseofulvin	Loss of OC effectiveness	Use alternative contraceptive or titrate OC dose to avoid breakthrough bleeding; consider use of BUM
Hydantoins (phenytoin—Dilantin, mephenytoin—Mesantoin)	Loss of OC effectiveness	Use alternative contraceptive or titrate OC dose to avoid breakthrough bleeding; consider use of BUM
Modafinil (Provigil)	Loss of OC effectiveness	Use alternative contraceptive or use BUM during therapy and for 1 mo after discontinuation of modafinil
Penicillins	Potential reduction in OC effectiveness, rare	Use BUM during short-course therapy or for first 2–3 wk of chronic antibiotic therapy
Rifampin	Loss of OC effectiveness	Use alternative or additional contraceptive
Tetracyclines	Potential reduction in OC effectiveness, rare	Use BUM during short-course therapy or for first 2–3 wk of chronic antibiotic therapy
Theophyllines	Decreased elimination of theophylline	Adjust theophylline dose
Topiramate (Topamax)	Loss of OC effectiveness	Use alternative contraceptive or titrate OC dose to avoid breakthrough bleeding; consider use of BUM
Troglitazone (Rezulin)	Loss of OC effectiveness	Use alternative contraceptive or titrate OC dose to avoid breakthrough bleeding; consider use of BUM
Troleandomycin (TAO)	Increased risk for cholestatic jaundice	Avoid concurrent use
Vitamin C ≥1 g/day	Increased serum level of EE (patient may experience spotting when vitamin is discontinued—similar to switching from high-dose pill to low-dose pill)	Take vitamin C and OC 4 h apart Limit vitamin C dose to ≤ 100 mg/d

ABBREVIATIONS: BUM, backup method; EE, ethinyl estradiol.

Figure 2-1

Choosing a combined oral contraceptive with less than 50 μg of estrogen. (From Hatcher et al.[17])

Start by determining if the woman can safely use estrogen

STEP 1	STEP 2
Is this person a good candidate for a pill with estrogen? ⟶	YES, she can use an estrogen. ⟶
In general, avoid prescribing a pill with estrogen to women with: ⟶	NO, it would be best if she did not use an estrogen. Therefore, you can consider:
<ul><li>Current or a history of circulatory diseases due to blood clots (including heart attack, stroke, or blood clots in deep veins) or cardiovascular disease due to diabetes.</li><li>Structural heart disease with complications such as atrial fibrillation or subacute bacterial endocarditis.</li><li>Blood pressure of 160/100 or greater.</li><li>Age of 35 or more who are smokers.</li><li>Breast cancer or history thereof (exceptions may be made if no evidence of disease in past 5 years).</li><li>Active hepatic disease including symptomatic viral hepatitis, severe or mild cirrhosis, or benign or malignant liver tumors.</li><li>Past history of jaundice (cholestasis) related to oral contraceptives.</li><li>Migraine headaches with neurologic impairment such as blurred or lost vision, seeing flashing lights or zigzag lines, trouble speaking or moving.</li><li>Diabetes and damaged vision (retinopathy), kidneys (nephropathy) or nervous system (neuropathy), or women who have had diabetes for 20 years or longer.</li><li>Plan to undergo major surgery or any leg surgery requiring immobilization for several days or more. Estrogen-containing pills should be discontinued 4 weeks before major surgery.</li></ul>	<ul><li>Progestin-only pills, such as:<ul><li>Micronor (0.35 mg norethindrone daily)</li><li>NOR QD (0.35 mg norethindrone daily)</li><li>Ovrette (0.075 mg norgestrel daily)</li></ul></li><li>Norplant (5-year levonorgestrel implants)</li><li>Depo-Provera (150 mg medroxyprogesterone acetate injection every 3 months)</li><li>Intrauterine device<ul><li>Copper T 380-A</li><li>Levonorgestrel IUD</li><li>Progestasert System</li></ul></li><li>Condoms (male or female)</li><li>Diaphragm, cervical cap, Reality female condom</li><li>Foam, VCF film, suppository</li><li>Fertility awareness</li><li>Male or female sterilization</li></ul>

Breastfeeding women, in general, should avoid estrogen until they start weaning the baby from breastfeeding.

Exceptions may be made in specific cases and occasionally pills may be prescribed for women in the above categories, provided that the specialized (individualized) grounds are well documented in the record.

© Robert A. Hatcher, MD, MPH
April 1993

The following individuals assisted in the development of this flow chart:
Marcia Angle, MD, MPH, Program for International Training and Health (INTRAH)
James Bellinger, PAC, Emory University School of Medicine
Willard Cates, Jr., MD, MPH, Family Health International (FHI)
John Guillebaud, MA, FRSCE, FRCOG, MFFP, Margaret Pyke Center, London
Robert A. Hatcher, MD, MPH, Emory University School of Medicine
Michael Policar, MD, MPH, Solano Partnership Health Plan
Sharon Schnare, CNM, MSN, FNP, DHHS/PHS–Region 10
Gary S. Stewart, MD, MPH, Planned Parenthood of Sacramento Valley
Susan Wysocki, RNC, BSN, NP, National Association of Nurse Practitioners in Reproductive Health

Figure 2-1 (continued.)

Most women may use any of the sub-50-µg pills

STEP 3	STEP 4

STEP 3

If there is no reason to avoid estrogen, you may choose between any of the following OCs based on:
- Number of micrograms of ethinyl estradiol
- Availability of pill
- Ease of understanding packaging of pills
- Price of pills to clinic**
- Price of pills to client**
- Prior experience of this individual woman or the clinician caring for this woman with a special pill

Pills are listed from the lowest to the highest number of micrograms of ethinyl estradiol:

Combined Pill	Estrogen (µg)	Availability/Cost In Your Clinic	Company
Loestrin 1/20	20	_____	Parke-Davis
Alesse	20	_____	Wyeth
Estrostep 21	20/30/35	_____	Parke-Davis
Loestrin 1.5/30	30	_____	Parke-Davis
*Desogen	30	_____	Organon
Lo-Ovral	30	_____	Wyeth
Nordette	30	_____	Wyeth
Levlen	30	_____	Berlex
*Ortho-Cept	30	_____	Ortho
Tri-Levlen	30/40/30	_____	Berlex
Triphasil	30/40/30	_____	Wyeth
Ovcon 35	35	_____	Mead Johnson
Demulen 1/35	35	_____	Searle
Ortho-Cyclen	35	_____	Ortho
Ortho-Tri-Cyclen	35	_____	Ortho
Ortho Novum 777	35	_____	Ortho
Ortho-Novum 1/35	35	_____	Ortho
Modicon	35	_____	Ortho
Brevicon	35	_____	Syntex
Norinyl 1/35	35	_____	Syntex
Tri-Norinyl	35	_____	Syntex
**Norcept-E 1/35	35	_____	Syntex
**Nelova 0.5/35	35	_____	GynoPharma
**Nelova 1/35	35	_____	Warner-Chilcott
NEE 0.5/35	35	_____	Lexis
NEE 1/35	35	_____	Lexis
**Genora 0.5/35	35	_____	Rugby
Genora 1/35	35	_____	Rugby
Jenest	35	_____	Organon
NEE 10/11	35	_____	Lexes
Norethin 1/35E	35	_____	Schiaparelli-Searle

*Women using pills containing desogestrel may have an increased risk of venous thrombosis.

**The four pills costing pharmacists less than $10.00 per cycle: Norcept E ($5.72); Nelova 0.5/35, Nelova 1/35 ($6.25); and Genora 0.5/35 ($8.23). Cost of most pills to pharmacists was $17.00 to $22.33 per cycle. In some clinics, pills may be purchased at prices as low as $0.50 to $1.00 per cycle. SOURCE: Anonymous: Drug Topics Red Book. Average wholesale price listing. The Medical Letter 1992; December 11.

STEP 4

Other clinical considerations that might help in OC choice

A. To minimize the risk potential for *thrombosis* due to estrogen in a woman 40–50 years of age, or any woman at increased risk for thrombosis due to another cause (e.g., diabetic, very overweight woman, or a young woman who is a heavy smoker), prescribe:
- Loestrin 1/20
- Alesse

B. To minimize *nausea, breast tenderness, vascular headaches*, and estrogen-mediated side effects, prescribe:
- Loestrin 1/20
- Alesse
- Estrostep
Or a 30-µg pill, such as:
- Levlen
- Loestrin 1.5–30
- Lo-Ovral
- Nordette

C. To minimize *spotting and/or breakthrough bleeding*, prescribe:
- Low-Ovral, Nordette, or Levlen
- Estrostep
- Ortho-Cyclen or Ortho Tri-Cyclen
- Desogen or Ortho-Cept

D. To minimize androgen effects such as *acne, hirsutism, oily skin, sebaceous cysts, pilonidal cysts, or weight gain*, prescribe
- Ortho-Cyclen or Ortho Tri-Cyclen
- Desogen or Ortho-Cept
- Ovcon-35, Brevicon, or Modicon
- Demulen-35

E. To produce the most *favorable lipid profile*, prescribe:
- Ortho-Cyclen or Ortho Tri-Cyclen
- Desogen or Ortho-Cept
- Ovcon-35, Brevicon, or Modicon

F. To use a combined pill as an emergency contraceptive:
- Ovral (2 within 72 h, repeat in 12 h)
- Lo-Ovral (4 within 72 h, repeat in 12 h)
- Levlen, Nordette (4 within 72 h, repeat in 12 h)
- Triphasil, Tri-Levlen (4 yellow pills within 72 h, repeat in 12 h)

side effects. For safety reasons, it is best to start with an OC preparation containing less than 50 μg estrogen; for cost reasons, the generic 35-μg estrogen pills (such as Genora) should be considered initially.

Packets of OCs are available in 28-day and 21-day regimens. The 28-day regimen has seven placebo pills that allow pills to be taken every day. The 21-day regimen does not contain placebo pills, and users take a 7-day pill break after completion of the active pill cycle. Options for starting the pill include the first day of the menstrual period, the first Sunday after the menstrual period begins, or immediately.

POSTPARTUM PERIOD For women in the postpartum period, the OC should be started no sooner than 2 to 3 weeks after delivery to avoid problems with hypercoagulability and the initiation of breast-feeding. No adverse effects on infant growth and development have been reported. For postpartum women who are not lactating, OCs should begin no later than the third week after delivery because ovulation resumes on average around 45 days. Among women who exclusively breast-feed, ovulation rarely occurs before the third month postpartum. Some authors suggest delaying initiation of OCs in lactating women until this time both because of the efficacy of lactational amenorrhea in preventing conception and because of studies indicating a decreased duration of breast-feeding among OC users. Alternatively a progestin-only pill may be considered. The OC may be started immediately after an abortion. Although women who begin the pill by the fifth day of the menstrual cycle are likely fully protected against pregnancy, many practitioners suggest use of a backup method during the first week of use.

PATIENT EDUCATION Women should be instructed to take the OC at the same time every day. Suggesting that the woman associate taking the pill with another activity carried out at the same time each day (meals, bedtime, brushing teeth, removing contacts) may be helpful. For women who

may be exposed to STDs, condoms should be advised in addition to the oral contraceptive.

Missed Pills. Women should receive instructions, both verbal and written, about steps to take when active pills (first 21 days of a cycle) are missed. If pills are missed, it is always safest to use a backup form of contraception for the next 7 days.

If it is less than 24 h from the missed pill, women should take the missed pill right away and take the next day's pill at the usual time. If it is more than 24 h, she should take both the missed pill and current day's pill at the same time. If more than 24 h and late for the second pill, take that pill right away, discard the first/other missed pills, and continue with the rest of the pills at the usual time.

If any pills are missed from the third week of pills (days 15 to 21), Hatcher et al.[17] recommend that women finish the rest of the pack as described above, but refrain from taking a week off pills (or the seven placebo pills of the 28-day packs). Rather, women should begin a new pack immediately to provide greater contraceptive protection. Women should be made aware that they may not have a withdrawal period until the second pack is completed and that this will not harm them.

Two new OC formulations that contain less than 35 μg of EE daily are Alesse® and Estrostep®. Although these products provide low-dose estrogen options, they resemble the progestin-only oral contraceptives in the increased likelihood of pregnancy if tablets are taken late (> 24 h between doses).

BENEFITS AND SIDE EFFECTS

The benefits of OCs are many. As a contraceptive it is highly effective, reversible, and safe. Noncontraceptive benefits are listed in Table 2-1 and include protection against endometrial and ovarian cancer, potentially beneficial effects on the menstrual cycle, lowered risk of ectopic pregnancy, decreased risk of benign breast disease (progestin effect), and improvement in acne and hirsutism. Medical illnesses that may be improved or prevented through use of OCs are osteoporosis, atherogenesis (estrogen increases high-density lipids and lowers low-density lipids), endometriosis, uterine fibroids, and possibly rheumatoid arthritis, peptic ulcer disease, and thyroid disorders.

Potential side effects are summarized in Table 2-1. Common side effects can be divided into groups based on the hormone associated with the effect. This grouping may assist in selecting an alternate OC if the particular side effect persists beyond the initial 3 months of therapy.

COMMON SIDE EFFECTS Common estrogenic side effects include nausea, increased breast size, fluid retention, and leukorrhea. Cyclic weight gain has also been a reported concern, but a recent report demonstrates only minimal midcycle gain and no overall weight change during a 4-month period for women taking OCs.[18] Breast tenderness and headache may be attributed to either or both estrogen and progestin. Common androgenic side effects include acne/oily skin, depression, fatigue, increased appetite and weight gain, increased breast size and tenderness, decreased libido and sexual enjoyment, and pruritus. Management of common side effects is discussed in the final section of this chapter.

SERIOUS SIDE EFFECTS The most serious side effects are related to the enhanced coagulation effects of estrogen; these include thrombophlebitis, thromboembolic disease, and rare cerebrovascular accidents or myocardial infarction (MI). The risk of MI is primarily increased among women who smoke cigarettes. For women without other risk factors, the use of OCs is associated with a risk of MI of 1/100,000 OC users; among smokers over 35 years of age the risk increases sevenfold. OC formulations using the new progestins may demonstrate favorable lipid changes, thereby lowering cardiovascular risk; however, it will be many years before outcome studies can confirm the benefits to women with cardiovascular disease or the safety of these preparations for women who smoke.

Encouraging information comes from the Royal College of General Practitioners OC study.[19] Although the results confirm a small increase in the risk of cerebrovascular disease, pulmonary emboli, and venous thromboembolic disease among women who use OCs (RR = 1.17, 95 percent CI 1.09 to 1.25), the risk was seen only among women less than age 50 who used the older OCs containing 50 μg estrogen or more. The use of low-dose OCs was not a risk factor overall for either ischemic or hemorrhagic stroke among current users in a recent population-based case-control study.[20] However, there was an increase in hemorrhagic stroke among current users of OCs containing norgestrel or levonorgestrel (OR 3.23, 95 percent CI 1.24 to 8.41).[20]

Hypertension is a rare complication of OC use. One large study of over 2500 African American women in the southeastern United States did not find significant blood pressure changes in pill users that differed from changes in nonusers.[21] When blood pressure elevations do occur, they are usually mild and resolve within a few weeks of discontinuing the pills.

The OCs may increase the risk for breast cancer, but the risk is small and the tumors tend to be less aggressive. Current users have a 24 percent increase in risk; the risk declines to that of nonusers about 10 years after discontinuing the pills.

CONTRAINDICATIONS

Contraindications are related to side effects and are listed in Table 2-3. In addition, a number of potential drug interactions may occur among women on OCs. The drug interactions and appropriate action to take are listed in Table 2-2.

Progestin-Only Contraceptives

Progestin-only contraceptives include Norplant, Depo-Provera, and progestin-only pills (POPs). The Norplant system is a subdermal implant of levonorgestrel (see Fig. 2-2). It was approved by the FDA in 1990. The system provides 5 years of effective, reversible contraception. Depo-Provera is a long-acting depot form of the progestin medroxyprogesterone acetate (DMPA) that is administered by intramuscular injection at 3-month intervals. This synthetic progestin has been used

Table 2-3

Precautions in the Provision of Combined Oral Contraceptives (OCs)

REFRAIN FROM PROVIDING combined oral contraceptives for women with the following diagnoses (World Health Organization [WHO] category #4):

PRECAUTIONS	RATIONALE/DISCUSSION
Deep vein thrombosis (DVT) or pulmonary embolism (PE) or a history thereof	Estrogens promote blood clotting. Thromboembolic events related to known trauma or an IV needle are not necessarily a reason to avoid use of pills.
Cerebrovascular accident (stroke), coronary artery or ischemic heart disease, or a history thereof	Estrogens promote blood clotting.
Structural heart disease, complicated by pulmonary hypertension, atrial fibrillation, or history of subacute bacterial endocarditis	Estrogens promote blood clotting.
Diabetes with nephropathy, retinopathy, neuropathy, or other vascular disease; diabetes of more than 20 y duration	Estrogens promote blood clotting
Breast cancer	Breast cancer is a hormonally sensitive tumor. In theory, the hormones in OCs might cause some masses to grow.
Pregnancy	Current data do *not* show that hormonal contraceptives taken during pregnancy cause any significant risk of birth defects. However, hormonal contraceptives should not be given to pregnant women.
Lactation (< 6 wk postpartum)	There is some theoretical concern that the neonate may be at risk due to exposure to steroid hormones during the first 6 wk postpartum. OCs can diminish the volume of breast milk.
Liver problems: benign hepatic adenoma or liver cancer, or a history thereof; active viral hepatitis; severe cirrhosis	OCs are metabolized by the liver and their use may adversely affect prognosis of existing disease.
Headaches, including migraine, with focal neurologic symptoms	Focal neurologic symptoms such as blurred vision, seeing flashing lights or zigzag lines, or trouble speaking or moving may be an indication of an increased risk of stroke.
Major surgery with prolonged immobilization or any surgery on the legs	Increased risk for DVTs and PE.
Over 35 y old and currently a heavy smoker (≥ 20 cigarettes a day)	Smoking increases the risk for cardiovascular disease.
Hypertension, 160+/100+ or with vascular disease	Hypertension is an important risk factor for cardiovascular disease.

EXERCISE CAUTION if combined OCs are used or considered in the following situations and carefully monitor for adverse effects (WHO category #3):

PRECAUTIONS	RATIONALE/DISCUSSION
Postpartum < 21 d	There is some theoretical concern regarding the association between OC use up to 3 wk postpartum and risk of thrombosis.
Lactation (6 wk to 6 mo)	In the first 6 mo postpartum, use of OCs during breast-feeding diminishes the quantity of breast milk and may adversely affect the health of the infant.
Undiagnosed abnormal vaginal/uterine bleeding	Although OCs are often used to manage heavy bleeding, clinicians should be sure that the cause of the bleeding is known before prescribing OCs.
Over 35 y of age and light smoker (< 20 cigarettes/day)	Smoking increases the risk for cardiovascular disease. All smokers should be warned of this risk and should be encouraged and advised to stop smoking.
Past history of breast cancer but no evidence of recurrence for 5 y	Breast cancer is a hormonally sensitive tumor.
Use of drugs that affect liver enzymes: rifampicin, rifabutin, and griseofulvin; anticonvulsants such as phenytoin, carbamazepine, barbiturates, topiramate, and primidone	OCs are metabolized by the liver. Drugs that affect liver enzymes could reduce the contraceptive effectiveness of OCs.
Gallbladder disease: medically treated and current biliary tract disease and history of OC-related cholestasis	Recent reports show that OCs may be weakly associated with gallbladder disease. There is also concern that OCs may worsen existing gallbladder disease.

worldwide for over 30 years and was approved by the FDA for contraceptive use in the United States in 1992. The POP, sometimes referred to as the minipill, contains a small amount of a progestational agent (0.35 mg norethindrone [Micronor or NOR-QD]) or 0.075 mg norgestrel (Ovrette) and is taken daily.

MECHANISM OF ACTION

Progestin-only contraceptives prevent pregnancy via several mechanisms that differ by type of delivery system (i.e., implant, intramuscular, or oral). Although inhibition of ovulation, primarily through suppression of LH, occurs consistently with Depo-Provera, about 30 to 40 percent of women using either Norplant or the POP continue to ovulate. The latter two methods have marked effects on cervical mucus. The mucus thickens and decreases in amount, impeding sperm penetration. In addition, the endometrium becomes thin and atrophic. The endometrial effect appears less important for women using Norplant because fertilization has not been detected in Norplant users. Premature luteolysis may also be an important mechanism with POPs.

The Norplant system acts by diffusing levonorgestrel through six tubular silicone elastic capsules that are surgically implanted beneath the skin of the upper arm (Fig. 2-2). Each capsule contains 36 mg levonorgestrel. The release rate of the progestin during the first 6 to 18 months averages 50 to 80 μg/d (similar to the levonorgestrel in POPs). After this time the rate of release declines to 25 to 30 μg/d and remains there for the remainder of the 5 years. At the end of 5 years, the implants are removed through a small incision under local anesthesia. Replacement capsules may then be implanted. The system is completely reversible, with blood levels of levonorgestrel returning to normal within 96 h after removal and ovulatory cycles resuming within 7 weeks.

Depo-Provera is delivered as microcrystals of DMPA suspended in aqueous solution. A deep intramuscular injection of 150 mg DMPA is given every 3 months. The microcrystals dissolve slowly and release the progestin. A delay in return of

Figure 2-2

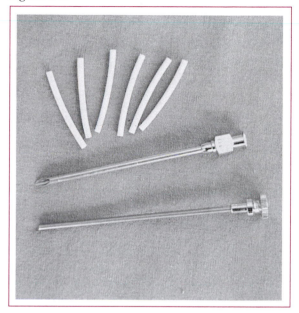

Norplant. The Norplant system consists of six progestin-impregnated rods that are inserted under the skin of the upper arm in a fan-shaped distribution. The trocar apparatus used for insertion consists of a hollow-bore insertion needle and a stylet.

fertility of about 9 months is observed after discontinuing injections; by 18 months 90 percent of users attempting pregnancy will become pregnant.

The POPs contain a small amount of a progestin and are taken every day with no pill-free interval. Although POPs contain two different progestins, there is no evidence of a clinically significant difference between them.

EFFICACY

The published failure rates for Norplant range from 0.04 to 0.2 pregnancies per 100 women in the first year of use with a cumulative rate of 3.7 percent over 5 years. There is some concern about an increased failure rate among obese women, but the extent of the problem is unclear. Depo-Provera has a probability of failure of 0.3 percent. The POPs are generally less effective than the combined OCs. In the first year of typical use 1.1 to 13.2 percent of users will become pregnant. In lactating women, however, the POP is nearly 100 percent effective.

PRESCRIBING INFORMATION

Norplant and Depo-Provera are excellent options for women who have difficulty remembering to take pills daily. The POPs should be strongly considered for women who have relative contraindications to combined OCs and for lactating women who are able to take the medication at a consistent time every day. Some studies suggest that milk volume may actually increase in POP users, and no deleterious effects on infant growth or development have been documented.[22]

Norplant insertion is a minor surgical procedure done under local anesthesia. Each Norplant kit comes with detailed step-by-step instructions. Wyeth Laboratories also produces two videotapes at no cost, one for patients and one for providers. In addition, the company will provide a refund if the device is removed within the first 6 months. Continuation rates for the first year are 88 to 95 percent, but by 3 years (the duration necessary to be cost-effective when compared with OCs) only 50 percent of women are still using this method.

The six implants are inserted on the inside of a woman's upper arm in a fanlike configuration within the first 7 days of the menstrual cycle or immediately after an abortion or delivery to avoid undetected pregnancy. When inserted under these circumstances, contraception is immediate. If inserted at other times a backup contraceptive is recommended if intercourse occurs within 24 h after insertion. The Norplant must be replaced after 5 years.

Depo-Provera is packaged in vials of 150 mg in each 1 cc. Deep intramuscular injections are made into the deltoid or gluteus maximus muscles. A 21- to 23-gauge needle 2.5 to 4 cm in length should be used. The area of injection should not be massaged because this may lower the effectiveness of DMPA. Injections in the deltoid are usually slightly more painful than those in the gluteus

maximus. Injections are scheduled every 3 months but may be given up to 2 weeks late. Satisfaction with this method may increase if patients are told to anticipate menstrual irregularity during the first year (70 percent). An increasing likelihood of amenorrhea is seen in subsequent years (80 percent of users by 5 years). An additional contraceptive should be used for the first week after the initial (or a delay > 2 weeks) injection, unless it is given within the first 5 days after beginning menses.

The POPs should be started within the first 5 days of the menstrual cycle or immediately postabortion or postpartum. The pill is taken every day (at 24-h intervals) for 28 days, then a new pack is started. It is critically important that POPs be taken at the same time every day for optimal contraceptive efficacy. If a woman is more than 3 h late in taking her pill, she should take it as soon as she remembers and use a backup method for 48 h. If two pills are missed, double the dose for 2 days and use a backup method for several days. In the case of two or more missed pills, consider emergency contraception.

BENEFITS AND SIDE EFFECTS

The progestin-only contraceptives share many advantages including lack of estrogen complications and reversibility (although return to fertility is delayed with DMPA) and the noncontraceptive benefits of scanty or absent menses, decreased menstrual cramping, and decreased anemia. There is also a decreased risk of developing endometrial and ovarian cancer and pelvic inflammatory disease. These agents can be useful in managing pain associated with endometriosis. Unlike POPs and Norplant, Depo-Provera has *not* been shown to interact with antibiotics or enzyme-inducing drugs; in fact, its use in women with seizure disorders has decreased the frequency of seizures. Women using these methods also have a lower risk of ectopic pregnancy.

Possible side effects are listed in Table 2-1. Disadvantages to all progestin-only contraceptives are menstrual cycle disturbances, weight gain, lack of STD protection, breast tenderness, and depression.

With respect to weight gain, POPs have a minimal effect, but weight gain with Norplant is on average 5 lb over 5 years and with DMPA it is significant— 5 lb in the first year, 8 lb by the second, and an average total of 14 lb after 4 years. Additional disadvantages of Norplant are risks of local pain, bleeding and infection with insertion and removal, relatively high initial cost, and drug interactions. The effectiveness of both Norplant and the POP is reduced when used concomitantly with antiepileptic medications (carbamazepine, phenytoin, phenobarbital, and primidone), rifampin, and phenylbutazone. Risks specific to DMPA are decreased bone density with long-term use (2 to 10 percent lower in one study, depending on site),[23] adverse lipid changes (high-density lipoprotein-C levels decrease), and the delay in return of fertility (6 to 12 months). The main side effects of POPs are acne and irregular bleeding. The incidence of other side effects is low.

CONTRAINDICATIONS

Absolute contraindications to progestin-only contraceptives are listed in Table 2-4. DMPA should be used with caution in women with cardiovascular disease or women with complications of diabetes because of the unfavorable lipid effect.

Barrier Contraceptives

Male condoms are the most commonly used of the barrier contraceptives. Other methods include the diaphragm, cervical cap, and the female condom. The contraceptive sponge had been taken off the market, based on a manufacturer decision after FDA recommendations for changes in the production process, but it may soon be marketed once again.

The diaphragm and cervical cap are believed to be most effective when used in combination with spermicides. Spermicides can also be used alone. In addition to pregnancy prevention, these methods all protect against most STDs. The effectiveness of these methods is highly user dependent, and most failures occur in the first year of use. Continuance rates at 1 year with these methods are 45 to 58 percent. The effectiveness, benefits, and potential side effects of these methods are listed in Table 2-1.

Table 2-4

Major Contraindications to the Use of Specific Methods of Contraception

Progestin-only contraceptives
  Active thrombophlebitis
  Undiagnosed genital bleeding
  Acute liver disease or liver tumors
  Breast cancer
Barrier devices
  History of latex or spermicide allergy, toxic
    shock syndrome,* or recurrent UTIs*
  Abnormalities of the vaginal anatomy
    or uterine prolapse
  Inability of the woman to place and
    remove it correctly
  †Cryosurgery, cauterization, or conization
    of the cervix within the past year, DES
    exposure, < 6 wk postpartum or
    postabortion, recent abnormal Pap smear,
    and cervical lacerations or erosions noted
    on physical examination
Intrauterine device
  Active or recurrent pelvic infection
  Known or suspected pregnancy
  Distorted uterine cavity
  Prior history of PID or current risk factors
    for PID‡
  Impaired response to infection
    (corticosteroid use, HIV)
  Undiagnosed or dysfunctional
    vaginal bleeding

*Not contraindications for the female condom.
†Contraindications for the cervical cap only.
‡Current risk factors include prior sexually transmitted diseases, multiple partners.
ABBREVIATIONS: DES, diethylstilbestrol; PID, pelvic inflammatory disease; UTI, urinary tract infection.

MECHANISM OF ACTION

MALE CONDOM   Male condoms, used for centuries, were initially made from animal tissue and are now made from latex or polyurethane, although a few animal "skin" or natural membrane condoms are still available. Condoms work by preventing sperm from entering the vagina and protect against disease by preventing direct contact between mucosal surfaces during intercourse. "Skin" condoms *do not* protect against STDs because of small pores present, which permit the passage of viruses. Some condoms are prelubricated and some contain small amounts of spermicide. The addition of spermicide does not appear to improve efficacy, and there has been a report of increased urinary tract infections in women associated with spermicide-coated condoms.[24]

FEMALE CONDOM   The Reality Female Condom is a thin sheath made of polyurethane, which is 7.8 cm in diameter and 17 cm long. The sheath is prelubricated on the inside and contains two flexible polyurethane rings; one lies inside the sheath attached to the closed end and the other forms

Figure 2-3

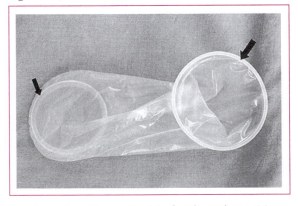

Female condom. The sheath of the female condom is 7.8 cm in diameter and 17 cm long and contains two flexible polyurethane rings. One ring lies inside the sheath, attached to the closed end of the condom (*small arrow*). It is used for insertion and sits in the posterior vagina. The other ring (*large arrow*) remains outside of the vagina and serves as the external opening of the device.

the external open edge of the device (Fig. 2-3). The former ring is used for insertion and sits inside the vagina similar to a diaphragm, and the external ring remains outside the vagina, covering part of the perineum and providing protection to the labia and base of the penis during intercourse. It should not be used with a male latex condom; friction from combined use causes the condoms to become dislodged. The female condom appears to offer similar protection against STDs, but has a higher reported failure rate (see Table 2-1). Experience with this method is limited; however, a recent study from China found high acceptance (90 percent) among 30 couples using the female condom.[25] Eighty-seven percent of the couples reported that the condom was easy to use, 80 percent of the women and 73 percent of the men reported no difference or improved sexual pleasure compared to the male condom, and 55 percent preferred the female condom over the male condom.

DIAPHRAGM AND CERVICAL CAP   The contraceptive effectiveness of the diaphragm and cervical cap is due to dual actions; they act as physical barriers to sperm and also hold spermicide near the cervix. The diaphragm is a circular latex cup that is inserted into the vagina and lies covering the cervix from the posterior fornix of the vagina to 1 to 2 cm behind the pubic bone, where the anterior rim fits snugly in place (Fig. 2-4). It comes in three types, arching, coil and flat spring, which refers to the construction of the inner edge of the rim. Sizes range from 50 to 95 mm (diameter of the cup), but most women are fitted with a size 60 to 85 mm. The cervical cap is a small latex rubber cup that fits directly over the cervix (Fig. 2-5). It is available in four sizes: 22, 25, 28, and 31 mm. The cap is held in place by suction between the cap's rim and the cervix and proximate wall of the vagina.

Both devices are to be used with a spermicidal cream, jelly, or gel. Although some data indicate a nearly twofold difference in pregnancy rates for diaphragm use without spermicide, several efficacy studies on the cap found no differences in

Figure 2-4

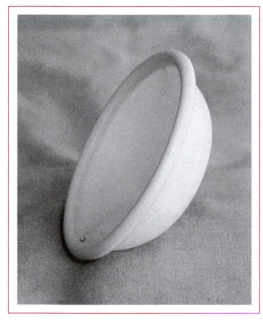

Diaphragm. The photograph shows an arching-spring rim type contraceptive diaphragm.

accidental pregnancy rate for women consistently using spermicide compared to those who did not.[26] Both the diaphragm and cervical cap require fitting by an experienced provider.

SPERMICIDE Spermicidal preparations are composed of a base or carrier and nonoxynol-9, an active spermicidal chemical. The action of spermicide is to kill sperm on contact by inhibiting sperm motility and survival. Spermicides come in a variety of formulations including foams (which add a physical bubble barrier produced by shaking the can prior to foam insertion), jellies, creams, gels, films, suppositories, and vaginal tablets; the first five methods are effective virtually immediately and the remaining two products are active 10 to 15 min after insertion. Used as a single agent, the contraceptive protection lasts about 1 h; when used with a cap or diaphragm, the jellies and creams last 6 to 8 h. Additional spermicide should be inserted vaginally for repeated acts

of intercourse; the diaphragm and cervical cap should not be removed for at least 6 h following intercourse.

EFFICACY

The failure rate of the male condom is typically in the range of 4 to 12 percent (see Table 2-1). Failure is often attributed to slippage and breakage, but these events are relatively uncommon (2 to 3 percent for breakage and 1 to 6 percent for slippage). Higher failure rates are associated with age (25 to 34 years old), years of sexual activity (5 years or more), use of a condom for less than 5 years, and high frequency of sexual intercourse. Use of a condom with a water-based lubricant has been reported to decrease failure rates. Polyurethane condoms appear to have equal efficacy to latex condoms (6-month pregnancy rates with typical use 4.8 percent and 6.3 percent, respectively; 6-month pregnancy rates with consistent use 2.4 percent and 1.1 percent, respectively).[27] In

Figure 2-5

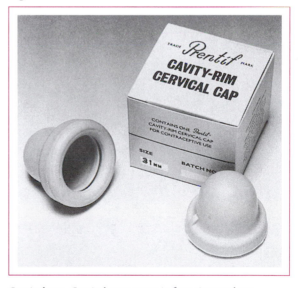

Cervical cap. Cervical caps come in four sizes and are packed individually. They must be ordered directly from the manufacturer. (Telephone 408-395-2100.) (*Courtesy of Cervical Cap, Ltd.*)

this randomized clinical trial, however, the polyurethane condoms were more likely to break or slip (8.5 percent versus 1.6 percent for latex condoms) and men randomized to use of the latex condom were more satisfied with the method.

Reported efficacy for the diaphragm and the cervical cap is similar (see Table 2-1); however, efficacy of the cap appears to be lower for parous women in whom accidental pregnancy rates are between 26 percent and 36 percent. The use of spermicide only has a reported accidental pregnancy rate of 21 percent. This relatively low rate may be due to the timing of use; spermicide offers the best protection when inserted into the vagina shortly before intercourse. When used only 15 to 30 min prior to intercourse 0 to 2 percent of sperm remain mobile; at longer intervals between spermicidal application and intercourse, less inhibition of sperm motility is noted.

PRESCRIBING INFORMATION

Both men and women should be offered written and oral descriptions of the method selected for use. Some products, such as the female condom, come with package inserts that provide directions for insertion. All oil-based lubricants (Table 2-5) and vaginal medications (e.g., antifungal preparations) should be avoided when using latex-based barrier methods because these lubricants can destroy the integrity of the latex. Polyurethane condoms can be used with oil-based lubricants and are not adversely affected by vaginal medication, which can damage latex.

The importance of counseling to enhance knowledge and use of barrier methods has been demonstrated in a number of studies; the counseling need not be extensive. For example, a study using brief interventions in waiting areas of public health clinics demonstrated a significant impact in helping women consistently use spermicide and condoms.[28] In this study, the best predictor of spermicide/condom use was knowledge about how to use spermicides correctly (OR = 3.2, 95 percent CI = 2.0, 5.0). Fear of AIDS or STDs did not predict spermicide use.

MALE CONDOM   The male condom is applied over the erect penis. The condom should be unrolled a short distance over a finger to be certain that it is

Table 2-5

Examples of Products that Can and Cannot Be Used as Lubricants with Latex Barrier Contraceptives*

SAFE	UNSAFE
Egg whites	Baby oil
Glycerine	Cold creams
Spermicide (nonoxynol-9)	Edible oils (olive, peanut, corn, sunflower)
Saliva	
Water	Hand and body lotions
	Massage oil
Examples of products:	Petroleum jelly
• Aloe-9 • K-Y Jelly	Rubbing alcohol
• Aqua Lube • Prepair	Suntan oil and lotions
• Astroglide • Probe	Vegetable or mineral oil
• ForPlay Lubricants • Ramses Personal Spermicidal	Vaginal yeast infection
• Gynol II • Touch Personal Lubricant	medications in cream
• H-R Lubricating Jelly • Wet	or suppository form

*All lubricants, including oil-based products, may be used with polyurethane condoms.
SOURCE: From Hatcher et al.[17]

unrolling properly and to allow a half-inch of empty space to remain at the tip of the condom to hold the ejaculate. This step is unnecessary with reservoir-tip condoms. The condom is then gently rolled down the shaft to the base of the penis. Additional lubrication (natural or artificial) is recommended before insertion because condoms are more likely to tear if the vagina or anus is dry. Suggested water-based lubricants are listed in Table 2-5.

The penis should be withdrawn soon after ejaculation while still erect, holding the rim of the condom against the base of the penis to prevent slippage. When the penis is away from the part-ner's genitals, the condom is removed without spilling the semen, checked for visible damage, and discarded.

Because this method is highly user dependent, motivation to use condoms should be increased by relating its use to important consequences. In addition to prevention of pregnancy and STDs, intention to use condoms among adolescents is associated with the following beliefs:

1. It enables one to have sex on the spur of the moment
2. It is easy to use
3. It is clean
4. It is popular with peers
5. It requires males to participate/have responsi-bility for using contraception.[29]

Providers should stress these as additional motivating factors. Because pain or discomfort with use is a common barrier reported by men, this should be openly discussed. Men who expe-rience this problem should consider the use of polyurethane condoms. These condoms were reported in a recent review of premarketing stud-ies to be preferred over latex in appearance, lack of smell, likelihood of slippage, comfort, sensitiv-ity, and natural look and feel (one study).

If a condom has torn or slipped off during use, spermicidal foam or cream should be inserted immediately. If this is not available, wash the vagina with soap and water. Emergency contra-ception should be considered.

Patients should also be informed that exposure to heat, inappropriate storage (long periods of time in a wallet), use with oil-based lubricants (see Table 2-5), and exposure to vaginal antifungal prepara-tions can reduce the reliability of this method.

FEMALE CONDOM   The female condom is inserted into the vagina by pinching together the upper ring, introducing the device into the vagina, and then pushing it into place with the first finger inserted inside the condom to ensure placement over the cervix (similar to the diaphragm). It is higher in cost than male condoms. Problems with slippage have also been reported. If a condom has torn or slipped off during use, spermicidal foam or gel should be inserted immediately. If this is not available, wash the vagina with soap and water. Emergency contraception should be considered.

Unlike male latex condoms, female (poly-urethane) condoms may be used with oil-based lubricants (see Table 2-5) or vaginal antifungal preparations. Reality condoms should not be used together with male condoms; this may cause slip-page of one or both condoms.

DIAPHRAGM   Of the three basic types of dia-phragms (arching, coil, and flat spring), most providers use the arching spring (Allflex [Ortho], Koroflex [Holland Rantos], and Ramses Bendex [Schmid]) in sizes 60 to 80 mm. An estimate of the correct size can be obtained by measuring the dis-tance along the examiner's index finger from the posterior vaginal wall to about 1 cm before the inside of the pubic arch. This estimate would cor-respond to the diameter of the device.

The diaphragm is inserted by pinching the sides together and gently inserting it into the vagina with a small amount of lubricant on the leading edge. Once inserted, it should cover the cervix and fit snugly in place with the rim in contact with the posterior and lateral vaginal walls and the anterior edge about one fingerbreadth before the pubic arch. It should be comfortable and easily removed by hooking the anterior rim with the examiner's index finger and gently pulling the device out of the vagina. If the diaphragm is too small, it will be very easy to remove and will sit well back from the symphysis; it will also be more likely to become dislodged during intercourse. If it is too large, it may cause discomfort and may bow or extend beyond the pubic symphysis and not under it.

Spermicide cream should be applied to the side of the diaphragm facing the cervix, covering the "cup" and rim, before insertion. The device may be inserted up to 6 h before intercourse, but additional vaginal spermicide (the diaphragm should not be removed for this purpose) may be inserted if intercourse does not occur soon after insertion or for repeated intercourse within 6 h. The diaphragm should be left in place for about 6 h after intercourse and removed within 24 h.

Women (or their partners) can insert the diaphragm while standing, squatting, or lying down. Women usually find it easiest to insert the diaphragm by pinching it between the thumb and third finger of their dominant hand, introducing the device into the introitus, and using the first finger (or the opposite hand) to push the back edge inside the vagina. The device should slide easily in place, but it may spring out of a woman's hand on initial attempts; she should be warned that this may happen and to not be discouraged. A plastic inserter or introducer can also be used to insert the coil and flat spring types of diaphragms. Removal is accomplished by inserting the first finger under the rim and pushing forward or by rotating the wrist (so that the knuckles of the hand are visible) allowing the device to be hooked by the index finger and pulled out of the vagina.

Women or their partners should be encouraged to practice inserting and removing the device in the office, after the initial fitting, until they are comfortable with the procedure. Women should be advised to inspect the device before each use for wear or tears and to replace them if these problems are identified or if odor is a problem. As with condoms, contact with oil-based lubricants can cause deterioration, and water-based lubricants are suggested if needed for additional lubrication with intercourse; spermicides can be used as lubricants (see Table 2-5). The diaphragm should be replaced every 2 years.

Women selecting a vaginal barrier method should also be advised to use the device *every time* she has intercourse. Sign and symptoms of toxic shock syndrome (TSS) should be reviewed; they are sudden high fever, vomiting and diarrhea, dizziness, faintness or weakness, rash (like a sunburn), and aching muscles or joints. Symptoms of urinary tract infections (UTIs) may also be discussed. If any problems arise, she should know whom to call and be encouraged to call for assistance.

CERVICAL CAP   The approximate size of the Prentif cavity-rim cervical cap, the only FDA-approved cervical cap available in the United States, is assessed by estimating the diameter of the cervix during the bimanual examination. Nulliparous women usually take the small sizes (22 or 25 mm).

The cap is inserted in the same manner by patients and providers, first folding the rim and compressing the dome so that when it is placed over the cervix, the expanding dome creates suction. The cap is then introduced into the vagina and placed over the cervix. Suction may be enhanced by inserting the cap at least 30 mins before intercourse. When the cap is in place, it should cover the cervix and fit snugly against the cervix at the fonices 360° around the rim. The examiner should check around the entire circumference to be sure that no gaps are detected. The cap should not become dislodged with gentle attempts of pushing forward and downward with the examining fingers, and when the dome is gently pinched, it should remain collapsed and resist tugging. Once in place, the anterior rim of the cap should be covered by the anterior wall of the vagina and should be as deep as possible from the introitus to avoid dislodgment by the penis. The cap is removed by probing with the index finger, tipping the cap to break the seal, and gently removing.

The cervical cap should be inserted about 30 mins before intercourse; the longer time (compared with the diaphragm) is suggested because this will improve suction. Additional spermicide may be inserted vaginally if intercourse does not occur soon after insertion. The cap should be left in place for at least 6 h after intercourse, but it may be left in place for 1 to 2 days.

The cervical cap can be inserted by the woman or her partner while standing, squatting, or lying down. Although a diaphragm can be prescribed for most women requesting one, only 50 to 70 percent of women requesting the cervical cap can use it due to inability of the provider to find a suitable fit, inability of the woman to insert or remove the cap, or contraindications to use. For this reason, it is particularly important to have the woman and her partner practice inserting and removing the device in the office until they are comfortable with the procedure. The cap should be replaced yearly.

Women selecting this method should also be advised to use the device *every time* she has intercourse. Signs and symptoms of TSS should be reviewed as above. If any problems arise, she should know whom to call and be encouraged to call for assistance.

BENEFITS AND SIDE EFFECTS

Advantages and disadvantages of barrier methods are listed in Table 2-1. All offer immediate contraceptive protection and protection against STDs and cervical dysplasia and neoplasia. Spermicides alone, however, may not reduce the risk of STDs. A recent controlled trial of use of latex condoms plus either nonoxynol-9 film versus placebo film by female sex workers in Cameroon found no decreases in the rate of new HIV, gonorrhea, or chlamydia infection.[30]

Although systemic side effects are absent for barrier methods, the diaphragm and cervical cap do increase the risk of TSS (2 to 3 cases per 100,000 users of vaginal barriers). Spermicides are also important as a backup method, as an adjunct used with other methods for additional protection, or as an emergency method if a condom breaks. At this time, condoms are the most effective choice to prevent HIV infection.

Allergy is the only adverse effect noted with male condoms, and this problem may be related to the spermicide because nonoxynol-9 appears to increase the release of natural rubber. There is also some concern that spermicide-mediated vulvovaginal microabrasions caused by the male condom may increase the risk of HIV.

Side effects of spermicides include skin irritation and allergy (rare). They are also messy to use and taste unpleasant. Bacterial colonization of the applicator may occur, increasing the risk of vaginitis and UTI; the applicator should be cleaned with plain soap and water after use. There appear to be no systemic effects or adverse effects even if accidentally used during pregnancy.

CONTRAINDICATIONS

Contraindications or cautious use for these devices are listed in Table 2-4. The listed contraindications for the cervical cap stem from a controversy over the whether the cap induces cervical dysplasia. The cap is not recommended for use during menstruation because of concern with obstruction to flow and interference with the cap's suction.

Intrauterine Device

The IUDs have long been an important method of birth control and, in many countries such as China, are the most commonly used method. During the mid-1980s many of these devices were taken off the U.S. market for a number of reasons including lack of profitability and lawsuits charging that IUDs were responsible for injuries to their users. Despite the fact that most of the cases that went to trial were won by the pharmaceutical company, legal fees and lack of insurance led to further withdrawal of IUDs from the U.S. market. Today, only two IUDs are available in the United States, the Cu T 380A (Paragard) and the Intrauterine Progesterone Contraceptive System (Progestasert).

MECHANISM OF ACTION

It is important to inform patients that the research evidence indicates that IUDs act primarily by inhibiting fertilization through multiple effects on sperm and ova. Although the inflammatory response created in the endometrium from the presence of the IUD inhibits implantation, few fertilized ova actually reach the endometrium.[31] In addition, with the hormone-containing IUD, thickening of cervical mucus interferes with sperm motility as well.

The Paragard is a T-shaped device made of polyethylene with barium sulfate added for visibility on x-rays (Fig. 2-6). It has copper wire on the vertical stem and on each transverse arm (total surface area 380 mm²) and two monofilament threads attached to the base of the stem for removal. The copper IUD prevents pregnancy primarily by preventing fertilization in the majority of instances; using human chorionic gonadotropin assays, fertilization was detected in less than 1 percent of menstrual cycles in IUD users. The copper also acts locally on the endometrium, creating a sterile inflammatory reaction (foreign body response) that prevents sperm from reaching the fallopian tubes; ovulation is not affected. White blood cells may also consume sperm in the uterus. The copper is not absorbed systemically to any significant degree, and the amount of copper released each day is less than the amount consumed daily in a regular diet.

The Progestasert is also a T-shaped device made of ethylene vinyl acetate copolymer containing a reservoir of 38 mg progesterone (and barium sulfate for visibility on x-ray) in a silicone oil base. The progesterone, released at 65 µg/d, acts primarily by thickening cervical mucus, impeding sperm penetration, and through a decidual reaction, resulting in glandular hypertrophy. This action, in addition to the local foreign body response, prevents implantation.

EFFICACY

The Paragard is highly effective. Rates of accidental pregnancy are between 0.5 percent and 1.5 percent, the latter figure after 7 years of use. The Paragard is currently approved for 10 years of continuous use. The effectiveness of the Progestasert IUD is slightly lower than that of the Paragard; 1.5 percent to 2 percent accidental pregnancies are reported in first-year clinical trials. The Progestasert must be replaced yearly.

Continuation rates are high for the IUD, about 70 percent in most studies after 1 year. This may be contrasted with a rate of about 40 percent among users of oral contraceptives.

PRESCRIBING INFORMATION

The role of the provider in prescribing the IUD is to screen interested women for risk factors, review important information about the device, obtain written informed consent for placement, provide careful insertion under sterile conditions, and arrange for regular follow-up and quick access to medical care if complications occur.

SCREENING Identifying the best candidate for the IUD is the most important step in reducing IUD-related complications. Women at low risk of STDs (such as those in mutually faithful relationships), women who have had children and do not want more in the near future, and women who have difficulty with other methods of contraception should strongly consider this method. An IUD should not be placed in a woman with active or recurrent pelvic infection, a prior history of pelvic inflammatory disease (PID), or current risk factors for PID (prior STDs, multiple partners, impaired response to infection such as chronic steroid use

Figure 2-6

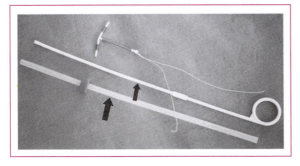

Intrauterine device. The photograph shows a copper IUD, along with the inserter device. The inserter device consists of a hollow barrel (*large arrow*) and a solid rod (*small arrow*).

or AIDS). Women with a history of ectopic pregnancy are not candidates for the Progestasert but may use the Paragard because of its protective effect against ectopic pregnancy and infrequent need for replacement. Women with menorrhagia or anemia should consider the Progestasert.

INSERTION   IUDs may be placed immediately or up to 48 h postpartum or immediately after a first trimester abortion. Advantages of immediate postpartum placement include lower cost, less pain and bleeding, and certainty of no pregnancy. Disadvantages include higher expulsion rates and higher rates of missing strings. Expulsion rates are much higher after second trimester abortions; IUD placement should be deferred in these cases. For other women, IUDs are often inserted during menses, taking advantage of the increased size of the cervical os and confirming that pregnancy is unlikely. Expulsion rates, however, are higher during this time of the cycle, and greater continuation rates are obtained when IUDs are inserted from day 12 to 17 of the menstrual cycle.[32] Complete information on insertion technique is available elsewhere[17] and will not be presented in this chapter.

PATIENT EDUCATION   Women should be instructed to check periodically for the IUD string to make sure that the device is in place, particularly over the first few menstrual cycles. Expulsion of the IUD occurs in between 1 and 10/100 women in the first year after insertion. It is more common among younger women and those who have never been pregnant. Women should also be counseled to report any symptoms of pelvic pain, bleeding, malodorous discharge, fever, or a missed period.

At the scheduled follow-up visit, the woman's questions should be addressed and any side effects noted should be discussed. Changes in her medical condition or sexual relationship(s) should be discussed. A bimanual examination may be considered to determine that the IUD is in place and that there is no evidence of infection or perforation. The date for scheduled removal should

be noted, keeping in mind that changing IUDs unnecessarily is to be avoided because most complications, including pregnancy, occur just after insertion. Finally, warning signs of serious complications (e.g., late period, abnormal spotting or bleeding, abdominal pain especially associated with fever or chills, pain with intercourse, or abnormal discharge) and what to do about them should be reviewed.

BENEFITS AND SIDE EFFECTS

Benefits of the IUD include high efficacy, safety, reversibility, and ease of use. In addition, the IUD does not interfere with lactation and these devices have no systemic side effects. Progestasert IUDs have the advantage of decreasing menstrual blood flow by as much as 40 percent. The number of days of light bleeding and spotting, however, may be increased. Copper IUDs lower the risk of ectopic pregnancy by about 50 to 90 percent compared to women using no contraceptive method; however, if pregnancy occurs, there is an increased risk of ectopic versus intrauterine pregnancy. The Progestasert, however, has a rate of ectopic pregnancy 50 to 80 percent higher than in women using no birth control method.

One of the most serious complications of IUD insertion is perforation of the uterus. Fortunately, this complication is rare (approximately 1.2/1000 insertions). A transient increased risk of PID is seen in the first 4 months after the procedure, likely due to the introduction of bacteria into the uterine cavity during the insertion. The risk is fourfold greater in the first month, returning to baseline by 5 months after insertion. A number of factors influence the risk of infection including the type of IUD (the Dalkon shield had the highest risk of infection), exposure to STDs, age (younger women, likely related to these women being less likely to be in monogamous relationships), and duration of use. The risk of contracting severe PID, requiring hospitalization, increases after 5 years of use to about five times the risk of nonusers of IUDs.[34] These infections appear to be caused primarily by *Actinomyces*. IUDs as well as oral contraceptives appear to alter the vaginal flora, with significantly more anaerobic bacteria isolated compared with barrier method users who maintained a lactobacilli-dominated flora. The significance of this finding is uncertain.

To reduce the incidence of postinsertion pelvic infection, some investigators advocate the use of antibiotics (single 200-mg oral dose of doxycycline, most commonly, or 500 mg erythromycin if breast-feeding or allergic to tetracycline) just before IUD insertion. Although studies show a decreased incidence of infection (31 percent in one large study) with this approach, the number of women who developed PID is too small to confer adequate power to detect a significant difference.

A disadvantage of the Paragard is the increased volume of bleeding per cycle (50 to 100 percent increase), which may result in anemia.[33] In clinical trials, this abnormal bleeding resulted in 4 to 15 percent of women discontinuing this method during the first year of use; the higher rates of removal were seen primarily among younger women who may be less tolerant of this side effect.

CONTRAINDICATIONS

Absolute contraindications to insertion of an IUD are active or recurrent pelvic infection, known or suspected pregnancy, and a distorted uterine cavity. Cautious use is advised for the other conditions listed in Table 2-4. Women with previous problems with an IUD and difficulty obtaining follow-up or emergency care for complications may also wish to consider another method.

Women with a history of ectopic pregnancy are not candidates for the Progestasert, but may use the Paragard because of its protective effect against ectopic pregnancy and infrequent need for replacement.

Natural Family Planning

A number of natural methods have been used since the 1950s for contraception. The earliest of these was the calendar method, which determined periods of fertility based on previous cycles over a 1-year period. Fertile days were determined by subtracting 18 days from the length of the shortest cycle (first fertile day) and 11 days from the longest cycle (last fertile day). Intercourse was avoided during this time period. High variability in cycles, however, led to a wide range of efficacy rates for this method. The temperature method used the body temperature rise just after ovulation (0.4° to 1.0° F), and the ovulation method used changes in cervical mucus (from thick and dry to clear, thin, and sticky) to predict ovulation. Intercourse was avoided during the presumed fertile period. Today, a combination of these methods, the symptothermal method, is recommended for use (Fig. 2-7) and is reviewed in detail elsewhere.[34]

MECHANISM OF ACTION

The symptothermal method is based on female reproductive anatomy and physiology. After a variable number of days after the onset of menses, an estrogen surge followed by a surge of LH triggers ovulation. The estrogen surge causes the columnar cells of the endocervical crypts to produce a clear thin stretchy mucus (type E, estrogenic). Type E mucus allows increased sperm penetration and longer sperm survival (3 to 5 days versus hours) and filters out morphologically defective sperm. Several studies have shown that this mucus, detected externally at the vaginal introitus, correlates closely with the time of ovulation; by 3 days following peak mucous production, ovulation occurs in nearly all women. An unfertilized egg can survive 12 to 24 h. Following ovulation, progesterone becomes the dominant hormone. Progesterone is thermogenic, causing the body temperature to rise, and the cervical mucus is changed to an opaque, thick sticky type (type G, gestagenic). The average length of the postovulatory phase is 13.7 days (range 9 to 17 days, but usually consistent within a given woman).

EFFICACY

Efficacy rates for this method vary greatly (see Table 2-1). Differences in reported rates may be

Figure 2-7

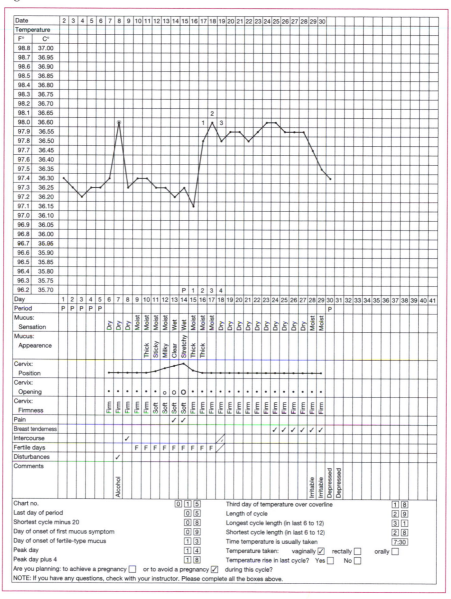

Example of chart used in the symptothermal method of natural planning. Note that the encircled dot represents an aberrant rise in temperature that is most likely the result of consumption of alcohol and not related to fertility.

due to different systems of natural family planning being evaluated, differences in instructors, classification of pregnancies as accidental or intended (ovulation methods are also used as a means of achieving conception), and consistency of use by couples.

PRESCRIBING INFORMATION

Couples need careful instruction in this method, often over several sessions, by a trained instructor to achieve optimal efficacy. Charting temperatures and symptoms also appears to be an important part of using this method effectively (see Fig. 2-7). Body temperature measurements should be obtained on awakening before rising from bed. Special thermometers (basal body temperature thermometers) are available to assist in documenting the temperature rise following ovulation. Women should begin checking cervical mucus following menses, paying special attention to the onset of sticky mucus. Intercourse should then be avoided. When the mucus changes to slippery, resembling raw egg white, a woman is entering her most fertile period, which continues until 3 days after the last day that slippery mucus appears (peak day). Women may also be aware of other symptoms of ovulation including adnexal pain (mittelschmerz), low backache, abdominal bloating, vulvar swelling, and intermenstrual spotting. Women may also be able to feel a widening of the cervical os on internal self-examination. Ovulation test kits are available, which can detect the LH surge, but these add greatly to the expense of this method. Use of one of these commercial kits, however, can narrow the time period of abstinence. After the third day following the peak day, couples may resume intercourse until onset of the menses. Intercourse should also be avoided during menses because women with short cycles may enter their fertile period during the last days of bleeding.

Providers should stress that absolute compliance with this protocol is vital to its efficacy. Trussel and Grummer-Strawn noted that the probability of pregnancy increased from 0.2 percent per cycle to 28 percent per cycle when any of three crucial rules were broken: no intercourse (1) during mucous days, (2) within 3 days after the peak day, or (3) during times of stress.[35] A summary of the rules for this method is shown in Table 2-6.

Lactational Amenorrhea

MECHANISM OF ACTION

The precise mechanism for lactational infertility is unknown. It is believed that suckling has a direct effect on the hypothalamus, which reduces the pulsatile secretion of gonadotropin-releasing hormone, thereby suppressing the LH release and ovulation.

EFFICACY

Women who exclusively breast-feed (no supplements are used to feed the infant) and who do not have a return of menstruation have failure rates of only 0.5 to 2 percent. Unfortunately, ovulation may resume before the first menses, and the probability that this will happen increases

Table 2-6

Key Events and Rules for Symptothermal Method of Natural Family Planning

CYCLE EVENT	DAYS	SIGNS	INTERCOURSE PERMITTED
Menstruation	1–5	Bleeding	No
Safe (dry) days	6–9	No cervical mucus	Yes
Fertile period begins	10	Sticky or stretchy mucus begins	No
Peak fertility	16	Last day of slippery mucus	No
Fertility ends	20	4 d after peak fertility	Next day
Safe days	20–29	Until menses begin	Yes

SOURCE: Adapted with permission from Hatcher et al.[17]

with time (from 33 to 45 percent during the first 3 months to 64 to 71 percent during the next 9 months).[17]

PRESCRIBING INFORMATION

Women using this method should be advised to feed on demand, avoid bottle-feeding or other food supplements, and begin using another method of birth control on return of menses or by 6 months for greatest efficacy.

Withdrawal

Chapter 2

MECHANISM OF ACTION

Withdrawal, or coitus interruptus, is when a man withdraws his penis from the vagina before ejaculation. This method of contraception works by preventing contact between the sperm and ovum. It is frequently used and, although widely criticized, provides contraceptive efficacy similar to the vaginal barrier methods.

EFFICACY

The accidental pregnancy rate with this method is 19 percent, although rates as low as 7 percent have been reported.

PRESCRIBING INFORMATION

To effectively use this method, a man must be able to determine when he is about to ejaculate and withdraw his penis from the vagina so that sperm do not come in contact with his partner's genitalia. Although there is some concern that the pre-ejaculate, the lubricating secretion from the Cowper's glands that occurs before ejaculation, contains sperm, several small studies found no sperm present in the pre-ejaculate of HIV-seronegative men. Because sperm have been detected in pre-ejaculates of HIV-positive men and this method does not protect against HIV,

couples should consider other methods of contraception, particularly with new partners. This method, however, should be encouraged at times when other methods are not available.

Emergency Contraception

Emergency contraception is the use of a drug or device to prevent pregnancy following intercourse. Options for emergency contraception include OCs, levonorgestrel, high-dose estrogen, mifepristone (RU 486), danazol, and insertion of a copper IUD. Of these, the combination of estrogen and progestin (often referred to as the Yuzpe regimen) is the method most commonly used in the United States.

This form of contraception is greatly underutilized, partially due to ignorance on the part of providers and the women they serve. It has been estimated that each year in the United States, widespread use of emergency contraception would prevent over 1 million abortions and 2 million unintended pregnancies carried to childbirth.[36] This form of contraception, whether given at the time of the emergency or in advance, has been shown to be cost-effective.[37] In addition, nearly one-half of women with unintended pregnancies report that they would have considered emergency contraception if they had known that it was available.[38]

MECHANISM OF ACTION

It is important to stress to patients that emergency contraceptive methods are forms of contraception (preventing pregnancy before implantation) and not abortifacents. Mechanisms of action include inhibition or delay of ovulation if given before ovulation (estrogen/progestin, mifepristone, danazol), interference with fertilization (IUD due to toxic effects on sperm), interference with function of the corpus luteum (mifepristone and possibly estrogen/progestin, danazol, and high-dose estrogen), and prevention of implantation (mifepristone delays endometrial maturation).[38]

EFFICACY

The efficacy rates for the methods of emergency contraception along with the timing of use, status of method, and source of data are listed in Table 2-7. With respect to efficacy, available data on mifepristone show that this method is more effective than the Yuzpe regimen (100 percent versus 75 to 80 percent of pregnancies prevented) with fewer reported side effects.[39] Unfortunately, this drug is not available in the United States for use as a contraceptive.

In a recent randomized clinical trial of levonorgestrel for emergency contraception versus combined estrogen/progestin, investigators found levonorgestrel to be more effective (85 percent versus 57 percent of expected pregnancies prevented; crude RR for pregnancy 0.36, 95 percent CI .18 to .70).[40] This method also had fewer side effects. The major limitation to use of this drug is the lack of availability of a 0.75-mg tablet. Using current preparations, women would have to take 20 tablets of Ovrette for two doses, 12 h apart, resulting in a large pill burden and high cost (approximately $52).

PRESCRIBING INFORMATION

Information on emergency contraception *should be provided to all patients*, particularly for those selecting barrier methods. In fact, providing emergency contraception to patients *in advance* appears to be the optimal strategy because women often find themselves in need on weekends or after the typical office hours. Glasier and Baird found that women randomized to receiving a replaceable supply of hormonal emergency contraceptive pills (N = 553) versus by physician prescription experienced fewer pregnancies (18 versus 25 unintended pregnancies, NS).[40] Although more women in the treatment group reported using emergency contraception once (47 percent versus 27 percent), they were not more likely to use it repeatedly. A pilot program in Washington, established in 1997, allows pharmacists to prescribe emergency contraception under protocol.[41]

In the first 4 months of the program, more than 500 participating, trained pharmacists wrote and filled more than 2700 prescriptions. In addition, a satisfaction survey found that inter-action with the pharmacists was rated highly and half of the women reported receiving the pills on a weekend or after 6 PM.

DOSE AND REGIMEN The estrogen/progestin regimen consists of two tablets of Ovral or four to five tablets of several other OCs given twice, with 12 h between doses (Table 2-8). The tablets must be given within 72 h after unprotected intercourse, although the highest efficacy occurs with dosing within 24 h of unprotected intercourse. This regimen is currently available by prescription as the product Preven (about $20). This packet includes the tablets with instructions and a pregnancy test kit.

Levonorgestrel is given as 0.75 mg given twice with 12 h between doses. There is no product containing this amount of medication, and this regimen as noted above must be dosed as 20 tablets of a norgestrel-containing POP for each dose.

Insertion of a copper IUD (Paragard) within 5 to 7 days after ovulation in a cycle when unprotected intercourse has occurred is also extremely efficacious in preventing pregnancy. The insertion procedure does not differ from the usual one. This option is used much less frequently than hormonal treatment in this country and is not an approved indication for the IUD.

BENEFITS AND SIDE EFFECTS

Emergency contraception is safe and effective for preventing pregnancy following unprotected intercourse. The major side effects of the estrogen/progestin regimen are nausea (in up to 50 percent) and vomiting (in up to 20 percent). Subsequent menses may be heavier than usual but should occur when expected. Some women have mild mastalgia for a few days after treatment.[39] Rare cases of venous thrombosis have also been reported, but the rates are far less than the risk of venous thrombosis associated with pregnancy.

Table 2-7

Methods of Emergency Contraception

Regimen	Time After Intercourse*	Status of Method	Reported Efficacy†	Source of Data
Estrogen and progestin (100 µg ethinyl estradiol and 0.5 mg levonorgestrel given twice, with 12 h between doses)	72 h	Licensed in some countries since early 1980 (e.g., United Kingdom, the Netherlands); available unlicensed in the appropriate combination of oral contraceptive pills	75–80% of pregnancies prevented	Meta-analysis of 10 trials involving >5000 women
Levonorgestrel (0.75 mg given twice, with 12 h between doses)	48 h (possibly up to 72 h)	Licensed in some countries in Eastern Europe and Asia	Equivalent to estrogen–progestin	One randomized trial involving 350 women
High-dose estrogen (e.g., 5 mg ethinyl estradiol daily for 5 d)	72 h	Licensed in the Netherlands; little used elsewhere	Equivalent to estrogen–progestin	Randomized trial involving 250 women; early trials suggested failure rates <1%
Mifepristone (a single 600-mg dose)	72 h	Widely used in China in a variety of lower doses; not licensed anywhere else for emergency contraception	100% effective	Two randomized trials involving a total of 600 women
Danazol (400–800 mg given twice 12 h apart or 400 mg given 3 times at intervals of 12 h)	72 h	Used only under research conditions	Reports vary from failure rates of <1% to ineffective	Two randomized trials, one involving >1700 women and suggesting failure rates of about 1%, and the other involving 193 women and suggesting little or no effect
Copper intrauterine device	Up to 5 d after the earliest estimated day of ovulation	Available worldwide, but not licensed for emergency contraception	Failure rates <1%	Meta-analysis of 20 published studies involving >8000 women

*The times given are for the first dose.

†Data on efficacy are not comparable because not all are based on exposure during the fertile phase of the cycle (see the text).

Source: Reprinted with permission from Glasier.[38]

Table 2-8

Oral Contraceptives Effective for Emergency Contraception

(First dose within 72 h of unprotected sex; second dose exactly 12 h later.)	
Brand Tablets	Per Dose
Preven kit	2 light blue
Ovral	2 white
LoOvral	4 white
Nordette	4 orange
Levlen	4 orange
Levora	4 white
Trilevlen	4 yellow
Triphasil	4 yellow
Trivora	4 pink
Alesse	5 pink
Levlite	5 pink
Ovrette (progestin only)	All 20

Note: Preven costs about $20 and is the only product packaged with directions for emergency contraception. Some facilities repackage pills from samples to reduce cost. Clinicians who do so should follow state regulations for repackaging pharmaceutical products. Source: Reprinted with permisssion from Judge.[56]

In a recent report of emergency contraception with an IUD used in 515 Chinese women, there were no cases of pelvic infection.[42] Efficacy was 92.4 percent (two pregnancies) and subsequent removal was requested in 14.9 percent of nulliparous and 3.5 percent of parous women, primarily due to pain and bleeding.

Medical Abortion

The availability of legal abortion has resulted in a large decrease in maternal mortality and morbidity, primarily from causes such as sepsis, hemorrhage, and trauma.[43] Unfortunately, there are still 20 million unsafe abortions performed annually worldwide and 200,000 women in developing countries die annually of complications after illegal abortion.[44] Even in the United States, many women do not have access to legal/safe abortion; in a 1990 review of abortion services, 83 percent of counties in the United States had no identified abortion provider.[45] Medical abortion, especially for women with pregnancies under 42 days of gestation, is a safe and effective alternative to surgical abortion and should be considered as an alternative for pregnant women who desire pregnancy termination. Blood loss may be greater with medical abortion, although differences in blood loss do not appear to be clinically important. Although medical abortion is 90 to 95 percent successful, success rates with surgical abortion are higher (98 to 99 percent).

Medical Options

As noted in a recent review of the literature on medical abortion in early pregnancy, either methotrexate or mifepristone (RU 486) plus a prostaglandin (most often misoprostol) are safe and effective medications for this purpose.[46] Mifepristone, however, is not an FDA-approved agent in the United States.

Methotrexate

Methotrexate is a dihydrofolate reductase inhibitor that is believed to act by damaging the connection of the trophoblast to the endometrium and also by decreasing trophoblast production of human chorionic gonadotropin.

efficacy   In the first randomized clinical trial of methotrexate (given intramuscularly) followed by misoprostol, investigators found the combination to be more effective than misoprostol alone with a reported efficacy of over 90 percent.[47] Since that time, this group of investigators documented an equally high success rate with oral methotrexate (50 mg),[48] higher success rates with earlier (up to 49 days' gestation) versus later pregnancies,[48] and higher success rates with higher-dose misoprostol (800 μg versus 600 μg) given at 7 days rather than 3 days following the methotrexate. Completed abortion rates from case series are 88 to 100 percent.[47] In the randomized trial of oral methotrexate, efficacy was decreased with increasing body surface area and the authors suggest that the intramuscular route or higher oral doses be considered for larger women.[49]

REGIMEN, PROGRESS OF ABORTION, AND SIDE EFFECTS
Regimens and side effects for methotrexate and misoprostol are provided in Table 2-9. Few abortions (7 percent) occur before administration of misoprostol. Cramping usually begins within hours after the misoprostol and bleeding within 5 h for women with immediate success (75 to 84 percent of women). Pain can usually be controlled with oral analgesics. Approximately 17 percent of women have delayed success, with abortion occurring within 10 to 45 days (median 23 days); these women did not require further intervention. The duration of bleeding regardless of whether abortion is immediate or delayed averaged 9 days total. Bleeding is rarely heavy enough to require transfusion.

Side effects overall are lower with intramuscular administration of methotrexate, with the exception of oral ulcers. Side effects with combination therapy (methotrexate and misoprostol) are similar to those with drug therapy with methotrexate alone.

MIFEPRISTONE

Mifepristone is a glucocorticoid antagonist and an antiprogestin and acts by antagonizing progesterone receptors in the uterus, thereby causing decidual breakdown and detachment of the embryo. Mifepristone also enhances myometrial contractions by increasing both uterine production of prostaglandins and uterine sensitivity to their effects.

EFFICACY   The aggregate success rates, based on randomized clinical trials, for the regimen of mifepristone and misoprostol is 93.7 percent (91 to 96 percent).[47] As with methotrexate, success rates are best for women with pregnancies

Table 2-9

Regimens and Efficacy and Safety Information for Medical Abortion

REGIMEN	EFFICACY	SIDE EFFECTS*	COMMENTS
Methotrexate 50 mg/m² IM or 50 mg orally once	88–100%[47]	Nausea (19–37%) Vomiting (10%) Diarrhea (7–12%) Dizziness (4–14%)	Avoid folate-containing vitamins for 1 wk after methotrexate administration
Followed in 6–7 d by Misoprostol 800 μg (4 tablets intravaginal)		Hot flushes (3–15%) Headache (9–13%) Fever/chills† (31%) Oral ulcers‡ (<1%)	
Mifepristone 600 mg orally once	91–96%	Nausea (33–70%) Vomiting (19–40%) Diarrhea (20–26%)	Not yet available in the United States
Followed in 2–4 d by Misoprostol 800 μg (4 tablets intravaginal)		Dizziness (12–37%) Headache (19–32%) Fever/chills† (4–37%)	

*Side effects and percentages shown are based on a summary estimate of published reports; abdominal pain, cramping, and bleeding were experienced by virtually all women.
†Side effect following misoprostol administration only.
‡Side effect seen after IM methotrexate only.

at lower gestational age ($\leq$ 49 days), but efficacy from case series reports continues to be over 90 percent for women with pregnancies of up to 63 days' gestation or less.

REGIMEN, PROGRESS OF ABORTION, AND SIDE EFFECTS
The currently recommended regimen is shown in Table 2-9. In the most recent report of a large case series of mifepristone (600 mg orally once) and misoprostol (400 μg 2 days later), termination of pregnancy occurred in 4 percent of women prior to administration of misoprostol, within 4 h after misoprostol insertion in 49 percent of women, and within 24 h in 75 percent of women.[49]

Side effects are listed in Table 2-9. Side effects were rated as severe in some women (30 percent for nausea, 10 percent for vomiting, 3 percent for diarrhea), increased with increasing gestational age, but rarely resulted in hospitalization or need for transfusion.

Advantages

Medical abortion can be offered earlier than surgical abortion and affords a woman making this difficult decision both privacy and autonomy. Most women will be able to avoid surgical intervention. Despite the high rate of reported side effects, most women report satisfaction with the procedure, and 64 to 95 percent of women would select the method again.[50]

Disadvantages

In addition to higher rates of side effects compared to surgical abortion, medical abortion is delayed in a substantial minority of women, particularly for single-drug therapy with methotrexate. There is also a higher failure rate than with surgical abortion and the added inconvenience of several visits that are often required to confirm termination or for further intervention. Women also need to be aware that they will need a suction procedure if abortion is incomplete or pregnancy continues. Misoprostol has been associated with fetal anomalies.

Contraindications

Medical abortion is contraindicated in women whose pregnancies are more advanced than those reported as resulting in successful termination in the clinical trials (within 49 days for use of methotrexate and 63 days for mifepristone). Medical abortion is also contraindicated for women who have suspected ectopic pregnancy and for women with asthma, cardiovascular disease, heavy smoking, or severe anemia. Some investigators have excluded women aged 35 and older, and less is known about the safety and efficacy of these regimens for these women. Medical abortion should not be attempted in settings where there is not immediate access to surgical abortion.

Protocol

The protocol proposed by Gold and colleagues offers guidance for clinicians who wish to provide medical abortion.[51] Because efficacy of medical abortion decreases rapidly with increasing gestational age, a vaginal ultrasound is recommended to ensure accurate dating and to exclude ectopic pregnancy. A baseline serum β-human chorionic gonadotropin (β-HCG), hematocrit, blood type, and Rh factor should be obtained and a pelvic examination performed to assess uterine size. Women who are Rh-negative should receive Rh immunoglobulin along with the initial abortifacient.

Women are then given one of the regimens shown in Table 2-9. Vaginal insertion of the misoprostol tablets may be completed by women at home or can be performed in the office with women remaining for 4 h after insertion (the time when approximately half the women will be expected to abort with the mifepristone protocol). Women should be seen by the clinician within 1 to 2 weeks to determine whether complete abortion has occurred either using vaginal ultrasound or checking serial β-HCG levels (falling levels of > 59 percent decrease).

If the initial attempt at medical abortion fails, steps to follow are shown in Fig. 2-8. Women

Figure 2-8

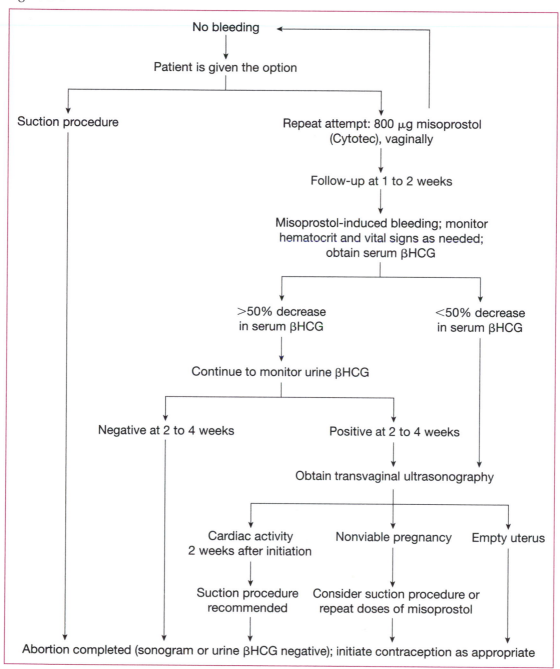

Steps to follow when initial attempt at medical abortion fails. βHCG, beta human chorionic gonadotropin.
<small>SOURCE:</small> Reprinted with permission from Gold et al.[51]

whose ultrasounds show fetal cardiac activity at 2 weeks' follow-up should be offered a suction procedure. Women whose ultrasounds show a nonviable pregnancy should be offered either another trial of misoprostol or a suction procedure.

For pain control, women may be offered either oral acetaminophen or acetaminophen with codeine. Nonsteroidal anti-inflammatory drugs should be avoided because they reduce the synthesis of prostaglandins. Antiemetics and antidiarrheal drugs (e.g., prochlorperazine and diphenoxylate hydrochloride) may be offered but are of unknown efficacy in this setting.

Choosing a Birth Control Method: Screening for Safety and Optimal Decision-Making

Providing information ahead of time on all available methods of contraception may be the most useful strategy in enhancing use of contraception. In a study conducted in an STD clinic using video presentations and group discussion with three

Figure 2-9

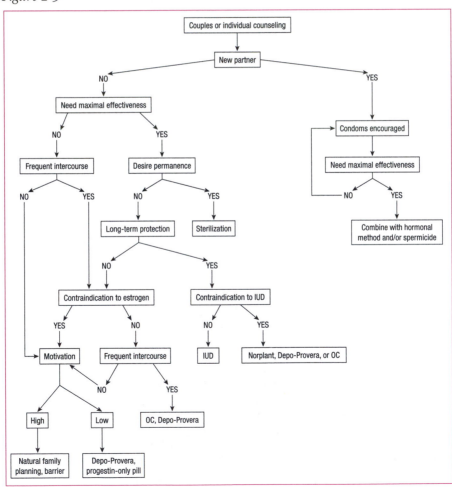

Algorithm providing a guide to the overall selection of a contraceptive method. IUD, intrauterine device; OC, combined oral contraceptive.

different counseling messages (full choice of women's barrier methods, female condom counseling only, or enhanced male condom counseling), the reduction in number of unprotected acts of intercourse at 2 weeks (N = 233) was greatest in the full choice arm, as compared with female condom and male condom arms (83 percent, 54 percent, and 39 percent, respectively).[52]

During the initial office examination, the following aspects of the history and physical examination will assist the clinician in providing important risk information for women and their partners to consider in making their initial decision.

Key History

Aspects of the medical, menstrual, and sexual history are important in considering birth control options. Contraindications for individual methods are reviewed in Table 2-4. Because menstrual patterns may be altered in positive or negative ways by hormonal methods, a review of a woman's current menstrual pattern is often helpful. Women should be asked whether they have a new partner and a monogamous relationship with a partner. This information is used to determine the need for protection against STDs. It is also important to consider the frequency of intercourse, how effective the method needs to be for the individual, and any contraindications to the specific method chosen. Questioning the patient about the desired length of contraception needed will also aid in the decision. Figure 2-9 incorporates many of these questions in an algorithm.

Physical Examination

All sexually active women should undergo periodic health examinations for primary and secondary prevention screening and advice (see Chap. 1). With respect to birth control advice and prescription, a blood pressure measurement should be performed (and repeated if blood pressure is elevated) to identify uncontrolled hypertension, a contraindication for the combined OC. Women should undergo a cardiac examination to rule out valvular heart disease (excluding mitral valve prolapse), which is a relative contraindication to IUD insertion. A clinical breast examination is useful in identifying breast cancer, a condition that precludes use of combined OCs, and women should be instructed in breast self-examination techniques.

A pelvic examination is performed looking for evidence of STD on the skin, vulva, and cervix (see below). A Pap smear should be obtained and cultures for chlamydia and gonorrhea should be considered, based on the history or examination findings. Testing of patients in nonexclusive relationships should be encouraged and testing offered to others (including serum HIV testing if the history is suggestive of risk). Although a bimanual examination of the uterus has not been found efficacious in the identification and management of ovarian cancer, an initial examination should be performed to assess for abnormalities of the vagina and uterus such as a vaginal septum, cervical abnormalities (postpartum or exposure to diethylstilbestrol), uterine fibroids, or a bicornuate uterus. These abnormalities may make vaginal barrier contraceptives and the IUD less appropriate. Women with uterine and cervical abnormalities may not be able to be adequately fit with a diaphragm or cervical cap, and an abnormal Pap smear is a contraindication to use of the cervical cap. Women with uterine fibroids, endometrial polyps, cervical stenosis, bicornuate uterus, or a very small uterus may not be candidates for an IUD because of difficulty with insertion and a greater chance of expulsion. Certain disabling conditions may also influence the choice of birth control, such as severe arthritis of the hands making the insertion of vaginal barrier devices difficult.

Physical findings of common STDs are listed in Table 2-10. The presence of an STD is a contraindication to IUD placement. Methods that protect against STDs (barrier, spermicide) should be strongly encouraged for all patients diagnosed with STDs, especially for patients with viral STDs where eradication of the disease is not possible. When cure is possible, patients should abstain from sexual intercourse until treatment is completed. Partners of patients with STDs should be notified and

Table 2-10

Physical Examination Findings That May Indicate a Sexually Transmitted Disease

Skin

Maculopapular skin rashes (secondary syphilis)

Vesicles or ulcers that are painless (primary syphilis, granuloma inguinale) or painful (genital herpes, chancroid) on the anus, mouth, labia, or cervix, often with associated inguinal lymphadenopathy

Flesh-colored to brownish exophytic, hyperkeratotic papules (warts) on the skin of the genital or perianal area (human papillomavirus [HPV])

Genitalia

Flesh-colored to brownish exophytic, hyperkeratotic papules (warts) on mucosal surfaces of the genital or perianal areas (HPV)

Nonpurulent (primary genital herpes), frothy (trichomoniasis), or purulent (gonorrhea, chlamydia) vaginal discharge

Pelvic examination

Inflamed cervix that bleeds easily (gonorrhea, chlamydia)

Tenderness of the uterus or adnexal areas on examination (gonorrhea, chlamydia, pelvic inflammatory disease)

Rectal examination

Tenderness or bleeding on rectal examination

referred for treatment and counseling. Assistance with partner notification may be found within local STD programs. Suspicion or confirmation of AIDS, positive HIV, syphilis, gonorrhea, chancroid, lymphogranuloma venereum, and granuloma inguinale must be reported to the local health department within 3 days of the patient visit.

For adolescents, it may be more important to start a method of contraception and defer the pelvic examination, if the examination itself appears to be a barrier. The examination may be performed on follow-up, once the adolescent is more comfortable with the provider.

Ancillary Tests

Some practitioners recommend a lipid profile prior to use of OCs in all women in whom individual risk is not known or who have a family history of hyperlipidemia, a first-degree relative with a history of MI before age 50, or for women over the age of 35. Kjos et al.,[53] however, found no significant adverse metabolic markers (lipids or carbohydrate) in women over the age of 35 who were long-term users of combined OCs. An author of this chapter (MS) does not perform routine screening beyond annual Pap smears for sexually active women, but reserves laboratory investigation (such as culture for STDs, blood tests for hemoglobin or hematocrit, liver function, VDRL, rapid plasma reagin, HIV) for patients with risk factors; this is established on an individual basis.

Algorithm

The algorithm presented in Fig. 2-9 may be useful in assisting couples or individuals selecting a method of birth control. Condoms should be strongly encouraged for new partnerships, teenage partners, patients with a history of STDs, and for couples where one partner has a viral STD and the other partner is not infected. When maximal pregnancy protection also is needed, patients should combine condoms with a hormonal method such as the OCs or Depo-Provera. For the majority of women selecting an OC, the appropriate initial dose of EE is 30 to 35 μg; lower-dose OCs or stepped-estrogen products can be used for women at risk of thrombotic complications and for those who do not tolerate standard doses of estrogen. Rarely would a 50-μg product be necessary.

For couples in stable relationships who desire maximal protection from pregnancy, sterilization can be considered along with the IUD, Norplant, Depo-Provera, or the OC if long-term protection is needed. Women engaging in frequent intercourse who desire short-term protection should consider OCs or Depo-Provera. For those who have less frequent intercourse (or in cases where a woman has contraindications to estrogen use) and are highly motivated, vaginal barrier methods or natural family planning may be most appropriate. The cap, however, is not as effective for parous women, and the diaphragm should be encouraged. For less motivated couples or individuals, Depo-Provera may be optimal. Finally, the POP is another option for women with contraindications to estrogen and for lactating women.

Alternatives

ABSTINENCE

It is helpful to mention that periods of abstinence from intercourse may be desired or needed based on medical or social situations. Women may need information on other forms of sexual expression and help in enforcing this decision. Deciding what one wishes to do about sexual intimacy in advance, informing one's partner (in advance), and avoiding high-pressure situations are helpful techniques to discuss. Additional techniques, particularly for adolescents, to reinforce a decision for abstinence include saying "no" clearly and repetitively, providing reasons for the decision ("I'm not ready," "I am concerned about infections"), leaving the situation, double-dating or keeping friends nearby, and threatening to call someone with authority for help.

COMBINED METHODS

In discussing efficacy of the patient's chosen method of contraception, several points should be mentioned. First, all methods may fail and there may be times when two methods should be considered. Even if two methods are deemed unnecessary, a backup method should be discussed. Also for most methods, failure is directly related to consistency of use, and time should be spent exploring patient motivation and potential barriers. In this regard, peer counselors, particularly for adolescent patients, are critical to improving compliance and should be used when possible.

With respect to HIV prevention, all patients, regardless of method of birth control, should be advised to use a male or female latex condom with each act of intercourse. Although use of a male and female condom together is not advised, two male condoms can be used for added protection in case of breakage. Very few cases of HIV transmission have been reported following oral-genital contact; however, mouth to penis contact can transmit most other STDs and hepatitis B. Condoms (nonlubricated and nonspermicide containing) can be used during oral-penile contact for protection. For mouth to vulva contact, female condoms may not provide sufficient barrier protection. Plastic wrap can be tried to create a barrier, but this has not been tested for efficacy. If a condom is not available, a vaginal spermicide will offer protection against bacterial infections, but not HIV. In addition, spermicides may cause tender, red, or raw tissue that can increase the risk of HIV transmission. Because any genital lesion will increase susceptibility to HIV, intercourse should be avoided until lesions are healed.

Management of Contraceptive Side Effects

Oral Contraceptives

Common side effects with combined OCs and their management are listed in Table 2-11. The most common side effect of POPs is menstrual irregularities. If menstrual irregularities are bothersome, bleeding patterns may be improved by the administration of prostaglandin inhibitors (NSAIDs). This side effect often decreases over time.

Diaphragm and Cervical Cap

To prevent odor and deterioration, these devices should be cleaned after each use with a mild soap

Table 2-11

Common Side Effects of Oral Contraceptives (OCs) and Their Management

SYSTEM OR SITE	TYPE OF PROBLEM	OPTIONS
General		
Physical	Weight gain	Increase exercise and decrease intake
	Fluid retention	Decrease estrogen or progestin or both
	Subcutaneous fat	Decrease estrogen potency
	Increased appetite	Decrease androgen potency
Psychological	Depression	Consider discontinuing OC and reassess symptoms
		Lower progestin or estrogen or both
		Add pyridoxine (B$_6$) 20–25 mg/d
		If cyclic and prior to menses, try "tricycling"*
Breast	Tenderness	Decrease estrogen or progestin or both
		Add vitamin E 400 IU daily
CNS	Headache	If at initiation of OC, decrease estrogen or progestin potency and reevaluate in 1–2 cycles
		If during pill-free interval try "tricycling"*
		If worsening, discontinue
Gastrointestinal	Nausea	Take the OC with food or at bedtime
		Switch to a pill with less or no estrogen
Gynecologic	Amenorrhea	Provide a pill with higher potency progestin
		Switch to a product containing a newer progestin
		Switch to a triphasic pill
	Bleeding	If within the first 3 months of beginning, wait
		If excessive menstrual bleeding, try an NSAID
		Explore possibility of missed pills, erratic timing, or drug interactions
		Provide a pill with higher potency progestin
		Switch to a product containing a newer progestin
		Increase the estrogen content or use a stepped-estrogen product

*Tricycling refers to continuous use of active pills (3-wk cycle with immediate restart of next pack); this is generally done for 3 mo at a time followed by a week off active pills to allow menses.
ABBREVIATIONS: CNS, central nervous system; NSAID, nonsteroidal anti-inflammatory drug.

or detergent (avoid deodorant or perfumed soap) and stored in a clean and cool place.

Intrauterine Device

Table 2-12 reviews common problems with the IUD and recommended management strategies. If pregnancy should occur with the IUD in place, women should be advised to have it removed immediately. When the IUD is left in place, spontaneous abortion occurs in 50 to 60 percent of intrauterine pregnancies, half during the second trimester, and the risk of premature delivery, stillbirth, and infants of low birth weight are increased. The risk of a septic abortion, while rare, is 26 times more common when the IUD is left in place. The risk of miscarriage is greatly lessened and the risk of septic abortion is eliminated once the IUD is removed.

Table 2-12

Management Strategies for Selected Intrauterine Device (IUD)-Related Complications

COMPLICATION	COMMENTS	SUGGESTIONS
Heavy periods	Usually decreases over time. If persistent, check for pathology (e.g., fibroids, cervicitis, cancer)	Monitor hemoglobin, provide iron (food and/or supplements), try ibuprofen (400–600 mg tid) during the first few days of the cycle.
Cramping/pain		
Immediately	Consider uterine perforation	If strings are present, remove IUD and treat as PID; if absent, ultrasound or x-ray/consult
Later	Consider pregnancy or infection	If fever, cervical motion or uterine tenderness, purulent cervical discharge, likely PID. Remove IUD, treat with appropriate medications. If normal examination and negative pregnancy test, try symptomatic treatment, follow-up or remove.
Vaginal bleeding with pain	Must rule out ectopic pregnancy	Bimanual examination for PID or adnexal mass Sensitive urine or serum pregnancy test
Pregnancy	Discuss patient's wishes Warn of risk of miscarriage	If strings present, remove IUD, assess for ectopic pregnancy, institute prenatal care or refer for abortion (per patient decision) if intrauterine. If strings absent, ultrasound, watch for infection, recover IUD at delivery. If signs of infection, refer or manage with uterine evacuation and antibiotic treatment.
Expulsion	Evaluate for pregnancy	
Partial		Remove IUD and may reinsert giving doxycyline (100 mg bid or *every* 12 h for 5–7d)
Complete	May need ultrasound or x-ray	Reinsert if desired
String problems		
Too long	May report partner discomfort	Sound cervix to check for presence of IUD, if IUD in place, cut string shorter
Too short	Rule out partial expulsion	Cut shorter and record length or replace IUD
Missing	Rule out pregnancy/expulsion	Consider ultrasound or x-ray versus examine during next menses; if string is within cervical canal bring though os, if not, explore cervix and uterus with plastic sound or alligator forceps.

ABBREVIATION: PID, pelvic inflammatory disease.

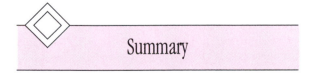

Summary

The newest barrier method awaiting approval is called Lea's Shield. It is a bowl-shaped silicone device, 55 mm in diameter, thicker posteriorly (to fill the posterior fonix of the vagina) that is resistant to petroleum-based lubricants, does not absorb odors, and does not cause allergic reactions in users with latex sensitivity. It has an anterior loop for ease of removal and a one-way flutter valve to prevent pressure buildup over the cervix. In a phase I trial, no motile sperm were found in the cervical mucus in any cycle in which Lea's Shield or the diaphragm was used with spermicide. In a phase II trial, 6-month life table pregnancy rates among the 185 women enrolled was 5.6 for spermicide users and 9.3 for nonspermicide users ($P = .086$).[54]

Newer spermicides are also being developed. Unlike nonoxynol-9, which acts as a detergent degrading sperm as well as some of the natural protective vaginal microorganisms, these new agents are far more specific in action and are designed to interrupt sperm maturation. Chemicals impeding the release of cholesterol from the plasma membrane encasing the sperm head (preventing the membrane from achieving a more fluid state), blocking the calcium channels in the sperm membrane (preventing the acrosome reaction where enzymes are released, allowing penetration of the egg's coat), and preventing protein binding between the sperm and the zona pellucida are being developed.[55] These should offer greater safety and high efficacy.

Hormonal alternatives for men include a long-acting (3-month duration) intramuscular injection of testosterone and progestin or injection of nonpeptide inhibitors, which halt sperm production by reducing the secretion of gonadotropin-releasing hormone.[55] For women, progestin-releasing vaginal devices, with or without estrogen, and dual-rod Norplant devices, which may be biodegradable, are being tested.

A new levonorgestrel-releasing IUD awaiting release has the advantage of the Progestasert in reducing menstrual blood loss but can be left in place up to 10 years. Due to suppression of the endometrium, 83 percent of users in one study had no bleeding or spotting after 1 year of use. No adverse effects on lipids were demonstrated. The efficacy rate is comparable to the Cu T 380A (0.5 percent).

Finally, vaccines for men and women (immuno-contraceptives) are undergoing phases I and II trials. The use of these agents results in the development of antibodies to selected proteins (FSH and LH-releasing hormone for men, human chorionic gonadotropin for women, or sperm antigens)

involved in reproduction. These vaccines will need to be reversible and demonstrated to be safe, particularly with respect to inducing unwanted immune responses against other tissues, before they are likely to be released.

References

1. Wilcox AJ, Weinberg CR, Baird DD: Timing of sexual intercourse in relation to ovulation: effects on the probability of conception, survival of the pregnancy, and sex of the baby. *N Engl J Med* 333:1517, 1995.
2. National Center for Health Statistics, Abma JC, Chandra A, Mosher WD, et al: Fertility, family planning, and women's health: new data from the 1995 Survey of Family Growth. *Vital and Health Statistics*. Series 23. No. 19. DDHS publication no. (PHS) 97, 1995.
3. Braverman PK, Strasburger VC: Contraception. *Clin Pediatr* 32:725, 1993.
4. Alexander B, McGrew MC, Shore W: Adolescent sexuality issues in office practice. *Am Fam Physician* 44:1273, 1991.
5. Landry DJ, Forrest JD: Private physicians' provision of contraceptive services. *Fam Plann Perspect* 28:203, 1996.
6. Peterson LS: Contraceptive use in the United States: 1982–90. *Adv Data* 260:1, 1995, February 14.
7. Savonius H, Pakarinen P, Sjoberg L, Kajanoja P: Reasons for pregnancy termination: negligence or failure of contraception? *Acta Obstet Gynecol Scand* 74:818, 1995.
8. Shivo S, Hemminki E, Kosunen E: Contraceptive health risks—women's perception. *J Psychosom Obstet Gynaecol* 19:117, 1998.
9. Forrest JD: Epidemiology of unintended pregnancy and contraceptive use. *Am J Obstet Gynecol* 1485, 1994.
10. Frost JJ: Family planning clinic services in the United States, 1994. *Fam Plann Perspect* 28:92, 1996.
11. Forrest JD, Samara R: Impact of publicly funded contraceptive services on unintended pregnancies and implications for Medicaid expenditures. *Fam Plann Perspect* 28:188, 1996.
12. Schenker JG, Rabenou V: Family planning: cultural and religious perspectives. *Hum Reprod* 8:969, 1993.

13. Steiner MJ, Hertz-Picciotto I, Schulz KF, et al: Measuring true contraceptive efficacy. A randomized approach—condom vs. spermicide vs. no method. *Contraception* 58:375, 1998.

14. Trussell J, Vaughan B: Contraceptive failures, method-related discontinuation and resumption of use: results from the 1995 National Survey of Family Growth. *Fam Plann Perspect* 31:64, 1999.

15. Magnani RJ, Haws JM, Morgan GT, et al: Vasectomy in the United States, 1991 and 1995. *Am J Public Health* 89:92, 1999.

16. Peterson HB, Xia Z, Hughes JM, et al: The risk of pregnancy after tubal sterilization: findings from the U.S. Collaborative Review of Sterilization. *Am J Obstset Gynecol* 174:1161, 1996.

17. Hatcher RA, Trussel J, Stewart F, et al: *Contraceptive Technology*, 17th ed. New York: Irvington Publishers; 1998.

18. Rosenberg M: Weight change with oral contraceptive use and during the menstrual cycle. Reports of daily measurements. *Contraception* 56:345, 1998.

19. Hannaford PC, Kay CR: The risk of serious illness among oral contraceptive users: evidence from the RCGP's oral contraceptive study. *Br J Gen Pract* 48:1657, 1998.

20. Schwartz SM, Siscovick DS, Longstreth WT, et al: Use of low-dose oral contraceptives and stroke in young women. *Ann Intern Med* 127:596, 1997.

21. Blumenstein BA, Douglas MB, Hall WD: Blood pressure changes and oral contraceptive use: a study of 2,676 black women in the southeastern United States. *Am J Epidemiol* 112:539, 1980.

22. McCann MF, Moggia AV, Higgins JE, et al: The effects of a progestin-only oral contraceptive (levonorgestrel 0.03 mg) on breast-feeding. *Contraception* 40:635, 1989.

23. Scholes D, Lacroix AZ, Ott SM, et al: Bone mineral density in women using depot medroxyprogesterone acetate for contraception. *Obstet Gynecol* 93:233, 1999.

24. Fihn SD, Boyko EJ, Normand EH, Chen CL, et al: Association between use of spermicide-coated condoms and *Escherichia coli* urinary tract infection in young women. *Am J Epidemiol* 144:512, 1996.

25. Xu JX, Leeper MA, Wu Y, et al: User acceptability of a female condom (Reality) in Shanghai. *Adv Contracept* 14:193, 1998.

26. Lauersen NH, Wilson KH, Graves ZR, et al: The cervical cap: effectiveness, safety, and acceptability as a barrier contraceptive. *Mt Sinai J Med* 53:233, 1996.

27. Frezieres RG, Walsh TL, Nelson AL, et al: Evaluation of the efficacy of a polyurathane condom: results from a randomized, clinical trial. *Fam Plann Perspect* 31:81, 1999.

28. Cohen D, Reardon K, Alleyne D, et al: Influencing spermicide use among low-income minority women. *J Am Med Womens Assoc* 50:11, 1995.

29. Kegeles SM, Adler NE, Irwin CE: Adolescents and condoms: associations of beliefs with intentions to use. *Am J Dis Child* 143:911, 1989.

30. Roddy RE, Zekeng L, Ryan KA, et al: A controlled trial of nonoxynol 9 film to reduce male-to-female transmission of sexually transmitted diseases. *N Engl J Med* 339:504, 1998.

31. Alvarez F, Brache V, Fernandez E, et al: New insights on the mode of action of intrauterine contraceptive devices in women. *Fertil Steril* 49:768, 1988.

32. White MK, Ory HW, Rooks JB, et al: Intrauterine device termination rates and the menstrual cycle day of insertion. *Obstet Gynecol* 55:220, 1980.

33. *Population Reports. Intrauterine Devices.* Series B, Number 5, March 1988, p.1–31.

34. Geerling JH: Natural family planning. *AFP* 52(6): 1749, 1995.

35. Trussell J, Grummer-Strawn L: Contraceptive failure of the ovulation method of period abstinence. *Fam Plann Perspect* 16(1):5, 1990.

36. Trussel J, Stewart F: The effectiveness of postcoital contraception. *Fam Plann Perspect* 24:262, 1992.

37. Trussell J, Koenig J, Ellerston C, Stewart F: Preventing unintended pregnancy: the cost-effectiveness of three methods of emergency contraception. *Am J Public Health* 87(6):932, 1997.

38. Glasier A: Emergency postcoital contraception. *N Engl J Med* 337(150):1058, 1997.

39. Task Force on Postovulatory Methods of Fertility Regulation: Randomized controlled trial of levonorgestrel versus the Yuzpe regimen of combined oral contraceptives for emergency contraception. *Lancet* 352:428, 1998.

40. Glasier A, Baird D: The effects of self-administering emergency contraception. *N Engl J Med* 339:1, 1998.

41. Exploring new territories in pharmacy practice. EMC prescribing progressing in Washington State. *Rx Ipsa Loquitur* 25:1, 1998.

42. Liying Z, Bilican X: Emergency contraception with the intrauterine device. *Adv Contracept* 14:161, 1998.

43. Singh K, Ratnam SS: The influence of abortion legislation on maternal mortality. *Int J Gynaecol Obstet* 63(suppl 1):S213, 1998.

44. Singh K, Ratnam SS: Induced abortion: a world review, 1990. *Fam Plann Perspect* 22:76, 1990.

45. Henshaw SJ, Van Wort J: Abortion services in the United States, 1987 and 1988. *Fam Plann Perspect* 22:102, 1990.

46. Grimes DA; Medical abortion in early pregnancy: a review of the evidence. *Obstet Gynecol* 89:790, 1997.

47. Creinin MD, Vittinghoff E, Keder L, Darney PD: Methotrexate and misoprostol for early abortion: a multicenter trial: I. Safety and acceptability. *Contraception* 53:321, 1996.

48. Creinin MD, Vittinghoff E, Schaff E, et al: Medical abortion with oral methotrexate and vaginal misoprostol. *Obstet Gynecol* 90:611, 1997.

49. Spitz IM, Bardin CW, Benton, L, Robbins A: Early pregnancy termination with mifepristone and misoprostol in the United States. *N Engl J Med* 338:1241, 1998.

50. Winikoff B: Acceptability of medical abortion in early pregnancy. *Fam Plann Perspect* 27:142, 1995.

51. Gold M, Luks D, Anderson MR: Medical options for early pregnancy termination. *Am Fam Physician* 56:533, 1997.

52. Gollub EL, French P, Latka M, et al: The women's safer sex hierarchy: initial responses to counseling on women's methods of STD/HIV prevention at an STD clinic (abstract no. Mo.D.583). *Int Conf AIDS* 11:52, 1996.

53. Kjos SL, Ballagh SA, La Cour M, et al: The copper T380A intrauterine device in women with type II diabetes mellitus. *Obstet Gynecol* 84:1006, 1994.

54. Mauck C, Glover LH, Miller E, et al: Lea's Shield: a study of the safety and efficacy of a new vaginal barrier contraceptive used with and without spermicide. *Contraception* 53:329, 1996.

55. Alexander NJ: Future contraceptives. *Sci Am* 273:136, 1995.

56. Judge DE: Emergency Contraception: it's not too late. *J Watch Women's Health* 4:24, 1999.

Margaret R. Helton

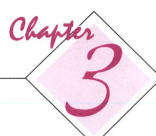

Chapter 3

Prenatal Care

Overview

Few events in a woman's life are as anticipated as the birth of a child. With the availability of birth control options, women today have the ability to control their fertility choices as never before. Women can continue to have choice and control when it comes to decisions made during the course of the pregnancy, even if the pregnancy is unplanned. These choices form the basis for modern prenatal care.

The first choice a woman makes is whether to seek preconception care. There is a recent emphasis on preconception counseling because a woman's medical condition, medications, occupational exposures, or social practices may have consequences in the earliest weeks of pregnancy, well before awareness of pregnancy or the traditional initiation of prenatal care. Optimizing health, controlling chronic illness, altering medications, updating vaccinations, and giving advice to supplement the diet with folic acid before conception can have a positive effect on a subsequent pregnancy. Family history should be reviewed to identify any genetic risks and a social and lifestyle history should be elicited. Preconception health care is an important opportunity to practice preventive medicine.[1]

Most women seek care early in a pregnancy. In 1993, 79 percent of American women initiated prenatal care in the first trimester, with less than 5 percent waiting until the third trimester or receiving no prenatal care at all.[2] It is the goal of the United States Public Health Service (USPHS) that at least 90 percent of American women initiate prenatal care in the first trimester.[3]

Efficacy of Prenatal Care

The recommendation for early initiation of care is based on the belief that early prenatal care will increase the chances of having a healthy pregnancy and a healthy baby, an outcome that most families now take for granted. In the past, such an outcome was far from guaranteed. In the United States, the maternal mortality rate was 582 deaths per 100,000 births in 1935,[4] but has fallen to 7.5 deaths per 100,000 births in 1993.[5] The infant mortality rate has fallen from 47 deaths per 1000 births in 1940[4] to 8.4 deaths per 1000 births in 1995.[5] Prenatal care has likely played a role in this dramatic decline in maternal and infant mortality, although other advances such as antibiotics, safe anesthesia, and better treatments for hemorrhage have also made a significant contribution.

It is difficult to measure the efficacy of prenatal care. For one reason, there is a great deal of disagreement on what constitutes a good outcome. Should the goal be to ensure that the woman has a "good" experience or should a good outcome be measured by Apgar scores? There is general agreement, however, that the infant mortality rate is a reasonable measure to use when assessing systems of care. More than 20 countries have lower infant mortality rates than the United States (Table 3-1).[6] Every one of these countries has an organized system of prenatal care that is readily available. In the United States, women with poor access to prenatal care have the worst outcomes, although analyses are confounded by the coexistence of poverty, poor social supports, and substance abuse that is also found in such populations.

Despite limitations in the ability to prove that prenatal care is effective, there is wide agreement among women and health providers that it is important. Most people also assume that it is safe, although this has not always been the case. The catastrophic fetal malformations caused by thalidomide, which was given to pregnant women as a sleep aid during prenatal care in the 1950s and 1960s, and the long-term problems afflicted on women whose mothers took diethylstilbestrol for the prevention of miscarriages are just two examples of harm caused by prenatal care. Given that most women will have healthy babies, any intervention introduced into that natural course should

Table 3-1

Infant Mortality Rates by Country

COUNTRY	INFANT MORTALITY RATE* (1994)
Japan	4.25
Singapore	4.34
Hong Kong	4.43
Sweden	4.45
Finland	4.72
Switzerland	5.12
Norway	5.23
Denmark	5.45
Germany	5.60
The Netherlands	5.64
Ireland	5.93
Australia	6.05
Northern Ireland	6.05
England and Wales	6.20
Scotland	6.20
Austria	6.25
Canada	6.30
France	6.47
Italy	6.63
Spain	6.69
New Zealand	7.24
Israel	7.80
Greece	7.93
Czech Republic	7.95
United States	8.02
Portugal	8.06
Belgium	8.20
Cuba	9.40

*Number of deaths of infants under 1 year per 1000 live births.
SOURCE: Health, United States, 1998 with Socioeconomic Status and Health Chartbook. U.S. Department of Health and Human Services, Centers for Disease Control and Prevention. DHHS Publication Number (PHS) 98–1232, p. 197.

be proved effective and safe. Fortunately, the past 15 years have seen an impressive growth in medical literature that critically appraises aspects of prenatal care. In the realm of childbirth, this effort has been pioneered by a group of British authors who conduct systematic reviews of the evidence of care related to pregnancy and childbirth. Their work, known as the Cochrane pregnancy and childbirth database,[7] was first published in 1989[8] and is now regularly updated and available on computer disk. Similarly, the United States Preventive Services Task Force Guide to Clinical Preventive Services Report[9] is an established reference source for evidence-based recommendations, including many components of prenatal care.

Seeking a Health Care Provider

Family physicians, midwives, obstetricians, nurse practitioners, and physician assistants provide prenatal care. Just as there is no general agreement about what constitutes a good outcome to a pregnancy, women vary widely in their needs and desires during the course of their pregnancy. One woman will determine that what is most important to her is preparation for natural childbirth in a setting outside of a hospital, whereas another will seek every technologic intervention available.

Significant within-specialty practice differences exist among practitioners and even greater variation is seen across disciplines with respect to the number and types of interventions used during prenatal care and childbirth. These differences have been shaped, in part, by patient preferences, hospital and state credentialing policies, medical malpractice issues, and the economics and politics of medicine. Understandably, most providers believe passionately that their approach is best. Research suggests that for low-risk women, there are no significant differences in maternal or neonatal health outcomes or patient satisfaction among patients cared for by different types of providers, although some studies have suggested that midwives use fewer obstetric interventions and have a lower rate of cesarean section.[10] The practice environment may have a more profound effect on style of practice and use of interventions than a provider's specialty. Because obstetric care is a major health expenditure in our country, issues related to outcomes and resource use need to be studied further.

Given that there is strength in diversity, the consumer will benefit from a health care system that offers a wide range of choices regarding practice style with respect to prenatal and delivery care. Patients are served best by collegial relationships among providers in the community with appropriate referrals to obstetricians or perinatologists, as needed, for high-risk patients.

All women agree on two issues, however: they want a healthy outcome to the pregnancy, for themselves and for the baby, and they must trust their health care provider. The belief that one approach is better than another is based on personal experience and previous teaching. Such impressions are sometimes right, but sometimes not. It is incumbent on the medical profession to continue looking at clinical practice with a critical eye and only adopt interventions that are proven to be safe and effective.

Prenatal Care

Although prenatal care focuses on medical surveillance for conditions such as preeclampsia and preterm labor, it should also include psychological and social support as well as patient education. In addition to clinicians, other health care providers such as social workers, nutritionists, and counselors often play an important role.

The frequency of prenatal care visits varies widely in different countries, from a low of three or four visits in Switzerland to a high of 14 in the United States.[11] In 1989, the USPHS convened an expert panel to review the content and timing of prenatal care.[12] The group concluded that more resources should be directed toward high-risk women and fewer visits provided to women with low-risk pregnancies. Such an approach has been shown to maintain good outcomes and patient satisfaction for women with low-risk pregnancies.[13]

Prenatal Screening

One of the first tasks is to establish that the woman is indeed pregnant. Through the ready availability of home pregnancy tests and recognition of a missed menstrual period, many women have already self-diagnosed a pregnancy. Pregnancy tests (urine or blood) are so sensitive that they are positive 6 to 8 days after fertilization, well before a missed menstrual period.[14]

HISTORY

MEDICAL HISTORY Prenatal care usually begins with a complete medical history taken at the first visit, including use of medications (both prescription and nonprescription), vitamins, and any alternative/complementary medicines (e.g., herbs).

The medical interview should also reveal any history of hypertension, diabetes, or other significant medical problem that could affect the pregnancy. Such women will require special surveillance during their pregnancy. A history of exposure to infectious diseases such as tuberculosis, toxoplasmosis, or rubella should be noted.

PREGNANCY HISTORY One of the most important predictors of success in a pregnancy and delivery is a good outcome in a previous pregnancy. The past pregnancy history should be carefully reviewed, with special attention directed toward the previous method of delivery and any obstetric or medical problems that developed. Women who previously experienced preterm labor, cervical incompetence, gestational diabetes, hypertension, or postpartum hemorrhage are at risk for a recurrence of these problems.

HEALTH BEHAVIORS Behaviors that affect pregnancy must be assessed. Tobacco use during pregnancy increases the risk of premature delivery or a baby with a low birth weight and perinatal death.[15,16] The consumption of alcohol is also harmful, causing mental retardation, microcephaly, growth retardation, and facial deformities, a constellation of symptoms known as fetal alcohol syndrome.[17] The threshold at which alcohol consumption causes these effects is not known, so a pregnant woman should be advised that the safest approach is abstinence.

Caffeine is widely consumed by pregnant women, in coffee as well as other beverages. No strong evidence links caffeine use to birth defects or miscarriage; however, there remains a concern that excessive caffeine use increases the risk of a low birth weight baby.[18] It seems prudent to recommend that pregnant women limit caffeine intake to less than 3 cups of coffee (300 mg caffeine) a day.

A history of drug abuse is often associated with a poor outcome to the pregnancy, but the specific impact of the drug abuse is difficult to measure because it is often associated with other harmful behaviors or conditions such as poverty, poor nutrition, alcohol consumption, tobacco use, poor psychosocial support, and limited access to care.[19] Health care providers should attempt to help women stop their drug use or seek treatment, while providing them with confidential, accessible prenatal care.

SOCIAL SUPPORT   Social support and relationship issues are assessed, with appropriate referrals to social workers, counselors, and nutritional support programs such as the Women, Infant and Children's program where appropriate. The quality of the primary relationship and sexual concerns should be assessed. Unless there is a medical complication, sexual relations are safe in pregnancy and, in fact, pleasure can be enhanced by new feelings of intimacy.

Unfortunately, domestic violence is all too common and can start or escalate during pregnancy (see Chap. 7). An effort should be made to assess the woman's risk of domestic violence through direct questions, and victims of violence should be assisted in creating a plan for safety.

FOLLOW-UP HISTORY   On subsequent visits, smoking, diet, medication use, and health habits are again reviewed, in addition to an ongoing assessment of the woman's social situation. Women should be questioned about the presence or absence of symptoms such as nausea, vomiting, headache, abdominal pain, and vaginal bleeding or discharge. Her attitude toward birth and breast-feeding should be explored as well.

PHYSICAL EXAMINATION

FIRST VISIT   The first prenatal visit should include a thorough physical examination, with special attention directed toward the size of the uterus and the shape of the pelvis, along with establishing the patient's baseline blood pressure and weight. A bimanual examination of the uterus can help determine the gestational age, as shown in Table 3-2. The clinician should also attempt to listen to the fetal heartbeat, which can be heard with a Doppler ultrasound device at 10 to12 weeks and with a fetoscope at 18 to 20 weeks.

SUBSEQUENT VISITS   On subsequent visits, the physical examination usually is limited to checking weight and blood pressure and looking for peripheral edema. A sustained blood pressure of

Table 3-2

Physical Examination Methods to Assess Gestational Age

UTERINE SIZE
7 wk gestation: size of a large hen's egg
10 wk gestation: size of an orange
12 wk gestation: size of a grapefruit, palpated at the pubic symphysis
16 wk gestation: palpated midway between symphysis and umbilicus
20 wk gestation: palpated at the umbilicus
21 wk and on: expected growth 1 cm per week

FETAL HEART TONES
10 to 12 wk: audible with Doppler ultrasound device
18 to 20 wk: audible with fetoscope

greater than 140 mmHg systolic or 90 mmHg diastolic suggests a hypertensive disorder of pregnancy, which will require intensive surveillance and possible early induction. Preeclampsia is hypertension associated with peripheral edema and protein in the urine.

After the first trimester (weeks 0 to 13), uterine growth is measured from the pubic symphysis to the top of the fundus (see Table 3-2). At 20 weeks the uterus is palpated at the level of the umbilicus; expected growth from 21 weeks on is about 1 cm/wk. A uterus that is greater than 2 cm larger than anticipated, particularly over several visits, means that the pregnancy is farther along than expected, the woman is carrying twins, or an obstetric problem such as polyhydramnios or macrosomia is present. A smaller than expected uterus (> 2 cm less than expected) can mean that the pregnancy is less advanced than presumed or an obstetric problem such as oligohydramnios or intrauterine growth retardation is present. The fetal status is further assessed by verifying a fetal heartbeat and, in the third trimester, by ascertaining the baby's position of presentation in the uterus, that is, determining where the head is in relation to the cervix. This is important because a breech or transverse lie has a profound impact on the method of delivery, often mandating a cesarean section. However, if such a malpresentation is discovered before the last 2 to 4 weeks of pregnancy, it is often possible to turn the baby (version) to a vertex (head down) position, giving the woman a significantly improved chance for a vaginal delivery.

Neonatal herpes is a devastating infection for a newborn, often causing neurologic impairment or death.[20] If a woman has a history of genital herpes, the genital area should be inspected if the woman reports symptoms of an outbreak near her due date. It is standard practice in most settings to deliver the infant by cesarean section if the mother has an active herpes lesion when she goes into labor, because it is thought to lower the exposure of the baby to the herpes virus. This approach has never been proven effective by randomized clinical trial. Because most babies infected with the herpes virus at birth are born to asymptomatic mothers, strategies for prevention that focus on symptomatic mothers have limited impact. The chance of a baby acquiring this infection from the mother during childbirth is significantly greater for primary herpes compared with recurrent herpes. Although there is general agreement that women who present with their first clinical case of genital herpes at delivery should have a cesarean section performed, the current practice of cesarean delivery for women with a history of genital herpes lesions that recur at delivery remains controversial; some argue that the high maternal morbidity and mortality and substantial financial expense is not justified.[21] The use of acyclovir to suppress recurrence near delivery is being explored as the search for alternative management strategies continues.

LABORATORY SCREENING

BLOOD TYPE   Several laboratory tests are routinely drawn during prenatal care (Table 3-3). At the initiation of prenatal care, a pregnant woman's blood type is determined to see if her red blood cells carry the A or B antigen and/or the D (formerly Rh) antigen. Only about 15 percent of people are negative for the D antigen. When a D-negative woman has a D-positive fetus (inherited from the father), the woman may develop an antibody to the infant's D antigen that crosses the placenta into the fetal circulation, destroying the fetal red blood cells leading to anemia, hyperbilirubinemia, or fetal hydrops. The incidence of this problem, known as erythroblastosis fetalis, has dropped dramatically in the past 30 years for two reasons. First, women are not having as many babies, and the incidence of isoimmunization increases with each subsequent pregnancy in a D-negative woman. Secondly, the availability of anti-D gammaglobulin, known as RhoGAM, has been one of the major obstetric achievements of the past 30 years. RhoGAM is given anytime there is a risk of fetomaternal bleeding, such as after an amniocentesis, and is given routinely at 28 weeks.

Table 3-3

Routine Laboratory Tests in Prenatal Care

TEST	PURPOSE	*SENSITIVITY %	*SPECIFICITY %	LEVEL OF EVIDENCE[†]
FIRST TRIMESTER				
Blood type and antibody screen	Determine likelihood of blood antigen incompatibility	99–100	99–100	A
Hematocrit or hemoglobin	Screen for maternal anemia	90	44	B
Hemoglobin electrophoresis[‡]	Screen for hemoglobinopathies	99–100	99–100	B
Rubella titer	Determine maternity immunity status	92–100	71–100	B
Hepatitis B surface antigen	Screen for maternal infection, acute or chronic	98	98	A
Syphilis test (VDRL or RPR)	Screen for maternal syphilis infection	62–100	75–99	A
HIV[§]	Screen for maternal infection	95	99.5	A
Urine culture	Screen for asymptomatic bacteriuria	98	94	A
Gonorrhea culture	Screen for maternal infection	80–95	99–100	B
Chlamydia	Screen for maternal infection	70–90	97–99	B
Pap smear	Screen for cervical cancer	60–80	90–99	A
SECOND TRIMESTER				
Serum multiscreen[#]	Screening for congenital malformations	48–91		B
Vaginal wet prep	Screen for bacterial vaginosis in women at risk for preterm delivery			
THIRD TRIMESTER				
Diabetes testing**	Identify mothers with gestational diabetes	71–83	78–87	C
Group B strep culture	Identify carriers	70	90	B
Hematocrit/Hemoglobin	Screen for maternal anemia			
Repeat gonorrhea, syphilis, chlamydia, hepatitis, and HIV tests	Repeat in women with behaviors that place them at high risk for acquiring these diseases.			A

*These numbers taken from U.S. Preventive Services Task Force.
[†]Level of evidence: A = strong or moderate research-based evidence (consistent across several studies, including at least 2 randomized controlled trials), B = limited research-based evidence (less consistent or extensive evidence, but preponderance of evidence supports use of treatment), C = common practice with little or no research-based evidence.
[‡]Performed in women found to be anemic who have risk factors for hemoglobinopathies.
[§]Offered to those with risk factors.
[#]Routinely offered to women between 15 and 19 weeks' gestation.
**No longer recommended routinely but reserved for women with risk factors for gestational diabetes.

After delivery, the baby's blood type is determined and if D-positive, the mother will be given another dose of RhoGAM within 72 h of birth. These practices are effective and safe, so these protocols are highly recommended.[22]

HEMOGLOBIN Hemoglobin or hematocrit is also determined early in pregnancy because evidence suggests that significant anemia can be associated with poor birth outcomes.[23] Cutoff values for anemia in pregnancy are listed in Table 3-4.[24] Women whose hemoglobin or hematocrit fall below these levels should be treated with iron; a follow-up test should be performed later in pregnancy to document a response to treatment. Unfortunately, the normal drop in hematocrit that occurs during pregnancy, due to expansion of the plasma volume, is frequently misinterpreted as iron deficiency. There is no evidence that iron supplementation is beneficial unless there is true iron-deficiency anemia. In fact, some evidence indicates that iron supplementation can even worsen outcomes, possibly by increasing the viscosity of the maternal blood.[25,26] Women who develop significant anemia and are at risk for hemoglobinopathies such as sickle cell disease and certain thalassemias (women with a family history or who are of African, Mediterranean, Middle Eastern, Southeast Asian, or Latin American descent) should have hemoglobin electrophoresis.

RUBELLA Rubella immunity is determined by assessing for antibodies to rubella, although ideally this is done before pregnancy when there is the opportunity to vaccinate nonimmune women. Maternal rubella infection in early pregnancy can lead to miscarriage, stillbirth, and the devastating effects of congenital rubella syndrome. The nonimmune pregnant woman should be advised to stay away from individuals with known outbreaks of rubella and should be vaccinated in the postpartum period.

HEPATITIS B Hepatitis B surface antigen is part of initial screening. A positive result indicates active (acute or chronic) hepatitis B infection, and babies born to these mothers need hepatitis B immunoglobulin and vaccination at birth.[27]

HIV AND SYPHILIS Pregnant women are now strongly encouraged to consider voluntary HIV testing, especially women with behaviors or partners that place them at increased risk for contracting HIV.[28] Promotion of this test in pregnant women has taken on a sense of urgency because the risk of transmitting HIV to the baby can be significantly reduced by prenatal treatment with zidovudine (azidothymidine or AZT) beginning at 14 weeks of gestation.[29,30] Congenital syphilis can be prevented with antibiotic treatment given to the afflicted pregnant mother, so testing for syphilis is also a routine part of prenatal care.

GENITOURINARY INFECTION Gonorrhea and chlamydia infections are often asymptomatic infections associated with poor outcomes such as premature

Table 3-4

Cutoff Values for Anemia in Women

PREGNANCY STATUS	HEMOGLOBIN (g/dL)	HEMATOCRIT (%)
Nonpregnant	12.0	36
Pregnant nonsmokers		
Trimester 1	11.0	33
Trimester 2	10.5	32
Trimester 3	11.0	33
Pregnant smokers (≥10 cigarettes/day)		
Trimester 1	11.3–11.5*	34–34.5
Trimester 2	10.8–11.0	33–33.5
Trimester 3	11.3–11.5	34–34.5

*Higher values for women who smoke 21–40 cigarettes per day.
SOURCE: From Centers for Disease Control and Prevention.[24]

delivery and neonatal infection, so pregnant women are screened for these infections. Cultures are obtained from a swab of the endocervix.

Asymptomatic bacteriuria in pregnancy is associated with an increased risk of maternal pyelonephritis, preterm delivery, and low birth weight, but recognition and treatment can reduce the incidence of these problems significantly.[31] Screening with a urine culture is recommended for all pregnant women at 12 to 16 weeks of gestation.

Bacterial vaginosis, an overgrowth of predominantly anaerobic bacteria, has been associated with preterm birth.[32] Randomized trials involving women at high risk for preterm delivery (history of preterm delivery, a low prepregnant weight of < 50 kg, or both) showed that treatment of bacterial vaginosis with metronidazole either alone or with erythromycin substantially reduced the rate of preterm birth.[33,34] Hence, women at high risk for preterm delivery who have a positive screen or symptoms of bacterial vaginosis should be treated with metronidazole administered orally (vaginal treatment does not appear to be as effective as oral). There is no evidence at this time that this strategy should be adopted for women at low risk for preterm delivery.

It is now routine to screen pregnant women at 34 to 37 weeks with a rectovaginal culture (and not a cervical culture) to identify those who are carriers of group B streptococcus (GBS).[35] Neonatal GBS infection can be devastating and is usually acquired by the baby during childbirth. In the United States, GBS sepsis occurs in 1.8/1000 live births with a case-fatality rate of 5 to 20 percent, leading to about 310 newborn deaths per year. Women who are identified as GBS carriers are offered treatment with antibiotics during labor, which can significantly lower the risk of transmission. An alternative strategy is to omit the prenatal screening but treat with antibiotics during labor any women who develop fever, have ruptured membranes more than 18 h, deliver before 37 weeks' gestation, had GBS bacteriuria in the pregnancy, or had a previous infant with significant GBS disease.

GESTATIONAL DIABETES Women at risk for gestational diabetes (obesity, hypertension, previous poor pregnancy outcome, or a strong family history of diabetes) should be screened with a 1-h 50-g glucose challenge at 26 to 28 weeks' gestation. A positive screen with a blood sugar level above 135 to 145 (depending on the laboratory) should lead to a 3-h 100-g oral glucose tolerance test (GTT), which, if positive, is diagnostic for gestational diabetes. Cutoff values for the 3-h GTT are: fasting blood sugar (FBS) greater than 105, 1-h blood sugar greater than 190, 2-h blood sugar greater than 165, and 3-h blood sugar greater than 145. The test is considered abnormal if the FBS or two of the remaining three values are elevated. Women with gestational diabetes should receive dietary counseling and glucose monitoring. Neither the Preventive Services Task Force[9] nor the American College of Obstetricians and Gynecologists[36] recommends routine screening of all pregnant women.

REPEAT TESTING Other laboratory tests performed in the third trimester include repeat testing for syphilis, gonorrhea, chlamydia, HIV, and hepatitis in women with behaviors that place them at increased risk for acquiring these infections.

PRENATAL DIAGNOSIS OF CONGENITAL MALFORMATIONS

It is the hope of every pregnant woman and her family that the expected baby is born healthy. However, congenital malformations occur in about 3 percent of newborns. Although most of these malformations are minor, some are life-threatening and congenital anomalies are now the leading cause of infant mortality in the United States. Infants with congenital malformations who survive may require lifelong special care, which has a tremendous impact on families. Many pregnant women want the opportunity to minimize the chance of this happening to their families and choose prenatal diagnosis, which is now routinely offered in some form to all pregnant women. Assessment of genetic risk should begin even before a women is pregnant, with a careful history of familial genetic defects or any risks related to ethnicity, such as sickle cell disease in people of African descent or Tay-Sachs disease in those of Jewish heritage. Other defects can be detected through antenatal screening.

It is the standard of care to offer prenatal diagnosis to every pregnant woman, but each woman should be thoroughly counseled as to the limitations of these tests and that there is always the risk of a false-positive test, which can lead to tremendous anxiety along with a cascade of further testing. Counseling by the health care provider should be accurate, thorough, and nonbiased, with each couple's individual preferences respected. Referral to genetic counselors is often useful when women and their families are faced with these decisions.

Women may wish for testing even if they know that they will not choose to terminate the pregnancy. Because there is no evidence that early detection of congenital anomalies improves outcome, the rationale for prenatal testing in such families is questionable. Some parents, however, may feel that the opportunity to prepare for the arrival of a child with malformations is important to them. In some situations, knowledge about a physical deformity before birth, such as a cardiac or abdominal defect, will allow for delivery at an institution with skilled personnel and appropriate facilities to maximize the chance for survival. The possibility of organ donation, in the case of a child with lethal anomalies (e.g., anencephaly) may be another option for a family.

NEURAL TUBE DEFECTS   Screening for neural tube defects such as spina bifida, anencephaly, and encephalocele is offered during the early second trimester of care. These defects occur in 4/10,000 live births.[37] A test measuring the maternal serum α-fetoprotein (MSAFP) between 15 and 19 weeks' gestation is used to predict neural tube defects.[38] About 1 to 5 percent of women will have an elevated (abnormal) MSAFP, but 90 to 95 percent of these women actually have babies without a neural tube defect, and the falsely elevated level is

due to underestimated gestational age, multiple gestation, or other anomalies. An ultrasound should be performed to assess for any of these causes. Amniocentesis should be offered to those women still without an explanation for the elevated MSAFP.[39]

DOWN SYNDROME   Trisomy 21, or Down syndrome, is the most common chromosome abnormality with a birth prevalence of 0.9/1000 live births.[40] The true incidence is much higher, but 65 percent of affected fetuses abort spontaneously. Children with Down syndrome are mentally retarded and have characteristic facies including upward-slanting eyes with epicanthal folds, protruding tongue, and finger and toe anomalies; 45 percent have a congenital heart anomaly. Screening for this syndrome is focused on the mother because in 95 percent of cases, the extra chromosome linked to the disorder comes from the mother. The risk of having a baby with trisomy 21 increases with advancing maternal age,[41] as illustrated in Table 3-5. Amniocentesis (performed at 15 to 19 weeks' gestation) or chorionic villus sampling (performed at 10 to 12 weeks' gestation) with karyotyping of the chromosomes is routinely offered to women who will be 35 or older at the time of delivery. The age of 35 is selected as the threshold for routinely offering karyotyping of the fetus because that is the age at which the risk of a chromosomal abnormality (1/179) approximates the iatrogenic fetal loss rate of these procedures (0.5 to 1 percent).[42]

Although the risk of trisomy 21 is highest in older mothers, because the vast majority of pregnancies are in younger women, most children with trisomy 21 are born to mothers under the age of 35, to whom amniocentesis or chorionic villus sampling is not routinely offered. In an effort to detect these younger mothers whose fetuses have trisomy 21, all women are routinely offered a screening blood test for trisomy 21 that involves measuring MSAFP, unconjugated estriol levels, and human chorionic gonadotropin levels. Reduced levels of MSAFP and estriol, with elevated levels of human chorionic gonadotropin, have been

Table 3-5

Incidence of Chromosomal Defects Relative to Maternal Age (Live Births)

MATERNAL AGE	RISK FOR DOWN SYNDROME	TOTAL RISK FOR CHROMOSOME ABNORMALITIES
20	1/1667	1/526
25	1/1250	1/476
30	1/952	1/385
35	1/312	1/179
40	1/90	1/63
45	1/25	1/17
49	1/9	1/7

SOURCE: Data taken from Hook.[83]

associated with trisomy 21, and it is estimated that 62 percent of cases can be detected with a false-positive rate of 5 percent.[43] A definite diagnosis via amniocentesis is then offered to women with a positive screen.

ULTRASOUND

Ultrasonography has had a profound effect on prenatal care, and it is accepted widely and even expected by many pregnant women. It is most commonly used to estimate the due date. A scan in the first trimester predicts the due date within a week of reliability; a scan in the second trimester can predict the estimated date of confinement within 2 weeks of reliability.[44] Ultrasonography is also used to detect multiple gestations or malformations, assess fetal growth, evaluate vaginal bleeding, and provide reassurance of fetal health in late pregnancy.

Although there is no doubt that ultrasound is useful when clinically indicated, routine ultrasound of all pregnancies is not recommended. The largest clinical trial to date studied 15,151 low-risk pregnant women and reported that routine ultrasound (ultrasound performed without a clinical indication) does not affect maternal or fetal outcomes.[45] The National Institutes of Health,[46] the

American College of Obstetricians and Gynecologists,[47] and the Preventive Services Task Force[9] all have taken the position that ultrasound should be used only when there is a specific medical indication. Indications for ultrasonography during pregnancy are listed in Table 3-6.

Despite these recommendations, many pregnant women expect and desire an ultrasound examination. Due to cost concerns and evidence that routine ultrasound does not improve outcomes, the use of this technology does not appear warranted, but it remains a popular procedure among pregnant women and clinicians alike.

Management Strategies

PROMOTING GOOD HEALTH IN PREGNANCY

A woman's body undergoes marked physiologic changes during pregnancy. Her blood volume increases by almost 50 percent, her endocrine system undergoes dramatic alterations, and her organs adjust to the profound anatomic and metabolic changes of pregnancy. In addition to these remarkable physiologic changes, most women are committed to taking good care of themselves during pregnancy.

NUTRITION AND WEIGHT GAIN It is presently recommended that an average-sized woman should gain 25 to 35 lb during pregnancy.[48] Underweight women and adolescents (who may still be growing themselves) require a 28- to 40-lb weight gain to reduce their risk of having a low birth weight baby. Women who are overweight at the onset of pregnancy, or who gain excessively during the pregnancy, have an increased incidence of hypertension and diabetes along with a tendency to produce large babies that can lead to difficult labors and operative delivery. Data are insufficient to demonstrate exactly how much weight obese women should gain. Because some have found an increased risk of intrauterine growth retardation in obese women with little weight gain,[49] it is generally recommended that obese women gain

Table 3-6

Indications for Ultrasonography During Pregnancy

Estimation of gestational age for patients with uncertain clinical dates or verification of dates for patients
  who are to undergo scheduled elective repeat cesarean delivery, indicated induction of labor, or other
  elective termination of pregnancy
Evaluation of fetal growth
Vaginal bleeding of undetermined etiology in pregnancy
Determination of fetal presentation
Suspected multiple gestation
Adjunct to amniocentesis
Significant uterine size/clinical dates discrepancy
Pelvic mass
Suspected hydatidiform mole
Adjunct to cervical cerclage placement
Suspected ectopic pregnancy
Adjunct to special procedures
Suspected fetal death
Suspected uterine abnormality
Intrauterine contraceptive device localization
Biophysical evaluation for fetal well-being
Observation of intrapartum events
Suspected polyhydramnios or oligohydramnios
Suspected abruptio placentae
Adjunct to external version from breech to vertex presentation
Estimation of fetal weight or presentation in premature rupture of membranes or premature labor
Abnormal serum α-fetoprotein value
Follow-up observation of identified fetal anomaly
Follow-up evaluation of placental location for identified placenta previa
History of previous congenital anomaly
Serial evaluation of fetal growth in multiple gestation
Evaluation of fetal condition in late registrants for prenatal care

SOURCE: Adapted from U.S. Department of Health and Human Services. Diagnostic ultrasound in pregnancy. National Institutes of Health
Publication No. 84-667. Bethesda, MD: National Institutes of Health, 1984.

at least 15 lb. It is often observed anecdotally that some obese women have healthy babies with lower gains.

VITAMIN AND MINERAL SUPPLEMENTS Most women are encouraged to take a prenatal vitamin during pregnancy. These are multivitamin preparations containing iron (usually 60 to 90 mg); zinc; copper; calcium (usually 250 mg); vitamins B_6, B_{12}, C, and D; and folate (usually 1 mg). If vitamin A is included, β-carotene is preferred over retinol to reduce the risk of toxicity. Because calcium and magnesium may interfere with iron absorption, upper limits of 250 mg and 25 mg per dose, respectively, are recommended as part of the vitamin supplement. Because many women experience nausea and vomiting during the first trimester, and vitamins may worsen these symptoms, supplemental minerals and vitamins can be started in the second trimester.

Folic Acid.   Folic acid reduces the risk of neural tube defects (spina bifida, anencephaly, or meningomyelocele), and dietary supplementation with 0.4 to 1 mg daily should ideally begin before conception and continue through the first 3 months of pregnancy.[50]

Iron.   It is recommended that all pregnant women supplement their diet with 30 mg elemental iron daily during the second and third trimesters. There is no evidence that further supplementation with iron is beneficial to the mother or the baby, except in those women with true iron-deficiency anemia. In fact, concern has been raised that excess iron may lead to zinc depletion, which is associated with intrauterine growth retardation.[51] In addition, iron supplementation can cause stomach upset, nausea, and constipation, although sustained-release preparations can lower the incidence of these side effects. The best food sources for iron include meats, chicken, fish, legumes, leafy vegetables, and whole grain or enriched breads and cereals. Tea and coffee can limit the absorption of iron and should be avoided at meals at which good sources of iron are eaten.

If a woman is experiencing iron-related side effects (as noted above) from a standard prenatal vitamin, a preparation with 30 mg iron should be substituted. This can be accomplished by using a nonprescription prenatal vitamin or two children's chewable vitamins with iron.

Vitamin A.   Excess ingestion of fat-soluble vitamins should be avoided, particularly vitamin A, which can cause birth defects at dosages just three to four times higher than the recommended daily allowance.[52] Use of β-carotene, the precursor of vitamin A found in fruits and vegetables, has not been shown to produce vitamin A toxicity. Supplementation with 5000 IU vitamin A per day should be considered the maximum intake before and during pregnancy. This is well below the minimum human teratogenic dose, which is

probably at least 25,000 to 50,000 IU daily. Prenatal multivitamins in common use contain 5000 IU or less of vitamin A, but vitamin tablets containing 25,000 IU or more of vitamin A are available as nonprescription preparations, so care should be exercised.

Other Minerals.   It is generally recommended that women ingest 1200 mg calcium daily during pregnancy; many women's diets do not provide this amount. These and other supplements are currently being studied, but at this time there is no evidence that the addition of multivitamins, zinc, magnesium, calcium, or even fish oil is of any benefit to the mother or her baby. An exception can be made for those women who truly have a marginal nutritional status imposed by social or economic limitations.

BREAST-FEEDING

No discussion on nutrition is complete without mentioning breast-feeding, the optimal nutritional choice for the baby. Breast milk is rich in nutrients, is easily digested, is readily available and inexpensive, and promotes the mother-baby relationship. Breast milk furnishes the necessary immunologic protection while the infant's immune system is maturing. Breast milk contains antibodies against common bacteria, viruses, and other pathogens, as well as providing anti-inflammatory agents and immunomodulating factors.[53] It also decreases the risk for immunologic disorders such as atopy and allergies. The evidence in support of breast-feeding is so overwhelming that entire texts have been devoted to detailing the art and science of breast-feeding.[54]

Women need to maintain healthy lifestyle habits while breast-feeding because drugs, tobacco toxins, and alcohol will pass into the breast milk. Breast-feeding women should maintain an adequate intake of calcium, especially because bone density decreases during lactation.

Breast-feeding should be addressed during pregnancy because most women make their decision on infant feeding well before the baby is born. Providers should ask women whether they have considered breast-feeding the baby and ask specifically about what they know (or have heard) about it, any past experience, expectations, and perceived problems. There is, however, no evidence that a health care provider can influence the choice of whether or not to breast-feed; attitudes of the woman and her family and friends are much more influential in this decision than the advice of her provider. However, a discussion about a woman's thoughts, concerns, and experiences with breast-feeding may uncover misconceptions and provide an opportunity for education and support. Ultimately, it is important to respect the mother's choice. For women who do choose breast-feeding, information on strategies to increase the likelihood of success and efforts to minimize common problems can be helpful.

UNPLEASANT SYMPTOMS OF PREGNANCY

Most women experience unpleasant symptoms during pregnancy. There is no shortage of advice on how to alleviate these discomforts. A summary of suggestions for these problems is presented in Table 3-7.

NAUSEA AND VOMITING   Most pregnant women experience nausea during the first 3 months of pregnancy, with at least half of them vomiting as well. The causes of this are still unknown but nausea usually resolves after the third month of pregnancy. General recommendations to manage nausea include eating small, frequent bland meals. Ginger (soda, tea, tablets, or ginger snaps) has been somewhat helpful as has vitamin B_6 (25 mg three times a day).[55] Acupressure at the wrists has been shown to reduce the incidence of persistent nausea, a concept embodied in commercially available Sea-Bands®.

When these measures are not enough, medications may be prescribed. Antihistamines and piperazine phenothiazines are effective in alleviating nausea (see Table 3-7). Doxylamine (Unisom®) combined with vitamin B_6 is also helpful. This combination was previously sold as Bendectin®

until it was removed from the market due to concerns regarding teratogenicity. These concerns were subsequently shown to be unfounded.[56]

CONSTIPATION AND HEMORRHOIDS   Decreased motility of the gastrointestinal tract during pregnancy leads to constipation for many women. Physiologic approaches such as increasing fruits, vegetables, and fiber in the diet; increasing fluids; and exercising regularly can often relieve this problem. The next step is taking bulk-forming agents or stool softeners, both of which are safe for long-term use in pregnancy. If these preparations fail to provide relief, some laxatives can be used on a short-term basis; cathartics and mineral oil should not be used at all because of the side effect of cramping; mineral oil is also associated with the risk of aspiration. The need for iron supplementation should be reconsidered for women who are constipated because iron supplements can cause constipation. Providing a lower dose of iron (30 mg versus the 60 mg contained in most prenatal vitamins) may be sufficient to resolve the constipation and will still provide the recommended dose of iron. Some nonprescription prenatal vitamins or two children's chewable vitamins with iron contain this amount of iron.

Effective management of constipation will reduce the incidence of hemorrhoids, another common and painful symptom of pregnancy. Rest and warm soaks in the tub may also relieve the discomfort of hemorrhoids.

HEARTBURN   Most women will experience heartburn during pregnancy (usually in the later months) due to the effects of progesterone, causing relaxation of the gastroesophageal sphincter, and the enlarged uterus pushing the stomach upward. It can be distressing and worsens after eating or when lying down. Sensible measures such as avoiding spicy foods and minimizing lying flat after eating are helpful. For further relief, liquid or chewable antacids are useful. Calcium carbonate is the preferred antacid in pregnancy. Drugs such as Alkaseltzer® and Peptobismol®

should be avoided because they contain salicylates. Some of the H_2-blockers have also been approved for use in pregnancy (see Table 3-7).

LEG CRAMPS At least half of pregnant women experience painful spasms in the calf muscles during late pregnancy. Because the cause of this is

Table 3-7

Treatment Options for Pregnancy-Related Symptoms

		DRUG THERAPY	
	NONDRUG THERAPY	DRUG AND DOSE	PREGNANCY CATEGORY*
Nausea and vomiting	Small, frequent meals Bland food Ginger Vitamin B_6	Promethazine (Phenergan®) 12.5–25 mg q 4 h and prochlorperazine (Compazine®) 5–10 mg tid–qid	C
	Accupressure at wrists (Sea Bands®)	Metoclopromide (Reglan®) 5–15 mg tid	B
		Doxylamine (Unisom®) 12.5–25 mg tid	B
		Vitamin B_6 25 mg tid	A
		Trimethobenzamide (Tigan®) 250 mg tid–qid	C
		Ondansetron (Zofran®) 4–8 mg tid	B
Constipation	Increase fluids and dietary fruit, vegetables, and fiber	Bulk-forming agents such as psyllium preparations (Metamucil® or Fiberall®)	*
	Exercise	Laxatives such as magnesium hydroxide (Milk of Magnesia®)	*
	Reduce or eliminate iron supplementation	Stool softeners such as Docusate	C
Hemorrhoids	Reduce constipation Warm soaks/sitz bath	Anusol HC	*
Heartburn	Small, dry meals, avoid greasy or spicy food	Antacids such as calcium carbonate (Tums®)	*
		H_2-blockers such as cimetidine (Tagamet®) 400 mg qid, ranitidine (Zantac®) 150 mg bid, and famotidine (Pepcid®) 20 mg bid	B
Leg cramps	Massage Warm water Muscle stretching		

Category A = Adequate and well-controlled studies have failed to demonstrate a risk to the fetus in the first trimester in pregnancy (and there is no evidence of risk in later trimesters).
Category B = Animal reproduction studies have failed to demonstrate a risk to the fetus and there are no adequate and well-controlled studies in pregnant women.
Category C = Animal reproduction studies have shown an adverse effect on the fetus and there are no adequate and well-controlled studies in humans, but potential benefits may warrant use of the drug in pregnant women despite potential risks.
*These nonprescription drugs have not been assigned to a pregnancy category.

unknown, effective treatments are lacking. Calcium, salt, or magnesium supplements have all been suggested as remedies for this painful condition, but none has clearly been shown to be of benefit. Massage, daily calf muscle stretching, and soaking in warm water all afford some relief and are harmless measures that are worth trying.

COMMON NONPREGNANCY-RELATED PROBLEMS

Table 3-8 lists some symptoms that are common and often occur during pregnancy. These include colds, allergies, headaches, urinary tract infections, and vaginitis.

UPPER RESPIRATORY INFECTIONS Many popular remedies have been proposed for colds, from chicken soup to vitamin C. There is still no cure for the common cold, but Table 3-8 lists some drugs for symptomatic relief that can be used in pregnancy. Pharmacologic treatments for allergies and headaches are listed as well. Urinary tract infections usually require antibiotic treatment for eradication.

VAGINITIS Vaginal infections also occur in pregnancy (see Chap. 11). Yeast infections are common and can cause intense itching. There can be a white vaginal discharge, although it can be difficult to differentiate between this and the normal increase in discharge that occurs during pregnancy. Azole antifungals applied vaginally, such as miconazole (see Table 3-8), are usually the therapy of choice and can be used in the first trimester. Oral azole antifungal agents are contraindicated in pregnancy.

Bacterial vaginosis can cause a "fishy" odor, a white, yellow, green, or gray discharge, and itching caused by an overgrowth of anaerobic bacteria in the vagina. It is thought to be associated with miscarriage, premature rupture of membranes, and preterm delivery.[32,57] Oral or topical clindamycin or metronidazole can reduce the symptoms as well as the associated risks.[34] The use of metronidazole in early pregnancy remains controversial. Although some studies report it is

safe to use even in the first trimester,[58] it is probably prudent to avoid its use until the second and third trimester. Clindamycin is a safe and effective alternative.

Trichomonas is a protozoa that can cause itching and discharge, although women are often asymptomatic. It is unclear whether trichomonas itself causes adverse pregnancy outcomes. As a sexually transmitted disease, it is often associated with other sexually transmitted diseases that are of known significance during pregnancy, so thorough evaluation is warranted. The only known effective treatment for trichomonas is metronidazole. Clotrimazole is often suggested as an alternative in the first trimester, even though it is only effective in a minority of cases.

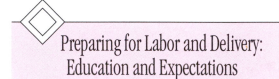

Preparing for Labor and Delivery: Education and Expectations

A wide range of approaches can be used to assist with delivery, and a woman should choose a provider whose philosophy on childbirth most closely reflects her own. Women choose every style from giving birth at home attended by a lay-midwife to delivering in a hospital using every technologic intervention available. There are passionate opinions on this, but because most women have good birth outcomes no matter what the style, it is difficult to ascertain which approach is best. In the United States, technologies and interventions have been routinely introduced into the management of labor before they have been demonstrated to be of benefit. Although a woman is unlikely to change the beliefs of her health care provider, it is helpful for her and her partner to be informed regarding basic care during childbirth, so that they can advocate for the approach they think is best for them. Birth plans, documents outlining the wishes of a pregnant woman and her partner, can be a useful way of understanding a woman's preferences. Sample birth plans can be

Table 3-8

Treatment Options for Nonpregnancy-Related Symptoms

	DRUG THERAPY		
		DRUG AND DOSE	**PREGNANCY CATEGORY***
Colds (viral upper respiratory infection) and allergy	Analgesic:		
	OTC	acetaminophen (Tylenol®)	B
	Decongestants:		
	Topical: OTC*	phenylephrine (Neosynephrine®, Sinex®)	No rating†
	OTC	naphazoline (Privine®)	No rating
	OTC	oxymetazoline (Afrin®)	C
	Oral: OTC	pseudoephedrine (Sudafed®)	C
	OTC	phenylpropanolamine (generic)	C
	Antihistamines:		
	OTC	chlorpheniramine (Chlor-Trimeton®)	B
	OTC	brompheniramine (Dimetane®, Dimetapp®)	B
	OTC	clemastine (Tavist®)	B
	OTC	diphenhydramine (Benedryl®)	B
	OTC	dexchlorpheniramine (Polaramine®)	B
		cetirizine (Zyrtec®)	B
		loratadine (Claritin®)	B
		astemizole (Hismanal®)	C
		azelastine (Astelin®)	C
		fexofenadine (Allegra®)	C
		hydroxyzine (Atarax®)	C
	Cough suppressant:		
	OTC	dextromethorphan (Robitussin DM®)	C
		benzonatate (Tessalon Perles®)	C
	Expectorant:		
	OTC	guaifenesin (Robitussin plain®)	C
Headache	OTC	acetaminophen (Tylenol®)	B
		butalbital (Fioricet®)	C
Urinary tract infection		nitrofurantoin (Macrodantin®, Macrobid®)	B
		ampicillin, amoxicillin	B
		sulfisoxazole (Gantrisin®)	C
		trimethoprim-sulfamethoxazole (Septra®)	C
Vaginitis: candida	Vaginal preparations:		
	OTC	clotrimazole (Gyne-Lotrimin®, Mycelex®)	B
	OTC	butoconazole (Femstat®)	C
	OTC	miconazole (Monistat®)	C
	OTC	tioconazole (Vagistat-I®)	C
		nystatin (Mycostatin®)	B
		terconazole (Terazol®)	C
	Oral agent:		
		fluconazole (Diflucan®)	C
bacterial vaginosis		metronidazole (Flagyl®)	B
		clindamycin (Cleocin®)	B
trichomonas vaginitis	OTC	clotrimazole (Gyne-Lotrimin®, Mycelex®)	B
		metronidazole (Flagyl®)	B

*OTC = over the counter/nonprescription
†Several of the nonprescription topical decongestants are not rated because information about use in pregnancy is limited and systemic effects of the agents are limited.
Category A = Adequate and well-controlled studies have failed to demonstrate a risk to the fetus in the first trimester in pregnancy (and there is no evidence of risk in later trimesters).
Category B = Animal reproduction studies have failed to demonstrate a risk to the fetus and there are no adequate and well-controlled studies in pregnant women.
Category C = Animal reproduction studies have shown an adverse effect on the fetus and there are no adequate and well-controlled studies in humans, but potential benefits may warrant use of the drug in pregnant women despite potential risks.

found on the Internet (e-mail address: www.child-birth.org).

Support in Childbirth

During the prenatal course, a pregnant woman should think about who she wants to be with her during labor. Companion support during childbirth, by either a partner or trained lay person has been shown to decrease the use of anesthesia, shorten the length of labor, and lower the rate of cesarean section.[59] Physical contact and group support has long been practiced in many cultures, and modern hospital policies should encourage this kind of support.

Nutrition During Labor

Many hospitals continue a policy of withholding food and drink from laboring women. The concern is that the woman might aspirate her stomach contents into her lungs if general anesthesia is needed for operative delivery. This is a rare but serious complication. Withholding food, however, does not guarantee an empty stomach and the skill and experience of the anesthesiologist in controlling the airway is a far more important factor with respect to maternal morbidity and mortality.[60]

INTRAVENOUS FLUIDS

Withholding food and drink can cause dehydration, ketosis, hunger, and thirst, especially in prolonged labors. In an effort to minimize these problems, the use of intravenous fluids became widespread. However, this can lead to fluid overload, restriction of movement, and increased perception of pain.[61] Given that there are little data about the nutritional needs of laboring women, a reasonable approach seems to be to allow the oral intake of fluids of the woman's choice along with light snacks.

Pain Management

Most women are willing to withstand some pain during childbirth, but the threshold of tolerance for pain varies tremendously. Preparation for childbirth, attitudes toward the father of the baby, and an individual woman's life experiences will affect her approach to dealing with the pain of childbirth. Many options are available to alleviate labor pain and these should be discussed during prenatal care.

NONPHARMACOLOGIC METHODS

Many women express a desire to avoid pharmacologic pain relief, and this preference should be supported, within reason. Prenatal care should include education to familiarize women with the choices available to reduce labor pain. Although the overall effects of prenatal classes cannot be generalized because of variation in the quality of the instruction and the attitudes conveyed, the existing evidence does suggest that they are associated with less use of analgesic medication during labor.[62]

Touch (e.g., stroking, massage) and movement (ambulation, position change, etc.) can be therapeutic during labor and are widely practiced in many cultures. Although the effectiveness of these measures has not been extensively studied, most experienced caregivers have found that counterpressure on the low back applied by a support person can alleviate back pain in some laboring women. Experience also shows that laboring women experience less pain in some positions than in others and can be trusted to select the positions that they find the most comfortable. Position changes can enhance the progress of labor as well; movement by the laboring woman should not be restricted.

Observational evidence suggests that the use of heat (hot-water bottles, hot towels, baths, and showers) and cold (ice packs and cool towels) can alter the perception of pain. These measures can be applied to the face, belly, perineum, and low back.

Focused concentration, visualization, relaxation techniques, music, and hypnosis have all been touted as being helpful in managing pain. Data on their effectiveness are limited, but there are no known adverse outcomes from these approaches.

Transcutaneous electrical nerve stimulation is a noninvasive method of pain control that transmits low-voltage electrical current to the skin, resulting in a "buzzing" sensation. The results of a few clinical trials were inconclusive,[63] and the use of such a device is not widespread.

PHARMACOLOGIC METHODS

Opiates, alcohol, and various other concoctions and potions have been used since ancient times. The challenge is to find a method that is effective in relieving pain while not compromising the health of the mother or the baby.

NARCOTICS Narcotics are widely used and reasonably effective (Table 3-9). Unwanted maternal side effects include hypotension, nausea, vomiting, dizziness, and delayed stomach emptying. Of even more concern is the respiratory depression and decreased alertness that can be observed in the newborn. This can be minimized by judicious dosing and avoiding use within an hour or two of delivery. Respiratory depression at birth due to maternal narcotic use can be reversed with intramuscular naloxone given to the newborn.

REGIONAL ANESTHESIA Regional anesthesia is widely used in labor. Epidural anesthesia is the most popular form of regional anesthesia and is effective in providing pain relief. However, a number of adverse outcomes are associated with its use including increased need for oxytocin,[64,65] prolonged labor, increased rates of instrumental deliveries, and possibly increased rates of cesarean section.[66] In a recent randomized trial of epidural versus patient-controlled meperidine analgesia during labor, however, there was no difference between groups in rates of cesarean section.[67] Epidurals frequently cause maternal temperature

elevation[68] that is difficult to distinguish from maternal infection and can lead to unnecessary testing and treatments in the newborn.[69]

Spinal (i.e., intrathecal) analgesia is gaining in popularity because it usually provides effective analgesia with an opioid without needing to use a local anesthetic. Unfortunately, it commonly has the side effects of nausea, pruritus, and headache. Spinal anesthesia can be used for operative deliveries because it has a rapid onset of action and is relatively easy to administer.

Paracervical block provides adequate analgesia but has fallen out of favor due to reports of fetal bradycardia, acidosis, and fetal death associated with its use. A pudendal nerve block and local perineal anesthesia are both effective methods of pain management in the second stage of labor.

Inhalation anesthesia (nitrous oxide) used to be a popular method of pain relief but is no longer used due to side effects of nausea and vomiting as well as concern for the medical staff repeatedly exposed to such gases.

Labor Management Decisions

Position in Labor and Delivery

When allowed to choose any position without interference or instruction, most women frequently change position in labor, using an average of 7.5 different positions.[70] The squatting position may offer an advantage because it enlarges the pelvic outlet by about 25 percent and makes use of gravity. Some studies have found that labor is shorter with a vertical position (sitting, standing, squatting, or kneeling).[71,72] Side-lying, or the lateral Sims' position, allows the clinician good visualization and results in a reduced need for episiotomy.[73] There is no evidence that the supine position confers any advantage to the laboring woman, and because the

Table 3-9

Narcotic Medications for Pain Relief During Labor

DRUG	DOSE	ROUTE	ONSET*	DURATION
Butorphanol (Stadol®)	1–2 mg	IM or IV	5–30 min	2–4 h
Fentanyl (Sublimaze®)	0.5–2 cc	IM or IV	1– 2 min	0.5–1 h
Meperidine (Demerol®)	50–100 mg	IM, IV, or SQ	5–15 min	1–3 h
Morphine	2–10 mg	IM or IV	5–30 min	3–5 h
Nalbuphine (Nubain®)	10 mg	IM or IV	2–15 min	3–6 h
Pentazocine (Talwin®)	10–20 mg	IM or IV	2–20 min	2–3 h

*The shorter time is the onset of action after IV administration of the drug, while the longer time is the onset of action after IM administration.

uterus may compress the woman's aorta and vena cava in this position, hypotension and fetal compromise may occur.

Women should be allowed to labor freely in the positions they choose, with birth attendants displaying flexibility and competence using different positions for delivery.

Continuous Electronic Fetal Monitoring

Electronic fetal monitoring is a classic example of applying a technology originally intended for high-risk patients to the general population before it is of proven benefit. When adequate studies were finally conducted, it was found that routine use of continuous electronic fetal monitoring compared to intermittent auscultation does not improve fetal outcomes but does increase the incidence of cesarean sections.[74] This technology may be helpful when used to monitor suspected fetal distress; in this situation, a fetal scalp capillary sample for blood pH can be used to confirm fetal compromise. A scalp pH value of less than 7.20 requires intervention (usually cesarean section), a pH of 7.20 to 7.25 requires repeat evaluation within 20 mins, and a pH of above 7.25 is reassuring. Internal scalp electrodes for monitoring the fetal heart rate should be considered when heart tones cannot be adequately detected with an external Doppler device or to evaluate beat-to-beat variability of the fetal heart rate.

Episiotomy

An episiotomy, or incision of the perineum just before delivering the head, is still performed by many clinicians who believe that it prevents damage to the perineum, anal sphincter, and rectum; is easier to repair than a tear; and prevents pelvic relaxation or urinary incontinence in later years. Studies, however, find either no difference in the rates of severe perineal lacerations or more severe lacerations among women who received episiotomies.[75,76] No data support the contention that episiotomy prevents pelvic relaxation, and the only randomized trial found no differences in urinary incontinence or dyspareunia.[77] Episiotomy should be limited to situations where it is needed to expedite delivery in cases of fetal distress.

Amniotomy

Amniotomy, or deliberate rupture of the fetal membranes, is a procedure performed for the purpose of inducing or augmenting labor, evaluating amniotic fluid for the presence of meconium, for placing a fetal scalp electrode, or obtaining fetal scalp blood to assess the baby's pH status. Amniotomy can shorten labor by 1 or 2 h,[78] but it can also occasionally result in increased uterine forces, cord prolapse, and increased potential for maternal or fetal infection.

Other Choices in Labor

Whether a woman delivers in a hospital, birth center, or at home, she should be given choices in labor. Although hospitals need policies for efficient functioning, they must allow flexibility toward individuals, especially because many rules and routines are of no proven benefit and may actually do more harm than good. For example, it is important to remember that the newborn baby belongs to the parents, not to the hospital, and policies that separate the baby from the mother should be abandoned. Women and their families should be treated with dignity, afforded privacy, and approached as individuals. Choice regarding who is in the room, what food and drink is consumed, and what clothing is worn by the laboring woman are small efforts that can help a woman feel in control during this major life event.

No evidence justifies the routine use of enemas or shaving pubic hair. These are uncomfortable procedures that can be embarrassing for a woman and they have no role for routine use in modern childbirth.

Postdate Pregnancy

For a woman and her family who see the long anticipated due date come and go, pregnancy can begin to look like a permanent state. Patience usually pays off, and in 90 percent of cases, spontaneous onset of labor will occur before the 42nd week. A postdate pregnancy is one that exceeds 42 weeks since the first date of the last menstrual period. The most common explanation is incorrect dating of the pregnancy, which again underscores how important it is to establish accurate dates early in the pregnancy. Of concern in the truly postdate pregnancy is the increased risk of uteroplacental insufficiency, oligohydramnios with umbilical cord compression, and the increasing size of the baby, which can make delivery more difficult.

It is common practice to assess fetal health in the postdate pregnancy by performing a nonstress test. This is performed using electronic fetal monitoring to assess the baby's heart rate and expected acceleration with movement (reactivity). This test is reassuring if it shows the expected reactivity (at least two fetal heart rate accelerations of at least 15 beats/min lasting at least 15 sec over a 20-min period), but the specificity is low (lack of fetal heart rate reactivity does not always indicate a compromised fetus).[79] Another common way to assess fetal health is a biophysical profile by ultrasound. This test assesses fetal movement and the amount of amniotic fluid present (Table 3-10). It is a fairly reliable way of predicting fetal health.[80] A modified biophysical profile,

Table 3-10

Components of the Biophysical Profile*

1. Reactive nonstress test
2. Fetal breathing movements (one or more episodes of rhythmic fetal breathing movements of 30 sec or more within 30 min)
3. Fetal movement (three or more discrete body or limb movements within 30 min)
4. Fetal tone (one or more episodes of extension of a fetal extremity with return to flexion)
5. Amniotic fluid index (the largest vertical pockets of fluid in each of the four quadrants are measured and added together; < 5 cm is oligohydramnios, 5–8 cm is borderline oligohydramnios, 8–20 cm is normal, > 20–25 cm is polyhydramnios)

*A score of 2 (normal) or 0 (abnormal) is assigned to each of these five components, they are then added together. A sum of 8 or 10 is normal; a sum of 6 is equivocal (consider retesting in 12–24 h); and a sum of 4 or less is abnormal.[82]

which is an ultrasound assessment of amniotic fluid in combination with the nonstress test, is as effective as a full biophysical profile in predicting fetal well-being.[81]

Concerning findings with any of these antenatal tests may suggest that labor should be induced. In many settings it is common practice to induce labor at 42 weeks, even in the absence of concerning findings about fetal health. Factors including the "ripeness" of the cervix and the preferences of the pregnant woman should be considered in the decision to induce labor.[82]

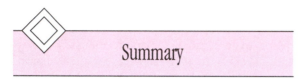

Summary

Prenatal care has played a role in reducing infant and maternal mortality and should be available to all pregnant women. Although the foundation of prenatal care is medical surveillance, attention should also be paid to psychosocial health, healthy behaviors, and preparation for labor and delivery. The philosophy toward prenatal care and childbirth is culturally dependent. The approach to childbirth can range from home births with little medical intervention to hospital births with use of multiple technologies. Regardless of the approach, two tenets should be followed: (1) women's choices should be honored as much as possible, and (2) any interventions should be proven effective before use.

References

1. Cefalo RC, Moos MK: *Preconceptional Health Care: A Practical Guide,* 2nd ed. St Louis: Mosby; 1995.
2. Ventura SJ, Martin JA, Taffel SM, et al: Advanced report of final natality statistics, 1993. *Monthly Vital Statistics Report 44, No. 3*(suppl), 1995.
3. Public Health Service: Healthy People 2000, National Health Promotion and Disease Preventing Objectives. Rockville, MD: U.S. Department of Health and Human Services, Public Health Service; 1992:381.
4. Dunn HL: *Vital Statistics of the United States*, 1941, Part 1. Washington, DC: U.S. Government Printing Office; 1943:27.
5. Gardner P, Hudson BL: Advanced report of final mortality statistics, 1993. *Monthly Vital Statistics Report 44* (suppl), 1996.
6. *The State of the World's Children* 1996. New York: Oxford University Press for UNICEF; 1996:81.
7. The Cochrane Database of Systematic Reviews. Available in The Cochrane Library. The Cochrane Collaboration, Issue I. Oxford: Update Software; 1998.
8. Chalmers I, Enkin M, Keirse M: *Effective Care in Pregnancy and Childbirth.* New York: Oxford University Press; 1989.
9. *U.S. Preventive Services Task Force: Guide to Clinical Preventive Services*, 2nd ed. Baltimore: Williams & Wilkins, 1996.
10. Rosenblatt RA, Dobie SA, Hart G, et al: Interspeciality differences in the obstetric care of low-risk women. *Am J Public Health* 87:344, 1997.
11. Blondel B, Pusch D, Schmidt E: Some characteristics of antenatal care in 13 European countries. *Br J Obstet Gynaecol* 92:565, 1985.
12. Public Health Service Expert Panel on Prenatal Care: Caring for our future: the content of prenatal care. NIH Publication No. 90-3182. Washington, DC: Public Health Services, U.S. Department of Health and Human Services; 1989.
13. McDuffie RS, Beck A, Bischoff K, et al: Effect of frequency of prenatal care visits on perinatal outcome among low-risk women. *JAMA* 275:847, 1996.
14. Chard T: Pregnancy tests: a review. *Hum Reprod* 7:701, 1992.
15. U.S. Department of Health and Human Services: Reducing the health consequences of smoking: 25 years of progress. A report of the Surgeon General. Publication No. DHHS (CDC) 89-8411. Rockville, MD: U.S. Department of Health and Human Services; 1989.
16. U.S. Department of Health and Human Services: The health benefits of smoking cessation: a report of the Surgeon General. Publication No. DHHS (CDC) 90-8416. Rockville, MD: U.S. Department of Health and Human Services; 1990.
17. Rosett HL, Weiner L, Edelin KC: Treatment experience with pregnant problem drinkers. *JAMA* 249:2029, 1983.
18. Martin TR, Bracken MB: The association between low birth weight and caffeine consumption during pregnancy. *Am J Epidemiol* 126:813, 1987.

19. Mayes LC, Granger RH, Bornstein MH, et al: The problem of prenatal cocaine exposure. A rush to judgment. *JAMA* 267:406, 1992.

20. Whitley R, Arvin A, Prober C, et al: Predictors of morbidity and mortality in neonates with herpes simplex virus infections. The National Institute of Allergy and Infectious Diseases Collaborative Antiviral Study Group. *N Engl J Med* 324:450, 1991.

21. Randolph AG, Washington EW, Prober CG: Cesarean delivery for women presenting with genital herpes lesions. *JAMA* 270:77, 1993.

22. American College of Obstetricians and Gynecologists: Prevention of D isoimmunization. Technical Bulletin 147. Washington, DC: American College of Obstetricians and Gynecologists; 1990.

23. Murphy JF, O'Riordan J, Newcombe RG, et al: Relation of haemoglobin levels in first and second trimester to outcome of pregnancy. *Lancet* 1:992, 1986.

24. Centers for Disease Control and Prevention: CDC criteria for anemia in children and childbearing-aged women. *MMWR* 38:400, 1989.

25. Paintin DB, Thomson AM, Hytten FE: Iron and haemoglobin level in pregnancy. *J Obstet Gynaecol Br Commwlth* 73:181, 1996.

26. Taylor DJ, Mallen C, McDougall N, Lind T: Effect of iron supplementation on serum ferritin levels during and after pregnancy. *Br J Obstet Gynaecol* 89:1011, 1982.

27. Wong VCW, Ip HMH, Reesink HW, et al: Prevention of the HBsAg carrier state in newborn infants of mothers who are chronic carriers of HBsAg and HBeAg by administration of hepatitis-B vaccine and hepatitis-B immunoglobulin: double-blind randomized placebo controlled study. *Lancet* 1:921, 1984.

28. Centers for Disease Control and Prevention: U.S. Public Health Service recommendations for HIV counseling and voluntary testing for pregnant women. *MMWR* 44:1, 1995.

29. Connor EM, Sperling RS, Gelber R, et al: Reduction of maternal-infant transmission of HIV-1 with zidovudine treatment. *N Engl J Med* 331:1173, 1994.

30. Fiscus SA, Andaora A, Schoenbach VJ, et al: Perinatal HIV infection and the effect of zidovudine therapy on transmission in rural and urban counties. *JAMA* 275:1483, 1996.

31. Romero R, Oyarzun E, Mazor M, et al: Meta-analysis of the relationship between asymptomatic bacteriuria and preterm delivery/low birth weight. *Obstet Gynecol* 73:576, 1989.

32. Hillier SL, Nugent RP, Eschenbach DA, et al: Association between bacterial vaginosis and preterm delivery of a low-birth weight infant. The Vaginal Infections and Prematurity Study Group. *N Engl J Med* 333:1737, 1995.

33. Hauth JC, Goldenberg RL, Andrews WW, DuBard MB, Copper RL: Reduced incidence of preterm delivery with metronidazole and erythromycin in women with bacterial vaginosis. *N Engl J Med* 333:1732, 1995.

34. Morales WJ, Schorr S, Albritton J: Effect of metronidazole in patients with preterm birth in preceding pregnancy and bacterial vaginosis: a placebo-controlled, double-blind study. *Am J Obstet Gynecol* 171:345, 1994.

35. Centers of Disease Control and Prevention: Prevention of perinatal group B streptococcal disease: a public health perspective. *MMWR* 45(RR-7):1, 1996.

36. American College of Obstetricians and Gynecologists: Diabetes and pregnancy. *Technical Bulletin 200*, 1994.

37. Flood T, Brewster M, Harris J, et al: Spina bifida incidence at birth—United States, 1983–1990. *MMWR* 41:497, 1992.

38. Maternal serum alpha-fetoprotein screening for neural tube defects: results of a consensus meeting. *Prenat Diagn* 5:77, 1985.

39. American College of Obstetricians and Gynecologists: Alpha-fetoprotein. *Technical Bulletin 154*, 1991.

40. Centers for Disease Control and Prevention: Down syndrome prevalence at birth—United States, 1983–1990. *MMWR* 43:617, 1994.

41. Hansen JP: Older maternal age and pregnancy outcome: a review of the literature. *Obstet Gynecol* 41:726, 1986.

42. NICHD National Registry for Amniocentesis Study Group: Midtrimester amniocentesis for prenatal diagnosis: safety and accuracy. *JAMA* 236:1471, 1976.

43. Haddow JE, Palomaki GE, Knight GJ, et al: Prenatal screening for Down's syndrome with use of maternal serum markers. *N Engl J Med* 327:588, 1992.

44. Campbell S, Warsof SL, Little D, et al: Routine ultrasound screening for the prediction of gestational age. *Obstet Gynecol* 65:613, 1985.

45. Ewigman BG, Crane JP, Figoletto FD, et al: Effect of prenatal ultrasound screening on perinatal outcome. The RADIUS Study Group. *N Engl J Med* 329:821, 1993.

46. National Institutes of Health Consensus Development Conference: The use of diagnostic ultrasound imaging during pregnancy. *JAMA* 252:669, 1984.
47. American College of Obstetricians and Gynecologists: Ultrasonography in pregnancy. *Technical Bulletin 187*, 1993.
48. Institute of Medicine: *Nutrition during Pregnancy: Part I. Weight Gain; Part II. Nutrient Supplements.* Washington, DC: National Academy Press, 1990.
49. Edwards LE, Hellerstedt WL, Alron IR, Story M, Himes JH: Pregnancy complications and birth outcomes in obese and normal-weight women: effects of gestational weight change. *Obstet Gynecol* 87:389, 1996.
50. Milunsky A, Jick H, Jick SS, et al: Multivitamin/folic acid supplementation in early pregnancy reduces the prevalence of neural tube defects. *JAMA* 262:2847, 1989.
51. Hemminki E, Merilainen J: Long-term follow-up of mothers and their infants in a randomized trial on iron prophylaxis during pregnancy. *Am J Obstet Gynecol* 173:205, 1995.
52. Rothman KJ, Moore LL, Singer MR, Nguyen U.S., Mannino S, Milunsky A: Teratogenicity of high vitamin A intake. *N Engl J Med* 333:1369, 1995.
53. Slusser W, Powers NG: Breastfeeding update 1: immunology, nutrition, and advocacy. *Pediatr Rev* 18:111, 1997.
54. Lawrence RA: *Breastfeeding: A Guide for the Medical Profession*, 4th ed. St. Louis: Mosby-Year Book; 1994.
55. Fischer-Rasmussen W, Kjaer SK, Dahl C, Asping U: Ginger treatment of hyperemesis gravidarum. *Eur J Obstet Gynecol Reprod Biol* 38:19, 1991.
56. Kolata GB: How safe is Bendectin? *Science* 210:518, 1980.
57. McGregor JA, French JI, Parker R, et al: Prevention of premature birth by screening and treatment for common genital tract infections: results of a prospective controlled evaluation. *Am J Obstet Gynecol* 173:157, 1995.
58. Burtin P, Taddio A, Ariburnu O, Einarson TR, Koren G: Safety of metronidazole in pregnancy: a meta-analysis. *Am J Obstet Gynecol* 172(2 Pt 1):525, 1995.
59. Kennell J, Klaus M, McGrath S, et al: Continuous emotional support during labor in a U.S. hospital. *JAMA* 265:2197, 1991.
60. Moir DD: The contribution of anaesthesia to maternal mortality. *J Int Med Res* 6 (suppl 1):40, 1978.
61. Newton N, Newton M, Broach J: Psychologic, physical, nutritional, and technologic aspects of intravenous infusion during labor. *Birth* 15:67, 1988.
62. Simkin P, Enkin M: Antenatal classes. In: Chalmers I, Enkin M, Keirse M (eds): *Effective Care in Pregnancy and Childbirth*. New York: Oxford University Press; 1989:318.
63. Harrison RF, Woods T, Shore M, Mathews G, Unwin A: Pain relief in labor using transcutaneous electrical nerve stimulation (TENS). A TENS/TENS placebo controlled study in two parity groups. *Br J Obstet Gynaecol* 93:739, 1986.
64. Eggertsen SC, Stevens N: Epidural anesthesia and the course of labor and delivery. *J Fam Pract* 18:309, 1984.
65. Niehaus LS, Chaska BW, Nesse RE: The effects of epidural anesthesia on type of delivery. *J Am Board Fam Pract* 1:238, 1988.
66. Thorp JA, Hu DH, Albin RM, et al: The effect of intrapartum epidural analgesia on nulliparous labor: a randomized, controlled, prospective trial. *Am J Obstet Gynecol* 69:851, 1993.
67. Sharma SK, Sidawi JE, Ramin SM, Lucas MJ, Leveno KJ, Cunningham FG: Cesarean section. A randomized trial of epidural versus patient-controlled meperidine analgesia during labor. *Anesthesiology* 87:487, 1997.
68. Fusi L, Maresh MJA, Steer PJ, Beard RW: Maternal pyrexia associated with the use of epidural analgesia in labour. *Lancet* 1(8649):1250, 1989.
69. Lieberman EL, Lang JM, Frigoletto F, et al: Epidural analgesia, intrapartum fever, and neonatal sepsis evaluation. *Pediatrics* 99:415, 1997.
70. Carlson JM, Diehl JA, Sachtleben-Murray M, McRae M, Fenwick L, Friedman EA: Maternal position during parturition in normal labor. *Obstet Gynecol* 68:443, 1986.
71. Flynn AM, Kelly J, Hollins G, Lynch PF: Ambulation in labour. *Br Med J* 2:591, 1978.
72. Mitre IN: The influence of maternal position on duration of the active phase of labor. *Int J Gynaecol Obstet* 12:181, 1974.
73. Kirkwood CR, Clark L: Lateral Sims' deliveries: a new application for an old technique. *J Fam Pract* 17:701, 1983.
74. Leveno KJ, Cunningham FG, Nelson S, et al: A prospective comparison of selective and universal electronic fetal monitoring in 34,995 pregnancies. *N Engl J Med* 315:615, 1986.

75. Gass MS, Dunn C, Stys SJ: Effect of episiotomy on the frequency of vaginal outlet lacerations. *J Reprod Med* 31:240, 1986.

76. Green JR, Soohoo SL: Factors associated with rectal injury in spontaneous deliveries. *Obstet Gynecol* 73(5 Pt 1):732, 1989.

77. Sleep J, Grant A: West Berkshire perineal management trial: three year follow up. *Br Med J* (Clin Res) 295:749, 1987.

78. Franks P: A randomized trial of amniotomy in active labor. *J Fam Pract* 30:49, 1990.

79. Freeman RK, Anderson G, Dorchester W: A Prospective multi-institutional study of antepartum fetal heart rate monitoring: I. Risk of perinatal mortality and morbidity according to antepartum fetal heart rate test results. *Am J Obstet Gynecol* 143:771, 1982.

80. Manning FA, Morrison I, Harman CR, et al: Fetal assessment based on fetal biophysical profile scoring: experience in 19,221 referred high-risk pregnancies: II. An analysis of false-negative fetal deaths. *Am J Obstet Gynecol* 157(4 Pt 1):880, 1987.

81. Miller DA, Rabello YA, Paul RH: The modified biophysical profile: antepartum testing in the 1990s. *Am J Obstet Gynecol* 174:812, 1996.

82. Manning FA, Harman CR, Morrison I, Menticoglou SM, Lange IR, Johnson JM: Fetal assessment based on fetal biophysical profile scoring: IV. An analysis of perinatal morbidity and mortality. *Am J Obstet Gynecol* 162:703, 1990.

83. Hook EB: Rates of chromosome abnormalities at different maternal ages. *Obstet Gynecol* 58:282, 1981.

Leslie A. Shimp
Mindy A. Smith

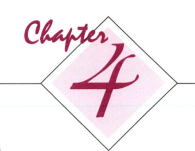

Chapter 4

Menopause

Overview

Menopause is an important transition in a woman's life. Over the past decade, the lay press and medical literature have been flooded with reports of the many adverse health events after menopause, events that are purported to need prevention or treatment with hormonal therapy. Information provided to both clinicians and their patients is frequently biased and opinion is often stated as fact. For example, an analysis of lay literature on menopause over a 3-year period found few articles written by those with credentials or expertise in women's health.[1] In addition, only

1 of the 42 articles written about hormone replacement therapy (HRT) discussed complications of therapy. In the medical literature, strong statements are made about the benefits of hormone therapy despite the fact that the vast majority of literature is based on observational studies, the use of unopposed estrogen replacement therapy (ERT), and selection of healthy, compliant women as candidates for therapy.

The predominant view of menopause as an estrogen-deficient state that heralds the onset of aging and illness has many negative connotations for women, in the way they view themselves, in the information they receive, and in their willingness to consider ERT/HRT. Menopause is not an illness to be treated, but a transitional state for which therapies are available to address symptoms and strategies can be implemented to prevent illness associated with both menopause and aging.

During the perimenopause (transition to menopause), many women interact with health care providers regarding management of symptoms (e.g., vaginal dryness, hot flashes, depressed mood) and for education and emotional support.[2] Although a recent clinic population study found that 71 percent of responding postmenopausal women were using HRT,[3] less than 20 percent of population samples of postmenopausal women in the United States have ever had ERT or HRT prescribed. In addition, less than 40 percent of women who begin therapy continue it after 1 year,[4] and less than 25 percent are still using postmenopausal hormones after 3 years.[5] This signals a need to understand and address the concerns of women when approaching treatment decisions.

How, then, do women view menopause? In a 1994 report of a random population sample of women from the Netherlands ($n = 234$, aged 45 to 65), nearly all women regarded the absence of menstruation with relief and most preferred a natural approach to the problems encountered.[6] Attitudes toward the use of HRT were neutral, but the level of knowledge about menopause, as judged by the investigators, was poor, and most women obtained their information from the media.

Similarly, in a U.S. survey conducted by the North American Menopause Society (NAMS), women cited the media as a source of information about menopause more often than they cited health professionals.[7] Reasons why women obtain information from sources other than health care providers may include the feeling that physicians are too distracted to take their concerns seriously[8] or that physicians tend to incorrectly estimate women's attitudes toward aspects of menopause and HRT. For example, in the NAMS survey, women reported that physicians underestimated women's desire for information, underestimated factors that women perceived as barriers to use of HRT, and overestimated their concern about cardiovascular disease and breast cancer.[9] Further, for women preferring a nonhormonal approach

to symptom management, clinicians may not be knowledgeable about alternatives or may convey a judgmental attitude that prohibits effective patient-provider communication.

Women are very interested in information about menopause, and health care providers should take advantage of opportunities presented to them (i.e., during annual examinations, when women ask about menopausal symptoms, or when women present to the pharmacy with a prescription for postmenopausal hormones) to discuss this condition. Because women may vary in their concerns about HRT, soliciting this information and seeking to understand the individual woman's risk factors and her viewpoint is critical to imparting adequate information and supporting her decision.

Typical Presentation

Definition

By definition, menopause is the final menstrual period, but a woman is not considered postmenopausal until she has had 1 year of amenorrhea. Menopause marks the end of a woman's reproductive phase of life. Menopause occurs due to a depletion of ovarian follicles and a resistance of remaining follicles to gonadotropin stimulation. This resistance results in increasing follicle-stimulating hormone (FSH) levels and a decline in the production of estrogen (most endogenous estrogen, estradiol, is produced by the follicles). Eventually the production of estrogen is so low that endometrial proliferation does not occur and menses cease.

Prevalence

The number of postmenopausal women in the United States is estimated at over 40 million; in the next decade the number of postmenopausal women is expected to increase to about 60 million.[10] The average age of menopause for U.S. women is 51 years; 95 percent of women reach menopause between 44 and 55 years of age. The average age of menopause has been remarkably stable since medieval times. Factors known to affect age at menopause for individual women include genetics (the age at onset and the symptoms experienced are similar between mothers and daughters), nutrition, and environmental factors such as tobacco smoking. The onset of menopause is, on average, 2 years earlier for smokers than for nonsmokers. If the average life expectancy of women is considered, about one-third of a woman's life will be lived after menopause.

Perimenopausal Physiologic and Biochemical Changes

A number of physiologic and biochemical changes occur during the perimenopause and the early postmenopausal years, independent of the effects of aging. Ovarian function begins to decline about 10 years before the cessation of menses. Hormonal changes include decreases in estrogen and progesterone. Estrogen levels decline by about 60 percent.[11] A decrease in androgen levels is also seen, but this precedes menopause and appears related to aging; total circulating testosterone levels in women in their forties is half that of women in their twenties. The decrease in all ovarian hormone levels, however, can be quite precipitous for women undergoing surgical menopause (bilateral oophorectomy), and symptoms of androgen deficiency (particularly reduced sexual desire and coital frequency) in addition to estrogen-related symptoms (such as hot flashes) may be seen.

Several biochemical changes with adverse cardiovascular consequences include a reduction in high-density lipoprotein (HDL) cholesterol and an increase in low-density lipoprotein (LDL) cholesterol (longitudinal data)[12]; an increase in triglycerides, apolipoprotein B, and apolipoprotein A-I;

higher diastolic blood pressure (cross-sectional data)[13]; and higher levels of serum ferritin (longitudinal data).[14] Premature menopause and surgical menopause are considered risk factors for cardiovascular disease.

The early period of postmenopause is also a time of rapid bone loss related to decreased gastrointestinal absorption of calcium and an increased bone turnover (greater bone resorption than formation) favoring bone loss (see Chap. 20).

Common Symptoms of Menopause

Symptoms typically associated with the perimenopause and menopause include menstrual changes (irregular or change in flow), hot flashes/hot flushes (sometimes resulting in insomnia and fatigue), sexual dysfunction (changes in libido and dyspareunia), urinary tract symptoms (urgency, frequency, dysuria, urinary tract infections [UTIs], stress incontinence), psychological symptoms (nervousness, irritability, depression, emotional lability), and cognitive symptoms (concentration, memory problems). It is difficult to ascribe all of these symptoms to menopause when few studies have correlated symptoms with hormonal status in population-based samples.

One of the few studies examining this issue, a survey of 850 British women aged 45 to 65, found that vasomotor symptoms (hot flushes and night sweats), difficulty falling asleep, decreased sexual interest, and vaginal dryness were significantly associated with menopause when controlling for the effects of age.[15] Sexual satisfaction, however, did not change with menopausal status; other symptoms commonly attributed to menopause, such as cognitive difficulties, depression, irritability, and various somatic symptoms were more strongly predicted by social class and employment status.

Table 4-1 presents a list of symptoms reported by more than 6000 menopausal women over a 6-month period.[10] Although many of these symptoms were experienced, far fewer women (about one-third) found the symptoms particularly bothersome.[16]

IRREGULAR MENSTRUAL PERIODS

One of the first symptoms of a decline in estrogen levels is irregular menses; this irregular pattern can precede menopause by 2 to 8 years.[17] The patterns of irregular menses vary from shortened to prolonged cycles and from oligomenorrhea to excessive bleeding.

Surprisingly little has been written about changes in the menstrual bleeding pattern of women as they transition into menopause. A recent report, based on menstrual diaries of 139 white women (39.5 percent of eligible women) ages 50 to 60, followed for 3 years, provides observational data on 1898 cycles.[18] Both cycle length (time between bleeding episodes) and duration (length of menses) tended to be longer compared to their cycles as younger women. Cycle length was found to range from 2 to 537 days with a median of 28 days. Only 45 cycles were separated by 2 days or less (0.2 percent) and 42 cycles were over 150 days between bleeding episodes. The duration of bleeding was from 1 to 46 days with a median of 5. Seven percent of bleeding episodes lasted only 1 day and only 6 cycles lasted longer than 29 days. Most cycles (77 percent) were of normal duration (defined as 3 to

Table 4-1

Menopausal Women's Experience of Symptoms over 6 Months

SYMPTOMS	% EXPERIENCING SYMPTOM (N = 6084)	% EXPERIENCING AS PROBLEM (N = 6084)
CLASSIC		
Hot flashes	57	22
Night sweats	55	24
Sleep problems	66	33
Dry/sore vagina	34	14
SOMATIC		
Aching/painful joints	67	29
Headaches	60	23
Sore breasts	51	14
Nocturia	48	16
Palpitations	37	13
Dizziness	35	11
PSYCHOLOGICAL		
Irritability	72	25
Concentration/memory problems	64	30
Anxiety	58	26
Depression	51	22
Feeling unable to cope	43	19

SOURCE: Modified from Porter M, Penny GC, Russell D: A population-based survey of women's experience of the menopause. *Br J Obstet Gynaecol* 103:1025, 1996.

8 days) and 48 percent were of normal length (defined as 22 to 35 days).

Several patterns of bleeding could be distinguished. Women who were in early perimenopause at baseline (those who had a single report of cycle irregularity) had the highest percentage of short-length cycles and short menses. Women who were in perimenopause at baseline (those reporting 3 to 11 months of amenorrhea or two or more consecutive reports of increased cycle length) had a tendency toward longer length cycles with normal menses. Finally, women who became postmenopausal during the study period had the highest percentage of cycles with short menses and a higher percentage of either short- or long-length cycles. This information may be helpful to women trying to judge where they may be in transition to menopause. There are no similar data on women of other races, and the women in this study, being older, more highly educated, and less likely to smoke than the population from which they were enrolled, may not represent the experience of most women.

HOT FLASHES/HOT FLUSHES

Hot flashes/hot flushes are the classic symptoms of menopause. The increase in body temperature and feeling of heat (hot flash) followed by a flushing or erythema and sweating of the head, neck, and upper thorax (hot flush) is experienced by 75 to 85 percent of European and North American women. Most commonly hot flashes persist for 2 to 5 years. However, only about 10 to 15 percent of women describe the hot flashes/hot flushes as significant enough to warrant therapy. Hot flushes that occur during the night (night sweats) and awaken women can lead to insomnia and fatigue; the resulting sleep deprivation can be severe enough to lead to symptoms of irritability, impaired memory, and poor concentration.

SEXUAL DYSFUNCTION

A decrease in estrogen levels can result in atrophic vaginal symptoms including vaginal dry-ness, vaginal itching or burning, and dyspareunia (pain with intercourse). Vaginal atrophy can occur as early as 3 to 6 months after menopause, and vaginal symptoms are often experienced within 5 years of menopause. After menopause, there are few vaginal secretions and lubrication with sexual arousal is lessened. In addition, the vaginal walls become thinner and less elastic and the vagina becomes shorter and narrower, which may lead to discomfort or pain during sexual activity.

When asked, many women report a decline in sexual interest and sexual activity with aging. The reasons for this are many and include physical, psychological, and social factors as listed in Table 4-2. Age-related changes in the sexual response cycle include a delay (from 10 to 15 sec to 5 min) and decrease in the quantity of vaginal vasocongestion and lubrication, a prolongation of the plateau phase, and a reduction in the number and intensity of vaginal and rectal contractions with orgasm.[19] These findings are less pronounced among women who remain sexually active. Most postmenopausal women report little change in the subjective feelings of sexual arousal and orgasmic response. Although a number of studies have confirmed a decrease in sexual fantasy and sexual interest from perimenopause to postmenopause,[20,21] this finding is not universal and some women (6.6 percent in one study[21]) report an increase in sexual interest.

URINARY TRACT SYMPTOMS

The atrophy that affects the vagina can also affect the lower urinary tract, resulting in detrusor irritability, urinary urgency, incontinence, and an increase in the frequency of UTIs.

PSYCHOLOGICAL SYMPTOMS AND COGNITIVE FUNCTIONING

Although emotional changes and lability (e.g., depression, irritability, headaches, and anxiety) and cognitive symptoms (e.g., forgetfulness, diffi-

Table 4-2

Factors Associated with Sexuality and Sexual Function Following Menopause

PHYSIOLOGIC CHANGES

Reduced hormone levels (estrogen, progesterone, androgen)
Decreased pelvic vascularity (blood flow decreases by up to 60%)
    Reduction in pubic hair
    Reduced fat and subcutaneous tissue from mons pubis
    Atrophy of labia majora, Bartholin glands, uterine cervix, and ovaries
    Loss of elasticity of vaginal barrel
    Vaginal epithelial thinning (loss of glycogen and lactobacilli, increased pH)*

PHYSICAL FACTORS
Gynecologic[†] or breast surgery Illness (arthritis, diabetes mellitus, renal failure) Medication use (antidepressants, antipsychotics, neuroleptics, diuretics, clonidine) Urinary incontinence Decreased vaginal lubrication and dyspareunia Menopausal symptoms (hot flashes, sleep disturbance) Depression

PSYCHOLOGICAL FACTORS
Nature of the interpersonal relationship (intimacy, communication problems, etc.) Death of partner New partner (anxiety, guilt) Loss of job Loss or deterioration of support network Financial struggles False expectations about sexual function Concerns about appearance

*Thinning of the vaginal epithelial layer from 8–10 cells to 3–4 cells can lead to postcoital bleeding and burning sensation, and changes in the vaginal microflora can result in bacterial infection.

†Hysterectomy results in absence of uterine contractions that may diminish sexual pleasure. However, relief from bleeding and pain may improve sexual function.

culty concentrating) have long been considered an aspect of menopause, clinical trials have not been able to demonstrate that either menopause or estrogen deficiency is a cause of emotional disturbances. Studies in four countries were not able to statistically link menopause and depression.[22] At the age of menopause, many physical and psychosocial changes can confound the relationship between estrogen levels and psychological functioning. However, there are also case reports of improved psychosocial and cognitive functioning in response to estrogen therapy.

Evidence is accumulating that changes in circulating estrogen levels after menopause may affect cognitive function. Estrogen affects functioning of the cholinergic system (e.g., promotes the growth and survival of cholinergic neurons), the most important system for memory and cognitive functions. Cognitive function studies comparing the performance of postmenopausal women using estrogen to nonusers found that users performed better on some tests such as those of verbal memory, conceptualization, and learning.[23,24] However, the effect is modest and no evidence indicates that women who do not take estrogen are impaired to the extent that daily functioning is compromised.[25]

However, women comprise the majority of persons with Alzheimer's dementia. It is hypothesized that the decrease in estrogen level with menopause may increase a woman's risk for dementia.[25] Several effects of estrogen (e.g., increased cholinergic system functioning, decreased amyloid deposition, and increased cerebral blood flow) may prevent or delay the onset of dementia.[25,26] Two studies have found that the risk for Alzheimer's disease was less among estrogen users compared to nonusers.[27,28] Investigators in a study of New York City residents found that the risk for Alzheimer's disease was reduced by 60 percent (RR 0.40, 95 percent CI 0.22 to 0.85) and the onset of disease was delayed among estrogen users. The Leisure World study found that, in addition to a 30 percent reduction in risk for developing Alzheimer's disease (odds ratio .69; 95 percent CI 0.46 to 1.03), higher estrogen doses and longer duration of use were most strongly associated with a decrease in the rate of dementia. Although the data accumulated to date are intriguing, they are also limited by the fact that estrogen users tend to differ from nonusers on a number of life-style characteristics. Thus, further study is needed to understand potential cognitive protective effects or the usefulness of estrogen therapy for persons with dementia.

Ethnic and Cultural Differences in Symptom Experiences

HEALTH CONSEQUENCES AND SYMPTOM REPORTING

There is significant disagreement about which health consequences and symptoms can be attrib-

uted to aging and which are specific to the lowered serum estrogen concentration and absence of menses that defines menopause. For example, despite lower serum estrogen levels, which may be less cardioprotective, Japanese women have lower rates of cardiovascular disease than white women.[29]

Even the presence of vasomotor symptoms is highly variable and strongly influenced by culture, including diet. Population surveys of women aged 45 to 55 performed in different countries demonstrated marked differences in reported rates of symptoms, with 12.3 percent, 31 percent, and 34.8 percent of Japanese, Canadian, and U.S. women reporting vasomotor symptoms, respectively.[30] Severity of vasomotor symptoms appears to have a major impact on the perception of other "menopausal" symptoms such as tenseness and irritability, with women with severe vasomotor complaints reporting higher percentages of somatic and psychological symptoms and poorer overall well-being regardless of whether or not they were still menstruating.[31] In short, although menopause is a universal biologic phenomenon among women of all racial and ethnic groups, its meaning, and even the associated symptoms, appears to be highly individual and influenced by both race and culture.

PHYSIOLOGIC DIFFERENCES

The issue of race and its effect on women's experience of menopause is complicated by the fact that there is no consensus of definition for race; measuring race by skin color alone may ignore a woman's biology, culture, behavior, and values. There are indications of physiologic differences between white and black women that should be considered in weighing decisions about the use of hormone therapy. Black women have significantly lower levels of serum cholesterol,[32] slower rates of decline in bone mineral density (BMD),[33] and greater breast cancer risks for those undergoing a natural menopause than white women.[34] This may reduce benefits and increase risks of HRT for black women.

Data also demonstrate that fewer black women have HRT prescribed for them compared to white women. In a secondary analysis of the National Health Interview Study data, 32 percent of white women reported previous use of estrogen pills compared to 13.6 percent of black women.[35] Black women, however, were more likely to begin ERT at an earlier age.

Menopause-Related Conditions (Late Consequences of Menopause)

The decline in circulating estrogen may be associated with the long-term potential adverse effects of osteoporosis and cardiovascular and cerebrovascular disease.

OSTEOPOROSIS

Over 90 percent of patients affected by osteoporosis are postmenopausal women. It is estimated that between 25 and 44 percent of postmenopausal women develop osteoporosis-related fractures, most commonly fractures of the vertebrae, hip, and distal forearm. Among white women, about 8/1000 experience an osteoporotic fracture; for black women the rate is 3/1000.[36] Although white and Asian women have an increased risk for osteoporosis-related fractures, black women have higher rates of death within the first 6 months after a hip fracture compared to white women (20 and 11 percent, respectively).[37]

Studies have clearly demonstrated that estrogen therapy can slow the development of osteoporosis and decrease the risk for osteoporosis-related fractures. The pooled estimate from studies suggests that women who have ever taken estrogen have a relative risk of 0.75 for hip fractures (95 percent CI, 0.68 to 0.84) compared to nonusers. Fractures of the distal forearm are decreased by about 50 percent among women who have taken estrogen for 10 years or more, and decreased rates of vertebral fractures were reported in three prospective studies.[38]

CORONARY HEART DISEASE AND CEREBROVASCULAR DISEASE

Coronary heart disease (CHD) is the leading cause of death for women in the United States (over 53 percent of postmenopausal women will die of cardiovascular disease) and the incidence of cardiovascular disease increases markedly after menopause. A number of epidemiologic studies have demonstrated a cardioprotective effect of estrogen. The cardiovascular benefits of estrogen include a decreased rate of CHD, a decreased death rate from both CHD and cardiovascular disease, reduced coronary artery occlusion, improved survival of women with coronary stenosis, decreased risk of myocardial infarction, and a decrease in all-cause mortality.[39] Most of these studies reported a 50 percent reduction in CHD among estrogen users. A large retrospective case-control study of women hospitalized over a 3-year period with acute myocardial infarction compared with age-matched controls, however, failed to demonstrate a reduced odds ratio for current users of either ERT or HRT.[40]

The Postmenopausal Estrogen/Progestin Intervention (PEPI) trial, a large randomized clinical trial ($n = 875$), measured four end-points relevant to cardiovascular disease over 3 years: HDL cholesterol, systolic blood pressure, serum insulin, and fibrinogen.[41] The investigators found that both ERT and HRT improve HDL cholesterol (the best predictor of heart disease in women) and lower LDL cholesterol, but the study was not designed to detect the occurrence of cardiovascular disease.

Recent evidence from the largest randomized placebo-controlled trial, the Heart and Estrogen/Progestin Replacement Study (HERS), indicates that HRT therapy for women with CHD may be associated with cardiovascular risk as well as cardiovascular benefit.[42] In this trial over 2000 women younger than 80 with known coronary disease were randomized to either placebo or combination conjugated equine estrogen (0.625 mg) and medroxyprogesterone acetate (MPA; 2.5 mg) daily. Over an average of 4 years of follow-up, there was a lack of an overall effect on cardiovascular outcomes (relative hazard [RH], 0.99; 95 percent CI, 0.88 to 1.22), despite a beneficial effect on lipids. More women in the hormone group experienced venous thromboembolic disease (34 versus 12) and gallbladder disease (84 versus 62). There was a significant time trend, however, with more CHD events in the hormone group in the first year of therapy and fewer in years 4 and 5. It may be true that in subsequent years a beneficial effect on cardiovascular disease may be seen. The authors concluded that HRT should not be used for secondary prevention of CHD, although women with CHD who are currently taking HRT may continue.

With regard to stroke, data are inconclusive. The pooled estimate of relative risk of stroke in a meta-analysis of 15 studies was 0.96 (95 percent CI, 0.65 to 1.45) for users of estrogen compared to nonusers, suggesting no beneficial effect on stroke incidence from using estrogen.[43]

Women's Concerns about Hormone Replacement Therapy

For perimenopausal and postmenopausal women, HRT is a salient issue. At menopause (or for some women, later in life) women face the decision about whether to use HRT. Many women are unsure about the risks and benefits of therapy for themselves. The decision about using HRT is one where possible benefits from therapy must be weighed against the possible risks of therapy.

DECISION-MAKING ABOUT ERT/HRT

In deciding about HRT, women and their health care providers need to consider many factors listed in Table 4-3. In an attempt to understand this decision, Schmitt et al. studied 265 women who estimated their likelihood of taking ERT/HRT to alleviate menopausal symptoms when faced with hypothetical cases.[44] They identified four groups with respect to their approach to this decision: (1) one group ($n = 120$) for whom the predominant factor was severity of hot flashes; (2) a second group ($n = 83$), the most highly educated women, who were influenced by both vasomotor symptoms and osteoporosis risk; (3) a third group ($n = 40$) influenced both by severity of hot flashes and by concern about resumption of menses with HRT; and (4) a fourth group ($n = 9$) for whom cancer risk most influenced choice. Addressing a woman's predominant concerns may result in greater success in assisting women with this decision.

COMPLIANCE WITH THERAPY

Once HRT is prescribed, many studies indicate poor compliance with therapy. The reasons include lack of understanding of the reasons for taking hormones, fear of breast cancer, reactivation of uterine bleeding, and medication side effects.

PERCEIVED VULNERABILITY AND RISKS   In a survey of female graduates of Stanford, respondents indicated a much greater concern about breast cancer than about heart disease, with 65 percent rating the risk of breast cancer as the most important concern compared to 27 percent rating the benefit on heart disease to be most important. In general, women perceived their risk of heart disease as low (73 percent rated risk of developing heart disease by age 70 as < 1 percent) and their risk of breast cancer high (52 percent perceived risk of developing breast cancer by age 70 as > 10 percent).[45] Although more accurate information on actual risk may be useful to women considering HRT, women are likely indicating value judgments and personal preferences, which may more strongly inform treatment choices than population prevalence rates and risks.

SIDE EFFECTS EXPERIENCED   Side effects from HRT are common. About one-third of women who take ERT/HRT experience troublesome side effects that may result in discontinuing therapy. Women

Table 4-3

Factors Relevant to Decision-Making about ERT/HRT

- Current symptoms: type and severity (how bothersome)
  Hot flashes and night sweats
  Difficulty falling asleep
  Decreased sexual interest
  Vaginal dryness

- Personal risk factors* for disease
  Coronary heart disease: hypertension; diabetes mellitus; obesity; high cholesterol, low-density
    lipoprotein, or triglycerides; smoking; sedentary; left ventricular hypertrophy; family history
  Osteoporosis: mother's history of hip, wrist, or spine fracture; hyperthyroid; thin; smoking;
    chronic/prolonged steroid use; white or oriental race; sedentary; low calcium diet; low bone
    mineral density
  Breast cancer: older age; family history in first-degree relative; diagnosed breast, uterine, or ovarian
    cancer; early menarche; late menopause; no pregnancies or first pregnancy after age 30

- Feelings about preventive care
  Interest in risk minimizing
  Interest in health promotion

- Attitudes about interfering with the natural process of menopause
  Desire for natural approaches
  Desire for alternative/complementary therapy

- Ability to take medication and tolerate potential side effects
  Commitment to chronic therapy
  Previous experience with hormones
  Concern about potential side effects
    Adverse health effects (breast cancer, thrombosis)
    Vaginal bleeding
    Breast tenderness
    Weight gain, bloating

*Risk factors listed add to the woman's risk of disease.

should be counseled about side effects that are likely to occur and what measures can be used to alleviate or minimize them. Side effects from therapy were the major reason for discontinuing therapy for 16 percent of past users of HRT.[46]

Between 30 and 80 percent of women who stop HRT do so because of vaginal bleeding; a reactivation of bleeding and irregular bleeding patterns may be the least tolerated of hormone side effects. About 85 percent of women who receive sequential regimens (intermittent progestin; see Selection of a Regimen) will experience withdrawal bleeding toward the end of or immediately after the progestin phase and most will continue a monthly withdrawal bleeding pattern. It is estimated that about 3 percent of younger women and 40 percent of women over the age of 65 develop amenorrhea on sequential therapy.

Forty percent of women on continuous regimens will bleed irregularly during the first 4 to 6 months of therapy. After this time, 62 to 100 percent of women become amenorrheic and most (90 percent) will continue to have amenorrhea for the subsequent 12 months (few studies continue beyond this time period). The exact number is difficult to predict because of high drop-out rates (up to 65 percent) in these studies. Amenorrhea is more common if a woman is at least 12 months beyond menopause before starting on a continuous regimen.

Acknowledging the possibility of side effects and offering strategies for managing them should they be encountered (as outlined in the section on Management of the Side Effects of HRT) will likely improve compliance. Greater attention to a woman's desire for a natural progression through menopause and a better understanding of her perceptions of risk, vulnerability, and values will likely improve both treatment choices as well as compliance.

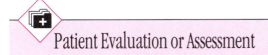

Patient Evaluation or Assessment

Diagnosis of Menopause

The diagnosis of menopause is a retrospective event diagnosed after 1 year of amenorrhea. However, certain tests can determine if menopause has been reached. After several months of amenorrhea, measurement of the FSH level can be done. FSH levels above 30 to 40 mIU/mL indicate that menopause has likely occurred; monthly fluctuations in FSH levels may occur during the perimenopause. If a woman is using an oral contraceptive, FSH levels should be taken at the end of the week off active pills. Another option for a woman who has experienced several months of amenorrhea is the progestin challenge test. A progestin, typically MPA (Provera), is administered for 10 days. If bleeding occurs after the progestin is discontinued, the

woman is not menopausal; conversely if no bleeding occurs, she has reached menopause. For women who have not reached menopause but who are also not having menses, progestin therapy should be continued monthly for 10 days to ensure shedding of the endometrial lining and protection against endometrial hyperplasia.

HISTORY

The medical history should address menopause-related symptoms including alterations of the menstrual cycle (e.g., length of cycles, bleeding patterns), vasomotor and related symptoms (e.g., hot flashes/hot flushes, night sweats, sleep disturbances), sexual functioning (e.g., changes in sexual activity or libido, vaginal dryness, irritation, or dyspareunia), urinary tract symptoms (e.g., dysuria, urinary frequency, incontinence), and psychological and cognitive symptoms (e.g., irritability, emotional lability, depression, forgetfulness). In addition, relevant family history (e.g., mother's menopause experience, risk factors for osteoporosis, heart disease, and cancer) should be obtained. Information can also be elicited about health behaviors that may modify the woman's risk for certain menopause-related medical conditions (e.g., exercise, tobacco use, ethanol consumption, dietary fat and cholesterol intake, calcium ingestion). For perimenopausal women, contraceptive needs should be assessed (see Chap. 2).

PHYSICAL EXAMINATION

The purpose of the physical examination is twofold: first, to detect menopausal changes (e.g., vaginal atrophy) and second, to help ascertain what benefits or risks may accrue from use of postmenopausal hormones (e.g., decrease in height may indicate vertebral fracture and osteoporosis). The second purpose will be addressed later.

Physical examination findings that suggest menopause are primarily atrophic changes in the breast and genitourinary system.[47] Breast changes, in response to the decline in ovarian hormones, include shrinkage of glands, increases in fat, and weakening of fibrous tissues. These changes reduce firmness and support, causing the breasts to sag. Aging causes the bladder to be smaller, with an increase in fibrous material in the bladder wall reducing the ability of the bladder to stretch and contract. These changes necessitate more frequent emptying. In addition, the urethra becomes thinner and more susceptible to injury. Thinning of the skeletal muscle causes weakening of the external urinary sphincter, reducing control of urination. These changes are greater in women and seem to result from the decrease in estrogen after menopause.

Shrinkage of the labia majora causes the labia to remain separated more of the time, allowing microbes to enter the vagina more easily. This increases the risk of vaginal infections. Atrophic vaginal changes that may be seen include partial loss of rugal folds, pain or bleeding during the speculum examination from mucosal tears, and increased vaginal pH. After menopause, the uterus is smaller (decreases in size by 50 percent within 15 years after menopause) and the ovaries are generally too small to be palpable.

Skin changes of redistribution of fat deposits and loss of elastic tissue with wrinkling, as well as reduced muscular strength, are likely due to aging and not reduced estrogen levels. However, women who are current estrogen users do not demonstrate a change in muscular strength, as measured by handgrip.[48]

LABORATORY TESTS

No routine tests are done to diagnose menopause (see above). Additional tests (e.g., lipid profile, BMD measurement) may be performed to evaluate common menopause-related symptoms or to assess patient factors relevant to the decision about whether to use postmenopausal hormones (see section below).

For women who complain about vaginal irritation or dryness, a wet prep should be performed to search for evidence of vaginitis (e.g., white blood cells, yeast, clue cells; see Chap. 11). For women with urinary symptoms (e.g., dysuria, frequency), a urinalysis will assist in diagnosis of a UTI.

Evaluation of Common Menopause-Related Symptoms

VASOMOTOR SYMPTOMS

There is considerable discrepancy in the numbers of women who report difficulty with hot flashes. This is due both to the location of the women who were surveyed (highest rates reported in specialty and general medical or family practice clinics [80 to 95 percent] and lowest in general population samples [34 percent]) and the ethnicity of the sample (lowest rates among Asian women [10 to 12 percent]). Because this symptom is common and troublesome in clinic populations of women, questions about hot flushes, their frequency and severity, should be asked at annual examinations of women from about age 45 to 55. This can lead into a discussion of menopause and provides an opportunity to address the therapeutic options available for both prevention and, depending on an individual woman's illness history and risk factors, treatment.

Questions about sleep disturbance are also important in judging not only the severity of the vasomotor symptoms, but the likelihood of other symptoms (such as mood disturbance), which are more common among women who are sleep deprived.

DYSFUNCTIONAL UTERINE BLEEDING

Menstrual abnormalities appear to be common and increase during the perimenopausal period (see Chap. 13). Irregularly timed cycles (shorter or longer) during the perimenopause do not often require a diagnostic workup and may be attributed to fluctuating hormone levels and managed as discussed below. For women who report heavy or frequent menses, a hemoglobin or hematocrit should be obtained to assess the presence and degree of anemia and need for intervention to control bleeding. When bleeding is irregular (frequent intermenstrual spotting or no discernible pattern to the bleeding), consideration should be given to the diagnosis of intrauterine or ectopic pregnancy. An endometrial biopsy may also be considered to assess the endometrial lining for hyperplasia or signs of cancer.

SEXUAL CONCERNS

Sexual concerns are not common presenting complaints among perimenopausal or postmenopausal women. However, because sexual concerns are pervasive and may not be brought to the attention of the provider, routine questions should be asked. Questions such as "Are you currently sexually active?" or "Do you or your partner have any sexual concerns or questions?" can initiate conversation and provide an opportunity to educate and inform women of options if problems are identified. At the time of an annual physical examination, specific questions about pain with sexual play or intercourse ("Do you have any pain with sex?"), changes in sex drive, vaginal lubrication, or orgasm can reveal additional concerns among women who may be reluctant to report these symptoms (see Chap. 5).

Assessment of Patient Factors Relevant to HRT Decision

In assessing the risks and benefits of ERT/HRT for the individual woman, several aspects of the history, physical examination, and laboratory test results are important (Table 4-4).

HISTORY

CANCER RISK   Cancer risk is perhaps the most concerning feature of prescribing ERT/HRT. A case-control study of women who developed breast cancer during HRT, however, is reassuring in that investigators found fewer locally advanced and more well-differentiated cancers in these women.[49] Theoretically, breast cancers that are

hormone-receptor-negative and presumably unresponsive to estrogen should not be considered contraindications to HRT. The question remains as to whether women, after removal of estrogen-receptor-positive tumors of the breast, will undergo progression of disease with HRT. The answer, at present, is unknown. If HRT is initiated, and breast cancer recurs, withdrawal from HRT has been shown in some cases to result in a temporary regression of metastatic disease.[50] The use of ERT/HRT for women with other types of cancer does not appear to be an added risk.

HYPERTENSION AND HEART DISEASE   Although the use of oral contraceptives typically results in a small rise in blood pressure, the use of estrogen for postmenopausal replacement therapy almost never raises blood pressure.[51] In addition, because the presence of hypertension increases the risk of cardiovascular disease, ERT/HRT may be even more important to consider in women with hypertension or other risk factors for heart disease, based on epidemiologic data showing a 50 percent decreased risk in heart disease among women on hormone therapy.

Investigators from the HERS trial found that HRT therapy for women with CHD was associated with an increase in venous thromboembolic disease and more CHD events in the hormone group than in the placebo group in year 1.[42] Although there were fewer CHD events in years 4 and 5, there was a lack of an overall effect on cardiovascular outcomes (RH, 0.99; 95 percent CI, 0.88 to 1.22), despite a beneficial effect on lipids. Women with CHD must weigh the increased risks in the first year of therapy with the potential benefits before making a decision about HRT use.

LIVER AND GALLBLADDER DISEASE   Estrogen is metabolized by the liver, and oral estrogen produces a pronounced hepatic response that alters bile composition and appears to lower the cholesterol saturation index.[52] For women with existing gallstones, estrogen administered by the transdermal route should be considered. Estrogen administered to

Table 4-4

Pretreatment Assessment for Hormone Replacement Therapy

PARAMETER	CONSIDERATION
HISTORY	
Cancer (breast, endometrium)*	Uncertain risk of worsening or recurrence of cancer
Cholelithiasis	Estrogen increases the risk of gallstones
Diabetes mellitus	Estrogen may slow progression of atherosclerosis
Hypertension	Estrogen in OCs raises blood pressure
Hyperlipidemia	Estrogen may precipitate pancreatitis
Ischemic heart disease	HRT increases risk of mortality (first year of therapy); benefit (lower risk of MI) may accrue after several years of therapy
Liver disease	Estrogen is metabolized by the liver, levels increase
Migraine headache	Possible increase in headache
Reactive airway disease	Potential exacerbation of disease
Smoking	Earlier menopause, predisposes to OP and CHD
Thrombosis (DVT/PE)	Estrogen predisposes to clotting
Vaginal bleeding[†]	If undiagnosed, may represent endometrial CA
FAMILY HISTORY	
Breast cancer	Estrogen increases risk of breast cancer*
Heart disease	Estrogen may decrease risk of heart disease
Osteoporosis	Estrogen decreases risk of bone loss
PHYSICAL EXAMINATION	
Height and weight	Obesity predisposes to endometrial/breast CA
Blood pressure	Theoretically, ERT/HRT may raise blood pressure
Breast examination	Estrogen may stimulate the growth of breast CA
Pelvic examination	Uterine fibroids predispose to excessive bleeding
LABORATORY TESTS (OPTIONAL)	
Clotting factors	Estrogen may have unfavorable effects
Lipid profile	Preexisting hypertriglyceridemia, pancreatitis risk
Liver function tests	As above
PROCEDURES/DIAGNOSTIC IMAGING	
Endometrial biopsy	ERT or continuous HRT may not prevent hyperplasia
Bone densitometry	This may be a deciding factor in initiating HRT
Mammography	May identify undetected breast cancer

*Considered contraindications to HRT.

[†]Data primarily for ERT.

ABBREVIATIONS: CA, cancer; DVT, deep vein thrombosis; CHD, coronary heart disease; MI, myocardial infarction; OCs, oral contraceptives; OP, osteoporosis; PE, pulmonary embolism.

women with active liver disease may result in increased circulating estrogen causing profound vasodilation. Caution should be exercised when considering ERT/HRT for these women.

MIGRAINE HEADACHE Migraine headache has been considered a relative contraindication to HRT because estrogens participate in the regulation of cerebral vasomotor tone and have been found to trigger or increase these headaches in about 3 percent of women initiating ERT.[53] Although migraines have been implicated in stroke, this association does not appear to be valid and ERT/HRT may be considered on an individual basis for these women. Because estrogen withdrawal can trigger migraine, continuous estrogen treatment is recommended. It may also be prudent to wait 4 to 12 weeks before initiating a progestin.[52]

REACTIVE AIRWAY DISEASE Reactive airway disease (asthma) may be another relative contraindication for prescribing HRT. Although exacerbation of bronchospasm during the luteal phase of the menstrual cycle is well known, exacerbation of reactive airway disease with the administration of exogenous estrogen had not previously been reported. A recent report of ERT use among postmenopausal women with mild to moderate asthma, however, found a subclinical worsening of disease activity as measured by peak expiratory flow and use of inhalers.[54] In this study, general feeling of well-being did not change during ERT.

SMOKING In addition to the known adverse health effects of smoking on lipids, coagulation factors, and the risk of ischemic heart disease and osteoporosis, smoking tobacco alters the metabolism and lowers the serum concentration of estrogen. Because of this, women who smoke, despite being in greater need of the preventive aspects of ERT/HRT, may not receive the same benefit as women who do not smoke. Smokers also have an earlier onset of menopause. These facts may provide additional motivation for women to stop smoking.

THROMBOEMBOLIC DISEASE The safety of ERT/HRT for women with previous thromboembolic dis-

ease is uncertain. The International Consensus Conference concluded that postmenopausal ERT does not increase the risk for thrombosis and, in low doses, ERT is not contraindicated in most women with a prior history of thrombosis or for women with collagen vascular diseases, such as lupus erythematosus.[55,56] They also concluded that ERT does not have to be stopped before surgery. However, some evidence indicates that high-dose estrogen may be thrombogenic in doses of 1.25 mg or more of conjugated equine estrogen (CEE),[39] and the results of the HERS trial (as noted above) raises further concerns about venous thromboembolic complications for women with CHD.[42]

ADDITIONAL FACTORS Additional factors of importance include a family or personal history of heart disease or osteoporosis as well as conditions such as hyperlipidemia or diabetes mellitus, which predispose a woman to accelerated ischemic heart disease. Inquiry into life-style factors is also important. Although preventive strategies in this area are covered elsewhere in this book, specific attention to dietary calcium, fat content, and food sources rich in phytoestrogens (soybeans, legumes) as well as exercise and smoking, may influence the perceived need for preventive treatment with HRT.

PHYSICAL EXAMINATION

Physical examination factors of importance in the decision to begin ERT/HRT include the height and weight, blood pressure, breast examination, and pelvic examination. Loss of height or thoracic kyphosis are indicators of osteoporosis. Blood pressure elevation may indicate hypertension, a risk factor for CHD and cerebrovascular disease, and one that may require caution or more intensive monitoring of blood pressure if ERT/HRT is selected.

A clinical breast examination also provides an opportunity to review breast self-examination and encourage women to perform these checks monthly. Pelvic examination is performed both for cancer screening (cervical/ovarian) and for the presence of an enlarged uterus that may indicate the presence of myomas. The latter may predispose women to excessive or irregular bleeding on HRT.

LABORATORY TESTING

LIPIDS   If not previously assessed, a lipid profile should be considered before the prescription of ERT/HRT. In women with severe hypertriglyceridemia, the precipitation of pancreatitis has been reported with ERT.[57] The use of medications known to alter lipid profiles, such as noncardioselective beta blockers and thiazide diuretics, might also prompt this test. In circumstances where liver disease is suspected, liver function tests should be obtained.

DIAGNOSTIC PROCEDURES

Routine screening for breast (clinical breast examination and/or mammography) and cervical cancer are encouraged before initiating ERT/HRT. Although the rationale for the former is clear, the recommendation for the latter, particularly if HRT is selected, is not justified beyond the prevention guidelines for cervical cancer screening in the general population. After age 65, the practice of regular Pap smears may be discontinued (see Chap. 1). HRT is not contraindicated for women with cervical, epithelial, ovarian, vulvar, or vaginal carcinomas.[58]

ENDOMETRIAL BIOPSY   The question of pretreatment endometrial biopsy is also controversial. There is good consensus that for women selecting cyclic HRT, pretreatment biopsy is unwarranted because the prevalence of hyperplasia in otherwise healthy postmenopausal women is small and this form of therapy (with 12 days of progestin) has been shown to reverse preexisting hyperplasia in 98 to 99 percent of cases.[67]

Among women selecting continuous treatment, some authors do recommend pretreatment biopsy because endometrial hyperplasia may persist and there appears to be a poor correlation between endometrial histology and bleeding pattern (i.e., the presence of amennorhea does not exclude endometrial pathology). Some authors suggest use of a progestin challenge test (12- to 13-day course of MPA [Provera] 10 mg/d or norethindrone [Norlutin] 2.5 to 5 mg/d) for all menopausal women being considered for ERT/HRT to identify the presence of estrogen-primed endometrium, reserving biopsy for women who have withdrawal bleeding.

For women selecting ERT who have not had a hysterectomy/oophrectomy, a pretreatment biopsy and yearly biopsies thereafter have been suggested because the risk of endometrial cancer on this regimen increases fourfold. As will be discussed below, a diagnostic endometrial biopsy (or vaginal sonography) should be performed with any heavy, irregular, or mistimed (deviation from usual pattern) bleeding after hormone replacement is initiated.

BONE MINERAL DENSITY   The need for and usefulness of measurements of bone density at menopause is a subject of debate. The authors of a recent overview on BMD measurement suggested its use, using dual-energy x-ray absorptiometry, in two situations: (1) when a woman's decision to begin HRT rests on her risk for osteoporosis and (2) for purposes of follow-up, perhaps to increase medication compliance.[59] Women at highest risk of osteoporosis are those with low baseline bone density and those experiencing high rates of bone loss, perhaps up to 30 percent of women[60] (see Chap. 20).

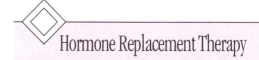

Hormone Replacement Therapy

The benefits of HRT are derived from the estrogen component. Estrogen relieves menopausal symptoms, maintains bone mass, and decreases the risk of cardiovascular disease. The purpose of the progestin component, for women with a uterus, is protection against endometrial cancer.

A progestin is unnecessary if a woman has had a hysterectomy.

Contraindications and Adverse Effects of Postmenopausal Hormones

CONTRAINDICATIONS

Not all women are candidates for HRT. Absolute contraindications to postmenopausal estrogen therapy are listed in Table 4-5. Prior complications from estrogen therapy, typically oral contraceptive use (e.g., cholestatic jaundice, migraine headache), are additional contraindications. In addition, there are other clinical situations (relative contraindications) where the risk of therapy might outweigh potential benefits. Estrogen should be used with caution in women with active endometriosis and uterine leiomyomata

Table 4-5

Contraindications to Postmenopausal Estrogen Therapy

- Absolute contraindications
  Presence of estrogen-related cancers
     (uterine, breast)
  Undiagnosed abnormal vaginal bleeding
  Active liver disease or chronic severe liver
     dysfunction
  Active thrombophlebitis or
     thromboembolic disorder
  Prior complications from estrogen therapy

- Relative contraindications
  Risk for thromboembolic disease
  History of gallstones
  Presence of conditions aggravated by fluid
     retention (e.g., congestive heart failure,
     seizure disorders, asthma)
  Active endometriosis
  Uterine leiomyomata (fibroid tumors)
  Acute intermittent porphyria
  Previous (treated) breast cancer

(estrogen use inhibits postmenopausal involution of these conditions) and acute intermittent porphyria (estrogen may cause attacks).

Hormone replacement therapy has generally been avoided in women with a history of breast cancer, but an assessment of the effect of estrogen exposure (e.g., pregnancy, oral contraceptive use, HRT use) on prognosis showed that estrogen exposure did not confer a worse prognosis.[61] The American College of Obstetricians and Gynecologists' Committee on Gynecologic Practice and the Eastern Cooperative Oncology Group have both examined this issue and suggested that for some women previously treated for breast cancer the use of postmenopausal estrogen may be appropriate.[62,63] These might be women with estrogen-receptor-negative tumors or women with extremely severe menopausal symptoms.

CANCER

The major limitation to use of postmenopausal hormones is the increased risk of cancer. Cancers known to be associated with use of postmenopausal estrogen are endometrial, ovarian, and breast cancer.

ENDOMETRIAL CANCER   Endometrial cancer is the third most common cancer in women in the United States. ERT substantially increases the risk for development of endometrial cancer. The pooled estimate of relative risk for endometrial cancer among ever-users of ERT, derived from 35 studies, was 2.31 (95 percent CI, 2.13 to 2.51).[64] All dosages of estrogen are associated with an increased risk, and risk increases with increasing dosage and duration of use. The relative risk for women who used estrogen for 10 years or longer was 9.5 (95 percent CI, 7.4 to 12.3). The risk of endometrial cancer also persists for 5 years or more after discontinuation of estrogen therapy.[65]

Progestins were added to ERT in the late 1970s after published reports of an increased risk of endometrial hyperplasia and carcinoma with use of ERT alone. Gambrell et al. were among the first to demonstrate the endometrial protective effect of adding a progestin.[66] This group and others found that the addition of progestin for 12 days to ERT lowered the rates of endometrial hyperplasia from more than 20 percent among users of ERT to less than 1 percent among users of HRT, with a concomitant rate reduction of endometrial cancer from 248/100,000 found in the general population to about 56/100,000.

Studies investigating shorter durations of progestin administration have failed to demonstrate complete reversal of estrogen-induced endometrial hyperplasia; when progestin duration was 7 days per month, hyperplastic endometrium was reversed to normal in 80.6 percent of patients.[67] Even 10 days of progestin therapy each month reversed hyperplasia in 98.4 percent of women compared with 100 percent reversal when the duration was increased to 13 days.

OVARIAN CANCER   The association between estrogen use and ovarian cancer is less clear. Of 10 case-control studies in the United States, none showed a significant association between estrogen use and ovarian cancer.[68] A recent meta-analysis, however, including 11 articles representing 12 analyses of 21 individual studies, found an increased risk of developing epithelial ovarian carcinoma with ever-use of HRT (OR 1.15; 95 percent CI 1.05 to 1.27).[69] The greatest risk was found among women taking HRT for more than 10 years (OR 1.27; 95 percent CI 1.00 to 1.61).

BREAST CANCER   Breast cancer is the most common cancer in women; a 50-year-old white woman has a 10 percent chance, and a 50-year-old black woman a 7 percent chance, of developing breast cancer during the remainder of her life. Women who have a mother or sister who developed breast cancer have an increased risk (about a 20 percent risk) of developing this cancer. Prolonged exposure to endogenous estrogen (early menarche, late menopause, nulliparity) is associated with an increased risk for breast cancer. The median age for breast cancer diagnosis is 69 years.[70]

One of the most significant questions regarding postmenopausal HRT is its possible association with breast cancer. Early data from individual studies and several meta-analyses indicated that ERT did little to increase the risk for breast cancer.[68,71] However, these studies were limited by their inability to address the risk of long-term therapy and the differential in risk for ever-users compared with current users.

Currently, the consensus opinion appears to suggest: (1) less than 5 years of use is associated with little increase in risk; (2) with a longer duration of use (e.g., 10 to 15 years or more) the risk is increased by 30 to 50 percent; (3) previous use seems to cause little increased risk, after therapy is discontinued for several (or up to 5) years; (4) older women, women who had a late menopause, and women with a previous history of breast cancer are at highest risk; and (5) doses greater than 1.25 mg conjugated equine estrogen (CEE) are associated with a higher risk than are lower doses (e.g., 0.3 to 1.25 mg CEE).[61,68,71,72]

The effect of the addition of progestin (i.e., HRT) on the risk of breast cancer is still controversial. Although some studies report a protective[73] or no effect on breast cancer risk,[74] others report a deleterious one.[75] Endogenous progesterone appears to act synergistically with estrogen on breast mitotic activity, which peaks when the progesterone level is highest. High doses of oral synthetic progestins have been used effectively in the treatment of breast cancer but little can be implied about the lower doses used in HRT. Long-term studies of HRT are clearly needed.

COMMON SIDE EFFECTS OF POSTMENOPAUSAL HORMONES

Side effects, often termed nuisance effects, of ERT and HRT are not a trivial matter for patients. Information on rates of individual side effects is difficult to find and primarily comes from older studies. In the Scottish study noted above, side effects were reported in 38 percent of the 101 current and previous users of hormones and included weight gain, nausea, depression, headache, and breast tenderness (regardless of hormone preparation).[76] In the PEPI trial, 210 women (24 percent) stopped their treatment prematurely; 60 percent because of symptoms including vaginal bleeding ($n = 25$), premenstrual-like symptoms ($n = 17$), vasomotor symptoms ($n = 11$), headaches ($n = 10$), anxiety-depression ($n = 10$), and breast tenderness ($n = 7$).[41] Twenty-four percent mandated a discontinuation of therapy by protocol (most due to endometrial abnormalities).

BREAST SYMPTOMS   One study reported that 9 of 31 women (27 percent) taking hormones (but no control subjects) had mammographic evidence of increased breast density and 7 of these women had moderate or severe breast pain after treatment.[77] A paradoxical improvement in breast pain has also been reported after initiation of HRT for women with frequent breast tenderness at baseline.[78] It seems reasonable that women should be counseled about the likelihood of some breast tenderness (13 to 32 percent) but that those with current breast tenderness may actually note some improvement.

PREMENSTRUAL SYMPTOMS   Premenstrual-type symptoms of bloating, headache, irritability, and fluid retention were reported by one author to be the most common side effects of HRT. The progestational side effects of mood alterations and bloating are thought to occur in about 15 percent of women. The issue of weight gain could not be substantiated from the literature reviewed; a prospective study, however, showed no increase over a 2-year period in central body fat among estrogen users compared to an increase among women in the matched control group.[79]

VAGINAL BLEEDING   Women who have not undergone hysterectomy should also be advised that they may experience more difficulty with bleeding than they would if they declined HRT. In a study of cyclic HRT, the incidence of abnormal vaginal bleeding necessitating gynecologic procedures for evaluation was significantly higher (RR, 3.1; 95 percent CI, 2.1 to 4.5), as was the rate of endometrial biopsy (RR, 3.4; 95 percent CI, 2.3 to 5.1) and possibly dilation and curettage (RR, 1.5; CI, 0.7 to 3.3) among women receiving HRT than among women not receiving HRT.[80]

Regular bleeding at the time of progesterone withdrawal should be expected with cyclic HRT, although 3 percent of younger women and 40 percent of women over the age of 65 develop amenorrhea. The number of women with regular bleeding, however, may be overestimated. Based on information obtained from menstrual diaries of women on HRT, Al-Azzawi and Habiba (using a variability in onset of bleeding of 2 days and in duration of bleeding of 1 day) were able to predict the bleeding patterns of less than one-third of their patients on various regimens.[81]

Options in Hormone Replacement Regimens

SELECTING THE TYPE OF THERAPY

Estrogen and progestin products that are commonly prescribed are listed in Table 4-6.

ESTROGEN THERAPY   Both synthetic and natural estrogens are available. Although synthetic estrogens (e.g., ethinyl estradiol) are most commonly used in oral contraceptives, the natural estrogens (e.g., conjugated equine estrogen, 17-β-estradiol) are preferred for estrogen replacement therapy because of their lower potency in stimulating liver proteins and fewer metabolic effects.[82] Ethinyl estradiol is estimated to be 1000 times as potent in stimulating liver proteins as CEE.

The estrogen with the strongest receptor affinity at the cellular level is estradiol. Transdermal estrogen (17-β-estradiol) produces the most physiologic ratio of estradiol to estrone; oral CEE results in higher estrone levels than estradiol levels. Therefore, with transdermal estrogen, total estrogen levels are lower when products are dosed to provide similar estradiol levels.[82] The clinical implications of these differences are unclear.

Premenopausally, the average minimal estradiol serum level is 40 pg/mL (25 to 75 pg/mL)

Table 4-6

Estrogens and Progestins Commonly Prescribed for Hormone Replacement Therapy

ESTROGENS	TRADE NAME	DOSAGE FORM	DOSES AVAILABLE	COMMON HRT DOSES
ESTRONES				
Conjugated estrogen	Premarin	Oral	0.3, 0.625, 0.9, 1.25, 2.5 mg	0.625 mg used most commonly 1.25 mg used for tobacco smokers, women on enzyme-stimulating drugs, or women who continue to lose bone density or experience menopause symptoms on lower doses 0.3 mg used for women who cannot tolerate higher dose
		Vaginal cream	0.0625% (0.625 mg/g)	Initial dose is 1/2–1 applicatorful once daily (2–4 g) Generally used short-term
Esterified estrogens	Estratab, Menest Ogen, Ortho-est, generic	Oral	0.3, 0.625, 1.25, 2.5 mg	Usual dose 0.3–1.25 mg daily
Estropipate		Oral	0.625, 1.25, 2.5, 5 mg	Usual dose is 0.625–1.25 mg daily
		Vaginal cream	0.15% (1.5 mg/g)	Initial dose is 1/2–1 applicatorful once daily (2–4 g)
ESTRADIOLS				
Estradiol	Estring	Vaginal ring	releases 7.5 µg/24 h over a 90-d period	One device is used for a 90-d period Symptomatic improvement seen in 3–12 wk
(micronized)	Estrace	Oral	1, 2 mg	Usual dose is 0.5–1 mg; 2 mg used for severe symptoms
		Vaginal cream	0.01% (0.1 mg/g)	Initial dose is 1/2–1 applicatorful once daily (2–4 g)
(17-β-estradiol)	Estraderm, Climara Vivelle	Transdermal	0.05, 0.1 mg/24 h 0.0375, 0.05, 0.075, 0.1 mg/24 h	Initial dose, 0.05 mg then titrate to response
Ethinyl estradiol	Estinyl, Feminone	Oral	0.02, 0.05 mg	Usual dose is 0.02–0.05 mg daily
NONSTEROIDAL ESTROGEN				
Dienestrol	Ortho-Dienestrol	Vaginal cream	0.01% (0.1 mg/g)	Initial dose is 1–2 applicatorsful (6–12 g) once daily, then reduce dose by 1/2 after 1–2 wk; after 2–4 wk switch to 1–3 time per week use.

PROGESTINS	TRADE NAME	DOSES AVAILABLE	COMMON HRT DOSES
Micronized progesterone 17-hydroxyprogesterone derivative	Prometrium	100 mg	200–300 mg daily
Medroxyprogesterone acetate	Provera, generic	2.5, 5, 10 mg	2.5, 5, 10 mg
Nortestosterone derivative			
Norethindrone	Micronor, Norlutin	5 mg	2.5 mg
Norgestrel	Ovrette	0.075 mg	0.15 mg
COMBINED ESTROGENS AND PROGESTINS			
Conjugated estrogen plus medroxyprogesterone acetate	Prempro (each tablet)	0.625 mg conjugated estrogen plus 2.5–5 mg medroxyprogesterone acetate	One daily
	Premphase	0.625 mg conjugated estrogen (days 1–28) plus 5 mg medroxyprogesterone acetate (days 15–28)	One daily
17-β-estradiol plus norethindrone acetate	Combipatch	0.050 mg estradiol plus 0.14 mg norethindrone acetate	Apply twice weekly

and, during the luteal phase, estradiol levels are about 100 pg/mL. These normal physiologic levels of estradiol can be used to guide the selection of estrogen doses for ERT.[82,83] A serum concentration of 40 to 60 pg/mL is the goal of therapy. A dose of 0.625 mg CEE, 50-μg transdermal estradiol, and a vaginal dose of 1.25 mg CEE result in serum estradiol levels within this range (see Table 4-6).[83,84]

Initial Dose.   The ability of estrogen to relieve menopausal symptoms and to maintain bone density depends on achieving an adequate serum concentration. The estradiol level achieved by a dose of 0.625 mg CEE is able to relieve menopausal symptoms in the majority of patients and is the lowest dose that is adequate to prevent osteoporosis in 90 percent of patients. This is also the dose commonly used by studies in which a cardiovascular benefit was demonstrated for women taking estrogen. Therefore, it is recommended that estrogen therapy be initiated with a daily dose of 0.625 mg CEE or an equivalent, if therapy is begun, to relieve menopausal symptoms or to prevent heart disease or osteoporosis.[85] The treatment of symptoms associated with urogenital atrophy can generally be accomplished with topical therapy administered only twice a week; however, topical therapy should be initiated with 3 to 4 weeks of daily administration.[86] Reevaluation of the dose should be done only after 3 months of therapy because it takes this long for the maximum effect to occur.

Persistent Symptoms.   If menopausal symptoms continue, the estrogen dose can be increased to 0.9 to 1.25 mg CEE. Higher doses of estrogen are rarely required to manage menopausal symptoms. However, higher estrogen doses (e.g., 1.25 mg CEE) might be needed to relieve symptoms in women just after surgical menopause or to treat a woman with osteoporosis-related fractures. If higher doses are initially required for relief of menopausal symptoms, the estrogen dose can often be decreased after 1 to 2 years of therapy.[87]

Discontinuing Therapy.   If therapy is begun solely to treat menopausal symptoms, it can be discontinued after several years when symptoms decrease. Tapering off of estrogen therapy, rather than abrupt discontinuation, is recommended to avoid provoking symptoms from a sudden decrease in estrogen levels.[88]

Dosage Forms.   Estrogen is usually administered orally or transdermally. In general, oral therapy is preferred because this dosage form has favorable effects on lipid levels.[85] There is controversy about whether the transdermal preparations will have the same cardioprotective effect as has been demonstrated for oral therapy.[82] However, transdermal therapy may be more appropriate for certain subgroups of patients.[89] Transdermal estrogen avoids the "first-pass effect" of liver metabolism and serum levels are more consistent. This may be useful for patients who notice estrogenic side effects at times of peak serum concentrations or menopausal symptoms when trough serum concentrations occur. However, some patients using the transdermal patch may notice an increase in vasomotor symptoms at the end of the dosing interval for the patch as estradiol levels begin to decline.[83] Similarly, because tobacco stimulates liver metabolism, it has been suggested that tobacco smokers may benefit from transdermal delivery of estrogen.[89]

Exposure of the liver to oral estrogen may cause greater effects on clotting factors, rennin substrate, and lipids.[83] Patients with a history of thromboembolism, migraine headaches, isolated hypertriglyceridemia, or gallbladder stones may be better candidates for transdermal therapy, whereas women with elevated cholesterol levels should receive oral therapy. It has also been suggested that transdermal therapy, because it provides lower serum levels of estrone, may be less likely to promote cystic breast changes.[89]

PROGESTIN THERAPY   Progestins are categorized into three types by the parent chemical compound—progesterone derivatives (e.g., micronized progesterone), 17-hydroxyprogesterone derivatives (e.g., MPA), and 19-nortestosterone derivatives (e.g., norethindrone, norgestrel) (see Table 4-6). Micronized progesterone is a natural progesterone but because of a large interpatient variability in absorption and metabolism, the synthetic progestins are more widely used in the United States.[83] MPA has properties similar to natural progesterone and a lesser potential for adverse lipid effects and androgenic side effects than the 19-nortestosterone derivatives.[82,83]

Gambrell has suggested that previous menstrual symptoms might help guide selection of a progestin.[90] The 19-nortestosterone derivatives might be a better choice for women who experience dysmenorrhea or heavy menstrual bleeding because menstrual flow is generally lighter and shorter with these androgenic progestins. Conversely, if a woman had previously experienced breast symptoms, such as tenderness, or had a history of fibrocystic disease, a 17-hydroxyprogesterone derivative would be more suitable.

Progestin therapy is indicated only for women who have not had a hysterectomy and need endometrial protection.[85] The protective effect of sequential HRT (various doses of progestin and lengths of progestin therapy) on the endometrium has recently been questioned. In a study of 413 women using sequential HRT for more than 6 months (mean duration 2.7 years), endometrial biopsies were performed before initiating continuous HRT.[91] Most women had bleeding starting around day 13 after starting the progestin. There was no correlation between endometrial histology and the time of onset of bleeding. Complex hyperplasia was found in 2.7 percent of women. The authors believe that while preexisting cystic and adenomatous hyperplasia has been found to revert to normal under the influence of progestins, patients who progress to complex or atypical hyperplasia may not revert to normal. Consequently it would be expected that 3 to 4 percent of these cases would progress to malignancy over the subsequent 13 years compared to a rate of endometrial cancer of about 5 percent among untreated postmenopausal women.

There are no cases of endometrial cancer reported among women using sequential HRT with 12 to 14 days of either MPA 10 mg or norethindrone 5 mg added monthly.[67]

SELECTION OF A REGIMEN

Patients who require only ERT should be provided daily dosing (oral or transdermal) without interruption.[85] Uninterrupted therapy has the advantages of avoiding estrogen deficiency symptoms, providing a continuous cardioprotective effect, and creating an easy regimen that promotes patient compliance.

If the combination of estrogen and a progestin therapy is used (HRT), one of four possible regimens might be prescribed. Selection of an HRT regimen for an individual patient can be accomplished by evaluating the potential benefits of each regimen and considering the patient's ability to tolerate both estrogen and progestins. Regimens can be either cyclic or continuous; cyclic regimens have hormone-free days (5 days) in the cycle. Regimens can also be referred to as sequential or combined, indicating whether the progestin is given intermittently (sequential) or daily with the estrogen. The estrogen component of therapy can be administered orally or via a transdermal patch. The regimens are described in detail by Gambrell and are shown in Fig. 4-1.[90]

CYCLIC SEQUENTIAL THERAPY Cyclic sequential therapy is the regimen with the longest history in the United States. This regimen provides estrogen for 25 days a month; progestin is added for the last 12 days of the month and from days 25 to 30 the patient does not receive any hormones. With this regimen, almost all women (97 percent) have withdrawal bleeding, usually light and painless, until at least age 60; after age 65 only 60 percent continue to bleed. This regimen has a low incidence of hormone-related side effects; 8 percent of patients experience side effects such as headache, irritability, depression, or lethargy compared to 14 percent of women on a continuous sequential regimen.[90] No cases

Figure 4-1

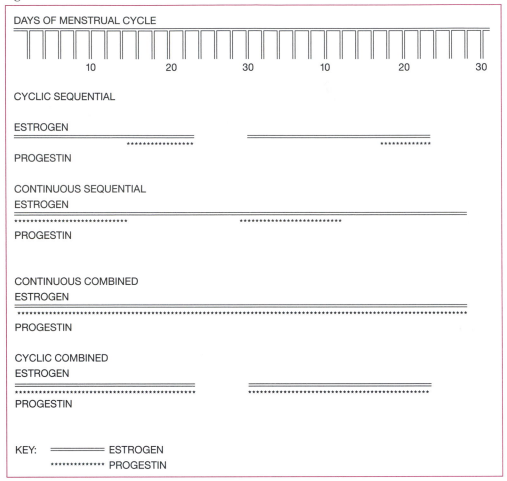

Treatment regimens for hormone replacement therapy.

of endometrial cancer have been reported using this regimen if an adequate dose (MPA 10 mg or norethindrone 5 mg) and duration (12 to 14 days) of progestin are used.[67]

CONTINUOUS SEQUENTIAL THERAPY   The continuous sequential regimen adds estrogen on the 5 days that were previously hormone free. This regimen was designed to avoid symptoms of estrogen deficiency for women who experience them on the days off estrogen. Progestins are then administered on the first 12 to 14 days of the cycle.

CONTINUOUS COMBINED THERAPY   Continuous combined therapy regimens were designed to promote amenorrhea to address one of the most common objections to HRT—continued menses. The most common continuous regimen and the one recommended by the American College of Physicians is 0.625 mg CEE daily plus MPA 2.5 mg daily.[85] During the first 4 to 6 months of this regimen, about 35 percent of women often experience unpredictable spotting and bleeding. By 6 months, however, 60 to 65 percent of women are amenorrheic.[83,90]

Unfortunately, there is a concern about the ability of this regimen to protect against endometrial cancer. Gambrell reports that he was able to identify 58 cases of endometrial cancer occurring during use of continuous combined HRT.[67]

Rosenfeld suggests that a dose of 5 mg MPA is necessary to achieve endometrial atrophy for the majority of women on a continuous combined regimen.[92] She suggests that women start on 2.5 mg MPA but, if bleeding is still present after 3 months, to increase the dose to 5 mg daily. If bleeding is present at 6 months, the dose should again be increased to 10 mg daily. This approach achieves amenorrhea in 85 to 95 percent of women by 9 months of therapy. It is not known whether this protocol will eliminate the concern about endometrial cancer.

CYCLIC COMBINED THERAPY The final type of regimen is cyclic combined. This regimen provides both estrogen and progestin for 25 days a month in the same doses used for continuous combined, but there is a 5-day hormone-free period in the cycle. The potential advantage of this regimen is greater endometrial protection, because stopping the progestin allows for shedding of the endometrium. In addition, there is less breakthrough bleeding after the first month of this regimen than is seen with the continuous combined regimen and a greater percent of women are amenorrheic by 4 months (75 percent of women on cyclic combined versus 60 to 65 percent on continuous combined at 6 months).[67] However, amenorrhea with this regimen is less common among women younger than age 55. Whether this regimen will be as endometrial protective as the cyclic sequential regimen with the higher dose progestin over 12 to 14 days is unknown.

WIDELY SPACED PROGESTIN THERAPY Another approach to reducing the side effect of bleeding with cyclic therapy is to use a progestin only every third to fourth month. The potential benefits cited for this approach are a lower annual dose of progestin, resulting in decreased progestin-type

side effects, and the avoidance of more frequent withdrawal bleeding.

The dose and duration of MPA used for these widely spaced progestin regimens is 10 to 20 mg MPA for 14 days. The withdrawal bleeding associated with these regimens is longer and heavier than that seen with more frequent dosing of progestins (5 to 8 days; heavy bleeding in 12 to 30 percent of women).[93,94] Despite this, the widely spaced regimen was preferred by 60 percent of women in one study.[93] These women preferred less frequent bleeding even if bleeding, when it occurred, was heavier and lasted longer. Unscheduled bleeding was experienced by some women and the recommended management was to shorten the time between MPA administration or to use the widely spaced regimen only for women who were menopausal for more than 3 years.[93,94] Both studies reported a low incidence of endometrial hyperplasia (1.5 to 3 percent); a rate consistent with the rate of hyperplasia seen with monthly cyclic MPA.

Unfortunately, many women are unable to avoid spotting in the interval period, and a Scandinavian study of quarterly progestin was terminated early because of a high rate of endometrial hyperplasia (6.2 percent) and one case of adenocarcinoma among study subjects.[95]

Management of Side Effects of HRT

A number of side effects are associated with the use of HRT. The management of these side effects was reviewed by Evans et al.[96] and is summarized in Table 4-7. Similar to advice with oral contraceptives nausea can be managed by taking the medication with food or at bedtime. Because nausea is attributed to initial sensitivity to estrogen, a gradual increase of dose to normal maintenance over the first 2 to 4 weeks may be useful. If nausea persists beyond the first few months, a different brand or formulation of estrogen may be better tolerated or transdermal patches may be offered.

Bloating may be managed by switching to a different progestational agent or by decreasing the

Table 4-7

Management of Common Hormone Replacement Therapy Side Effects

ADVERSE EFFECT	MANAGEMENT TECHNIQUE
Nausea	• Take medication with food or at bedtime • Gradually increase estrogen to maintenance dose • Switch to a different estrogen or different route of estrogen administration (transdermal)
Breast tenderness	• Reduce estrogen dose • Switch to transdermal estrogen • Switch to a different progestin • Use a C-21 progestin (MPA) • Limit caffeine • Add diuretic, vitamin E
Vasomotor symptoms	• Increase estrogen dose • Switch to transdermal estrogen
Heavy withdrawal bleeding	• Decrease estrogen dose • Switch to a continuous progestin dosing regimen • Use a 19-nortestosterone progestin (norethindrone or norethindrone acetate)
Headaches	• If migraine-like consider discontinuation of therapy • Switch to continuous estrogen therapy • Switch to transdermal estrogen
Bloating	• Switch to a different progestin • Lower progestin dose • Add diuretic on days of progestin or for 7–10 days before menses
Mood alterations	• Switch to a different progestin • Decrease the progestin dose • Switch to continuous progestin dosing • Add a diuretic
Decreased libido	• Add androgen to the regimen • Use of natural estrogen

SOURCE: Reproduced with permission from Evans et al.[96]

dose. A strategy of limiting progestin therapy to every 3 months can also be considered. Complaints of continued vasomotor symptoms can be managed by increasing the estrogen dose, changing to a different estrogen, or trying a different delivery system. For women who report difficulties with decreased libido, combined androgen-estrogen hormone replacement can be considered but may be associated with elevated serum testosterone, hirsutism, and virilism.

Breast tenderness may improve by using strategies of reducing the estrogen dose (by administering estrogen on a schedule of days 1 to 25 of each month or Monday through Friday) or trying a different progestin. Other avenues include limiting caffeine intake or adding a mild diuretic or daily vitamin E (200 to 400 IU/d). Underlying breast disease should be considered.

ABNORMAL BLEEDING ASSOCIATED WITH USE OF HORMONE THERAPY

ABNORMAL BLEEDING IN WOMEN WITH A UTERUS ON ERT Unpredictable uterine bleeding occurs in 35 to 40 percent of women with a uterus who are on ERT.[85] Bleeding in these women is most often due to endometrial hyperplasia (20 to 62 percent, depending on duration of therapy). Endometrial hyperplasia may progress to endometrial cancer, particularly if the type of hyperplasia identified is atypical (29 percent may progress).[97] A meta-analysis of 30 case-control and cohort studies reported a relative risk of developing endometrial cancer with unopposed estrogen therapy of 2.3 (95 percent CI 2.1 to 2.5), with a risk ratio of 9.5 with 10 or more years of use.[64] This risk remained elevated even after discontinuing unopposed estrogen. Any bleeding that occurs in a woman on ERT should be evaluated. Most authors and clinicians begin the investigation with an endometrial biopsy.

ABNORMAL BLEEDING IN WOMEN ON HRT Abnormal bleeding for women on cyclic HRT is bleeding that is either prolonged, but at the appropriate time, or that does not occur at the normal time (breakthrough bleeding). Abnormal bleeding for women on continuous regimens is bleeding that occurs after 6 months of therapy; this type of bleeding is most commonly caused by unstable or atrophic endometrium. One author suggested that evaluation for irregular bleeding should be considered if the bleeding is heavy (heavier than a normal menstrual period), prolonged (longer than 10 days at a time), or persists beyond the first 10 months of therapy.[85] Others proceed with continued bleeding after 6 months of therapy.

Although regular bleeding at the time of progesterone withdrawal is expected with cyclic HRT, the number of women with regular bleeding appears to be overestimated. Based on information obtained from menstrual diaries of women on HRT, Al-Azzawi and Habiba (using a variability in onset of bleeding of 2 days and in duration of bleeding of 1 day) were able to predict the bleeding patterns of fewer than one-third of their patients on various regimens.[81]

Causes. A recent review by Spencer et al. summarizes the current literature in this area.[98] Causes of abnormal bleeding while on HRT include problems with adherence to the HRT regimen, failure to synchronize exogenous hormone treatment with continued endogenous activity (most important for pre- and perimenopausal women who continue to cycle), gynecologic disorders (responsible for about 27 percent of cases of abnormal bleeding on HRT), and use of certain drugs (tamoxifin) or drug interactions potentially causing enhanced estrogen metabolism (e.g., griseofulvin, rifampin, phenytoin).

Investigation. Abnormal bleeding (as defined above) in women on HRT requires investigation. Common gynecologic disorders identified include (in order of prevalence) submucous fibroids, endometrial polyps, and endometrial hyperplasia; the latter uncommon in women taking progesterone for 10 or more days each month.[99] Options for investigation include endometrial biopsy, transvaginal ultrasonography, and hysteroscopy. Akkad, in an investigation using endometrial biopsy of 106 women with abnormal bleeding on HRT, found no cancers and only 1 woman with endometrial hyperlasia.[100] Twenty-four percent of these women, however, had submucous myomas and two women had endometrial polyps. These investigators concluded that hysteroscopy should be considered the optimal diagnostic approach because biopsy alone fails to detect submucous myomas, ultrasound can often not distinguish between these tumors and polyps, and hysteroscopy allows the entire surface of the endometrium to be visualized.

Spencer et al., in their review of the literature, suggested use of endometrial biopsy during the latter half of the cycle for women on cyclic therapies who have heavy withdrawal bleeding, prolonged bleeding, or breakthrough bleeding during two or more cycles.[98] Because only a limited amount of endometrium is sampled, however, they recommend hysteroscopy if bleeding continues and no etiology is found.

For women on combined continuous therapies, transvaginal ultrasound is considered a good option because most of these women will have an atrophic endometrial lining. An endometrial lining measuring more than 5 mm thickness or showing irregularities would warrant biopsy or hysteroscopy. In a review of vaginal sonography in assessing the endometrium in postmenopausal women, an endometrial thickness of less than 5 mm essentially excluded the diagnosis of endometrial cancer.[101] Submucous fibroids and endometrial polyps can be demonstrated more easily by ultrasound following infusion of saline.

Management.   Bleeding problems in women on HRT can often be managed by changes in dosing. Heavy withdrawal bleeding can be diminished by decreasing the estrogen dose, if possible, or by switching to a continuous regimen. Bleeding that occurs early in the progestin phase may be due to lack of secretory activity and is managed by increasing the dose of progestin. This lack of activity can be documented on endometrial biopsy taken during the progestin phase, if there is confusion about the diagnosis.

Bleeding, especially menorrhagia, may be due to uterine fibroids. If this is suspected (or suggested on ultrasound), use of the lowest dose of estrogen to control symptoms should be considered. Other approaches include changing from a sequential to a continuous regimen or changing the type of estrogen preparation used. A 1-month period of no hormone use (wash-out period) may assist in avoiding irregular bleeding prior to switching.

Treatment

Understanding Treatment Options

Selection of therapy for an individual patient is based on the goals of therapy and the patient's medical history. Duration of therapy is determined by whether the goal is to relieve symptoms such as hot flushes and insomnia or to prevent cardiovascular disease or osteoporosis. Similarly, the route of administration and dose are determined partially by the goal of therapy—symptoms associated with urogenital atrophy can often be managed with intermittent low-dose topical therapy, whereas relieving hot flushes or preventing osteoporosis is generally treated with oral or transdermal therapy and higher doses of estrogen. The woman's personal medical history (e.g., blood pressure, history of venous thrombosis during pregnancy or while taking an oral contraceptive), family history (e.g., breast cancer, heart disease, osteoporosis), and a pretreatment assessment (e.g., lipid profile, BMD measurement) will also provide a useful framework for determining optimal therapy.

Alternatives to hormone therapy can be useful when a woman is reluctant to use hormone therapy or if a contraindication or intolerance to either estrogen or progestin therapy exists. It is estimated that estrogen is intolerable or unsafe for about 10 percent of women.[102] Alternative therapy is generally not as well studied and may not be as efficacious as hormone therapy.

Table 4-8 may be a useful guide for assisting peri- and postmenopausal women in selecting among the pharmacologic therapies available, based on their major personal risk factors. General measures for the prevention and management of heart disease and osteoporosis, such as smoking cessation, diet, and exercise, should also be discussed (see Chaps. 17 and 20).

Relief of Vasomotor Symptoms

HORMONE THERAPY

ESTROGEN   Both ERT and HRT provide relief from vasomotor symptoms in about 90 percent of women. These symptoms usually diminish over the first 5 years of the menopausal transition and continued use of hormone therapy for this indication beyond 5 years may be unnecessary. This is true for the following treatment options as well.

Table 4-8

Assisting Women with the Selection of Pharmacologic Therapy: Hormone Therapy and Other Drug Alternatives

Risk Factors (Personal)	Options*
Cardiovascular disease	HRT/ERT (oral)[†]
	Raloxifene[†]
	Aspirin, vitamin E
	Phytoestrogen
Osteopenia/osteoporosis	HRT/ERT (oral or transdermal) or Alendronate or raloxifene
	Calcium, vitamin D
	Calcitonin
	Fluoride
Menopausal symptoms	HRT/ERT (oral, vaginal, transdermal)
	Phytoestrogen
	Clonidine
	Black cohosh
	Lubricant products
Breast cancer	Tamoxifen[‡]
	Raloxifene[‡]
	Phytoestrogen

*Options listed from best evidence for effectiveness.
†Caution for women with known heart disease based on HERS trial data.[42]
‡May not be appropriate therapies for women experiencing hot flashes.

PROGESTIN ALONE Progestin therapy can be used alone to treat hot flushes. This is not a Food and Drug Administration (FDA)-approved indication for progestins. The progestin best studied is MPA; it has been used in both the oral form (10 to 20 mg/d) and the injectable, depo-medroxyprogesterone acetate (DMPA) (50 to 150 mg monthly). In a number of studies, MPA or DMPA was found to be superior to placebo in relieving hot flushes.[102] One trial comparing 150 mg DMPA to 0.625 mg CEE found the two drugs to be equally effective; the percentages of patients who initially experienced a decrease in the number of hot flushes on CEE or DMPA were 62 percent and 69 percent, respectively.[103] The efficacy of DMPA therapy appears to increase with increasing doses. One study of 50-, 100-, and 150-mg doses found that hot flushes were relieved in 65 to 80 percent, 80 to 95 percent, and 85 to 100 percent of patients,

respectively.[104] It may be appropriate to try a lower dose initially and titrate upward; the benefit is usually apparent after 2 weeks and maximal benefit is seen at 4 weeks. Common side effects from progestin therapy are irregular bleeding, headache, and vaginal dryness. One study also reported a 10 percent incidence of depression in women treated with DMPA, but it was unclear how strongly this symptom was related to the drug therapy.[102]

OTHER MEDICATIONS

CLONIDINE Clonidine has also been studied for the treatment of hot flushes. The efficacy of clonidine is controversial.[102] Both oral and transdermal dosage forms have been studied. Doses that were effective were in the range of 0.1 to 0.2 mg twice a day. However, it is recommended that with oral therapy a patient initially be treated with

0.05 mg twice daily and the dose titrated upward; the maximum daily dose is 2.4 mg. Side effects including orthostatic hypotension, sedation, fatigue, dizziness, and weakness are common with oral clonidine therapy. These symptoms may prompt many patients to discontinue therapy so it is important to warn patients taking clonidine not to suddenly stop the drug to prevent rebound hypertension. Transdermal clonidine is likely to be much better tolerated.

BELLADONNA　Bellergal-S (40 mg phenobarbital, 0.6 mg ergotamine, 0.2 mg belladonna alkaloids) is another agent that has been studied. Little evidence supports its use and, given the potential adverse effects (habituation to phenobarbital, contraindications to ergots such as peripheral or coronary vascular disease, and clinically significant drug-drug interactions), the use of this agent is rarely indicated.

ALTERNATIVE THERAPIES

PHYTOESTROGEN　Phytoestrogens, compounds found in plants that are structurally or functionally similar to estradiol, have been suggested for relieving hot flushes. Classes of phytoestrogens shown to have biologic activity in humans include isoflavones (major dietary source is soy) and lignans (major dietary source is flaxseed). Extensive information can be found in two excellent recent reviews.[105,106] With respect to the management of hot flashes, phytoestrogen, given as a 60-g isolated soy protein supplement, was found to reduce hot flushes by 45 percent by week 12 compared to a 30 percent reduction obtained with placebo ($P < .01$).[107]

Several studies using foods containing dietary phytoestrogen (45 g soy flour, linseed, or bean curd) found a modest decrease in hot flushes of 40 percent, but this may not be significantly different from the placebo response. The incidence of hot flushes is clearly much lower among Asian women (12 and 18 percent among women in Japan and China, respectively)[30,108] than among their European or American counterparts, but it is not known how much of this difference to attribute to diet and what amount and types of food would produce comparable results in other populations of women. For example, the consumption of soy products is only as high as 200 mg/d in Japanese populations,[109] and the consumption of legumes throughout Asia is thought to supply between 25 to 35 mg total isoflavones each day.[110] The dietary sources highest in phytoestrogen are shown in Table 4-9.

BLACK COHOSH　Black cohosh is an herb widely used for management of premenstrual and menopausal symptoms; the German Commission E has approved black cohosh for these indications.[111] Several clinical studies, including one randomized trial, have shown a benefit of black cohosh in reducing menopausal symptoms. It is not known whether black cohosh can protect against osteoporosis or heart disease, and little is known about long-term use. The German Commission E recommends use for no longer than 6 months due to lack of clinical data. The suggested daily dose ranges from 40 to 200 mg. The active ingredient of black cohosh has not been elucidated and standardization of products is lacking. Black cohosh should not be confused with blue cohosh, a different plant that is potentially more toxic.

Dysfunctional Uterine Bleeding Associated with Menopause

Dysfunctional uterine bleeding (DUB) is a perimenopausal irregularity in bleeding that occurs when the action of estrogen, which results in growth of the endometrial lining, is unopposed by progestin. This can result in bleeding that is heavy and prolonged or irregular spotting. An endometrial biopsy may be indicated to rule out endometrial cancer (see Chap. 13).

Two approaches are often effective in managing DUB. Oral contraceptives can be used to promote regular withdrawal bleeding and sloughing of the endometrial lining. Use of the oral contraceptives often results in lighter and predictable

Table 4-9
Dietary Sources of Phytoestrogen

FOODSTUFF	SERVING SIZE	ISOFLAVONES
Tofu, tempeh	100 g	62–112 mg
Miso	120 g	40 mg
Soy milk	250 g	40 mg
Texturized soy protein	100 g	138 mg
Soy beans, roasted	100 g	162 mg
Green soy	100 g	135 mg

SOURCE: Taylor M: Alternatives to conventional hormone replacement therapy. *Comp Ther* 23:514, 1997.

bleeding. For perimenopausal women, a lower dose oral contraceptive (e.g., a 20-μg ethinyl estradiol product) may be appropriate, particularly for women who do not require contraception. Intermittent administration of a progestin (e.g., MPA) for 10 to 13 days per month can also be used to promote regular withdrawal bleeding. The progestin is administered monthly until the woman ceases to bleed following the progestin therapy, indicating menopause. Additional information on the management of DUB can be found in Chap. 13.

Atrophic Vaginal Symptoms

LUBRICANT PRODUCTS

Vaginal water-soluble lubricant products may offer some relief for symptoms of urogenital atrophy such as vaginal dryness, itching, and burning. Judicious use of the lubricant products (initially 2 tablespoons can be inserted vaginally several times daily; the dose can then be titrated in quantity and frequency to comfort) may provide relief of atrophic vaginitis. The effect of water-soluble lubricants may not be long-lasting; however, products containing polycarbophil (e.g., Replens®) may provide a longer duration of benefit. When lubricants are used for symptoms of dyspareunia, vaginal application plus application at the vaginal opening and to the penis should be used.

HORMONAL THERAPY

If vaginal dryness or discomfort with sexual intercourse occurs during the perimenopausal period, when pregnancy protection may still be needed, low-dose oral contraceptives may alleviate symptoms.[112]

Usually the vaginal symptoms of menopause are responsive to estrogen therapy, with a 50 to 70 percent improvement.[70] Estrogen therapy can either be administered orally or vaginally (cream or vaginal ring). The dose of oral estrogen is typically 0.625 mg CEE daily, but 0.3 mg CEE daily may be adequate for management of vaginal symptoms.

Topical therapy with a vaginal cream is initiated with daily therapy (2 to 4 g of 0.625 mg CEE cream) for 4 to 8 weeks; use is then tapered to application several times per week or several times monthly. In many cases women can discontinue the therapy after 6 months. With intermittent use of vaginal estrogen cream, progestin therapy is usually not prescribed, although if use is more frequent or is continued long-term then progestin therapy should be added for endometrial protection.

Estring®, a new vaginal estradiol delivery system, is inserted into the upper third of the vagina where it remains for 90 days. Minimal systemic absorption of estrogen occurs with Estring® and progestin therapy is not required for women with a uterus. The need for continued therapy can be assessed at 3-month intervals and the product can be inserted by the patient or a health care provider. If the product is dislodged from the vagina during use it can simply be rinsed with warm tap water and reinserted.

Sexual Concerns

Perhaps most important in treating sexual complaints is the recognition and validation of the woman's sexuality and her concerns about her current sexual functioning. Educating women about physiologic changes associated with menopause and aging and discussing her current relationship with her partner are important components of management. For women with difficulties in sexual arousal or enjoyment, discussing forms of noncoital activity such as mutual masturbation or oral sex and emphasizing direct clitoral stimulation and more time for love-making may be helpful. Referral to individual or couple family or sex therapy may be necessary (see Chap. 5).

Dyspareunia and related vaginal symptoms cause sexual intercourse to be uncomfortable for 8 to 25 percent of postmenopausal women. Continued sexual activity appears to lessen the severity of urogenital atrophy.[102] Vaginal water-soluble lubricant products may offer some relief for both dyspareunia and other symptoms of urogenital atrophy. Lubricant products can be applied at the time of sexual intercourse or can be used regularly to manage other symptoms.

ESTROGEN THERAPY

Dyspareunia due to urogenital atrophy can be managed with ERT/HRT. Topical estrogen therapy likely offers similar benefits for vaginal symptoms and lubrication, and the dose may be titrated

to produce symptom relief with minimal systemic effect. Dosing information is given above.

Although ERT/HRT are likely to have positive effects on adequacy of vaginal lubrication and postcoital spotting, the duration of this benefit and need for continued treatment for these symptoms is unclear. In addition, the impact on libido is limited at best. Most studies show that estrogen's effect on sexuality and sexual function is indirect, minimal, limited to some women, and related to the specific compound used.[113] For example, studies using conjugated equine estrogen (Premarin) have not demonstrated benefit in improving sexual interest.[114] In women reporting a decrease in libido when placed on HRT or for women in whom sexual concerns are of primary importance, natural estrogens or combination products of estrogen and testosterone can be tried, but benefit remains unproven.

ANDROGEN THERAPY

The role of androgens on sexuality in the menopause is also controversial. Although testosterone does play a role in sexual interest, the doses available in most replacement preparations far exceed physiologic levels. Some menopausal women do experience dramatic decreases in testosterone level, but replacement in these women appears to have only marginal benefit on sexual activity.

The strongest evidence for a positive effect of testosterone comes from a study of 53 women following oophorectomy. For women randomized to replacement with testosterone or combination therapy (with testosterone), sexual desire and arousal were enhanced.[115] Several randomized clinical trials using parenteral testosterone systems (injections or implants) that are not currently approved by the FDA for use in the United States have shown improvements in libido[116] and sexual activity,[117] and a 10-week trial of oral therapy (5 mg methyltestosterone) also found improvements in frequency of masturbation and orgasms and pleasure derived from masturbation.[118] The latter dose of testosterone is also higher than found in the available oral formulations (1.25 to 2.5 mg in combination with estrogens).

Testosterone, particularly in high doses, can result in androgenic side effects such as hirsutism (0 to 36 percent), acne (0 to 30 percent), and lower vocal pitch (percentage not specified). High doses can be associated with clitoromegaly (not always reversible on stopping medication) and liver dysfunction; these complications have not been seen with doses usually prescribed and liver changes are not expected to occur with parenteral preparations. Newer transdermal preparations may be ideal but are not yet approved for this indication. Recent studies using the adrenal androgen dehydroepiandrosterone (DHEA) found a positive association with overall well-being, but no association with measures of sexuality.

Urinary Urgency and Incontinence

Estrogen is believed to promote continence by enhancing the closure pressure of the urethra and by enhancing the responsiveness of urethral tissues to α-adrenergic stimulation; α-adrenergic stimulation causes contractions that close the bladder outlet. Estrogen therapy may also improve urinary stress, urge, or mixed (both stress and urge) incontinence (see Chap. 12) and reduce the likelihood of UTIs.[16]

Estrogen can be administered either orally (0.625 mg CEE daily) or topically. Topical estrogen may be more effective than oral estrogen at reducing urinary incontinence. Dosing of topical estrogen for the management of urinary symptoms is the same as the dosing used for treatment of atrophic vaginal symptoms (see above). More information on the management of urinary incontinence can be found in Chap. 12.

Prevention and Treatment of Osteoporosis

A complete discussion of this topic can be found in Chap. 20.

Prevention of Cardiovascular Disease

An abundance of data indicates that postmenopausal estrogen is likely to confer some protection against cardiovascular disease, particularly the development of CHD. However, as the HERS trial demonstrated, estrogen may be associated with risk for certain cardiovascular outcomes (venous thromboembolic disease). It does not appear appropriate to consider HRT as a therapy for prevention of cardiovascular disease, particularly secondary prevention, unless other reasons for use of HRT exist. Measures to reduce the risk of cardiovascular disease are discussed in Chap.1 and Chap.17.

The dose of estrogen used in most of the studies that have demonstrated a cardioprotective effect for estrogen has been 0.625 to 1.25 mg CEE.[38] Therefore the dose currently recommended for cardioprotection is the same as the dose recommended for the prevention of osteoporosis, 0.625 mg CEE or the equivalent.

The estrogen delivery system and the addition of progestin therapy both have a significant influence on the cardioprotective effect of postmenopausal estrogen. Transdermal estrogens do not appear to be as potent as oral estrogen in altering serum lipid levels. Although transdermal estrogen decreases LDL cholesterol there is little effect on HDL cholesterol, an important factor in cardioprotective effects in women. The difference in lipid effects is thought to be due to the higher concentration of estrogen in the portal vein after oral administration. The International Consensus Conference concluded that at this time data are insufficient to demonstrate a cardioprotective effect from nonoral estrogen.[55]

Progestins have an adverse effect on lipids—increasing LDL cholesterol and decreasing HDL cholesterol. The concern with adding progestin to estrogen therapy is that the cardioprotective effects might be diminished or lost. The recent PEPI trial, which compared the effect of estrogen alone and four estrogen-progestin regimens on heart disease risk factors, did show that the addition of progestin to estrogen attenuated but did not eliminate the cardioprotective effect of estrogen via lipid alterations.[41] With respect to the progestin component of HRT, micronized progesterone (Prometrium®) appears to have an advantage over other progestins in having no adverse effect on HDL cholesterol.

Raloxifene has recently been shown to exert a positive effect on biochemical markers of cardiovascular risk by lowering LDL, fibrinogen, and lipoprotein (a) and by increasing HDL_2 cholesterol without elevating triglycerides.[119] However, in contrast to estrogen therapy, total HDL is not increased. Further trials are needed with respect to cardiovascular outcomes before a recommendation can be made for prevention of heart disease.

Risk-Benefit Analysis

The topic of long-term HRT is commonly approached as a risk-benefit analysis. Despite a number of studies on this topic, significant controversy still exists regarding a number of aspects of HRT including the optimal types and doses of these hormones, the extent of risk and degree of benefit, appropriate duration of therapy, and even which patients should avoid or be encouraged to take HRT. Until more data become available, the decision to use postmenopausal HRT will be made with incomplete information. Therefore, it is important for women to be educated about the potential risks and benefits of HRT; the woman's health goals, risk profile, and concerns must be weighed, particularly when long-term therapy is considered.

Risk-benefit analysis is designed to provide insight into the consequences of long-term therapy by estimating the effect of therapy on longevity and the likelihood that patients will develop or avoid certain medical conditions. When this type of analysis is applied to postmenopausal HRT, the analysis usually includes possible increased risks for endometrial cancer and breast cancer and possible decreased risks for CHD and osteoporosis. In addition, some analyses include other risks or benefits, such as the risk of stroke, gynecologic procedures, hysterectomy, colon cancer, and myocardial infarction.

The basis for making decisions involves estimates published in the literature of alteration in risk as a result of exposure to HRT. These analyses, however, are based on population data and generally provide little guidance to individual women. Investigators have attempted to address which women would benefit to the greatest extent.[38,120] Still, the concern remains that published benefits may be overestimated if generally healthier women are more likely to be prescribed estrogen therapy and risks may be underestimated if higher-risk women (e.g., family history of breast cancer) are excluded from therapy.

The most commonly cited risks of postmenopausal hormone therapy are endometrial cancer and breast cancer (Table 4-10). The two benefits of postmenopausal estrogen routinely cited in risk-benefit analyses are a decreased risk for osteoporosis-related fractures and CHD. Although there is disagreement in the risk-benefit estimates, the estimates presented in the table reflect consensus from the literature.

Because CHD is the most common cause of death for postmenopausal women and these analyses measure risk-benefit in terms of mortality, the benefit of estrogen on decreasing cardiovascular mortality overshadows the number of deaths attributed to cancer, even if a 30 percent increase in the risk for breast cancer is included in the analysis. This has led many authors to conclude that HRT should be prescribed for almost all women. Although heart disease is a common condition, the percent of women affected by osteoporosis is only 10 to 20 percent,[121] so many women may not develop either condition. In addition, the benefit of ERT/HRT is often not differentiated from the benefits of other concurrent health behaviors (e.g., exercise, dietary changes). However, some data suggest that estrogen can offer cardiovascular benefits even when variables known to increase the risk for CHD (e.g., hypertension, diabetes mellitus,

Table 4-10

Risks and Benefits of Hormone Replacement Therapy

	RISK FOR UNTREATED WOMEN	RISK WITH ERT	RISK WITH HRT
Endometrial cancer	Lifetime risk 2.6%	Risk is increased 4–11-fold Higher dose and longer duration associated with greater risk 5-yr survival for low-grade early stage cancers is good	Little added risk if progestin is added for 12–14 d per mo Some regimens may provide greater protection than others
Breast cancer	Lifetime risk 10%	No increased risk with short-term therapy (≤ 5 yr); 30–50% increased risk with long-term therapy (> 10 yr)	Most data suggest the risk is similar to that for ERT
Osteoporosis	15% lifetime probability of hip fracture (white women) 10–20% of women develop osteoporosis	Estrogens reduce the incidence of fractures of the hip and wrist by 25% and spine by 50% after 6–10 yr of therapy The benefit of therapy is related to both dose and duration; a dose of 0.625 mg conjugated equine estrogen is the optimal dose for most women; 7 years is the minimum length of therapy for long-term effect on bone density	Progestins do not negate estrogen's effect on bone
Coronary heart disease (CHD)	46% lifetime probability of developing and a 31% probability of dying from CHD	Estrogen (current use) reduces risk of CHD by 50%; benefit may be greatest for women with risk factors for CHD	Progestins may reduce but do not negate benefit
	By age 60, 1 in 17 women have had a coronary event	For women with diagnosed CHD there is an increased risk for thromboembolic and CHD events during the first year of therapy	Progestins vary in the extent of lipid alterations; micronized progesterone may be a preferable agent
	After age 60 CHD is the primary cause of death for women; for women 50 years or older— average annual CHD mortality rate is 3.8%		

SOURCE: Adapted with permission from Smith MA, Shimp LA: Hormone replacement therapy. In: Rosenfeld J (ed): *Primary Care for Women.* Baltimore, MD: Williams & Wilkins Press; 1997.

tobacco use, elevated cholesterol, obesity) are considered.[122] Consistent with this idea is the recommendation that ERT or HRT is most appropriately prescribed for subgroups of women, particularly women with risk factors for CHD.[51,123] Caution must be used if beginning HRT in a woman with known CHD.[42]

The algorithm provided in Fig. 4-2 may be useful in assisting women with the decision about HRT. It is intended to identify women whose life expectancy is increased by at least 6 months by HRT.[46] Dr. Col has also published a guide that can be used by women to assess their individual risks and to make a more informed and personal decision about initiating or continuing therapy.[17] In addition, as more information is gathered about the selective estrogen receptor modulators like raloxifene, additional strategies may be offered. For example, after 2 to 5 years following menopause, vasomotor symptoms may no longer be a concern and raloxifene may offer continued bone protection without breast and uterine stimulation. Although recent information supports a benefit of raloxifene on fracture rates,[124] more information on raloxifene and cardiovascular disease will be needed before recommendations can be made with confidence.

The use of ERT or HRT provides a magnitude of benefit similar to other common preventive interventions such as treatment of high blood pressure or elevated cholesterol or recommending a patient stop smoking.[51,120] In addition, the extent of benefit is likely to be related to duration of use; decreased mortality or life-years gained is

Figure 4-2

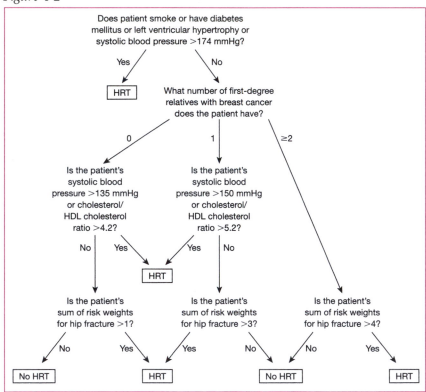

Partitioning diagram to identify patients whose life expectancy is increased by at least 6 months by HRT. (*Reprinted with permission from Col NF, et al: JAMA 277:1140, Copyright 1997.*)

most likely to be seen after at least 10 to 15 years of therapy.[120] Furthermore, ERT/HRT may provide benefits that improve the quality of life and decrease mortality. At this time, the data from the risk-benefit analysis can be a starting point for discussion, but risk factors for a particular individual should be carefully considered. Not all women are likely to benefit from ERT/HRT. Women with a family or individual history of breast cancer and women with known CHD may be at particular risk from therapy; for many women the optimal course of action will be unclear.[37,51]

References

1. Carlson ES, Holm K: An analysis of menopause in the popular press. *Health Care for Women International* 18:557, 1997.

2. Anderson E, Hamburger S, Liu JH, Rebar RW: Characteristics of menopausal women seeking assistance. *Am J Obstet Gynecol* 156:428, 1987.

3. Saver BG, Taylor TR, Woods NF: Use of hormone replacement therapy in Washington State. Is prevention being put into practice? *J Fam Pract* 48: 364, 1999.

4. Hammond CB: Women's concerns with hormone replacement therapy—compliance issues. *Fertil Steril* 62(6 suppl 2):157S, 1994.

5. Ettinger B, Li D-K, Klein R: Continuation of postmenopausal hormone replacement therapy; comparison of cyclic versus continuous combined schedule. Menopause: *Journal of the North American Menopause Society* 3:185, 1996.

6. Barentsen R, Foekema HA, Bezemer W, van Stiphout FL: The view of women aged 45–65 and their partners on aspects of the climacteric phase of life. *Eur J Obstet Gynecol Reprod Biol* 57(2):95, 1994.

7. Kaufert P: Women and menopause: Beliefs, attitudes, and behaviors. The NAMS 1997 Menopause Study. Menopause: *Journal of the North American Menopause Society.* 5(4):197, 1998.

8. Mansfield PK, Voda AM: Women-centered information on menopause for health care providers: Findings from the Midlife Women's Health Survey. *Health Care for Women International* 18:15, 1997.

9. Ghali W, Freund K: Menopausal hormone therapy: Physician awareness of patients' attitudes. *Am J Med* 103:3, 1997.

10. Witt DM, Lousberg TR: Controversies surrounding estrogen use in postmenopausal women. *Ann Pharmacotherapy* 31(6):745, 1997.

11. Payne PA, Curtis P: Promoting health for women at menopause. In: Sloane PD, Slatt LM, Curtis P, Ebell MH (eds): *Essentials of Family Medicine*, 3rd ed. Baltimore: Williams & Wilkins; 1998:179.

12. Matthews KA, Wing RR, Kuller LH, et al: Influence of the perimenopause on cardiovascular risk factors and symptoms of middle-aged healthy women. *Arch Intern Med* 154:2349, 1994.

13. Dallongeville J, Marecaux, N, Isorez D, et al: Multiple coronary heart disease risk factors are associated with menopause and influenced by substitutive hormonal therapy in a cohort of French women. *Atherosclerosis* 118:123, 1995.

14. Penckofer SM, Holm K, Schwertz D, Chandler P: The relationship of menopausal status and serum ferritin to cardiovascular risk. *Womens Health Issues* 7(1):55, 1997.

15. Hunter M, Battersby R, Whitehead M: Relationships between psychological symptoms, somatic complaints and menopausal status. *Maturitas* 8:217, 1986.

16. Porter M, Penny GC, Russell D: A population-based survey of women's experience of the menopause. *Br J Obstet Gynaecol* 103:1025, 1996.

17. Col NF: *Woman Doctor's Guide to Hormone Therapy.* Worcester, MA: Tatnuck Bookseller Press; 1997.

18. Johannes CB, Crawford SL, Longcope C, McKinlay SM: Bleeding patterns and changes in the perimenopause: A longitudinal characterization of menstrual cycles. *Clin Consultations Obstet Gynecol* 8(1):9, 1996.

19. Meston CM: Aging and sexuality. *West J Med* 167: 285, 1997.

20. McCoy NL, Davidson JM: A longitudinal study of the effects of menopause on sexuality. *Maturitas* 7:203, 1985.

21. Denerstein L, Smith AMA, Morce CA, et al: Sexuality and the menopause. *J Psychosom Obstet Gynecol* 15:59, 1994.

22. Rosenfeld JA: Menopause. In: Rosenfeld JA (ed): *Woman's Health in Primary Care.* Baltimore: Williams & Wilkins, 1997:787.

23. Schmidt R, Fazekas F, Reinhart B, et al: Estrogen replacement therapy in older women: A neuro-

psychological and brain MRI study. *J Am Geriatr Soc* 44:1307, 1996.

24. Sherwin BB: Estrogen effects on cognition in menopausal women. *Neurology* 48(suppl 7):S21, 1997.

25. Birge SJ: Is there a role for estrogen replacement therapy in the prevention and treatment of dementia? *J Am Geriatr Soc* 44:865, 1996.

26. Tang MX, Jacobs D, Stern Y, et al: Effect of oestrogen during menopause on risk and age at onset of Alzheimer's disease. *Lancet* 348:429, 1996.

27. Henderson VW: The epidemiology of estrogen replacement therapy and Alzheimer's disease. *Neurology* 48 (suppl 7):S27, 1997.

28. Paganini-Hill A, Henderson VW: Estrogen deficiency and risk of Alzheimer's disease in women. *Am J Epidemiol* 140:256, 1994.

29. Khaw KT: Epidemiology of the menopause. *Br Med Bull* 48:249, 1992.

30. Lock M: Menopause in cultural context. *Exp Gerontol* 29:307, 1994.

31. Oldenhave A, Jaszmann LJB, Haspels AA, Everaerd W: Impact of climacteric on well-being. *Am J Obstet Gynecol* 168:772, 1993.

32. Demirovic J, Sprafka JM, Folsom AR, et al: Menopause and serum cholesterol: Differences between African Americans and Caucasian Americans. *Am J Epidemiol* 136(2):155, 1992.

33. Meier D, Luckey M, Wallenstein S, et al: Racial differences in pre- and postmenopausal bone homeostasis: Association with bone density. *J Bone Miner Res* 7:1181, 1992.

34. Mayberry R, Stoddard-Wright C: Breast cancer differences among black and white women: Similarities and differences. *Am J Epidemiol* 136:1445, 1992.

35. Bartman BA, Moy E: Racial differences in estrogen use among middle-aged and older women. *Womens Health Issues* 8(1):32, 1998.

36. Jacobsen SJ, Goldberg J, Miles TP, et al: Hip fracture incidence among the old and very-old: A population-based study of 745,435 cases. *Am J Public Health* 80:871, 1990.

37. Jacobsen SJ, Goldberg J, Miles TP, et al: Race and sex difference in mortality following fracture of the hip. *Am J Public Health* 82:1, 1992.

38. Grady D, Rubin SM, Petitti DB, et al: Hormone therapy to prevent disease and prolong life in postmenopausal women. *Ann Intern Med* 117:1016, 1992.

39. Schwartz J, Freeman R, Frishman W: Clinical pharmacology of estrogens: Cardiovascular actions and cardioprotective benefits of replacement therapy

in postmenopausal women. *J Clin Pharmacol* 35:1, 1995.

40. Sidney S, Petitti DB, Quesenberry CP: Myocardial infarction and the use of estrogen and estrogen-progestogen in postmenopausal women. *Ann Intern Med* 127:501, 1997.

41. The Writing Group for the PEPI Trial: Effects of estrogen or estrogen/progestin regimens on heart disease risk factors in postmenopausal women. The Postmenopausal Estrogen/Progestin Interventions Trial. *JAMA* 273:199, 1995.

42. Hulley S, Grady D, Bush T, et al: Randomized trial of estrogen plus progestin for secondary prevention of coronary heart disease in postmenopausal women. *JAMA* 280:605, 1998.

43. Manson JE: Postmenopausal hormone therapy and atherosclerotic disease. *Am Heart J* 128:1337, 1994.

44. Schmitt N, Gogate J, Rothert M, et al: Capturing and clustering women's judgment policies: The case of hormonal therapy for menopause. *J Gerontol* 46:92, 1991.

45. Pilote L, Hlatky MA: Attitudes of women toward hormone therapy and prevention of heart disease. *Am Heart J* 129:1237, 1995.

46. Col NF, Eckman MH, Karas RH, et al: Patient-specific decisions about hormone replacement therapy in postmenopausal women. *JAMA* 277:1140, 1997.

47. Digiovanna AG: *Human Aging Biological Perspectives.* New York: McGraw-Hill; 1994.

48. Cauley JA, Petrini AM, LaPorte RE, et al: The decline of grip strength in the menopause: Relationship to physical activity, estrogen use and anthropometric factors. *J Chron Dis* 40:115, 1987.

49. Bonnier P, Romain S, Giacalone PL, et al: Clinical and biologic prognostic factors in breast cancer diagnosed during postmenopausal hormone replacement therapy. *Obstet Gynecol* 85:11, 1995.

50. Dhodapkar MV, Ingle JN, Ahmann DL: Estrogen replacement therapy withdrawal and regression of metastatic breast cancer. *Cancer* 75:43, 1995.

51. Kaplan NM: The treatment of hypertension in women. *Arch Intern Med* 155:563, 1995.

52. Berga SL: Hormonal management of the sick menopausal woman. *Obstet Gynecol Clin North Am* 21(2):231, 1994.

53. Kaiser HJ, Meienberg O: Deterioration or onset of migraine under oestrogen replacement therapy in the menopause. *J Neurol* 240:195, 1993.

54. Lieberman D, Kopernik G, Porath A, et al: Subclinical worsening of bronchial asthma during

estrogen replacement therapy in asthmatic post-menopausal women. *Maturitas* 21(2):153, 1995.

55. Lobo RA, Speroff L: International Consensus Conference on postmenopausal hormone therapy and the cardiovascular system. *Fertil Steril* 62(suppl 2):176S, 1994.

56. Arden NK, Lloyd ME, Spector TD, Hughes GR: Safety of hormone replacement therapy (HRT) in systemic lupus erythematosus (SLE). *Lupus* 3:11, 1994.

57. Glueck CJ, Lang J, Hamer T, Tracy T: Severe hypertriglyceridemia and pancreatitis when estrogen replacement therapy is given to hypertriglyceridemic women. *J Lab Clin Med* 123(1): 59, 1994.

58. Buller RE: Hormone replacement therapy following gynecologic cancer. *Postgrad Obstet Gynecol* 13(7):1, 1993.

59. Rozenberg S, Vandromme J, Kroll M, et al: Overview of the clinical usefulness of bone mineral measurements in the prevention of postmenopausal osteoporosis. *Int J Fertil* 40(1): 12, 1995.

60. Christiansen C: Selection of postmenopausal women for estrogen therapy. *Postgrad Med* 85 (Special Issue):10, 1989.

61. Hulka BS: Links between hormone replacement therapy and neoplasia. *Fertil Steril* 62(suppl 2): 168S, 1994.

62. ACOG Committee Opinion: Committee on Gynecologic Practice: Estrogen replacement therapy in women with previously diagnosed breast. *Int J Gynecol Obstet* 45:184, 1994.

63. Cobleigh MA, Berris RF, Bush T, et al: Estrogen replacement therapy in breast cancer survivors. *JAMA* 272:540, 1994.

64. Grady D, Gebretsadik T, Kerlikowske K, et al: Hormone replacement therapy and endometrial cancer risk: A meta-analysis. *Obstet Gynecol* 85:304, 1995.

65. Writing Group for the PEPI Trial: Effects of hormone replacement therapy on endometrial histology in postmenopausal women. *JAMA* 275: 370, 1996.

66. Gambrell RD Jr, Massey FM, Castaneda TA, et al: Use of the progestogen challenge to reduce the risk of endometrial cancer. *Obstet Gynecol* 55:732, 1980.

67. Gambrell RD Jr: Strategies to reduce the incidence of endometrial cancer in postmenopausal women. *Am J Obstet Gynecol* 177:1196, 1997.

68. Barrett-Connor E: Hormone replacement and cancer. *Br Med Bull* 48:345, 1992.

69. Garg PP, Kerlikowske K, Subak L, Grady D: Hormone replacement therapy and the risk of epithelial ovarian carcinoma: A meta-analysis. *Obstet Gynecol* 92:472, 1998.

70. Lindsay R, Bush TL, Grady D, et al: Therapeutic controversy: Eestrogen replacement in menopause. *J Clin Endocrinol Metab* 81:3829, 1996.

71. Colditz GA, Stampfer MJ, Willett WC, et al: Prospective study of estrogen replacement therapy and risk of breast cancer in postmenopausal women. *JAMA* 264:2648, 1990.

72. Colditz GA, Hankinson SE, Hunter DJ, et al: The use of estrogens and progestins and the risk of breast cancer in postmenopausal women. *N Engl J Med* 332:1589, 1995.

73. Gambrell RD: Role of progestogens in the prevention of breast cancer. *Maturitas* 8:169, 1986.

74. Stanford JL, Weiss NS, Voigt LF, et al: Combined estrogen and progestin hormone replacement therapy in relation to risk of breast cancer in middle-aged women. *JAMA* 274:137, 1995.

75. Colditz GA, Stampfer MJ, Willett WC, et al: Type of postmenopausal hormone use and risk of breast cancer: 12-year follow-up from the Nurses' Health Study. *Cancer Causes Control* 3:433, 1992.

76. Garton M, Reid D, Rennie E: The climacteric, osteoporosis and hormone replacement: Views of women aged 45-49. *Maturitas* 21:7, 1995.

77. McNicholas MM, Heneghan JP, Milner MH, et al: Pain and increased mammographic density in women receiving hormone replacement therapy: A prospective study. *Am J Roentgenol* 163(2):311, 1994.

78. Marsh MS, Whitcroft S, Whitehead MI: Paradoxical effects of hormone replacement therapy on breast tenderness in postmenopausal women. *Maturitas* 19:97, 1994.

79. Haarbo J, Marslew U, Gotfredsen A, Christiansen C: Postmenopausal hormone replacement therapy prevents central distribution of body fat after menopause. *Metabolism* 40:1323, 1991.

80. Ettinger B, Selby JV, Citron JT, et al: Gynecologic complications of cyclic estrogen progestin therapy. *Maturitas* 17(3):197, 1993.

81. Al-Azzawi F, Habiba M: Regular bleeding on hormone replacement therapy: A myth. *Br J Obstet Gynaecol* 101:661, 1994.

82. Sitruk-Ware R: Hormonal replacement therapy: What to prescribe, how and for how long. In: Sitruk-Ware R, Utian WH (eds): *The Menopause and Hormone Replacement Therapy.* New York: Dekker; 1991.

83. Jones KP: Estrogens and progestins: What to use and how to use it. *Clin Obstet Gynecol* 35:871, 1992.

84. Stenchever M: Hormone replacement. In: Stenchever MA, Aagaard G (eds): *Current Topics in Obstetrics and Gynecology: Caring for the Older Woman.* New York: Elsevier; 1991; Chap. 12.

85. American College of Physicians: Guidelines for counseling postmenopausal women about preventive hormone therapy. *Ann Intern Med* 117:1038, 1992.

86. Marsh MS, Whitehead MI: Management of the menopause. *Br Med Bull* 48:435, 1992.

87. Gambrell RD: Estrogen replacement therapy. *Drug Therapy* 17:68, 1987.

88. Birkenfeld A, Kase NG: The management of the postmenopausal woman. In: Glass RH (ed): *Office Gynecology*, 4th ed. Baltimore: Williams & Wilkins; 1993:Chap. 14.

89. Lufkin E, Ory S: Relative value of transdermal and oral estrogen therapy in various clinical situations. *Mayo Clin Proc* 69:131, 1994.

90. Gambrell RD: Guidelines for choosing the regimen—Managing attending problems. *Consultant* 34:1047, 1994.

91. Sturdee DW, Barlow DH, Ulrich LG, et al: Is the timing of withdrawal bleeding a guide to endometrial safety during sequential oestrogen-progestagen replacement therapy? *Lancet* 344:979, 1994.

92. Rosenfeld J: Update on continuous estrogen-progestin replacement therapy. *Am Fam Physician* 50:1519, 1994.

93. Ettinger B, Selby J, Citron JT, et al: Cyclic hormone replacement therapy using quarterly progestin. *Obstet Gynecol* 83:693, 1994.

94. Hirvonen E, Salmi T, Puolakka J, et al: Can progestin be limited to every third month only in postmenopausal women taking estrogen? *Maturitas* 21:39, 1995.

95. Cerin A, Heldaas K, Moeller B: Adverse endometrial effects of long-cycle estrogen and progestogen replacement therapy. (Letter) *N Engl J Med* 334:668, 1996.

96. Evans MP, Fleming KC, Evans JM: Hormone replacement therapy: Management of common problems. *Mayo Clin Proc* 70:800, 1995.

97. Kurman RJ, Kaminski PF, Norris HJ: The behavior of endometrial hyperplasia: A long-term study of "untreated" hyperplasia in 170 patients. *Cancer* 56:403, 1985.

98. Spencer CP, Cooper AJ, Whitehead MI: Management of abnormal bleeding in women receiving hormone replacement therapy. *BMJ* 315:37, 1997.

99. Paterson MEL, Wade-Evans T, Sturdee DW, et al: Endometrial disease after treatment with oestrogens and progestogens in the climacteric. *BMJ* 22:822, 1980.

100. Akkad AA, Habiba MA, Ismail N, et al: Abnormal bleeding on hormone replacement: The importance of intrauterine structural abnormalities. *Obstet Gynecol* 86:330, 1995.

101. Wikland M, Granberg S, Karlsson B: Assessment of the endometrium in the postmenopausal woman by vaginal sonography. *Ultrasound Quarterly* 10(1):15, 1992.

102. Miller KL: Alternatives to estrogen for menopausal symptoms. *Clin Obstet Gynecol* 35:884, 1992.

103. Lobo RA, McCormick W, Singer F, et al: Depomedroxypogesterone acetate compared with conjugated estrogens for the treatment of postmenopausal women. *Obstet Gynecol* 63:1, 1984.

104. Morrison JC, Martin DC, Blair RA, et al: The use of medroxyprogesterone acetate for relief of climacteric symptoms. *Am J Obstet Gynecol* 138: 99, 1980.

105. Knight DC, Eden JA: A review of the clinical effects of phytoestrogens. *Obstet Gynecol* 87:897, 1996.

106. Adlercreutz H, Mazur W: Phyto-oestrogens and western diseases. *Ann Med* 29:95, 1997.

107. Albertazzi P, Pansini F, Bonaccorsi G, et al: The effect of dietary soy supplementation on hot flushes. *Obstet Gynecol* 91:6, 1998.

108. Boulet MJ, Oddens BJ, Lehert P, et al: Climacteric and menopause in several south-east Asian countries. *Maturitas* 19:157, 1994.

109. Cassidy A, Bingham S, Setchell KDR: Biological effects of a diet of soy protein rich in isoflavones on the menstrual cycle of premenopausal women. *Am J Clin Nutr* 60:333, 1994.

110. Coward L, Barnes NC, Setchell KDR, Barnes S: The isoflavones genitein and daidzein in soybean foods from American and Asian diets. *J Agric Food Chem* 41:1961, 1993.

111. Blumenthal M (ed): *The Complete German Commission E Monographs: Therapeutic Guide to Herbal Medicines*. Austin, TX: American Botanical Council; 1998.

112. Bachmann GA: The changes before "the change." *Postgrad Med* 95:113, 1994.

113. Levine SB: The sexual consequences of peri-menopause and menopause. *Women's Health in Primary Care* 1:509, 1998.

114. McCoy NL: Sexual issues for postmenopausal women. *Top Geriatr Rehabil* 12:1, 1997.

115. Sherwin BB, Gelfand MM, Brender W: Androgen enhances sexual motivation in females. A prospective, crossover study of sex steroid administration in the surgical menopause. *Psychosom Med* 47:339, 1985.

116. Sherwin BB, Gelfand MM: The role of androgen in the maintenance of sexual functioning in oophorectomized women. *Psychosom Med* 49:397, 1987.

117. Davis SR, McCloud P, Straus BJD, et al: Testosterone enhances estradiol effects on postmenopausal bone density and sexuality. *Maturitas* 21:227, 1995.

118. Myers L, Dixen J, Morrissette D, et al: Effects of estrogen, androgen and progestin on sexual psychophysiology and behavior in postmenopausal women: A 10 week double-blind study. *J Clin Endocrinol Metab* 70:1124, 1990.

119. Walsh BW, Kuller LH, Wild RA, et al: Effects of raloxifene on serum lipids and coagulation factors in healthy postmenopausal women. *JAMA* 279:1445, 1998.

120. Zubialde JP, Lawler F, Clemenson N: Estimated gains in life expectancy with use of postmenopausal estrogen therapy: A decision analysis. *J Fam Pract* 36(3):271, 1993.

121. Breslau NA: Calcium, estrogen, and progestin in the treatment of osteoporosis. *Rheum Dis Clin North Am* 20:691, 1994.

122. Gambrell RD: The menopause: Benefits and risks of hormone replacement therapy. *Compr Ther* 20:580, 1994.

123. Daly E, Roche M, Barlow D, et al: HRT: An analysis of benefits, risks and costs. *Brit Med Bull* 48:368, 1992.

124. Cummings SR, Eckert S, Krueger KA, et al: The effect of raloxifene on risk of breast cancer in postmenopausal women: Results from the Multiple Outcomes of Raloxifene Evaluation (MORE) randomized trial (see comments). *JAMA* 281(23):2243, 1999.

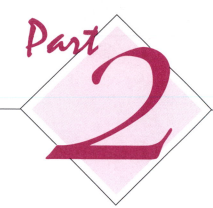

Part 2

Womanhood:
Choices and Challenges

Linda A. Bernhard
Robert W. Birch

Sexuality

Overview

Sexuality is one of the most complex and important aspects of a woman's life, both as an individual and as a partner within a relationship. Few women can fully describe their sexuality in simple terms, but if they could, it would probably include intimacy, caring, trust, respect, and a wide range of emotions, as well as a description of not only their own genital sexual behavior but that of their partner(s) as well. Furthermore, most women are unprepared to answer specific sexual questions, whether asked by a friend, partner, or health care provider. Clinical experience suggests that many women do not communicate openly about their sexuality, seeming to assume their experiences to be fairly typical. Only when women experience a change from their presumed normal sexuality or are made aware of a change or deficit by a partner, do they identify a problem—and not always then. Most sexual difficulties identified by women or their partners concern sexual functioning or sexual behavior within a significant relationship.

Describing Sexuality

Sexuality is much more than physiology; it is multidimensional, with psychosocial, attitudinal, cultural, situational, and political aspects, as well as biology. Sexuality is dynamic, affected by early life experiences and social learning and, within certain limits, subject to individual choice. An individual's sexuality changes across the life span, under changing social, physical, or environmental conditions, and with different sexual partners.

Levine[1] argues that there neither is, nor can be, a simple definition of sexuality. Instead, he describes sexuality as a collage of overlapping meanings that include sexual identity, an internal drive for pleasure (i.e., desire), the biologic capacity for sexual arousal and orgasm (often referred to as sexual functioning), and a repertoire of intimate physical behaviors (what a person does when "having sex"). Earlier, Money and Ehrhardt[2] distinguished between gender identity and gender role. Gender identity is the persistence of a self-awareness of being female, male, or ambivalent [sic]. Gender role is everything a person says or does to indicate to others the degree to which one is female, male, or ambivalent/transgendered. It includes, but is not restricted to, sexual arousal and response. Money and Ehrhardt consider gender identity as the private experience of gender role, and gender role as the public expression of gender identity.

Recently, Bockting[3] identified four aspects of sexuality, highlighting its complexity. Natal sex is that which is assigned at birth, based on the external appearance of a newborn's genitals. Gender identity is the subjective personal conviction one holds about being male or female, despite the appearance of genitalia. Social sex role includes one's behavioral characteristics, conformance with gender stereotypes, and general manner of dress and self-presentation. Finally, sexual orientation is identified by the gender of one's objects of affection and erotic attraction.

Considerable controversy exists about whether sexual orientation is biologic or developmental. Sexologists generally hold that the majority of women who consider themselves as lesbian or bisexual date this awareness to some of their earliest memories. Despite expectations of family, school, and church and the influence of predominantly heterosexual role models in the media, for lesbians, the objects of their affection and sexual attraction were always of the same sex. Money[4] states, ". . . homosexuality, like heterosexuality, is not a matter of preference, choice, or voluntary decision. It is a status, like being tall, dwarfed, or left-handed, and is not changed by desire, incentive, will power, prayer, punishment, or other motivation to change." However, for those growing up in a society intolerant of multiple forms of sexual expression, the "coming out" process (acknowledgement to oneself and others that one is homosexual) can be quite difficult for lesbian women.

Sexual orientation is part of sexual identity. People have multiple identities, such as race, ethnicity, class, and family, as well as sexuality. Many feminists believe that women consciously choose their sexual identity. To say that individuals have a choice about their sexual orientation and are capable of change is to challenge the notion that sexuality is a genetic, fixed part of existence. Some lesbians report changing their sexual orientation from heterosexual to lesbian, as part of a developmental process. A woman who thought she was heterosexual falls in love with a woman; her feelings may include shock and surprise, but if she becomes emotionally and sexually involved with women, she often describes the feelings as natural, pleasant, and even joyful. Sometimes gradually, sometimes suddenly, but as a result of the change in gender of her sexual partners, she will say that her sexual orientation is lesbian.[5]

Sexual identity is not always consistent with sexual orientation and sexual behavior. Some women engage in sexual activities with other women, but continue to identify themselves as heterosexual, rather than lesbian. Other women identify as bisexual but interact sexually with one gender only. Moreover, women have a sexual identity and sexual orientation, whether or not they engage in any sexual activities.

Female Sexual Response

In their pioneering book, *Human Sexual Response*, Masters and Johnson[6] described a four-phase sexual response cycle. Their model begins with the excitement (or arousal) phase. With continued and effective stimulation, arousal builds to a plateau phase of high sexual excitement. If stimulation is continued, the woman will reach the orgasm stage, followed by resolution. According to this model, women may experience one or multiple orgasms—returning to plateau between orgasms and entering the resolution phase only when sexual satiation occurs.

Masters and Johnson described the genitalia of the nonaroused female as the baseline from which the physical aspects of response can be observed. Shortly after entering the excitement phase, vasocongestion of the woman's genital tissue results in engorgement within the vaginal introitus and the secretion of a transudate, or vulvar lubrication. As excitement builds, the labia majora, and to a lesser extent the labia minora, increase in size and separate, affording greater exposure of the vaginal introitus. Vasocongestion of the clitoris results in increased size, as this exquisitely sensitive structure becomes tumescent and increasingly responsive to touch. For some women the tumescent clitoris, which is covered in the nonaroused state, emerges from beneath the clitoral hood.

With arousal the entrance to the vagina opens as the walls along the length of the vaginal barrel separate and become smooth. The vaginal barrel lengthens slightly, and during the plateau phase, the uterus elevates into the abdominal cavity, causing the inner two-thirds of the vaginal vault to balloon in what Masters and Johnson referred to as "the tenting effect."

As some women approach orgasm, Masters and Johnson describe a deepening of the coloration of the labia minora. The vaginal opening engorges and tightens, becoming the "orgasmic platform." Behaviorally, as most women approach orgasm, they quiet, closing their eyes to focus on the building erotic sensations. A woman's body is likely to tense reflexively and, with this involuntary hypertonicity, some women, voluntarily or involuntarily, arch their backs, tense their abdominal muscles, and tighten their legs. A woman with physical pain might consciously or unconsciously avoid high arousal and the associated hypertonicity, thus reducing her potential for reaching orgasm.

Masters and Johnson described the physical component of female orgasm as consisting of contractions in the musculature of the perineum, including the sphincters of both the vagina and anus. The subjective experience typically includes an awareness of these physical contractions, each accompanied by a wave of pleasure that sweeps throughout the body. The contractions may or may not be accompanied by pelvic thrusts or vocal sounds. Independent contractions occur within the uterus, rippling down from the fundus toward the cervix. These contractions are not in synchrony with the stronger pelvic floor contractions, and most women are unaware of them. However, after a hysterectomy some women report a perceptible change in their experience of orgasm, typically expressed as a loss.

Some women report a more subdued orgasmic experience, telling of a crescendo of excitement, leading to a warm pleasurable sensation deep within the pelvis, followed by a sense of sexual satisfaction. The intensity of the orgasmic experience differs from woman to woman and from episode to episode, depending on a multitude of psychological, biologic, and relational variables; descriptions of the personal experience will always include unique perceptions and associations.

The genital vasocongestion subsides as a woman enters the resolution phase. This final phase of physical and emotional relaxation and sense of physical satisfaction and psychological well-being is often referred to as the "afterglow."

Although he did not publish his ideas until later, Harold Lief[7] noted soon after Masters and Johnson published the sexual response cycle that it lacked a motivational drive for sexual expression. Lief conceptualized a response model for which he coined the acronym DAVOS: desire, arousal, vasocongestion, orgasm, and satisfaction.

Helen Singer Kaplan[8] developed a model including the desire phase of sexual response. Kaplan's model is a triphasic sexual response cycle, beginning with appetitive erotic desire, escalating into arousal (incorporating Masters and Johnson's plateau and Lief's vasocongestion), and with sufficient stimulation, ending in orgasm (including Masters and Johnson's resolution and Lief's satisfaction).

Today, the sexual response cycle is normalized in the *Diagnostic and Statistical Manual of Mental Disorders* (DSM-IV) as the norm or standard against which sexual dysfunctions are identified.[9] The DSM-IV sexual response cycle consists of four phases that are a combination of the work of Masters and Johnson, Leif, and Kaplan. The phases are (1) appetitive (desire), (2) excitement (arousal), (3) orgasm, and (4) resolution.

Sexual Behaviors

Women engage in a wide variety of sexual activities, alone or with one or more sexual partners. Most women value each sexual activity as an end in itself, and not necessarily as "foreplay" for something else. The form that a woman's sexual expression takes may depend on the number and gender of her partners.

Penile-Vaginal Intercourse

Nearly all sexually active heterosexual women identify penile-vaginal intercourse as their most frequent form of sexual expression; 97 percent of the women surveyed in the National Health and Social Life Survey[10] (NHSLS) reported engaging in penile-vaginal intercourse. The NHSLS was a national probability sample that included more than 1600 women, ages 18 to 59, of a variety of races and socioeconomic levels. Couples engage in penile-vaginal intercourse using a variety of positions. Although penile-vaginal intercourse may be the most common and most fulfilling form of sexual activity for many women, it is an approach that results in orgasm for only 25 percent of women.[11] When a woman (or her partner) has a physical disability that affects mobility or physical endurance or results in physical pain, a change in position may be required to maintain sexual pleasure for both partners. Health care providers can assist couples by inquiring about discomfort before and during intercourse and, when appropriate, suggesting possible alternative positions both for fondling and coitus.

Oral-Genital Stimulation

Most women also report engaging in oral sex—cunnilingus (oral stimulation of the female genital organs), fellatio (oral stimulation of the male genital organs), or both.[12] In the NHSLS[10] more than two-thirds of women had both given and received oral sex in their lifetimes, but only about one-fifth engaged in it regularly. Among lesbians, cunnilingus is one of the most common forms of sexual activity,[13] although clinical experience indicates that creative women find many ways to share physical intimacy.

Anal Stimulation

Anal sex is a less common sexual activity for women that may be performed, not by the woman's choice, but in response to a partner's desire. About 12 percent of the college women in a recent study reported having experienced anal intercourse.[12]

Strong societal taboos are associated with anal stimulation, despite the identification of the anal sphincter as an erogenous area. For many women, anal intercourse may be uncomfortable and degrading. In addition, if not prepared (i.e., relaxed, well lubricated, and dilated), physical injury may result. If not consensual, both physical and emotional injury may occur; however, with mutual consent and preparation, anal intercourse can be accomplished safely and with mutual pleasure.

Cleanliness is also an issue. Participants in anal play should be reminded not to engage in any activity that could transport bacteria from the anal region to the vulva. For the safety of both partners, condoms should be worn during anal intercourse and carefully discarded before continuing with other activities. Anal dildos, vibrators, or other sex toys should be cleaned with an antibacterial agent or, if possible, boiled for at least 5 mins before they are used again.

Analingus, or "rimming," is the stimulation of the anus with the tongue. Cleanliness is again a concern because bacteria, normally present in the lower gastrointestinal tract, can cause infections in the mouth. The entire anal area can be stimulated safely if covered with a latex barrier or plastic cling wrap. Plastic wrap is readily available and convenient. Latex gloves can be purchased in almost every pharmacy, and the hand portion can be cut open to use as a barrier. Even a latex condom when unrolled and cut lengthwise can be stretched to cover the anal area. Dental dams, available in dental supply stores, sex toy stores, and some pharmacies, can also be used as barriers.

Self-Stimulation

Despite the double standard that generally accepts masturbation by men, female masturbation is not openly acknowledged or endorsed. Still, masturbation, or self-stimulation, is commonly used by women to manage their sexual desire in a safe manner, to enjoy their physical response, to relax, and for a variety of other unique and personal reasons.[14] In a recent study 35 percent of women in a college sample reported masturbating alone.[12] Lesbians report a very high (90 percent) incidence of masturbation, both alone and with partners.[13] Women often report that orgasms experienced through masturbation are stronger and more easily reached than orgasms achieved through other forms of stimulation.

Masturbation helps women learn about their bodies, and a significant number of women can masturbate to orgasm, even if they are unable to achieve orgasm during sex with a partner. Moreover, masturbation can be performed alone, with a partner present and watching, or with a partner helping or masturbating simultaneously.

Many women use vibrators or dildos as part of their sexual activity. A diverse group of women in one recent study reported using vibrators, primarily during self-stimulation, but also during sexual activity with a partner, including penile-vaginal intercourse.[15] The use of vibrators may increase the duration of activity, as well as the intensity of orgasms.[15]

Fantasy is often combined with masturbation and other types of sexual activity. Although about one in five women engage in daily sexual fantasies,[10] almost every woman has erotic fantasies at one time or another.[16] Fantasies reflect women's thoughts and interests, although what is fantasized (e.g., rape or bondage) is not necessarily what women really want to do sexually.[16] Nonetheless, about 25 percent of women experience guilt feelings because of their fantasies.[17]

Although not technically fantasy, many women have very sexual and erotic dreams that include orgasms. In clinical practice, furthermore, a small number of women who have never experienced orgasms while awake, report orgasms during sleep with fair regularity.

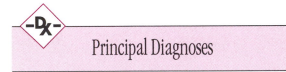

Principal Diagnoses

The DSM-IV[9] lists six types of sexual dysfunction in women: hypoactive sexual desire disorder, sexual aversion disorder, female sexual arousal disorder, female orgasmic disorder, dyspareunia, and vaginismus (Table 5-1) The DSM was developed to facilitate communication among clinicians and researchers by using a consistent set of criteria for various diagnoses.[9] A review of the literature, however, reveals that, despite DSM, there continues to be some confusion and ambiguity in the use of terms, making cross-comparisons between studies difficult at best. Medical researchers and behavioral scientists do not always differentiate between a sexual dysfunction and a sexual disorder, and indeed, the difference might be more one of semantics. In clinical practice, women occasionally report a sexual concern that does not fall neatly into the DSM criteria for the sexual dysfunctions. For example, a woman might report high desire and subjective arousal but inadequate lubrication, or a woman might cite high desire and good lubrication but no subjective sexual pleasure (anhedonia), or a woman might complain of an orgasm within seconds of being touched, cutting short her ability to experience (and share) a more prolonged sexual encounter. Problems that do not fit nicely into the diagnostic nomenclature, whether of physical or psychological origin, are nonetheless a valid concern for the woman.

The labeling of sexual dysfunction is based on the assumption that there is "normal" or "typical" sexual function. In this paradigm, dysfunction is perceived as a breakdown or disruption of the baseline "healthy" sexual response. It is this normalization of the sexual response cycle and the medicalization of sexuality[18] that are the basis for labeling sexual problems and dysfunctions, when virtually any experience of sexuality is considered normal by those who experience it and could also be considered normal by clinicians.

There are few existing data about the incidence or prevalence of sexual problems in either clinical populations or the general population, and the existing statistics vary greatly. Results of a clinical sample of women attending a gynecology clinic included 38 percent with anxiety or inhibition during sexual activity, 16 percent with lack of sexual pleasure, and 15 percent with difficulty achieving orgasm.[19] In the NHSLS population study,[10] 33 percent of women reported a lack of sexual interest, 24 percent reported inability to have orgasms, and 14 percent reported dyspareunia in the past year.

Sexual problems or difficulties are common in primary care. Shafer[20] reports that 15 percent of medical outpatients present with some form of sexual complaint, but that the incidence of sexual problems is related directly to the frequency with which clinicians take a sexual history.

Table 5-1

DSM-IV Female Sexual Dysfunctions

DYSFUNCTION	DEFINITION
Hypoactive sexual desire disorder	Lack of desire to engage in sexual activity
Sexual aversion disorder	Dislike and avoidance of genital sex with a partner
Female sexual arousal disorder	Lack of pelvic vasocongestion and vaginal lubrication
Female orgasmic disorder	Inability to have orgasms
Dyspareunia	Pain during or after vaginal sexual activity
Vaginismus	Involuntary contraction of muscles surrounding the introitus, such that vaginal penetration is impossible

Factors Affecting Sexuality

Almost anything can affect sexuality, but several important considerations will be presented here. Age is an important variable in understanding and assessing female sexuality. Sexuality begins at birth (or before), and little girls learn much about sexuality in their families and immediate subculture (e.g., religion or ethnic group). Cultural and parental expressions of love and affection and attitudes and beliefs about sex (e.g., sexual activity is only allowed within marriage, old people do not have sex, homosexuality is a sin, genitals are dirty, and nudity is never acceptable) influence girls as they develop their own concepts of intimacy and sexuality.

LIFE CYCLE AND PERSONAL CHARACTERISTICS

Adolescence is a time when young women often explore their sexuality and participate in a variety of sexual activities, both coital and non-coital.[21] The adolescent struggles with peer expectations and pressures, sometimes becoming sexual when emotionally immature and without adequate information about contraception and safer sex. The risk of unwanted pregnancies or of acquiring sexually transmitted infections (STIs) increases among unprepared young women. At this age young women may become overly concerned about their breast development, general physical appearance, and weight. When confronted with the unrealistic social standard of beauty, concerns about acceptance, and peer pressures, eating disorders are not uncommon and clinicians must inquire tactfully when a young woman appears to have undergone a dramatic weight loss. Questioning parents or family members is indicated when the patient is a minor and an eating disorder is suspected.

Adult women have usually established their own pattern of sexual activity. Factors that influence those patterns include childbearing and lactation, child care, and employment. Women who are mothers and also work outside the home often experience high levels of stress in response to the demands placed on them. When partners work on different time schedules or for long hours, they may both feel tired, with less energy, less time, and consequently, fewer sexual encounters. Research shows that women engage in sexual activity more frequently during weekends and holidays than on weekdays.[22]

In midlife, significant changes occur for women; many are related to their aging parents and growing children. Menopause is prominent among these life events. Menopause can positively influence sexuality for women who feel less concern about contraception or for those who view aging as a growing, changing time. For others, menopause can negatively influence sexuality both psychologically, for women who link sexuality with fertility or associate menopause with physical deterioration, and physically, if symptoms interfere with sleep or physical functioning including vaginal lubrication (see Chap. 4).

Older women usually continue the patterns of sexuality that they developed earlier in life. However, the physiologic effects of aging and the increasing likelihood of chronic illnesses in women themselves or in their sexual partners can alter those patterns. Although widowhood is expected by many old women, being alone can have a dramatic impact on sexuality, particularly for women who have continuing sexual needs, but who never learned to be comfortable with masturbation.

A woman's socioeconomic situation plays an important part in sexual function. Such factors as race, ethnicity, culture, and religion influence a woman's sexual comfort and the expectations she has of herself and of her partners.[23–25] The messages about love, sex, and intimacy that a woman learned in her family, religion, and culture often dictate what body parts are taboo, what sexual behavior is acceptable, and even the degree of pleasure that is allowed.

FERTILITY AND CHILDBEARING

Concerns about fertility greatly affect expressions of sexuality. There are issues of preventing pregnancy and issues of wanting it. Fear of pregnancy can produce extreme anxiety. Because most women expect to be able to conceive if they decide to have children, fertility and infertility are important aspects of their identity as women, role as partners, and sense of sexuality. In attempting to conceive, sexual encounters may be scheduled and sexual limits pushed in the attempt to have intercourse at the right time. Both partners may experience mild performance anxieties that are forgotten when conception occurs.

If a couple discovers their infertility, both partners may feel a tremendous impact on their sexual self-esteem. Infertile women may consider themselves less feminine, their partners may feel inadequate, and having sex becomes work, rather than pleasure.

Women's sexuality is greatly affected by pregnancy, childbirth, and lactation. Many variables,

including religion and cultural beliefs about sexual behavior during pregnancy and whether the pregnancy was planned or unplanned, affect sexuality during pregnancy. Research results are limited and conflicting, but it seems that most women experience a decrease in sexual desire and activity over the course of pregnancy, although there may be a return of desire in the second trimester when women feel better.[6,26] Explanations for decreases in sexual activity include physical discomforts, loss of desire, awkwardness of sexual positions, loss of feelings of attractiveness, and being told by others that sex should be avoided.[27] In early pregnancy, fatigue and morning sickness often result in a decrease in frequency of sexual activity. In the third trimester, women experience major changes in body image and become more uncomfortable. Many positions of intercourse become awkward or painful, and for some women orgasms in late pregnancy can result in uncomfortable uterine spasms. Some couples may avoid intercourse out of unfounded fear of either miscarriage or injury to the fetus. Clinicians should always talk with a pregnant woman (and her partner if possible) about sexual activity during and after pregnancy. Most couples resume sexual activity after childbirth, but concerns about perineal healing, lingering fatigue, and breast feeding can interfere.

The lactating mother may not experience erotic feelings when her breasts are fondled and might be psychologically conflicted about having her milk-producing breasts treated as sexual parts. Her nipples may be sore and there may be discomfort with breast engorgement. It might be uncomfortable for some lactating women to have her partner lie on top of her. Her partner might miss being able to involve the woman's breasts in sex play and, in the worse case, resent the newborn for taking over parts of the woman's body that were once sexual. Psychological or relational issues aside, the lactating woman may not lubricate as well, due to low estrogen levels. Temporary use of an artificial lubricant may be indicated. Postpartum follow-up assessments should always include questions about changes in sexual response, possibility of relationship problems, and thorough inquiries about any sexual pain. Improvement in sexuality usually accompanies cessation of breast feeding.[28]

RELATIONSHIPS

The history and chronology of a woman's relationship(s) or marital history are important components of her sexual health. A good relationship is important for relaxed and responsive sexual expression, particularly for women. Although the quality of a woman's emotional relationship may be crucial, sexual technique also plays a role, particularly in long-term relationships and with aging couples. Preferences about the frequency, time, place, and dress during sexual activity influence sexual expression and can cause sexual difficulties when they differ from those of a partner. Good communication between a woman and her partner(s), both in general and about sexual matters, is an important measure of the quality of a relationship and is essential to finding resolution or compromise for differing expectations.

Clinicians must evaluate a woman's experiences of violence and abuse because these can directly affect sexuality. This includes an entire range of violence, from emotional and physical partner abuse and marital rape to incest and date or acquaintance rape. Research shows that a large number of women who are battered by partners are also sexually abused, but the sexual abuse is much harder for women to acknowledge. Violence in a relationship often begins during pregnancy or may begin because a woman withholds sex. Women who survive incest may resist being touched or may report flashbacks associated with specific sexual activities. This topic is addressed in Chap. 7.

INJURY, ILLNESS, AND DISABILITY

Injury, illness, and disability can all affect women's sexuality (Table 5-2). Numerous research studies document sexual problems or difficulties among women with a wide range of health problems, physical and developmental disabilities, and diseases.[29–31] Moreover, it is not only the problem but also the treatment(s) for a problem that can affect sexuality. Chronic illnesses and sexually transmitted diseases (STDs), including HIV, can negatively affect sexual functioning as well as how a woman perceives herself as a sexual being. Radical surgery, radiation, or chemotherapy for treatment of breast, cervical, and other cancers may

Table 5-2

Selected Health Conditions and Possible Sexual Effects for Women

HEALTH CONDITION	POSSIBLE SEXUAL EFFECTS
Alcoholism	Decreased desire, decreased arousal
Breast cancer	Decreased desire, decreased satisfaction, altered body image
Diabetes	Decreased desire, decreased lubrication, decreased orgasm
Epilepsy	Decreased arousal, dyspareunia, decreased orgasm
HIV/AIDS	Decreased desire
Hypertension	Decreased desire, arousal, lubrication, and orgasm
Hysterectomy, oophorectomy	Decreased orgasm
Interstitial cystitis	Dyspareunia
Multiple sclerosis	Decreased arousal, lubrication, and orgasm
Premenstrual syndrome	Decreased desire, decreased orgasm, decreased satisfaction
Renal failure	Decreased desire, decreased satisfaction, altered body image
Spinal cord injury	Decreased orgasm, decreased satisfaction

Table 5-3

Selected Drugs/Medications and Their Sexual Side Effects

DRUG/MEDICATION	POTENTIAL SEXUAL SIDE EFFECTS
Alcohol	Initially increases sexual arousal, but higher doses impair orgasm
Antibiotics	May cause vaginitis, with dyspareunia as a consequence
Anticancer drugs	Decreased sexual desire
Antihistamines	Decreased lubrication with long-term use
Benzodiazepines	Decreased desire and orgasm
β-Adrenergic blockers	Decreased desire, decreased lubrication
Cimetidine	Decreased desire, decreased arousal
Cocaine	Inhibits orgasm; increases arousal
Lithium	Either increased or decreased desire and orgasm
Oral contraceptives	Decreased desire
SSRIs	Decreased desire, decreased orgasm
Fluoxetine	Vaginal anesthesia
Tamoxifen	Prolonged use may increase arousal
Tricyclic antidepressants	Decreased orgasm, decreased lubrication

ABBREVIATION: SSRI, selective serotonin reuptake inhibitor.

cause temporary or permanent alterations in sexual expression as the result of body image changes, surgically altered sexual anatomy, or decreases in estrogen. Psychiatric problems, such as depression or schizophrenia, are often associated with diminished sexual desire, as are some of the medications used in the treatment of these psychiatric disorders. Chronic pain is often associated with both depression and sexual difficulties related to the pain itself or to the medications prescribed.

Although many medications are not well studied in women, numerous prescribed medications, particularly antipsychotics and antidepressants negatively influence women's sexuality. Commonly used drugs and their potential sexual side effects are listed in Table 5-3. Crenshaw and Goldberg[32] provide an excellent review of the sexual side effects of medications and drugs. Illicit drugs, particularly crack cocaine, also can cause sexual difficulties.

Key History

Sexual health assessment should be a routine part of primary care, and it should not be taken lightly. The clinician must be prepared to deal with all kinds of information and responses from women during history taking. Many women, out of embarrassment, do not initiate discussion with clinicians about the sexual ramifications of their illness, disability, or the treatments they undergo. Other women who experience sexual difficulties secondary to a medical condition or treatment simply accept the diminished or altered sexual functioning as a part of the disease or treatment. They may assume that nothing can be done for them and that improvement is not possible. Thus, it is incumbent on clinicians to initiate discussion.

The clinician can often assist women in identifying and reporting sexual concerns through patient education. When a clinician knows that sexual difficulties may result from a diagnosed problem or treatment, educating her about this possibility will provide an opportunity for her to opt for another treatment. If there are no other treatment alternatives, at least she will understand what is happening if she does in fact experience difficulties.

Although some women may be uncomfortable, embarrassed, or fearful, the clinician can help by explaining that information about sexual functioning is necessary for a complete picture of the woman's health, providing a baseline for any problems that may develop in the future. Clinicians should also indicate that all information would be treated confidentially.

Complete Sexual History

Although it would be ideal for every patient to have a complete sexual history recorded, in most busy practices there is insufficient time to do a complete sexual history on every woman. A complete history includes assessment of any factors that might affect sexual function, including factors discussed in the previous section, and integrating those with many other factors that are already part of a complete health history. Nonetheless, some clinicians conduct the complete sexual history over several visits or schedule a visit whose only purpose is to obtain the sexual history.

Most clinicians, however, are able to conduct a shorter screening sexual history. Each clinician can develop a systematic and consistent set of questions to use. However, the questions in Table 5-4 provide a good screening sexual history. They address psychosocial and medical/biologic aspects of sexuality. Each clinician can add "prompts" after these questions to expand on what a woman might say, particularly if the response is neutral or negative. Such prompts also educate women and demonstrate the clinician's willingness to hear what a woman might think is not appropriate or acceptable. For example, when asked about frequency, a woman indicates that she never has sex. A prompt might be, "Kissing, masturbation, oral sex?" Women who think that "sexual activity" includes only vaginal intercourse, but who engage in many other sexual activities, may then be able to share this information.

Follow-Up Sexual Assessment

Ongoing sexual assessment can be incorporated into the general health assessment at return visits

Table 5-4

Screening Sexual History

Do you feel that you have a good sexual drive?
When you are sexual, do you feel adequately aroused? Do you lubricate sufficiently well?
How frequently do you engage in sexual activity? Are you OK with that?
What kinds of sexual activities do you usually do? Are you OK with that?
Do you experience any pain associated with your sexual activity?
Are you able to reach orgasm? Do you have any concerns about this ability?
Are your partners men, women, or both? (If multiple partners, how many partners do you have?)
How well do you get along with your partner(s)?
Have you ever had any sexual concerns related to illnesses or medical treatments?
Would you like to change anything about your sex life?
Are there any sexual concerns that you would like to discuss?

Table 5-5
Follow-Up Sexual Assessment Questions

> Have you made any changes in your sexual
>   practices or changed partners?
> Has the frequency of your sexual activity
>   changed?
> Are you having any difficulty with sexual
>   desire, lubrication, or orgasm?
> Are you having any pain before, during, or after
>   sexual activity?
> Do you have any sexual concerns that you
>   would like to discuss?

with a few simple questions, as shown in Table 5-5. A woman's answers to the screening or ongoing assessment questions will determine the need for a more in-depth history if specific problems related to sexuality are identified. However, no sexual problem should be diagnosed unless the woman confirms that it is a problem. Clinicians must avoid creating problems for women where they do not exist.

In-Depth Sexual Problem History

When a woman, or her clinician, identifies a sexual problem, an in-depth sexual assessment is indicated. It can begin in the same way as any health problem is assessed: subjective description of the problem, onset and duration, and attempts to solve the problem. The woman's own description of the problem is critical because it helps the clinician determine the scope and seriousness of the problem as the woman perceives it. Additional questions that may help to clarify the description of the problem include: What usually happens during sexual activity and how is it different now? When does the problem occur and what is associated with it? These questions help to determine whether the problem is generalized or situational.

A generalized, or global, problem is context-independent of specific circumstances, situations,

stimulation, and partners. A situational problem arises when the dysfunction occurs under specific situations, with (or without) certain forms of stimulation, or with a certain partner or partners. A situational problem is sometimes referred to as partner-specific dysfunction.[33]

Onset and duration of a sexual problem is sometimes classified as lifelong or acquired. Lifelong applies to a sexual concern that has been present throughout the individual's sexual history, and acquired refers to problems that occur after a period of satisfactory sexual function. Acquired problems may also be evaluated as rapid versus gradual onset and as having continuous or intermittent symptoms.[34]

Finally, the clinician may want to ask: Why do you think you have this problem and what do you want to do about it? The woman's explanation and her goals for treatment are important in management. The clinician needs to work collaboratively with the woman, her partner(s), and a qualified sex therapist, as necessary, to provide a treatment plan that will achieve the woman's desired outcomes or help her to adjust her goals to those that are realistically achievable.

Treatment

The goal of health care providers with regard to sexuality is the integration of sexual health into holistic care for women. Clinicians must be aware of their knowledge level about sexuality, as well as their attitudes and personal biases, including sexism, racism, heterosexism and homophobia, ageism, and ableism (i.e., preference for able-bodied, rather than disabled, persons). Among health care providers, ignorance about sexuality is common but not an acceptable excuse for lack of awareness and understanding of female sexuality and sexual problems.

The PLISSIT model[35] is a widely accepted schema for conservative intervention with sexual concerns. The PLISSIT acronym stands for permission, limited information, specific suggestions, and intensive therapy, which identify levels of patient education and counseling. Many clients need permission when they hesitate to try something that is not in their usual repertoire of behaviors or when what they are doing is no longer satisfactory or sufficient. Permission is not specific; it is permission to try something new, to talk openly about one's needs, to risk a new behavior, to be curious, to enjoy erotic pleasure, and so forth. It can be given in written form or verbally. When clinicians give permission, their authority gives the client the freedom to explore without guilt.

The provider of limited information must possess greater sexual knowledge. At this level of intervention the clinician provides limited information in answering, for example, a woman's spoken or unspoken questions about how this illness or treatment might affect her sexuality or about what is typical sexual behavior in a long-term relationship. The information may dispel myths or enhance understanding, for example, about safer sex. The giving of limited information is an educational process that may be all that is needed to enhance a sexual relationship, relieve unnecessary concern, or prevent future sexual difficulties. The clinician may provide reading materials or selected web sites where information can be obtained. These are extremely cost-effective strategies (Table 5-6).

Clinicians who intervene at the level of giving specific suggestions regarding sexual behavior should have a thorough knowledge of the biologic sexual response cycle and of individual and couple dynamics. They must be able to ask specific questions, make a differential diagnosis, and design a medical or psychological treatment plan that is specific to the concerns expressed. Specific suggestions may include activities to perform or avoid, specific positions to use for intercourse, or timing of sexual activities when a woman is most rested or comfortable.

An open mind and sex-positive attitude is required to be a good permission giver. To provide limited information the clinician must be a good listener and have enough general sexual knowledge to give basic sexuality education. A qualified sex therapist may be best able to accurately assess and treat sexual disorders and dysfunctions within the behavioral/cognitive sex therapy modality.

Intensive therapy, the highest, most costly, and longer level of treatment, should be reserved for those who cannot benefit from the other more conservative treatment interventions. Intensive therapy is appropriate for persons with serious mental disorders or intrapsychic problems that prevent working directly with a sexual concern, disorder, or dysfunction.

The health or mental health clinician must know when to refer to a qualified sex therapist,

---

Table 5-6

Selected Readings and Internet Sites

www.aasect.org	American Association of Sex Educators, Counselors, & Therapists
www.indiana.edu/~kinsey	The Kinsey Institute
www.plannedparenthood.org	Planned Parenthood Federation of America
www.sexologist.org	The American Board of Sexology
www.siecus.org	Sexuality Information and Education Council of the United States
www.ssc.wisc.edu/ssss	Society for the Scientific Study of Sex

Boston Women's Health Book Collective: *Our Bodies, Ourselves for the New Century: A Book By and For Women.* New York: Touchstone; 1998.
Cole E, Rothblum ED (eds): *Women and Sex Therapy.* Binghamton, NY: Haworth; 1989.
Kitzinger C: *Woman's Experience of Sex.* New York: GP Putnam's Sons; 1983.
Reichman, J: *I'm Not In The Mood: What Every Woman Should Know About Improving Her Libido.* New York: William Morrow & Company; 1998.

and the sex therapist must also recognize when to refer for another level of treatment (i.e., medical intervention or intensive psychotherapy). Referrals to other types of treatment should be explained and the woman should be involved in the decision-making and subsequent care.

Most of the sexual difficulties or problems in clinical practice are problems that can be identified by a primary care provider. The provider can often manage such problems using the PLISSIT levels of intervention.

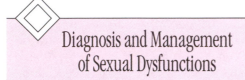

Diagnosis and Management of Sexual Dysfunctions

Epidemiologic data are scant with respect to the prevalence of sexual dysfunction in community populations of women. A recent analysis of data from the 1992 NHSLS found that 43 percent of women reported sexual dysfunction within the past 12 months (defined as a positive response to seven dichotomous items on desire for sex, arousal difficulties, inability to achieve climax, anxiety about sexual performance, climaxing too soon, physical pain during intercourse, and not finding sex pleasurable).[36] The most common category of dysfunction was a low sexual desire (22 percent prevalence), followed by arousal problems (14 percent) and sexual pain (7 percent). Women reporting emotional or stress-related problems were more likely to experience sexual dysfunction in each category; in contrast, women reporting poor health were only at increased odds of experiencing sexual pain.

The differential diagnosis for sexual dysfunction includes a purely psychological/relational cause (due to psychological factors), a purely biologic/pharmaceutical cause (due to a general medical condition or substance-induced), or a combination of psychogenic and biogenic (due to combined factors).[9] Historically, underlying cause was perceived simplistically as either psychological (psy-

chogenic) or organic (biogenic). A more holistic model portrays a continuum, along which there is a combination and interaction of mind and body. Dysfunctions of biologic etiology are quite likely to have both an emotional and a physical impact on each individual within a relationship and on the relationship itself. Medical intervention (e.g., testosterone injections) with one partner may not resolve relationship issues (e.g., emotional distancing or feelings of pressure) that existed in the relationship before or as a result of dysfunctional interactions during the course of the underlying physical problem. In addition, female sexual disorders, classified according to the diagnostic criteria in DSM-IV, may coexist with other mental or physical disorders and may be secondary to other nonsexual disorders.[9] A woman may have more than one sexual dysfunction, and in the assessment, the relationship between them must be carefully explored. Moreover, a woman may present with a sexual disorder in the company of a partner who also has a diagnosable sexual dysfunction.

Sexuality is an aspect of life that, for most women, is shared with one or more partners. The expression of her sexuality is both influenced by and influences these relationship(s). A partner-specific sexual concern most clearly points to the necessity for a careful evaluation of the emotional and physical aspects of a woman's relationship, as well as her own psychological nature and the psychology of her partner. However, even when the dysfunction is presented as more global, the impact on a partner and the impact of a partner's reaction to the woman is significant and cannot be ignored. The complex interactional dynamics of a relationship cannot be fully comprehended in a brief office visit. The planning of a treatment strategy must involve a judgment of where first to place the therapeutic emphasis.

To be diagnosed as a sexual dysfunction, an identified sexual problem must be causing the woman personal distress or interpersonal difficulties and must meet specific criteria, which are presented in the next section.[9] Although a woman may exhibit the defining criteria, if she does not have personal or relationship difficulties as a result, the sexual dysfunction cannot be diagnosed.

Sexual Desire Disorders

There are four important issues concerning sexual desire: what it is, how to measure it, sources of its deficiencies and excesses, and the line between normal and abnormal levels of desire.[37] Sexual desire has many definitions. It may be physical sensations that originate in the limbic system of the brain, specifically the hypothalamus, that are mediated through the spinal cord to the genitals. It may be emotional sensations of feeling sexy or "horny." Sexual desire is part memory and part expectation; it is cognitive. The sensations of desire cease after sexual gratification.[8] Positive sexual experiences can enhance desire, and negative sexual experiences can inhibit desire.

Sexual desire can also be defined in terms of the frequency of sexual activity and the individual's subjective interest in having participated in that act. With this definition, either the lack of internal motivation or the absence of overt activity could indicate diminished sexual desire. Spontaneous desire for sexual arousal can be differentiated from desire elicited from external stimulation.[38] With all of these definitions, diagnosing a desire problem is complicated, and clinicians must be careful to consider all potential causative factors.

HYPOACTIVE SEXUAL DESIRE DISORDER (DSM-IV DIAGNOSTIC CODE 302.71)

The diagnosis of hypoactive sexual desire (HSD) is based on persistent or recurrent absence of sexual fantasies and desire for sexual activity.[9] HSD is often referred to as the lack or loss of libido and was originally referred to as inhibited sexual desire (ISD).[7] The term hypoactive recognizes that some clients with low desire may be responding to biologic processes rather than purely psychological ones. Women with HSD may present in different ways. A woman might never have had sexual desire, might have lost desire after having felt it, or might feel desire for some object/person of attraction but not feel an attraction for a specific partner.

A common precipitating condition, bringing an individual or couple into therapy, is a desire discrepancy or disparity in the relationship. In this instance one partner (not necessarily the woman) experiences a lower sexual appetite (desire) than the other, causing psychological distress to one or both. It is possible, however, that one partner has a "typical" level of desire and the other is sexually hyperactive.[39] There is no DSM-IV diagnostic code for an unusually high sex drive.

DIAGNOSIS In the assessment, clinicians must consider all factors that might account for the desire deficit. Comprehensive evaluation must differentiate between lifelong/acquired and general/ situational subtypes. The history should reveal whether the sexual dysfunction is confined to the desire phase or whether there are also problems with arousal, orgasm, or sexual pain, and if there are, which occurred first.

Lifelong HSD requires evaluation of laboratory data, including complete blood count, fasting blood sugar, lipid levels, urinalysis, creatinine, thyroid function studies, as well as estrogen, progesterone, testosterone, prolactin, luteinizing hormone, and follicle-stimulating hormone studies (Table 5-7). A complete physical examination should also be performed to determine whether any physical problems, especially endocrine difficulties, are responsible.

When a woman has experienced a good sexual appetite but loses desire, the circumstances surrounding this loss must be explored. Was it after starting on an oral contraceptive or another medication (see Table 5-3) or after giving birth? Was it after discovering a partner's infidelity, after the death of a loved one, or after surgery that adversely altered her body image? Was it after a hysterectomy or chemotherapy?

MANAGEMENT If any physical problem is identified, that problem must be treated first. If the woman is taking a medication with sexual side effects, and the medication can be changed or stopped, that

Table 5-7

Laboratory Investigation of Lifelong Hypoactive Sexual Desire

TEST	SIGNIFICANCE
Complete blood count	Iron deficiency anemia
	High mean corpuscular volume (MCV) without anemia could suggest chronic alcoholism
	High white blood count could suggest leukemia or autoimmune disorders
Fasting blood sugar	Diabetes mellitus
Lipid levels	Cardiovascular disease or thyroid disorders
Urinalysis	Glucosuria suggests diabetes mellitus Proteinuria could suggest renal disease
Creatinine	Elevated level suggests renal disease; can be high with hypothyroidism
Thyroid function studies	Hypothyroidism (this can also be associated with depression)
Sex hormones (estrogen, progesterone, testosterone)	Low levels may indicate ovarian or adrenal failure (affects arousal and desire)
Pituitary hormones (prolactin, LH, FSH)	FSH controls the secretion of estrogen High prolactin could suggest a pituitary tumor

ABBREVIATIONS: LH, luteinizing hormone; FSH, follicle stimulating hormone.

should be attempted. Such approaches may resolve the desire disorder.

In women who have low androgen levels, particularly women who have had their ovaries removed, testosterone therapy can improve sexual desire.[40] Potential adverse effects include virilizing side effects (e.g., hair growth, deepening of voice, acne, decreased breast size, clitoral enlargement; 3 to 9 percent), adverse effects on serum lipids (increased low-density lipoproteins, decreased high-density lipoproteins; 3 to 9 percent), and hepatotoxicity (1 to 3 percent). These potential side effects must be weighed against possible benefit. Other drug therapies for desire disorders include yohimbine or antidepressants. However, the lack of demonstrated therapeutic effect of yohimbine[41] and the sexual side effects of antidepressants[42] make these therapies equivocal at best. Bupropion is one antidepressant that may improve libido.[42]

When difficulty with sexual desire appears to be partner specific, couples therapy is indicated. A woman in a relationship with an unreasonable and demanding partner first needs help with her relationship. A demanding partner who is uncooperative, impatient, or hostile will seriously impede the progress of therapy. Conversely, a more positive prognosis is seen when the partner is loving, respectful, and willing to devote the time to resolve the desire discrepancy.

In a behavioral/cognitive approach to couples therapy, the skilled therapist cooperates with the couple in developing a behavioral strategy to remove any performance demands. The behavioral prescriptions (i.e., "homework") involve specific suggestions to begin moving the woman into comfort with nonsexual touch and a focus on sensual experience. These stepwise behavioral assignments are called sensate focus exercises.[43]

The timing of each progressive step is negotiated with the couple, with assistance given to foster effective verbal and nonverbal feedback during the sensate focus sessions. If the woman becomes aroused and can reliably achieve orgasm, during the course of the therapy she learns to trust her body and her partner and without spontaneous desire will allow the stimulation that will trigger her excitement.

SEXUAL AVERSION DISORDER (DSM-IV DIAGNOSTIC CODE 302.79)

Sexual aversion disorder is the "aversion to and active avoidance of genital sexual contact with a sexual partner."[9] The woman with sexual aversion will report anxiety, fear, or disgust when confronted with a sexual opportunity or assertive sexual partner. There may be a specific aversion to genital contact, such as vaginal penetration, or to vaginal secretions. For some women, kissing, fondling, or even visual stimulation will engender an experience of revulsion. The aversion may also be an aversion to talking or reading about sex and even thinking about sex. The intensity of the subjective experience when exposed to the aversive stimulus may range from moderate anxiety and lack of pleasure to extreme anxiety, fear, or panic.

DIAGNOSIS In the history the clinician must first differentiate between sexual avoidance and sexual aversion. Avoidance is typically the reaction to performance anxiety or the fear of failure; it is less intense, more passive, and more subtle than aversion.[34] For the individual or couple, over time, it becomes "safer" to avoid a sexual attempt than to risk the embarrassment, frustration, or anger that is associated with a "failure."

The diagnosis of sexual aversion is problematic for the clinician because it may be a marker of early childhood sexual abuse. With a woman who is sexually aversive, this may be an extremely delicate topic to approach in a time-limited initial office visit; a scheduled follow-up visit or referral should be considered. Caution must be taken to be certain that a woman is ready and willing to discuss her history of abuse. Conversely, if there is no history, the woman may jump to the conclusion that the clinician knows something she does not know. She may begin worrying needlessly about a history that does not exist. Caution should also be taken not to suggest a history that the woman does not recall.

In addition, the woman with sexual aversion might be a lesbian who has not yet accepted or assimilated this identity. Growing up in a homophobic society with the expectation that every woman should be emotionally and physically attracted to men can make self-awareness/self-acceptance difficult. Internalized homophobia, the unconscious assimilation of anti-gay prejudice, can be devastating to a woman who is lesbian. However, for some women, it may be less traumatic to be sexually aversive than to be homosexual. Although abuse and homosexuality should be considered in the differential diagnosis of sexual aversion, it is wrong to assume automatically that a woman with sexual aversion has been sexually abused or that she must be a lesbian.

MANAGEMENT Lifelong (primary) sexual aversion is extremely difficult to treat. The aversion is likely to be related to deep-seated psychopathology requiring long-term intensive therapy. In fact, given the strength of a sexual aversion, the individual is unlikely to independently seek help for the sexual concern, but rather may appear as the resistive, hostile, or anxiety-ridden party coerced into the office by a distressed, bewildered, frustrated, or angry partner. For such women, the motivation around sex is to avoid it, not to work on it, and these women may have had difficulty maintaining relationships all their lives.

Most typically, individuals with deep-seated intrapsychic disorders are seen by clinicians for their other behavioral/emotional manifestations and it is only in the course of the initial assessment that the sexual aversion will be noted. Antianxiety and antipsychotic medications may facilitate access to a discussion of sexual concerns, but the aversion may remain unresolved. Given the complexity and deep-seated nature of sexual aversion, most women should be referred to a qualified mental health professional, skilled in the evaluation and treatment of the full range of sexual concerns, including sexual dysfunction, sexual abuse, and issues of sexual orientation.

Female Sexual Arousal Disorder (DSM-IV Diagnostic Code 302.72)

Sexual arousal can be described as a psychophysiologic state. Women's arousal has been studied in the laboratory, most often through evaluating the physiologic and subjective response to pornographic films. Female laboratory volunteers consistently have a physical, genital response, within seconds, to such stimuli. However, subjective arousal and physical arousal correlate poorly.[44]

The DSM-IV reflects the Masters and Johnson[6] description of female arousal as involving the mechanical processes of vasocongestion and vaginal lubrication. The diagnostic criteria, therefore, include the persistent or recurrent inability to attain or to maintain an adequate swelling-lubrication response that results in significant distress to the woman or her partner(s).

DIAGNOSIS   Female arousal disorder is often associated with a desire disorder or with an orgasmic disorder. It is more typically the absent or reduced subjective sense of sexual passion, rather than the absence of physiologic internal/external changes, that lead women to seek professional assistance.[45] Hence, attention to arousal problems is often lost in the greater attention paid by clinicians to problems of sexual motivation and orgasm. However, the absence of physical arousal is a significant problem that might result in sexual avoidance and sexual pain.

A woman who has problems of arousal, therefore, might report physical discomfort or pain with stimulation of her external genitalia or with vaginal intercourse. With a nonmenopausal woman, who is not lactating or taking a medication with lubrica-

tion side effects (see Table 5-3), an indication that an artificial lubricant is being used might suggest an underlying arousal disorder. Laboratory assessment may reveal low estrogen levels.

In the history, it is essential to differentiate between problems of desire and problems of arousal. When the problem is determined to be one of difficult or absent arousal, it is extremely important to differentiate between a persistent global problem and one that is situational or partner specific, because the precise diagnosis dictates the treatment direction. Global arousal disorder, especially when lifelong, is likely to have a biologic etiology.

MANAGEMENT   When the arousal problem is situational, understanding what is happening in the woman's life is most useful to help her plan a better strategy for coping with the stress in her life, so that she is less likely to compromise her ability to relax in the bedroom. Her job, children at home, a parent in an adjoining bedroom, a noisy neighborhood, or the telephone can all be sources of situational difficulty. The clinician can assist the woman and her partner to find creative ways for privacy and to see that they can take control and make time for their sexual play. With the motivation to be sexual and an artificial lubricant, such as K-Y Jelly (or Astroglide), comfortable penetration can be accomplished.

If the arousal problem is partner specific, non-sexual aspects of the emotional relationship might demand attention before turning to the sexual matters. In such instances, marital therapy must precede sex therapy. There are, however, couples in whom the relationship is sound, but there is sexual ignorance, poor sexual communication, or ineffective sexual techniques. It is only with a very detailed inquiry that the clinician can determine that the primary need is permission, general information, or creative individualized suggestions.

After giving suggestions and possibly some behavioral homework, it is advisable to have an early follow-up visit to determine whether or not the couple understood and followed the suggestions. Verbal compliance in the office does not always result in behavioral compliance in the bedroom. The clinician may not discover that an important piece of information in the history was missed until the couple reports an inability or unwillingness to do the homework. Sex therapists view the giving of behavioral prescriptions as a part of the ongoing assessment of a very complex multifaceted human problem. A sex therapist will inquire into the resistance to uncover dynamics (in the environment, in the woman's psyche, or within the relationship) that were not immediately apparent. Based on new and evolving information, the homework will be renegotiated, the direction of the therapy temporarily diverted, or the focus of the treatment completely changed.

If the problem is related to low estrogen levels, whether or not the woman is menopausal, application of a small amount of estrogen cream to the vaginal tissues twice a week can be helpful. A small amount of 2 percent testosterone ointment (which usually must be specially compounded by pharmacists) applied to the labia once a week will also enhance arousal in some women. Use of hormones in menopause is discussed in Chap. 4.

Female Orgasmic Disorder (DSM-IV Diagnostic Code 302.73)

Women expect that they will have orgasms. Moreover, women often believe that having one or more orgasms is the ultimate goal of sexual activity.[46] They may expect that it should happen with each sexual encounter, and failure to achieve orgasm is often perceived as a personal deficit, a lack of caring, or a reflection on the partner's sexual abilities. Nonetheless, most women do not consider orgasm as their most important source of sexual pleasure.[47]

Many studies have investigated women's experiences of orgasm. Although results vary considerably, the majority of women report having experienced an orgasm at some time. However, only 29 percent of women in the NHSLS reported always having orgasms with their primary sexual partner in the past year.[10] Some women feel pressured by a partner to have an orgasm. Still, many women do not have orgasms, have them inconsistently, or do not recognize the presence of an orgasm because they expect it to be more spectacular. The majority of women are not orgasmic with vaginal stimulation only, and many women are orgasmic with masturbation but are not with partner stimulation. Some women have orgasms in one coital position, but not in another. Some have orgasms with manual stimulation but not oral, but for others cunnilingus works and manual stimulation does not. Others will achieve orgasm exclusively with the intense stimulation of a vibrator.

When a sexual encounter becomes intensely focused on the goal of orgasm, the experience of intimacy and playfulness may be jeopardized. "Performance anxiety" was originally identified as a male problem, related to psychogenic erectile disorder.[43] However, when a woman loses her focus on pleasure and focuses on accomplishing a goal (for her partner or for herself), she is likely to experience anxiety and may actually limit her ability to reach orgasm.

Although occasional difficulty in reaching orgasm is fairly common, the total inability ("primary orgasmic dysfunction") to achieve orgasm is reported in about 10 percent of women.[47] Barbach[48] used the label "preorgasmic" for these women, reflecting the belief that all women are capable of learning how to achieve their orgasmic response. Such optimistic affirmations, despite the best of intent, reinforce the assumption that sexuality is about orgasm and that every woman should strive to reach this goal.

DIAGNOSIS A diagnosis of orgasmic disorder (or anorgasmia) is made when the woman reports a persistent or recurrent delay in, or absence of, an orgasm after having reached a high level of sexual excitement.[1] Sometimes the diagnosis of anorgasmia is made during an assessment of low sexual arousal.[49] The diagnosis of orgasmic disorder is laden with multiple subjective variables on the part of the woman, her partner(s), and the clinician. Clinical judgments must be made based, among other things, on the woman's age, physical condition, the nature of the stimulation, the quality of her relationship, and the woman's expectations.

It is always necessary to rule out medical explanations for an orgasmic dysfunction, especially if it is an acquired or sudden onset. With the increased use of antidepressant medications, specifically selective serotonin reuptake inhibitors (SSRIs), many women are developing orgasmic disorders, secondary to therapy (see Chap. 9). Some women develop difficulty with orgasms after hysterectomy, especially with oophorectomy.

Chambless and DeMarco[50] developed the Woman's Sexuality Questionnaire to assess the frequency and subjective experience of female orgasm, as well as the activities leading to orgasm. Birch[34] developed a comprehensive clinical assessment questionnaire for female sexual concerns. These published questionnaires are too detailed and time-consuming for initial screening in a primary care setting. However, the questions in Table 5-8 can be used to determine whether a concern about orgasm exists.

These questions may well open other avenues of inquiry and opportunities for education. Women have expectations that influence their perception of their sexuality as functional or dysfunctional. It is important to talk to these women to determine what it would mean psychologically if, for example, they were orgasmic during coital activity, capable of multiple orgasms, or able to climax simultaneously with a partner. Women

should be helped to understand the diversity of female sexual experience, and each woman must be assisted in seeing her uniqueness as valid. If the performance concerns are generated by the partner, that individual must be included in any attempts to bring the issues into clearer focus and arrive at a reasonable compromise. These questions also allow a clinician to determine whether a change of medication is indicated.

MANAGEMENT   In the evaluation of an orgasmic concern, the clinician often has an opportunity to provide permission for the variety of orgasmic experiences, as well as offer helpful information to the woman and her partner with regard to realistic expectations. Most of all the clinician must affirm the woman's choice of what she wants for herself with regard to her sexual response.

With adequate direction, the majority of women with primary or lifelong orgasmic disorders are capable of orgasm, although not necessarily easily, reliably, or multiply. The woman must learn to relax and to block out mental distractions. The use of sexual fantasy is recommended to facilitate an erotic focus, and women can be encouraged to learn about their bodies through masturbation.[51] Women need to practice letting go and claiming their right to pleasure. Once a woman becomes orgasmic on her own, she can help her partner (if in a relationship) understand what works best for her by giving verbal feedback and by guiding her partner's hands.

If progress is slow with manual stimulation or if arousal seems to plateau, vibrators are recommended to women who are comfortable using something that many see as "mechanical." Mechanical or not, many women have learned to be orgasmic with a vibrator and rely on them to gain their sexual satisfaction.

If the concern is with sporadic orgasms, an attempt should be made to assist the woman in identifying a pattern that might give clues to how best to be of help. For example, she might be more easily orgasmic at one point in her menstrual cycle than another, or with one partner than with another. If she is orgasmic alone, but not

Table 5-8

Questions for Detecting Orgasmic Disorder

Do you feel that you are having any problems reaching orgasm?

Has your ability to reach orgasm changed over time? When? How?

Have any medications (including birth control pills) interfered with your orgasms?

Has your partner expressed any concerns about your orgasms?

with any partner, can she identify the difference? Relaxation training, techniques for erotic focus, and masturbation may be involved in the specific suggestions given. Partner involvement is essential if the woman has a partner, particularly if the concern involves that relationship. Couples counseling allows the provider an opportunity to explore expectations, to discover personal taboos, to explore new options, and to guide the partnership into mutually satisfying encounters.

Treatment of acquired orgasmic dysfunction requires attention to the presumed causative problem. If the dysfunction can be related to a medication, the drug should be changed or stopped, if possible. Although Viagra is not yet approved for use in women, it is being tested in women who have had oophorectomies. Although it is too soon to assess the outcome of this research, one woman who had taken Viagra was quoted in an Associated Press newspaper article (May 1, 1998), as saying she had her "first orgasm since my hysterectomy five years ago." Such media attention may stir unrealistic expectations among women, their partners, and health care clinicians.

Sexual Pain Disorders

DYSPAREUNIA
(DSM-IV DIAGNOSTIC CODE 302.76)

Nearly two-thirds of all women who have been sexually active have suffered from dyspareunia at one time or another.[52] Dyspareunia is characterized by genital pain associated with sexual penetration, although pain may also occur with non-coital stimulation and may linger after sexual activity has ceased. Dyspareunia can be associated with pelvic or vulvar pathology, infection, atrophic changes, or psychological concerns. Insufficient lubrication is the most common cause of superficial dyspareunia in women 30 to 50 years of age and in lactating women.[53] Third- or fourth-degree episiotomy extension tears are likely to result in dyspareunia.[54] Vulvar vestibulitis syndrome (VVS), the major subtype of vulvar pain and dyspareunia, accounts for about 15 percent of all sexual pain complaints by women.[55]

DIAGNOSIS   The accurate assessment of female sexual pain is a serious challenge to clinicians of both medical and psychological professions. If there is not time for a detailed history, these two questions will likely signal any issues that require attention:

- Are you experiencing any pain or discomfort during sexual activity?
- (If yes) Is that with intercourse, other sexual activities, or both?

If there is an indication of dyspareunia, the clinician should inquire about the location of the discomfort—external genitalia, introitus, along the walls of the vagina, or deep within the vagina or lower abdominal area. Inquiry should include questions about the nature of the pain, whether sharp, dull, burning, shooting, pinching, or stretching. The assessment should also determine any pattern, such as is pain felt only in certain positions of intercourse, only at certain times of the month, related to the level of subjective arousal, or only with a certain partner but not another (past or present)?

Because difficulties of arousal can masquerade as pain, questions regarding sexual activities might reveal that intercourse is attempted prematurely, with discomfort the price of impatience. The skilled clinician can offer specific suggestions, tailor-made for the problem. Even if a physical problem is diagnosed, the woman should be questioned about the impact of the problem on her relationship(s) or on her sexual self-esteem. Because sexual problems may have a combination of biogenic and psychogenic components, a pharmaceutical prescription may not address all of the holistic concerns of a woman, living in the context of her significant relationships and stressful environment. Women who have dyspareunia, of whatever origin, often have emotional sequelae or feel inadequate as a sexual partner. Out of the fear of pain they may avoid sexual activities completely, which can disrupt existing relationships, or prevent the establishment of new ones.

"Deep" dyspareunia, at the cervix or lower abdomen, may indicate pelvic inflammatory disease or endometriosis. However, clinicians should not hesitate to ask about perceived size incompatibility (i.e., "Do you feel that your partner is too big for you?"). Dyspareunia at the introitus, sometimes called "superficial" dyspareunia, may be due to vaginitis or vaginismus (discussed later). Allergic reactions to contraceptives, douches, or soaps are also possible.

On pelvic examination the position of the uterus should be checked. If the uterus is retroverted or retroflexed, a change in position during intercourse, with the woman on top or on her side, for example, may resolve the problem. The clinician should examine the genitals and pelvic area in an attempt to identify the source and type of pain. Although findings are often unremarkable, the clinician can look for evidence of recurrent vaginal or urinary tract infection (vaginal, urethral, or vulvar erythema or abnormal discharge), scar tissue, adhesions, tumors, or any abnormality that may be causing pain. Insufficient lubrication, associated with postmenopausal vaginal atrophy or low levels of estrogen during lactation, may also be a cause. In vaginal atrophy the mucosa may appear thin, delicate, or pale.

Women with VVS experience chronic and persistent pain when the vaginal vestibule is touched or vaginal penetration is attempted. Extreme tenderness is generally reported with cotton-swab palpation of the vestibular area; physical findings may reveal vestibular erythema.

A Pap smear should be done, and office laboratory testing includes a vaginal smear for wet mount or culture, looking for white blood cells and pathogens (see Chap. 11). A urinalysis should also be considered, looking for evidence of a urinary tract infection (presence of white and red blood cells and bacteria).

MANAGEMENT   Most women with dyspareunia, if they seek care, do so in a primary care setting.

Referral to a qualified mental health professional should only occur when organic etiology has been diagnosed or ruled out. Physical problems, causing painful intercourse, must be diagnosed and treated medically when possible. However, not all causes of dyspareunia can be treated; skin sensitivity may not be cured, even with removal of scars.

If the woman reports deep pain related to her partner's penile thrusting, it is helpful to advise the woman to experiment with various coital positions. It may be helpful if, when on her back, she allows penetration, but then closes her legs. This prevents full penetration even during vigorous thrusting.

Reports of insufficient lubrication should elicit questions regarding adequacy of foreplay and level of arousal before initiating intercourse. If the woman reports prolonged and pleasurable foreplay and a subjective experience of arousal, a good water-soluble artificial lubricant should be recommended. Most pharmacies carry a variety of personal lubricant products (e.g., K-Y Jelly®, Replens®, and Astroglide®) (see Chap. 4).

When no physical etiology can be established by the primary care clinician, and if the woman or her partner are emotionally distressed by the pain, a referral to a behavioral health practitioner is indicated. It is helpful to maintain a file of community resources for referrals of sexually related concerns. Many university hospitals have sexual health clinics staffed by a multidisciplinary team. Often a chronic pain clinic will have a staff member with expertise in dealing with sexual pain. Behavioral health practitioners working in private practice or community mental health agencies and who specialize in sex therapy may be identified by their certification as a Sex Therapist by the American Association of Sex Educators, Counselors and Therapists (AASECT) or by the American Academy of Clinical Sexologists (AACS).

Success of behavioral treatment depends on the patient's motivation, partner cooperation, and an accurate diagnosis. For example, if there are severe relationship issues or if a partner demands intercourse despite the pain caused, the prognosis is dim. If the problem was superficially diagnosed as a sexual pain disorder when the issue was really absence of desire and insufficient arousal, therapeutic interventions must address these dysfunctions first.

VAGINISMUS
(DSM-IV DIAGNOSTIC CODE 306.51)

Dyspareunia and vaginismus may overlap, and care must be taken in the differential diagnosis. There are no reliable estimates of the prevalence of vaginismus in the general population, but reports comprise 12 to 17 percent of women in sex therapy clinics.[56] The essential diagnostic feature of vaginismus is the recurrent or persistent involuntary contraction of the perineal muscles that surround the opening of the vagina. Insertion, attempted insertion, or even the mere approach of a penis, finger, dildo, tampon, or speculum may trigger the muscular contraction.[57] The contraction may range from mild, including some tightness and discomfort, to severe, with penetration rendered impossible. As a result of the sexual pain, both the woman and her partners may contribute to the avoidance of sexual intimacy.

There is no single cause of vaginismus. Despite common assumptions that familial factors such as a sex-negative environment or psychological issues such as fear of intimacy, loss of control, or low self-esteem play a role, the picture is far from clear. Childhood abuse involving sexual penetration, particularly when physical force is used, can negatively affect a woman's adult sexuality; however, the impact of childhood sexual contact and later adult activity remains unclear.[58] Clinicians working with adults who have sexual dysfunctions should always inquire about the possibility of sexual abuse, but must recognize that abuse does not always precede later dysfunction.[59]

Vaginismus can be psychologically devastating, but is particularly traumatic for a couple when it is their intent to conceive. However, many loving couples continue to engage in a variety of noncoital sexual activities, and many women with vaginismus report no difficulty in reaching orgasm with clitoral stimulation.

DIAGNOSIS Unfortunately, some women with primary vaginismus do not seek medical or psychological attention, often believing that they are alone with a grossly abnormal vagina incapable of penile containment. These women are not easily convinced of their normal female anatomy and do not quickly engage in therapy. Women with primary vaginismus who avoid any form of penetration but are responsive to oral and manual stimulation offer a better prognosis. Often these women will come to a clinician when they want to conceive, begin intercourse with a partner, or are curious about what they feel they are missing. Women with vaginismus secondary to dyspareunia of an organic nature date the problem back to a time of persistent sexual pain. Women with vaginismus secondary to trauma offer a special treatment challenge because the posttraumatic stress usually must be addressed before attempting to resolve the sexual concern.

To determine whether the vaginismus is primary (lifelong) or secondary, specific questions such as the following can be asked.

- Are you able to insert a tampon?
- Have you ever had pelvic exams?
- Have you ever been able to experience complete penile penetration?
- Do you think that your vagina is too small to hold a penis?

The answers to these questions are likely to give many leads to follow. Vaginismus may also be diagnosed when the clinician tries to perform a pelvic examination and is unable to do so.

MANAGEMENT The majority of cases of vaginismus are psychogenic in origin and are an example of a true psychosomatic disorder. If in addition to vaginismus, there is sexual aversion, a long-term combination of sex therapy and psychotherapy is indicated.

When the specific symptoms of vaginismus can be addressed, the expedient approach is cognitive/behavioral in nature. The woman is encouraged to spend time doing relaxation exercises and is also instructed in Kegel exercises. It is important for the woman to be able to relax in a sexual encounter and practicing on her own and in private is of help. If she is to learn to relax the muscles that surround the opening of her vagina, it is helpful to first find these muscles with the Kegel exercises and begin gaining a sense of mastery over them.

As a woman learns to relax, she should begin to insert a series of graduated dilators, starting only with those that are easily introduced. An artificial lubricant, such as K-Y Jelly or Astroglide, should be recommended. The woman should hold the dilator at the opening of her vagina and squeeze her pelvic floor muscles three times, slowly tightening and relaxing them.[48] The dilator is then inserted as the woman relaxes from the third contraction. Vaginal dilators can be obtained from Milex Products, Inc. as single vaginal-hymenal dilators ($55.00) or in a set of four ($132.00). The address is 4311 N. Normandy, Chicago, IL 60634, or they can be reached at their website: http://www.milexproducts.com. Vaginal latex dildos may also be used; these can be obtained through Eve's Garden, 119 W. 5th Street, New York, NY 10019.

Dilator insertion should be practiced frequently at home with realistic schedules taken into consideration. Three or four times per week is ideal, but not always practical. If the woman is in a relationship, her partner must be involved in the therapy from the beginning. Initially, as the woman begins the self-insertion of the dilators, the partner needs to adhere to a moratorium on any attempt at penetration. As the therapy progresses, and with the woman, her partner, and the clinician working as a team, partner involvement can be gradually increased. With proper timing, the insertion of a small finger similar in diameter to a comfortable dilator, can be attempted, facilitated by sufficient arousal and extra lubrication if needed. With fingers as with dilators, the woman may find that it helps to tighten and relax three times before gentle insertion is made.

As the woman becomes comfortable with the dilation and confident that her partner will not rush, the partner can insert the appropriate dila-

tors during sex play. As dilators increase in size and penetration is found to be comfortable, larger fingers can be inserted. The care provider must caution the partner to be patient because treatment might extend over 6 months.

Only after there is comfort with dilators equal in size to the partner's penis should penile-vaginal penetration be attempted. The woman must feel in control; it is often helpful if her partner waits at the opening as she squeezes and relaxes three times. Initial penetration must be gradual with the woman controlling the depth. Thrusting must wait until a later time because initially the essential task is for the woman to be able to remain relaxed, accept the penis, and feel comfortable with that containment. In time she will signal her partner when he can thrust and when he must rest. Obviously a cooperative partner contributes significantly to the favorable prognosis of vaginismus.

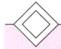

Summary

Sexuality is a central part of most women's lives. Incorporating a sexual history as part of routine examinations will assist clinicians in identifying potential and actual sexual difficulties and dysfunctions in women. Clinicians can evaluate their own knowledge and abilities for managing sexual problems, and in concert with patients, either provide needed interventions or refer to qualified specialists.

References

1. Levine SB: What is clinical sexuality? *Psychiatr Clin North Am* 18:1, 1995.
2. Money J, Ehrhardt AA: *Man & Woman, Boy & Girl.* Baltimore: Johns Hopkins University Press; 1972.
3. Bockting W: Presidential address: sex and sexuality on the transgender frontier. Midcontinent Region,

Society for the Scientific Study of Sexuality, Indianapolis, IN 1998.

4. Money J: *Lovemaps*. New York: Irvington; 1986;105.

5. Dancey CP: Sexual orientation in women. In: Choi PYL, Nicolson P (eds): *Female Sexuality: Psychology, Biology and Social Context*. New York: Harvester/Wheatsheaf; 1994;27.

6. Masters WH, Johnson VE: *Human Sexual Response*. Boston: Little-Brown; 1966.

7. Lief H: What's new in sex research? Inhibited sexual desire. *Medical Aspects of Human Sexuality* 11:94, 1977.

8. Kaplan HS: Hypoactive sexual desire. *J Sex Marital Ther* 3:3, 1977.

9. American Psychiatric Association: *Diagnostic and Statistical Manual of Mental Disorders*, 4th ed. Washington, DC: Author; 1994.

10. Laumann EO, Gagnon JH, Michael RT, Michaels S: *The Social Organization of Sexuality: Sexual Practices in the United States*. Chicago: University of Chicago Press; 1994.

11. Rosenbaum M, O'Hanlan KA: *The AMWA Guide to Sexuality*. New York: Dell; 1996.

12. Andersen BL, Cyranowski JM: Women's sexuality: behaviors, responses, and individual differences. *J Consult Clin Psychol* 63:891, 1995.

13. Schreurs KMG: Sexuality in lesbian couples: the importance of gender. *Annual Review of Sex Research* 4:49, 1993.

14. Dodson B: *Sex for One*. New York: Crown Trade Paperbacks; 1987.

15. Davis CM, Blank J, Lin H, Bonillas C: Characteristics of vibrator use among women. *Journal of Sex Research* 33:313, 1996.

16. Strassberg D, Lockerd L: Force in women's sexual fantasies. *Arch Sex Behav* 27:403, 1998.

17. Leitenberg H, Henning K: Sexual fantasy. *Psychol Bull* 117:467, 1995.

18. Tiefer L: The medicalization of sexuality: conceptual, normative, and professional issues. *Annual Review of Sex Research* 7:252, 1996.

19. Rosen RC, Taylor JF, Leiblum SR, et al: Prevalence of sexual dysfunction in women: results of a survey study of 329 women in an outpatient gynecological clinic. *J Sex Marital Ther* 19:171, 1993.

20. Shafer L: Approach to the patient with sexual dysfunction. In: Stern TA, Herman JB, Slavin PL (eds): *The MGH Guide to Psychiatry in Primary Care*. New York: McGraw-Hill; 1998:271.

21. Thompson S: *Going All the Way*. New York: Hill and Wang; 1995.

22. Silber M: Menstrual cycle and work schedule: effects on women's sexuality. *Arch Sex Behav* 23:397, 1994.

23. Daniluk JC: The meaning and experience of female sexuality. *Psychology of Women Quarterly* 17:53,1993.

24. House WC, Faulk A, Kubovchik M: Sexual behavior of inner-city women. *Journal of Sex Education & Therapy* 16:172, 1990.

25. Wyatt GE, Lyons-Rowe S: African American women's sexual satisfaction as a dimension of their sex roles. *Sex Roles* 22:509, 1990.

26. Engel NS: The maternity cycle and sexuality. In: Fogel CI, Lauver D (eds): *Sexual Health Promotion*. Philadelphia: WB Saunders; 1990; 179.

27. Solberg DA, Butler J, Wagner NM: Sexual behavior in pregnancy. *N Engl J Med* 288:1098, 1973.

28. Forster C, Abraham S, Taylor A, et al: Psychological and sexual changes after the cessation of breast-feeding. *Obstet Gynecol* 84:972, 1994.

29. Bambrick M, Fazio VW, Hull TL, et al: Sexual function following restorative proctocolectomy in women. *Dis Colon Rectum* 39:610, 1996.

30. Leiblum SR, Baume RM, Croog SH: The sexual functioning of elderly hypertensive women. *J Sex Marital Ther* 20:259, 1994.

31. LeMone P: The physical effects of diabetes on sexuality in women. *Diabetes Educator* 22:361, 1996.

32. Crenshaw TL, Goldberg JP: *Sexual Pharmacology: Drugs That Affect Sexual Functioning*. New York: Norton; 1996.

33. LoPiccolo J, Steger JC: The sexual interaction inventory: a new instrument for assessment of sexual dysfunction. *Arch Sex Behav* 3:585, 1974.

34. Birch RW: *A Sex Therapist's Manual*. Columbus, OH: PEC Publishing, 1996.

35. Annon JS: *Behavioral Treatment of Sexual Problems*. San Francisco: Harper & Row; 1976.

36. Laumann EO, Paik A, Rosen RC: Sexual dysfunction in the United States. Prevalence and predictors. *JAMA* 281:537, 1999.

37. Levine SB: Intrapsychic and individual aspects of sexual desire. In: Leiblum SR, Rosen RC (eds): *Sexual Desire Disorders*. New York: Guilford Press; 1988:21.

38. Garde K, Lunde I: Female sexual behavior: a study in a random sample of 40-year old women. *Maturitas* 2:240, 1980.

39. Beck J: What's love got to do with it? The interplay between low and excessive desire disorders. In: Rosen RC, Leiblum SR (eds): *Cases in Sex Therapy*. New York: Guilford Press; 1995;46.

40. Davis SR: The clinical use of androgens in female sexual disorders. *J Sex Marital Ther* 24:153, 1998.

41. Piletz JE, Segraves KB, Feng Y, Maguire E, Dunger B, Halaris A: Plasma MHPG response to yohimbine treatment in women with hypoactive sexual desire. *J Sex Marital Ther* 24:43, 1998.

42. Segraves RT: Antidepressant-induced sexual dysfunction. *J Clin Psychiatry* 59(suppl 4):48, 1998.

43. Masters WH, Johnson VE: *Human Sexual Inadequacy*. Boston: Little-Brown; 1970.

44. Laan E, Everaerd W: Determinants of female sexual arousal: psychophysiological theory and data. *Annual Review of Sex Research* 6:32, 1995.

45. Wincze JP, Carey MP: *Sexual Dysfunction: A Guide for Assessment and Treatment*. New York: Guilford Press; 1991.

46. Riley A: Helping people with sexual problems. *Fam Med* 2:8, 1998.

47. de Bruijn G: From masturbation to orgasm with a partner: how some women bridge the gap—and why others don't. *J Sex Marital Ther* 8:151, 1982.

48. Barbach LG: *For Yourself*. New York: Penguin; 1975.

49. Rosen RC, Beck JG: *Patterns of Sexual Arousal*. New York: Guilford Press; 1988.

50. Chambless DL, DeMarco D: Women's sexuality questionnaire. In: Davis CM, Yarber WL, Davis SL (eds): *Sexuality-Related Measures: A Compendium*. Lake Mills, IA: Graphic Publishing; 1988;110.

51. Heiman JR, LoPiccolo J: *Becoming Orgasmic*. New York: Prentice Hall; 1988.

52. Glatt AE, Zinner SH, McCormack WM: The prevalence of dyspareunia. *Obstet Gynecol* 75:433, 1990.

53. Sarazin SK, Seymour SF: Causes and treatment options for women with dyspareunia. *Nurse Pract* 16:30, 1991.

54. Klein MC, Gauthier RJ, Robbins JM, et al: Relationship of episiotomy to perineal trauma and morbidity, sexual dysfunction, and pelvic floor relaxation. *Am J Obstet Gynecol* 171:591, 1994.

55. Heiman JR, Meston CM: Empirically validated treatment for sexual dysfunction. *Annual Review of Sex Research* 8:148, 1997.

56. Spector IP, Carey MD: Incidence and prevalence of the sexual dysfunctions: a critical review of the empirical literature. *Arch Sex Behav* 19:389, 1990.

57. Beck JG: Vaginismus. In: O'Donohue W, Geer JH (eds): *Handbook of Sexual Dysfunctions: Assessment and Treatment*. Boston: Allyn & Bacon; 1993;381.

58. Browing CR, Laumann EO: Sexual contact between children and adults: a life course perspective. *American Sociological Review* 62:540, 1997.

59. Sarwer DB, Durlak JA: Childhood sexual abuse as a predictor of adult sexual dysfunction: a study of couples seeking sex therapy. *Child Abuse Negl* 20:963, 1996.

Elizabeth A. Alexander
Leslie A. Shimp
Mindy A. Smith

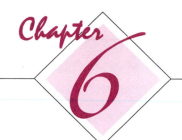

Chapter

6

Obesity and Eating Disorders

MANAGING MEDICAL COMPLICATIONS   *Bulimia Nervosa*
    CARDIAC COMPLICATIONS   HOSPITALIZATION
    GASTRIC COMPLICATIONS   NUTRITIONAL CARE
    AMENORRHEA   MANAGING DYSFUNCTIONAL EATING BEHAVIOR
    OSTEOPOROSIS   PSYCHIATRIC TREATMENT
NUTRITIONAL CARE   **Summary**
PSYCHIATRIC TREATMENT

Obesity

Definition

Obesity is a term that refers to excess body fat. Obesity is defined in several ways, with the standards being different for women than for men. Common methods used to define obesity include percentage of body fat, height and weight tables, and body mass index (BMI, see below), with the latter two measures being useful proxy measures for percentage of body fat. Most experts agree that for women, obesity is present when more than 30 percent of body weight is fat (25 percent for men).

Table 6-1

Body Mass Index Table

BMI	19	20	21	22	23	24	25	26	27	28	29	30	35	40
HEIGHT (INCHES)						BODY WEIGHT (POUNDS)								
58	91	96	100	105	110	115	119	124	129	134	138	143	167	191
59	94	99	104	109	114	119	124	128	133	138	143	148	173	198
60	97	102	107	112	118	123	128	133	138	143	148	153	179	204
61	100	106	111	116	122	127	132	137	143	148	153	158	185	211
62	104	109	115	120	126	131	136	142	147	153	158	164	191	218
63	107	113	118	124	130	135	141	146	152	158	163	169	197	225
64	110	116	122	128	134	140	145	151	157	163	169	174	204	232
65	114	120	126	132	138	144	150	156	162	168	174	180	210	240
66	118	124	130	136	142	148	155	161	167	173	179	186	216	247
67	121	127	134	140	146	153	159	166	172	178	185	191	223	255
68	125	131	138	144	151	158	164	171	177	184	190	197	230	262
69	128	135	142	149	155	162	169	176	182	189	196	203	236	270
70	132	139	146	153	160	167	174	181	188	195	202	207	243	278
71	136	143	150	157	165	172	179	186	193	200	208	215	250	286
72	140	147	154	162	169	177	184	191	199	206	213	221	258	294
73	144	151	159	166	174	182	189	197	204	212	219	227	265	302
74	148	155	163	171	179	186	194	202	210	218	225	233	272	311
75	152	160	168	176	184	192	200	208	216	224	232	240	279	319
76	156	164	172	180	189	197	205	213	221	230	238	246	287	328

NOTE: To use the BMI table, find the appropriate height in the left-hand column. Move across to a given weight. The number at the top of the column (in the BMI row) is the body mass index for that height and weight. Pounds have been rounded off from NIH tables.
(BMI = weight in kg/m^2.)
Normal 19–24; overweight 25–29; obese 30 and over.

BODY FAT

Methods for determining percentage of body fat include skinfold thickness measurement with a caliper at the triceps subscapular or suprailiac area. Additionally, most assessments of overweight people include the waist/hip ratio. The waist/hip ratio is an indicator of abdominal obesity as the pattern of fat distribution. In women, a waist/hip ratio greater than 0.8 results in additional risk for diabetes and cardiovascular disease, independent of the risks conferred by excess weight alone. The National Heart, Lung and Blood Institute (NHLBI) guidelines suggest use of the waist circumference alone (>88 cm or >35 inches) as an estimate of increased risk.[1]

BODY MASS INDEX

The BMI is probably the most reliable and clinically useful measure for overweight and underweight persons, with ranges related to clinical risks for increased morbidity and mortality. BMI is calculated by dividing weight in kilograms by the square of height in meters. For those more familiar with pounds and inches, BMI can be calculated by multiplying weight in pounds by 703 and then dividing by height in inches twice (e.g., for a 5′6″ woman who weighs 155 lb, the formula is 155 lb × 703 = 108,965; divided by 66 = 1650; divided by 66 = 25; BMI = 25).[2] According to both the NHLBI guidelines and the World Health Organization, overweight is defined as a BMI of 25 to 29.9 and obesity as a BMI of 30 or greater.

The BMI may serve as a proxy for percentage of body fat or obesity in most people. The only exception to this principle is in body builders, who have a much higher muscle mass density. Therefore, BMI and height and weight tables are not accurate measures of obesity in this group of people. Table 6-1 provides a conversion table for height and weight into BMI.[3]

EVALUATION OF RISK STATUS

Whatever the classification method of excess weight, it should have relevance primarily to health care providers and patients for health-related risks, rather than being some arbitrary number based on "ideal body type." This classification and risk relationship should be based on the best data available that relate obesity and weight status to chronic health problems. Using BMI as the best marker for obesity, Table 6-2 broadly outlines the categories of BMI related to adverse health risks and mortality that can be used with patients in the clinical setting to identify where they fall in terms of the relationship of weight to medical risk.[4-8]

Prevalence and Trends of Obesity Among U.S. Women

In the United States, 97 million people are either overweight or obese, including almost 51 percent of adult women and 60 percent of adult men.[1]

Table 6-2

Medical Risk Classification of Weight and Obesity, by BMI

BMI < 20	Associated with increased mortality from pulmonary and gastrointestinal disease; some disordered eating patterns (anorexia)
BMI 20–25	Range least likely to be associated with adverse health consequences or increased mortality
BMI 26–27	May lead to adverse health consequences for some people, depending on other comorbid factors
BMI > 27–32	Increasing risk of health problems related to obesity, particularly increased complications and mortality from cardiovascular disease and diabetes
BMI > 32	Risks for heart disease, diabetes, hypertension, premature death related to weight markedly increased

This represents an increase in obesity between 1980 and 1994 from 25 percent of the population to now over 33 percent of the population. Table 6-3 shows the prevalence of obesity among the U.S. population from 1960 to 1994.

The prevalence of obesity is greater among women of most racial-ethnic minority populations than among white women. Asian American women are an exception; they have a lower prevalence of obesity than the general adult U.S. population. Minority women with low incomes have an even higher prevalence of obesity than do minority women who are not poor. Data for Mexican American adult women living in the United States illustrate this trend; for this group, the age-adjusted prevalence of BMI greater than 27 is 46 percent for those living below the federally designated poverty line but only 40 percent for those women living above the poverty line. Additionally, a higher percentage of centripetal obesity in some ethnic groups results in additional cardiovascular and diabetes risks, most notably involving American Indian, African American, and Mexican American women.[9,10] Weight changes with age in women are heterogeneous, but on the whole, weight tends to increase until the age of 55, after which it decreases slightly.[11,12]

The economic costs of obesity are staggering—to individuals, to employers, and to insurers. The estimated direct medical cost of treating obesity in the United States is $51.6 billion, which accounts for 5.7 percent of the national health expenditures. The indirect costs ($47.6 billion), such as lost productivity due to morbidity and mortality, are similar in magnitude to the indirect cost associated with tobacco smoking. Executives at Dupont Chemical estimate that they spend over $400/employee for health problems due to obesity, *not including* hypertension, hyperlipidemia, or programs targeted at increasing exercise in employees. Women are the primary consumers of weight-reducing medications, weight loss clinics, and fad dieting approaches to weight loss. At any one time, as many as 40 percent of adult women are attempting to lose weight, often with the use of nonprescription products.[13–15]

Health Consequences of Obesity

Obesity is the second leading cause of preventable death (second only to tobacco smoking) in the United States, accounting for about 300,000 deaths yearly. The relationship between body weight and disease risk is continuous, and except for very underweight people, the risk of disease increases as weight increases. The consequences of obesity on health are many, particularly among women who are extremely obese. The NHLBI guidelines[1] document an increase in morbidity associated with overweight or obesity for individuals with hypertension, type 2 diabetes, coronary heart disease (CHD), stroke, gallbladder disease, osteoarthritis, sleep apnea, and some cancers. For example, in the United States, at least one-third of all hypertension is related to excess weight. The prevalence of high blood pressure among obese women is doubled, at 32.2 percent compared with a prevalence in normal-weight women of 16.5 percent; this translates into an increased risk for CHD and stroke for obese women. In addition, 88 percent to 97 percent of cases of type 2 diabetes occur in overweight persons, hyperlipidemia is one-and-a-half times more likely in overweight people compared with normal-weight persons, and there is a direct linear relationship between BMI above 27 and death from CHD.[16–18]

Similarly, obese women have three times the risk for CHD, twice the risk for ischemic stroke, twice the risk for colon cancer, and three times the risk for endometrial cancer as normal-weight women. Obesity also increases the risk of maternal and fetal adverse health consequences during pregnancy. Obese women are more likely to develop gestational diabetes (10 percent incidence among obese pregnant women) and hypertension during pregnancy. Obesity in pregnancy is also associated with an increased risk of congenital malformations, particularly neural tube defects. Table 6-4 shows the consequences of increasing weight on a person's health.[16–22]

The relationship between overweight and mortality is less certain than for obesity. The NHLBI guidelines suggest that mortality from all causes,

Table 6-3

Prevalence of Obesity (BMI ≥ 30.0 kg/m^2) Among Adults Age 20 to 80+ Years, by Gender, Race/Ethnicity, and Age:
United States, 1960–1994

	NHES I	NHANES I	NHANES II	HHANES	NHANES III
GENDER, RACE/ETHNICITY, AGE 20 YEARS AND OLDER, AGE ADJUSTED:	**1960–62** (AGE 20–74)	**1971–74** (AGE 20–74)	**1976–80** (AGE 20–74)	**1982–84** (AGE 20–74)	**1988–94** (AGE ≥ 20)
Both sexes	12.8	14.1	14.4		22.3
Men	10.4	11.8	12.2		19.5
Women	15.1	16.1	16.3		25.0
White men	10.1	11.4	12.0		20.0
White women	13.7	14.7	14.9		23.5
Black men	13.9	15.9	15.2		20.6
Black women	25.0	28.6	30.2		36.5
White, non-Hispanic men			12.0		19.9
White, non-Hispanic women			14.8		22.7
Black, non-Hispanic men			15.0		20.7
Black, non-Hispanic women			30.0		36.7
Mexican-American men				15.4	20.6
Mexican-American women				25.4	33.3
AGE AND GENDER-SPECIFIC CATEGORIES:					
MEN					
20–29	9.0	8.0	8.1		12.5
30–39	10.4	13.3	12.1		17.2
40–49	11.9	14.2	16.4		23.1
50–59	13.4	15.3	14.3		28.9
60–69	7.7	10.3	13.5		24.8
70–79	8.6	11.1*	13.6*		20.0
80+	N/A†	N/A†	N/A†		8.0
WOMEN					
20–29	6.1	8.2	9.0		14.6
30–39	12.1	15.1	16.8		25.8
40–49	17.1	17.6	18.1		26.9
50–59	20.4	22.0	22.6		35.6
60–69	27.2	24.0	22.0		29.8
70–79	21.9	21*	19.4*		25.0
80+	N/A†	N/A†	N/A†		15.1

*Prevalence for age 70–74 yrs.
†Not available.
SOURCE: Clinical guidelines on the identification, evaluation, and treatment of overweight and obesity in adults. The evidence report. National Institutes of Health: Heart, Lung, and Blood Institute. June 1998.

Table 6-4

Specific Health Risk Increase (by Percentage) by Increasing BMI, Compared to BMI Below 27

BMI	<20	20–26	27–28	29–31	32–35
Death, all causes	—	—	60%	110%	120%
Death, heart disease	—	—	210%	360%	480%
Death, from all cancers	—	—	—	80%	110%
Colorectal cancer	—	—	—	—	133%
Endometrial cancer	—	—	—	—	155%
Type 2 diabetes mellitus	—	—	>2-fold increase	>5-fold increase	>10-fold increase
Hypertension	—	—	180%	260%	330%
Arthritis	—	—	0%	400%	400%
Gallbladder disease	—	—	150%	270%	270%
Neural cord birth defects in offspring of mothers	—	—	None	90%	90%
Maternal mortality	—	—	None	—	200%
Anorexia nervosa	120%	—	—	—	—
Bulimia nervosa	—	—	—	—	—
Toxemia/eclampsia	—	—	—	—	700%

particularly cardiovascular diseases, is increased for obese individuals by 50 percent to 100 percent compared with normal-weight individuals; for overweight individuals there is little effect of weight on mortality. A recent German study (N = 6193; 4602 women) of the long-term effect (patients were followed an average of 14 years) of obesity on mortality found that the mortality of moderately obese women and men was not different from the mortality of the general population. However, for the gross or morbidly obese, mortality was increased and 57 percent of deaths of morbidly obese women could be attributed to their obesity.[23]

One of the goals of the *Healthy People 2000* report was to reduce the health consequences of poor nutritional and activity habits of the population. Despite the proliferation of health clubs, a 300-fold increase in work site health programs, better food labeling, and improved consumer awareness about the importance of healthy diets, progress toward the goals for both physical activ-

ity and dietary health has gone in a negative rather than positive direction. The rates of obesity for both adults and adolescents have continued to increase, while the percentage of adults and adolescents who engage in regular physical activity has declined.[24] Clearly, because of the health implications of weight problems and inactivity, health care providers must continue to find better ways to motivate patients to lose weight.

The Societal Influence on Disordered Eating: A Differential Influence on Women

One only has to watch a few television commercials, attend movies, or read popular magazines to grasp the cultural bias favoring thinness in the United States. Models and actresses are slender and lithe, beauty pageants define the "ideal" as extremely slim, advertisements enticing the public to buy products, whether it be cars or cigarettes, use svelte women to sell or seduce. The message is clear. If one wants to be loveable, successful, and considered beautiful, one should strive to be thin. The social consequences of obesity verify this social bias and pressure.

Because societal prohibitions on being overweight are stronger for women than for men, the social and personal costs of weight disorders have a more serious effect on women. Overweight individuals have lower rates of acceptance into college despite equal academic qualification. As adults, they earn an average of over $6000 a year less than nonobese individuals. They are more likely to live in poverty, independent of ethnicity. Overweight children are more likely to be viewed by peers as unacceptable friends; this starts a lifetime pattern of self-esteem issues that are difficult to overcome. Although the toll on self-esteem is difficult to quantify, it is significant and clearly appears to be higher for women and girls than for men and boys. Because of the discrimination against overweight persons, obesity has been identified as a disability protected by the Americans with Disabilities Act.[13]

Pathophysiology and Etiology

The ultimate problem for a woman with a weight problem is an imbalance between caloric intake (eating) and caloric expenditure (activity). Further, the weight of any particular individual is affected by a number of complex factors including genetics, environment, childhood feeding patterns, and emotions, in addition to eating and activity behaviors. For many years obesity was thought to be a result of undisciplined behavior, simply eating too much or exercising too little. Obesity is now known to be multifactorial in origin and to have a strong genetic component. It is estimated that up to 80 percent of body weight may be determined by genetic factors. In addition, fat content appears to be regulated by the body and a number of physiologic factors act to maintain the usual body weight, even when that body weight is high. Therefore, although the ready availability of calorically dense foods, a generally sedentary lifestyle, and environ-

mental factors (e.g., watching television) contribute to the development of obesity, behavior is not the only determinant of body weight.[25]

FAMILIAL AND GENETIC FACTORS

Twin and familial studies in obesity have documented the role of heredity in weight problems, with identical twins having consistently more similar weights than fraternal twins. When children come from families in which both parents are of normal weight, they have only a 9 percent chance of becoming obese as adults, whereas if one or both parents are obese, a child's odds of becoming an obese adult increase to 50 percent and 80 percent, respectively. Family eating patterns and food preferences are also learned at an early age, as are patterns of activity and enjoyment of and opportunity for exercise. Although the situation has improved in the past two decades, girls still remain disadvantaged in terms of opportunity for and encouragement of lifetime participation in sports and recreational activities compared with their male cohorts.[26–28]

ENVIRONMENTAL FACTORS

Although genetics is clearly a dominant force in the etiology of overweight and obesity, environmental factors are also important. Among various groups that are similar genetically, certain differences in weight can be explained better by demographic and environmental factors than by genetics. For example, there are differences in the prevalence of obesity among white women with high incomes compared to white women with low incomes. Similarly, population migration studies have shown that individuals moving into the United States tend to gain weight when exposed to the standard U.S. diet.[1]

Environmental influences that most strongly promote overweight and obesity are behaviors related to food intake and physical activity. High-calorie foods are widely available in the United States, and many social events involve consumption of these types of foods. Foods are aggressively marketed and eating in restaurants, where food portions are often large, is common for many people.

For many individuals, work is a relatively sedentary activity and even transportation to work usually involves inactivity (e.g., sitting in a vehicle of some type). Common leisure activities such as watching television and "surfing the web" are also sedentary. Therefore, most individuals must consciously choose to exercise or alter their usual behaviors (e.g., climb stairs at work rather than taking an elevator) to increase physical activity. Choices and behaviors that individuals make within the realms of food intake and physical activity can prevent undesirable weight gain and promote long-term weight management.

MEDICAL CAUSES OF OBESITY

Although many patients would prefer to believe that obesity is caused by a malfunction of the thyroid gland and thus is amenable to drug therapy, this is rarely the case. Table 6-5 details the major causes of obesity, with endocrine and

Table 6-5
Etiology of Obesity

- **Very Common**
  Genetic or familial
- **Common**
  Dietary
  Physical inactivity
- **Uncommon**
  Endocrine problems: Cushing's syndrome, polycystic ovary syndrome, growth hormone deficiency, gonadal insufficiency, hyperinsulinism
  Drug induced: tricyclic antidepressants, phenothiazines, glucocorticoids, synthetic progestins, insulin, anticonvulsants, sulfonureas, lithium
- **Rare**
  Hypothalamic

hypothalamic causes being extremely rare.[8] Of the endocrine causes of obesity, polycystic ovary syndrome is the most common among women (see Chap. 13). It includes in its presentation hyperinsulinism and hyperandrogenism, as well as obesity. However, none of the conditions listed in Table 6-5 should be routinely dismissed without a history and physical examination to eliminate suspicion about a specific cause.

With weight gain being more common than weight loss as a side effect of medication, it is advisable to consider this potential adverse effect when prescribing medication, particularly in women who are already overweight or in those who would view weight gain as a reason for stopping medication. Of the medications listed in Table 6-5, synthetic progestins and tricyclic antidepressants are the most common categories of drugs responsible for weight gain side effects. For most drugs that cause weight gain, however, the gains are modest, in the 5- to 15-lb range; they are generally not enough to be the sole cause of obesity in an otherwise healthy woman.

Diagnosis and Evaluation of Excess Weight

HISTORY

After discussion of risk status, the clinician should evaluate the woman for the presence of diseases that may be related to overweight or those that are worsened by the presence of obesity. This assessment will assist the clinician and patient in establishing treatment goals and approaches. The NHLBI guidelines suggest that the presence of heart disease (congestive heart failure [CHF] or ischemic heart disease), diabetes mellitus, or sleep apnea, in addition to obesity, place the patient at high risk for disease complications and mortality.[1] Cardiac risk factors to assess include tobacco smoking, hypertension, hyperlipidemia, and a family history of premature heart disease (see Chap. 17). Clinicians should also inquire about signs and symptoms of osteoarthritis (e.g., joint pain and swelling), gallstones (e.g., right upper quadrant abdominal pain after meals; see Chap. 19), and stress incontinence (e.g., leaking urine when coughing or sneezing; see Chap. 12); these conditions are more prevalent among women with obesity. The woman's motivation to enter weight loss therapy should also be assessed along with previous experience with weight loss attempts and exercise.

One of the most useful screening tools for eating patterns is to ask a woman to review what and how much she ate in the previous 24 h. This recall, if it represents a typical day, can be instructive in considering how best to help patients change their eating patterns. It will also provide instructive information for both patients and providers about long-standing food habits and preferences, hidden calories that are overlooked (e.g., beverages), and estimates of amounts of food that may be necessary to consider in planning for change. Exercise and activity histories may be similarly useful. These should include not only formal and recreational exercise but also data about stairs at home and at work and sedentary versus active jobs.

PHYSICAL EXAMINATION

The physical examination should be directed toward pertinent positives from the history. Height and weight should be obtained and BMI category determined. Blood pressure should be assessed and heart and lungs examined to look for signs of CHF and to assess respiratory status. A peak flow measure may be useful if shortness of breath is reported. Joints should be examined for evidence of restricted motion, pain, and swelling.

LABORATORY TESTS

The following tests may be considered based on the clinical findings, age, and weight:

- Lipid panel (women over age 45 and/or in the presence of diabetes mellitus, heart disease, or cardiac risk factors)
- Fasting blood sugar (women with a suggestive history for glucose intolerance, including symptoms of elevated blood sugar or history of gestational diabetes or the delivery of babies over 9 lb, or women who have a waist/hip ratio over 1 or BMI above 28)
- Thyroid-stimulating hormone (symptoms of hypothyroidism include fatigue, dry skin, loss of lateral eyebrows, and cold intolerance)
- Sleep study (history of daytime sleepiness and snoring)
- Exercise treadmill (history suggestive of cardiac disease or as needed to determine safety of planned exercise program)

Management of Obesity

PLANNING APPROACHES TO TREATMENT: THE CLINICAL INTERVIEW

Because weight problems can have a severe effect on long-term health, clinicians should address the issue directly during office visits. Just as one would not wait for a patient to spontaneously raise the issues of diabetes or hypertension, a provider should not hesitate about raising the subject of obesity. Several questions need systematic attention when working with patients on these issues. Table 6-6 lists the most important issues to be addressed with the patient in the initial stages of planning for change. A history of a women's typical eating and activity patterns forms the foundation for understanding which approaches are most likely to be successful; additionally, historical information indicates whether or not diagnostic studies should precede a plan for change. Components of this history include weight changes over time, previous successful and unsuccessful attempts at weight management, medication review, family history, current eating patterns, current exercise and activity patterns, and preferred eating and exercise patterns.[29]

GOALS OF THERAPY

When taking the initial history, it may be more productive to define the problem as one of health, rather than one of weight. The goal for change thus

Table 6-6

Planning Approaches to Treatment: Clinical Interview

Does the woman's BMI, combined with other risk factors, involve increased risk to health?
   (If No, reassure and educate)
   (If Yes, continue screening until all questions have been asked)
What is the woman's weight history (long-standing, recent)? If recent, do historical clues to cause of
   changes suggest appropriate intervention(s)?
   (If Yes, tailor an intervention)
Are there elements of the history or physical examination that suggest a medical or drug-related cause for
   obesity?
   (If Yes, evaluate or change medications)
Is there a family and genetic history involving obesity?
   (If Yes, educate)
What is the woman's dietary recall, with food preferences? Does she primarily eat and prefer a healthy diet,
   or does she prefer and select foods at the top of the food pyramid?
   (If Yes, consider further education and/or referral to a nutritionist)
Does this person understand the principles of a healthy diet?
   (If No, consider further education and/or referral to a nutritionist)
Are there ethnic and/or cultural factors that need consideration in planning nutritional changes?
Who does the shopping and meal preparation for this person?
What is the woman's exercise history?
If she does not exercise regularly, what are the options that she would consider possible and fun?
   If she does exercise, can she increase amount or intensity?
   Is this person motivated to lose weight?
   (If No, work toward weight maintenance and increasing activity)
Is it possible to establish sound short-term goals for eating, weight, and activity patterns for this patient?
   (If Yes, use the following as important elements of patient's plan:
      1. Realistic goals
      2. Most useful interval for follow-up
      3. Anticipation of obstacles and strategies to overcome them
      4. Individualized strategies for healthy eating, based on patient's food preferences
      5. Individualized strategies for increased activity or exercise based on patient's preferences
      6. Use of participation in formalized groups if they are likely to benefit this patient)

becomes one of healthy eating and activity habits rather than attaining an "ideal" weight. For years the goal of obesity management was to have the obese patient reduce her weight to "ideal" or a lean body mass. However, improved knowledge of obesity and the genetic factors that establish weight have altered the primary goal of obesity management. This change has occurred for four principal reasons. First, most obese individuals cannot, even with significant effort, reduce their body weight to "ideal." Second, given that weight is determined by a variety of physiologic factors and is resistant to change, altering just one factor (e.g., enhance satiety via drug therapy) is not likely to alter body weight dramatically. Third, most individuals who initially lose weight regain

Figure 6-1

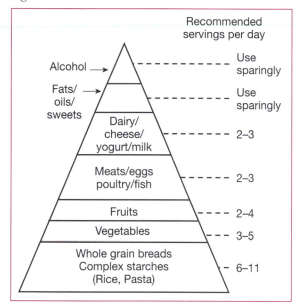

The food pyramid.

STRATEGIES FOR WEIGHT LOSS AND MAINTENANCE OF WEIGHT LOSS

DIET Instituting dietary change is the primary tool for weight loss; most weight loss results from dieting rather than increased physical activity. Dietary modifications focus on reducing the number of calories ingested daily as well as decreasing fat content of the diet and promoting healthy eating. It has been suggested that the diet create a daily deficit of 500 to 1000 calories in comparison to normal intake. In addition, ideally, less than 30 percent of total calories would be obtained from fat. Diets that can be used as models to plan this type of dietary change are the National Cholesterol Education Program's (NCEP) step I and step II diets.[1] Patients can be aided in the selection of foods that restrict fat and calories by use of the food pyramid (Fig. 6-1). The goal for food intake becomes consumption of more foods from the base of the food pyramid rather than from the top. This balance may actually result in a larger volume of different kinds of foods, rather than restrictive small amounts of food.

the lost weight; two-thirds of people who lose weight regain it within 1 year. Finally, improvement in health and reduction in risk for developing obesity-related diseases occur with just modest loss of weight.[2,25] Current recommendations from several medical organizations (Institute of Medicine of the National Academy of Science,[30] 1995 Dietary Guidelines for Americans,[31] NHLBI[1]) now advocate a reduction in baseline body weight of 5 to 10 percent. This modest weight loss has positive effects on risk for disease and is an attainable and sustainable goal for many patients.[32]

By definition, this reframing of goals defines the issue of obesity as long-term rather than short-term and is focused on alteration of eating and activity habits to maximize health rather than simply for appearance. Such an approach helps patients who have defined their weight problems as ones that are shameful and intricately tied up with self-esteem and self-worth and redirects it at promoting health.

PHYSICAL ACTIVITY/EXERCISE Increasing energy output through increased physical activity or exercise is a mainstay of successful weight loss and maintenance. The importance of working with patients toward this goal cannot be overemphasized.[33,34] Increased physical activity is of benefit because it helps to prevent weight regain.[1] In addition, exercise may help patients adhere to their diet modifications; exercise can increase the desire for high-carbohydrate foods and reduce the desire for high-fat foods.[25] Exercise has many other health benefits, including maintenance of muscle mass and tone, increasing bone mass, increasing a sense of well-being, and stress management. Half of all the people in the United States get no regular exercise at all, and most adults do not get enough exercise. More than half of adults who start exercise programs will quit within 6 months of initiating a program.

In general, patients will not maintain exercise over the long haul if it is unpleasant. People usually do best with forms of exercise that they consider to be fun. Additionally, an exercise plan has to be realistically integrated into the rest of a woman's life. For example, the options are very different for a woman who is a single mother of three small children, holding down two jobs and maintaining her family, than they are for someone with more discretionary time and income. Preferred patterns of exercise can be elicited simply by asking the question, "If you were to exercise regularly, what form of exercise would be most pleasurable to you and would fit with your schedule best?" Most women, in response to this question, will tell you what they would like to do. Strategies for assisting patients with increasing physical activity and exercise are listed in Table 6-7.

Exercise becomes more self-reinforcing when done regularly, preferably 5 to 6 days a week. The Centers for Disease Control and Prevention and the American College of Sports Medicine recommend that all adults engage in at least 30 mins of moderately intense physical activity daily.[2] Although any increase in activity is better than none, the length of time to gain cardiovascular benefit with aerobic exercise, as well as have a significant effect on weight, is 30 to 40 mins a day. For some women, this is not possible. The NHLBI guidelines recommend walking as an initial exercise, which is readily available, costs less, and avoids injuries. The intensity and duration of walking can then be increased over time to about 45 mins of intense walking at least 5 days a week. Exercise of this magnitude will result in the "burning" of 100 to 200 calories daily.[1] However, types of exercise may vary in weight loss benefit. Exercise that is of high intensity followed by low intensity may result in greater weight loss than sustained moderate level exercise.[25]

Finally, data suggest that the addition of activity that builds muscle mass, done twice a week, may help in weight loss because muscle tissue burns more calories than does fat. The use of free weights can be done either in the workplace or the home and is inexpensive and readily available. Apart from the metabolic benefits, the building and maintenance of muscle mass has additional benefits on bone density and on strength as women age.

The goal of these activity changes is to reduce sedentary time. For the group of women who do not see exercise as an option, either because of lack of conditioning, lack of time, or difficulty

Table 6-7

Successful Strategies for Increasing Activity and Exercise

STRATEGY	EXAMPLE
Set goals in terms of health, rather than weight	To gain endurance or muscle mass
Make it pleasant	Walking or dancing for people who do not like aerobic exercise
Consider social forms	Tennis, walking with friend
Find additional motivators	Listening to music or news while walking
Set goals within goals	If goal is to run a marathon, first start with 1K
Set specific times for exercise, ones most likely to be successful	Lunchtime walking, on way to or from work
Increase activity that is not formal exercise	Stairs instead of elevators; parking farther away from workplace
Avoid locking into an "all or nothing" mentality	"I missed exercise last week, and so I just gave up."

Table 6-8

Characteristics of Formal Weight Loss Programs

PROGRAM/OPTION	RELATIVE COST	SPECIAL FOODS, SUPPLEMENTS	USE OF EXERCISE	APPROACH
Weight Watchers	$	$	No	Group
Take off Pounds Sensibly (TOPS)	$	No	No	Group
Nutri-System	$$	$$	No	Group and individual
Health clubs/gyms	$$	Sometimes	Yes	Variable
Nutritionists	$$	No	Variable	Individual
Severe caloric restriction programs	$$$	$$	No	Group
Overeaters Anonymous	No cost	No	Variable	Group

NOTE: $ =   range of $10–20/wk
$$ =   range of $20–30/wk
$$$ =   over $30/wk

enjoying an increased activity level, the best approach may be to increase activity levels within their current daily routines, such as using stairs instead of elevators at work.

BEHAVIOR MODIFICATION   The NHLBI guidelines suggest that reinforcement activities be incorporated into the treatment plan. These activities promote adherence to diet and exercise and include stress management, stimulus control, and problem-solving. In addition, an understanding of the meaning of eating and circumstances of eating (when, where, and how an individual eats) will help to modify problematic behaviors. Another option is referral of the patient to a formal weight loss program.

Formal Weight Loss Programs.   A multitude of available programs provide structure, nutritional products, exercise programs, and behavioral modification strategies. One of the reasons that formalized weight loss programs are so popular is that they provide regular accountability and reinforcement for staying with a program or plan. Although some programs may be helpful to some patients, no clear evidence suggests that one approach is more beneficial than others or that

such programs are helpful over and above a plan for dietary modification with increased activity. Table 6-8 summarizes some of the more commonly used options, and Appendix 1 provides addresses for several weight loss and disordered eating organizations.[34]

Helping the Patient Who Gets "Stuck."   Many patients, in the course of trying to change diet and exercise habits, get "stuck" and are unable to achieve further weight loss. Although it is wise to take holidays away from some diet plans, ultimately patients need to learn to have a combination of intake of food and outlay of activity (exercise) that they can maintain as a lifelong pattern. For those who come in with concerns about being stuck, it is useful to update the history of recent diet and exercise habits, as well as the patient's understanding of why their efforts at change could not be maintained. Usually a patient knows what has happened. The role of the health care provider is to act as a coach in helping the woman identify strategies to get beyond the perceived obstacles. Often what is seen as no progress is simply slow, but realistic, progress. The health care provider can reinforce, reassure, and help the patient understand what is realistic.

This is particularly true for women whose BMI is greater than 30, in whom the initial weight loss may be more rapid, setting up expectations that are unrealistic for the long-term process.

PHARMACOLOGIC THERAPY When the patient is obese, with a BMI of 30 or above, and is working toward adopting healthy eating and exercise habits, it is sometimes useful to consider additional medical intervention. Medication or anorectic drugs are not indicated for those patients whose BMI is less than 27 and simply want to lose weight for cosmetic reasons for an upcoming event. Likewise, medication use is not appropriate for those who simply want a quick intervention without dietary and exercise changes. Data clearly show that medications used in this way do not have benefit either for long-term health or maintenance of weight goals. Table 6-9 lists indications for consideration of medication in addition to diet and exercise by BMI.[1, 35–37]

The appropriate role for drug therapy in the management of obesity is controversial and complicated. Drug therapy can produce modest loss of weight, but the effect is sustained only so long as therapy continues. Adverse reactions are a concern, particularly with the use of these agents as long-term therapy. Within the past 2 years two widely used agents (dexfenfluramine [Redux®] and fenfluramine [Pondimin®]) were removed from the U.S. market due to serious adverse effects (primary pulmonary hypertension and valvular heart disease). Therefore, key issues regarding drug therapy for obesity include selec-

tion of appropriate candidates for drug therapy, realistic expectations for pharmacologic therapy, and the potential for adverse drug effects.

Candidates for Weight Loss Drug Therapy. The NHLBI guidelines suggest that appropriate candidates for drug therapy are patients with a BMI of 30 or above without obesity-related diseases or risk factors or patients with a BMI of 27 or above with obesity-related risk factors or diseases.[1] Good candidates are patients who have instituted diet and physical activity modifications for at least 6 months but who have not been able to lose weight effectively (about 1 lb/wk). Weight loss drugs should be used in conjunction with a low-calorie diet and exercise. The role of medications is to help the patient continue with a diet and exercise plan while losing weight and then to maintain weight loss. Furthermore, drug therapy should be seen as a long-term therapy; obesity is a chronic disorder and drug benefit exists only as long as the patient continues to take the medication.

Drug Effects and Efficacy. Both single-drug use and combination therapy usually result in modest weight loss, in the range of 5 to 25 lb. However, in a number of studies with various agents, drug use resulted in a considerably higher number of patients achieving clinically significant ($\geq$10 percent baseline body weight) weight loss. Of the agents currently on the U.S. market, none appears to have superior efficacy.[32]

Loss of weight generally occurs within the first 6 months of therapy and then plateaus. If drug therapy is continued, the majority of agents allow for continued reduction in body weight (no weight regain) over at least a 1-year period. However, some weight regain is commonly seen after 1 year, even with continued drug use. The continuation of drug therapy should be determined by the improvement in obesity-related risk factors or diseases and the tolerability of therapy, along with consideration of the potential adverse effects of long-term therapy. Some patients (up to 15 percent in several recent studies of sibutramine) do

Table 6-9

Choice of Treatment Based on Risk (1 = First Choice)

RISK	DIET	EXERCISE	DRUGS	SURGERY
BMI <27	1	2	NA	NA
BMI 27–33	1	2	3	NA
BMI 34–39	1	2	1	3
BMI >39	1	2	1	2

not respond to weight loss drugs. If therapy has not demonstrated benefit within a month the agent should be discontinued.

Pharmacologic Agents.   The pharmacologic agents currently available on the U.S. market can be categorized into three groups: noradrenergic agents, which suppress appetite; a noradrenergic-serotonergic agent (sibutramine), which enhances satiety; and orlistat, an agent that reduces absorption of nutrients. Sibutramine and orlistat are approved by the Food and Drug Administration (FDA) for long-term use; the noradrenergic agents are approved for only 3 months of therapy.

Noradrenergic Agents   A number of noradrenergic agents are on the market (Table 6-10). Most of the noradrenergic agents act by releasing norepinephrine (mazindol blocks the reuptake of norepinephrine) and thereby suppressing appetite. One agent, phenylpropanolamine, is available as a nonprescription weight loss agent.

Dose/Regimen   The dose and regimen of agents are listed in Table 6-10. Tolerance to the effects of these agents may develop within several weeks of use. Therapy may be continued up to 6 months in patients who continue to lose weight and do not develop dependence (agents are chemically related to the amphetamines) or intolerable side effects. Studies have shown phenylpropanolamine to be most effective at inducing weight loss at the beginning of treatment; it is indicated for only 8 to 12 weeks of use.

Side Effects and Contraindications   Common side effects of the noradrenergic agents result from central nervous system (CNS) stimulation (e.g., insomnia, irritability, and nervousness). Less common side effects include dizziness, nausea, constipation, cardiovascular effects (e.g., palpitations, tachycardia), and depression.

These agents are contraindicated in patients with moderate to severe hypertension, cardiac arrhythmias, symptomatic cardiovascular disease, glaucoma, during or within 14 days of use of monoamine oxidase (MAO) inhibitors, hyperthyroidism, or a history of substance abuse. Diethylpropion and phentermine are not recommended for long-term use because of amphetamine-like effects on the cardiovascular system and CNS.[38] Mazindol was evaluated in one long-term trial, which showed a high drop-out rate (more than 50 percent of patients) due to side effects or lack of effect. However, no significant adverse side effects were noted. Common side effects included thirst, constipation, and fatigue.[38] The long-term safety of other prescription noradrenergic agents has not been evaluated; only short-term studies have been conducted.

Adverse effects from phenylpropanolamine are similar to other noradrenergic agents. Doses of this agent should be limited to 75 mg/d because increased blood pressure can result from higher doses, particularly if the agent is administered in conjunction with caffeine.[38]

Serotonergic Agents   Sibutramine (Meridia®), the newest of the serotonergic agents, inhibits eating (enhances satiety) by inhibiting both norepinephrine and serotonin reuptake within the hypothalamus. It does not affect release of dopamine or serotonin, thus acting differently than the noradrenergic agents. It may also effect weight by stimulating thermogenesis and increasing energy expenditure.[38]

Dose/Regimen   The recommended initial dose of sibutramine is 10 mg daily. It can be given with or without food. Long-term benefit from sibutramine can be predicted by a weight loss of 1.8 kg or more than 1 percent of initial body weight within the first 4 weeks of treatment. Up to 15 percent of patients may not respond to sibutramine, regardless of dose. If benefit is not seen after 4 weeks at 10 mg daily, then the drug should be discontinued or the dose should be increased to 15 mg daily. Weight loss with sibutramine is dose-related; however, doses greater than 15 mg daily should not be used.[39] Maximal weight loss

Table 6-10

Pharmacologic Agents Available for the Management of Obesity

NORADRENERGIC DRUGS

GENERIC	TRADE NAME*	DOSAGE RANGE/ DAY	COMMON SIDE EFFECTS	COMMON ABSOLUTE CONTRAINDICATIONS
Benzamphetamine HCl	Didrex	25–50 mg	Hypertension, cardiac arrhythmias, dependence, withdrawal on discontinuation, anxiety, insomnia, paranoia	Age >60
Diethylpropion HCl	Tenuate, Tepanil	25–75 mg	As above	BMI <27, anorexia
Mazindol	Mazanor, Sanorex	1–2 mg	As above	Uncontrolled hypertension and cardiac disease
Phentermine HCl	Fastin, Ionamin	15–37.5 mg	As above	History of addictive disease

SEROTONERGIC DRUGS

GENERIC	TRADE NAME*	DOSAGE RANGE/ DAY	COMMON SIDE EFFECTS	COMMON ABSOLUTE CONTRAINDICATIONS
Sibutramine HCl	Meridia	5–20 mg	Headache, dry mouth, insomnia, constipation, elevated blood pressure	MAO inhibitor therapy within 2 wk
Fluoxetine†	Prozac	10–60 mg	Pulmonary hypertension	MAO inhibitor therapy within 2 wk
Fenfluramine	Pondamin	60–120 mg	Seizures, hypertension, diarrhea, insomnia, dry mouth, depression on withdrawal, memory deficits	Anorexia, MAO inhibitor therapy within 2 wk

ANTIABSORPTIVE

GENERIC	TRADE NAME*	DOSAGE RANGE/ DAY	COMMON SIDE EFFECTS	COMMON ABSOLUTE CONTRAINDICATIONS
Orlistat	Xenical	120 mg tid with meals	Fatty/oily evacuation, abdominal pain, fecal incontinence	

Table 6-10

Pharmacologic Agents Available for the Management of Obesity *(Continued.)*

		NONPRESCRIPTION PREPARATIONS WITH SOME DEMONSTRATED EFFICACY AND SAFETY		
GENERIC	**TRADE NAME***	**DOSAGE RANGE/ DAY**	**COMMON SIDE EFFECTS**	**COMMON ABSOLUTE CONTRAINDICATIONS**
Phenylpropan-olamine	Dexatrim, Accutrim	25–75 mg	Nervousness, hypertension, insomnia, headache, arrhythmia	Anorexia, hypertension, cardiac arrhythmia, coronary heart disease, diabetes, thyroiditis
Very calorie liquid diets	Optifast, Slimfast	1–4 cans/day	Muscle wasting, fatigue	Anorexia

		NONPRESCRIPTION PREPARATIONS, UNSAFE†		
GENERIC	**TRADE NAME***	**DOSAGE RANGE/ DAY**	**COMMON SIDE EFFECTS**	**COMMON ABSOLUTE CONTRAINDICATIONS**
Guar gum‡	Cal Ban 3000	Variable	Electrolyte disturbances	All patients
Cascara sagrada, diuretics	Diet teas	Variable	Electrolyte disturbances	
Ephedra	Ma Huang Metabolife	Variable	Hypertension, psychosis, MI, seizures	All patients

		NONPRESCRIPTION PRODUCTS, WITHOUT EVIDENCE FOR EFFICACY, PROBABLY SAFE†		
GENERIC	**TRADE NAME***	**DOSAGE RANGE/ DAY**	**COMMON SIDE EFFECTS**	**COMMON ABSOLUTE CONTRAINDICATIONS**
Blue-green algae preparations	Spirulina			
Hydrophilic hemicellulose	Glucomannan		Diarrhea	
Chromium	Marketed in a variety of products	50–200 µg		

*Not exclusive list of trade names.
†Not approved by FDA for weight loss treatment.
‡Taken off market by FDA.
ABBREVIATIONS: MAO, monoamine oxidase; MI, myocardial infarction.

is seen after about 6 months of therapy. After 24 weeks, a clinically significant weight loss of 10 percent was seen in 16 percent of individuals taking 10 mg daily and 28 percent of those taking 15 mg daily. Women tend to lose less body weight than men.[39]

Side Effects and Contraindications   The most common adverse effects, occurring in more than 5 percent of users, are headache, dry mouth, insomnia, and constipation. Sibutramine increases blood pressure and heart rate among some patients; these effects are reversible when the agent is discontinued. In clinical trials, 2.6 percent or fewer patients experienced cardiovascular events such as elevated blood pressure, tachycardia, or palpitations. The mean increase in diastolic blood pressure seen with 10 mg given over 12 months was 1.6 mmHg and heart rate increased on average 3 to 4 beats/min. Blood pressure and heart rate should be monitored regularly, and if a sustained increase in blood pressure or heart rate is seen, particularly if the patient develops hypertension or tachycardia, the drug should be discontinued.

Sibutramine should be used cautiously in combination with agents that may increase blood pressure, including nonprescription sympathomimetics (e.g., phenylpropanolamine, pseudoephedrine). It should also be used with caution in patients with a history of hypertension or seizures (type not defined) and should be avoided in patients with narrow-angle glaucoma. Although this agent differs in mechanism of action from dexfenfluramine or fenfluramine in combination with phentermine (a combination of noradrenergic and serotonergic effects), there are concerns about the long-term safety of the agent given that it has both noradrenergic and serotonergic effects.[38]

Sibutramine is contraindicated in patients with a history of CHD, CHF, arrhythmias, or stroke. Moderate hepatic dysfunction (undefined) does not appear to alter sibutramine kinetics, but this agent is contraindicated in patients with severe hepatic dysfunction as well as patients with renal

dysfunction. This agent is also contraindicated in patients who have taken an MAO inhibitor within the previous 2 weeks or those patients taking a centrally acting weight loss drug. Sibutramine does not effect the efficacy of the combined oral contraceptives.

Antiabsorptive Agent   Orlistat (Xenical®) is an agent that inhibits pancreatic and other lipases in the gastrointestinal lumen, preventing the absorption of about one-third of dietary fat. This agent has limited systemic absorption. After 1 year of therapy, 25 percent of users lost more than 10 percent of body weight compared to 15 percent of those receiving placebo. An additional benefit is the decrease in serum cholesterol levels seen with this agent. In clinical trials, decreases of 6 to 10 percent were seen in total and low-density lipoprotein-cholesterol levels; levels of high-density lipoprotein-cholesterol, however, were also decreased about 8 percent.[40]

Dose/Regimen   Orlistat is administered three times daily, in a dose of 120 mg, with meals.

Side Effects and Contraindications   The side effects seen commonly with orlistat are a result of the inhibition of fat absorption rather than the drug itself. These include abdominal pain (5 percent of patients), fatty/oily evacuation (20 percent of patients), and fecal incontinence (13 percent of patients); these side effects were severe in only 2 to 6 percent of patients.[40] Side effects other than gastrointestinal were not different from placebo.

In theory, absorption of the fat-soluble vitamins (A, D, E, and K) might be decreased by orlistat. However, results of long-term trials (2 years' duration) found orlistat had little effect on the serum levels of these vitamins, and if decreased levels occurred, vitamin supplementation was adequate to reverse the changes in most instances.[2] Vitamin supplements should not be taken at the same dosing time as orlistat.

Orlistat is contraindicated for patients with chronic malabsorption syndrome or cholestasis.

Alternative Therapies. Alternative therapies are widely used by women attempting to lose weight, sometimes inappropriately and with risk to health. Caffeine and ephedrine combinations are one of the most commonly used alternative appetite suppressants. Diet products containing ephedrine are marketed under many names, including Ma Huang, Herbal Ecstasy, Ultimate Euphoria, Metabolife, and protein-containing body-building drinks. The FDA has set the safe 24-h dose of ephedrine as 24 mg, with no more that 8 mg/dose; yet in many unregulated diet programs, the dosage exceeds this amount, going over 100 mg in some cases. For example, one widely advertised product, Metabolife, contains 12 to 24 mg ephedrine per dose (1 to 2 caplets), and at the recommended four times daily dosing, a patient would ingest 96 mg/d.

Both ephedrine and caffeine increase blood pressure and heart rate and, in combination, raise the metabolic rate. In addition, these agents can cause CNS effects (e.g., anxiety, insomnia, restlessness, aggressive behavior). Because patients often believe that products touted as "natural" are safe, they may be less diligent in assessing side effects or adhering to recommended dosages.[35] Health care providers should inquire about the use of these agents when patients experience symptoms consistent with the adverse effects of ephedrine and caffeine.

TREATMENT ALGORITHM

The treatment algorithm, suggested by NHLBI and shown in Fig. 6-2, provides an overview of the assessment for overweight and obesity and diagrams the subsequent management decisions that can be made based on that assessment. Primary care providers are encouraged to identify and address this important and prevalent problem with their patients, provide education, and offer assistance in adopting improved patterns of diet and exercise and the achievement of reasonable weight loss goals.

Anorexia Nervosa and Bulimia Nervosa

Two other patterns of disordered eating—anorexia nervosa and bulimia nervosa—also have significant effect on the health of women. Both disorders tend to begin in young women, between the ages of 13 and 24, and they may occur concomitantly or sequentially throughout adulthood. They are characterized by seriously disturbed eating patterns, including restriction of intake and binge eating (excessive food consumption in a discrete period of time associated with a sense of loss of control over eating), and excessive concern over body shape and weight.

Epidemiology

Anorexia and bulimia affect about 5 million Americans each year and occur within all socioeconomic classes and major ethnic groups.[41] Both disorders are about 10 times more common in women than in men. It is estimated that 5 to 10 percent of adolescent girls in this country have one or both of these disorders, with the incidence of these disorders rising rapidly over the past 25 years. These disorders disproportionately affect girls and women from the majority culture and from middle and upper socioeconomic backgrounds. Alcohol and substance abuse disorders represent significant comorbid diagnoses, particularly among women with bulimia nervosa, as do mood disorders (e.g., obsessive-compulsive disorder among women with anorexia and depression and anxiety among those with bulimia).[42,43]

With respect to the etiology of these disorders, most authors support a multidimensional perspective including a biologic predisposition and many of the antecedents listed in Table 6-11.[44] The types of individual problems encountered and family and cultural pressures result in experiences of

Figure 6-2 Treatment algorithm

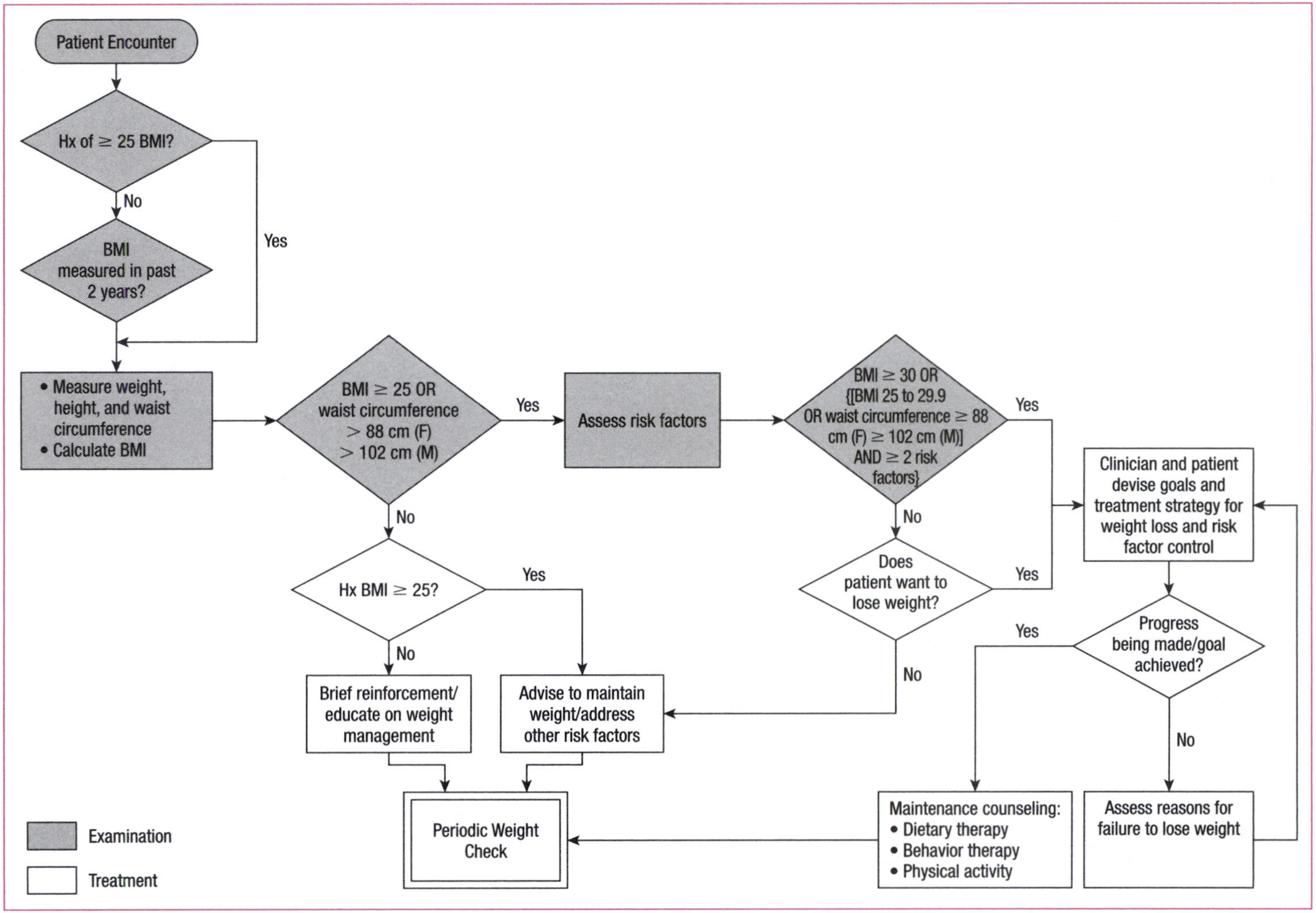

SOURCE: National Heart, Lung and Blood Institute.[1]

Table 6-11

Common Antecedents to the Development of an Eating Disorder

INDIVIDUAL
• Autonomy, identity, and separation concerns • Perceptual disturbances • Weight preoccupation • Cognitive disturbances • Chronic medical illnesses
FAMILY
• Inherited biologic predisposition • Family history of eating disorders • Family history of alcoholism, affective illness • Family history of obesity (bulimia) • Magnification of cultural factors • Parent–child interactions leading to problems with autonomy and separation
CULTURAL
• Pressures for thinness • Pressures for performance

SOURCE: Reprinted with permission from Woodside.[44]

diminished self-esteem or self-control to which the person responds by engaging in dieting behaviors.

The eating patterns in bulimia nervosa tend to be remitting and relapsing, characterized by binge eating followed by bulimia, purging, fasting, and inappropriate use of diuretics, laxatives, and emetics to clear the gastrointestinal tract of nutrients.[42,43] Both disorders have potentially serious medical consequences.

Medical Consequences

Evidence strongly suggests an increase in mortality rates among patients with anorexia nervosa; data are less clear for those with bulimia nervosa. In a quantitative summary of estimates of standardized mortality rates in eating disorders, investigators found that increases in mortality rates ranged from 25 to 240 percent.[45] Women had an increased risk of death that averaged 0.59 percent/years and the mortality rate was higher for those presenting at lower weights and for those over age 30 at presentation. For patients with anorexia, most studies show a mortality rate for the first 5 to 8 years of follow-up of 5 percent increasing to up to 20 percent by 20 years.[44] Among patients with bulimia, mortality rates of 5 percent are reported over 2 to 5 years.[44] However, there appear to be more deaths from suicide than from medical complications of the eating disorder. The mortality rate associated with anorexia is 12 times higher than the annual death rate for all causes of death among young women in the general population.[41] The profile of patients at high risk for death is presented in Table 6-12.[44]

ANOREXIA NERVOSA

Medical complications of anorexia are primarily those associated with starvation. For a complete review of these complications, the reader is referred to several recent reviews.[41,44,46] Major negative effects are seen within the cardiovascular, endocrine, and gastrointestinal systems (Table 6-13). Cardiac complications are the most common medical cause of death in patients with anorexia. A screening electrocardiogram (ECG) commonly shows sinus bradycardia, ST-segment depression, T-wave flattening, low-voltage, rightward QRS axis, and possibly a prolonged QT

Table 6-12

Profile of a Patient at High Risk for Death
(Each added behavior increases the risk of death.)

1. Chronic illness (>2 y) 2. Underweight (BMI <18) 3. Daily vomiting 4. Daily bingeing 5. Laxative abuse 6. Diuretic abuse 7. Ipecac use 8. Stimulant use (amphetamines, cocaine)

SOURCE: Reprinted with permission from Woodside.[44]

Table 6-13

Medical Complications of Eating Disorders

COMPLICATIONS	MANAGEMENT STRATEGIES
Anorexia Nervosa	Improve overall nutrition and moderate exercise (consider family therapy)
Cardiovascular system	Returns to normal following recovery
Hypotension	
Bradycardia	
Reduced left ventricular mass	Slow refeeding to prevent cardiac decompensation
Mitral valve prolapse (mild)	
QT prolongation (increases risk of arrhythmias and sudden death)	Avoid use of medications that also prolong QT interval (e.g., tricyclics), correct electrolyte abnormalities
Endocrine system	Recovery may not reverse all changes
Low levels of FSH, LH, serum estradiol, and testosterone	
Amenorrhea, oligomenorrhea	Consider oral contraceptives
Osteoporosis	Supplement with calcium (1500 mg/d) and vitamin D (400 IU/d)
Hypercortisolism	
Euthyroid sick syndrome	No treatment necessary
Partial diabetes insipidus	
Gastrointestinal system	Returns to normal following recovery
Prolonged intestinal transit time	Consider prokinetic agents (e.g., metoclopramide or cisapride)
Chronic constipation	Adequate fluid intake, increase fiber
Bulimia Nervosa	Normalization of eating behaviors and weight control (consider cognitive-behavioral therapy)
Oral complications	Most resolve except dental
Dental erosions	Cessation of induced vomiting, dental care
Enlarged salivary glands, oral trauma	Cessation of induced vomiting
Gastrointestinal system	
Esophageal injury, perforation	Urgent medical/surgical evaluation if gastric pain and hematemesis
Heartburn	Antacids
Reflux esophagitis	H_2 receptor antagonists, omeprazole
Metabolic	
Electrolyte abnormalities (depletions of hydrogen chloride, potassium, sodium, magnesium)	Correct (watch for fatigue, muscle spasms, palpitations, paresthesias, tetany, seizures)

ABBREVIATIONS: FSH, follicle-stimulating hormone; LH, luteinizing hormone.

interval. The latter finding may be a marker of patients at risk for ventricular tachycardia and sudden death, and closer surveillance is warranted. Other potentially serious cardiac findings are a pulse less than 40 beats/min, rhythms other than sinus, systolic blood pressure less than 60 mmHg, or evidence of CHF. The greatest period of risk for cardiac decompensation is during the first 2 weeks of refeeding; the reduced left ventricular mass and contractility may be unable to withstand the increased metabolic demand, particularly in the setting of hypophosphatemia associated with refeeding.

The etiology of amenorrhea, a cardinal manifestation of anorexia, is likely multifactorial including malnutrition, weight loss, and strenuous exercise in the setting of a hypothalamic abnormality. Studies on recovery of menses show variable rates of persistent amenorrhea from 5 to 44 percent.[46]

Bone loss is a serious clinical problem, and 50 percent of women with anorexia have bone mineral density measurements (both cortical and trabecular bone) that are more than 2 SD below normal.[47] Among young women who have not yet achieved their full growth, anorexia can impede maximal skeletal growth and mineralization. Contributing factors include estrogen deficiency, vitamin and micronutrient deficiency, cortisol excess, progesterone deficiency, and the inhibitory effect of malnutrition on bone formation and osteoblast function.

Gastrointestinal difficulties are primarily related to alterations in intestinal motility; prolonged transit time is present in up to 80 percent of patients with anorexia. This can lead to symptoms such as postprandial fullness and discomfort, sometimes prompting induced vomiting in an attempt to relieve the sensation. Chronic constipation is likely due to both starvation and reflex hypofunctioning of the colon; fecal impaction can result.

Other medical complications include cerebral atrophy, generalized muscle weakness, dermatologic changes (e.g., dry skin, brittle nails, and increased lanugo-like hair on the back and extremities), and hematologic changes (anemia, leukopenia, or pancytopenia).[41,46] Reported effects on the immune system are inconsistent. For women who are able to conceive, pregnancies are often complicated by poor weight gain and the delivery of low birth weight or premature infants.[41,48]

Psychological complications of starvation include impaired concentration, labile mood, and depressed mood to the point of severe psychomotor retardation with more severe starvation.[44] These side effects are often unrecognized or mistreated as depression without addressing food intake.

BULIMIA NERVOSA

Complications of bulimia are primarily related to the dysfunctional eating behaviors of bingeing and purging and are most commonly gastrointestinal (see Table 6-13). Binge eating alone rarely causes complications such as gastric or esophageal rupture, but it does cause a number of bothersome symptoms such as nausea, abdominal pain and distention, and weight gain. Purging behaviors (e.g., self-induced vomiting or use of enemas, laxatives, or diuretics) may result in perioral stomatitis and local irritation to the parotid gland from gastric acid or adverse effects on bowel function from chronic use of laxatives. A few patients develop gastroesophageal reflux as a result of induced vomiting that may be difficult to treat.[43]

Bingeing and purging behaviors can also lead to electrolyte abnormalities with accompanying symptoms of fatigue, muscle spasm, and palpitations. Cardiac dysrhythmias and seizures are potential serious complications requiring acute hospital care. Orthostatic hypotension and cardiomyopathy are other possible side effects of these behaviors. The use of ipecac, for example, is associated with direct toxicity to the myocardium and can cause clinical signs of heart failure.[49] Abuse of diuretics may cause renal impairment, hematuria, and pyuria.[50] The pathologic mechanisms responsible for these effects are not clear and may be related to direct toxicity and severe dehydration.

Menstrual irregularities are also seen in this disorder. Pregnancy complications include a higher risk of miscarriage if eating behaviors are not controlled.

The associated substance abuse and psychological disorders must be addressed as well (see Chaps. 8 and 9). Whether these may be managed as an inpatient or outpatient depends on the severity of the problem, the associated health consequences, and previous successful or unsuccessful interventions.

Natural History

Prognosis for those with anorexia nervosa is modest with about 50 percent of patients making a good recovery (normalization of weight, menstruation, and eating behavior) over a period of 20 years, although rates of recovery vary across studies from 15 to 76 percent.[41] About 30 percent have a fair outcome (improvement in one or two areas) and 20 percent show no improvement.[51] Among patients with bulimia nervosa, about 20 percent continue to have bulimia after 2 to 5 years and an additional 25 percent have some bulimic symptoms.[52] Recovery rates reported for this condition range from 44 to 100 percent.[41] Unfortunately, clearly identifiable predictors of outcome are not available.

Diagnosis of Eating Disorders

Underlying both anorexia nervosa and bulimia nervosa is an exaggerated concern with body image, the need to be thin, and self-rejection based on the assumed societal belief that thinness is a prerequisite for acceptability and beauty. Warning signs of developing eating disorders include various dieting behaviors that may begin even at very young ages. For example, investigators in one study found that 60 percent of 6- to 12-year-old girls thought they were too fat and 35 percent had been on at least one diet.[53] These dieting behaviors include dieting associated with decreasing weight goals, increasing criticism of the body, and increasing social isolation; dieting associated with amenorrhea; and evidence of purging.[44] The diagnostic criteria for both disorders are listed in Table 6-14.[54] Differential diagnosis of weight loss includes inflammatory bowel disease, diabetes mellitus, cancer, and thyroid disease.[41]

History

In taking a general dietary history, the provider should attend to cues that might suggest a diagnosis of anorexia or bulimia, or both. Patients with anorexia are often divided into two types: restricting and bulimic. If a patient with anorexia is early in the anorexia and is bulimic, she may be diagnosed initially with bulimia rather than anorexia. Table 6-15 outlines some of the diagnostic clues on history and physical examination that may raise the index of suspicion for anorexia and bulimia.

Useful questions to ask in eliciting a history of eating disorders are shown in Table 6-16. These questions should be considered whenever suspicion of an eating disorder is raised based on a woman's BMI or the clues listed in Table 6-15. A 24-h dietary recall may provide additional evidence of severe food restriction or overeating.

Because of the high incidence of mood disorders in patients with eating disorders, evaluation for concomitant psychiatric illness should be routine. This assessment should focus on establishing a diagnosis (see Chap. 9), evaluating the risk of suicide, and exploring the psychosocial context of the symptoms; the latter may assist the clinician in choosing appropriate individual, family, or behavioral therapy. Questions about substance abuse should also be part of routine assessment (see Chap. 8).

Physical Examination

Important vital signs include height, weight, temperature, blood pressure, and pulse. A body weight less than 85 percent of the expected value or a BMI of 17.5 or less are part of the diagnostic criteria for anorexia nervosa. Hypothermia, hypotension, and bradycardia may be seen in association with low weight.

In addition to the signs listed in Table 6-13, cardiac auscultation may reveal an arrhythmia or signs of mitral valve prolapse (midsystolic click and murmur) or mitral regurgitation (rare). Abdominal distention, diffuse tenderness, or palpable stool in the colon may also be found. It should be remembered that physical examination findings may be normal, particularly among women of normal weight with bulimia.

Table 6-14

DSM-IV Criteria

ANOREXIA NERVOSA	BULIMIA NERVOSA
• Refusal to maintain body weight at or above a minimal normal weight for age and height (e.g., weight loss leading to maintenance of body weight < 85% of that expected; or failure to make expected weight gain during period of growth, leading to body weight < 85% of that expected).	• Recurrent episodes of binge eating; an episode of binge eating is characterized by eating in a discrete period of time (e.g., within any 2-h period) an amount of food that is definitely larger than most people would eat during a similar period of time and under similar circumstances, and a sense of lack of control over eating behavior during the episode (e.g., a feeling that one cannot stop eating or control how much one is eating).
• Intense fear of gaining weight or becoming fat even though underweight.	• Recurrent inappropriate compulsory behavior to prevent weight gain, such as self-induced vomiting; misuse of laxatives, diuretics, or enemas; strict dieting or fasting; or excessive exercise.
• Disturbance in the way in which one's body weight, size, or shape is experienced; undue inflation of body weight or shape in self-evaluation or denial of the seriousness of the current low body weight.	• The binge eating and inappropriate compensatory behaviors both occur on average at least twice a week for at least 3 mo.
• In postmenarcheal women, amenorrhea in the absence of at least three consecutive menstrual cycles when otherwise expected to occur (primary or secondary amenorrhea); a woman is considered to have amenorrhea if her periods occur only following hormone, e.g., estrogen, administration.	• Self-evaluation is unduly influenced by body shape and weight.
• Restricting type: during the current episode of anorexia nervosa the person has not regularly engaged in binge eating or purging behavior (i.e., self-induced vomiting or the misuse of laxatives, diuretics, or enemas).	• The disturbance does not occur exclusively during episodes of bulimia nervosa.
• Binge eating/purging type: during the current episode of anorexia nervosa the person has regularly engaged in binge eating or purging behavior (i.e., self-induced vomiting or the misuse of laxatives, diuretics, or enemas).	• Purging type: during the current episode of bulimia nervosa the person has regularly engaged in self-induced vomiting or the misuse of laxatives, diuretics, or enemas.
	• Nonpurging type: during the current episode of bulimia nervosa the person has used other inappropriate compensatory behaviors such as fasting or excessive exercise.

SOURCE: Reproduced with permission from DSM-IV, *Diagnostic and Statistical Manual of Mental Disorders,* 4th ed.

Table 6-15

Historical and Physical Examination Clues to Diagnosis of Anorexia Nervosa or Bulimia Nervosa

ANOREXIA NERVOSA	BULIMIA NERVOSA
• History of sexual abuse (50%) • Onset in middle-late adolescence • Positive response on CAGE Screen (> 30%) • History of obsessive or compulsive behaviors • Perception that she is fat, when normal or underweight • Hypomenorrhea or amenorrhea, delayed sexual development if onset of disorder is early • Disturbed eating, with very low calorie intake on dietary recall. • Emaciation, with poor muscle tone and mass • Dry skin, lanugo-like body hair on back, arms, legs, and side of face; dry, nonlustrous hair • Low blood pressure, cold discolored feet and hands • History of fractures from decreased bone density	• History of sexual abuse (50%) • Onset in late adolescence to early adulthood • Positive response on CAGE Screen (30%) • History of obsessive or compulsive behaviors • History of frequent fluctuations in weight over 10 lb, usually slightly underweight • History of eating in secret • History of dissatisfaction with eating patterns • Participation in aggressive exercise programs • History of frequently missing meals, especially breakfast and lunch, on dietary recall • Dental erosion, periodontal disease • Skin lesions on the back of the hand from induced vomiting

LABORATORY ASSESSMENT

Routine laboratory assessment includes a complete blood count, serum electrolytes, and serum glucose.[41] Anemia, neutropenia, and thrombocytopenia have been described in patients with anorexia nervosa. Hypokalemia with an increase in the serum bicarbonate level may indicate frequent vomiting or use of diuretics. Laxative abuse may result in a nonanionic gap acidosis. Hyponatremia (from excess water intake or impaired release of vasopressin) is also common among patients with anorexia. Hypoglycemia is also common with low weight and may be asymptomatic.

A urinalysis should also be considered; dehydration and proteinuria are common findings in chronic starvation and hematuria may be seen in patients who use diuretics. In addition, a low specific gravity will be seen in patients using water loading to promote the illusion of higher weight or to eliminate the sensation of hunger. A thyroid screen may also be considered in the workup of amenorrhea, along with a serum prolactin, lutein-izing hormone, and follicle-stimulating hormone (see Chap. 13).

Although an initial ECG is recommended in a new patient, routine ECG surveillance is not supported by the literature if the initial ECG is normal.[46] Depending on severity of the disease, cardiograms may show arrhythmia and evidence of cardiomyopathy, which can be confirmed with echocardiogram.[42,43,55]

Measurement of bone density by dual energy x-ray absorptiometry may be of use in both the initial assessment and for monitoring response to treatment (see Chap. 20).

Treatment Considerations

The goals of treatment in eating disorders are to stabilize and treat medical complications, to regain nutritional health and energy balance, to initiate behavioral therapy, to identify and manage psychological comorbid conditions and precipitants, to identify and treat substance abuse, and to involve

Table 6-16

Questions for Use in the Assessment of Eating Disorders

REGARDING ATTITUDES TOWARD WEIGHT AND WEIGHT CONTROL MEASURES
What do you think you should weigh?
Many women try to control their weight, have you tried to control your weight? (If yes, what have you tried?)
Are you doing anything now to control your weight or lose weight?
Have you ever made yourself vomit? (If yes, how many times a day; over how many days/months/years? Was ipecac used?)
Have you ever had a binge (or "pig out")? (If yes, how often does this happen? What triggers a binge?)
Have you ever used laxatives? diuretics? diet pills or stimulants? (If yes, how often and how much?)
Do you exercise? (If yes, what do you do, how often, how much? How stressed do you feel if you miss exercising?)

REGARDING ATTITUDES TOWARD BODY SHAPE AND WEIGHT
How important is your weight or shape to you?
How do you feel about your current weight?
How would you feel if you gained 2 lb?

REGARDING ATTITUDE TOWARD FOOD
How much are you bothered by thoughts of food?
Does thinking about food keep you from doing other things that interest you?

SOURCE: Adapted from references 45 and 52.

the patient in taking responsibility for her own plan of treatment. The role of the primary care practitioner depends on the level of interest and expertise, the availability of specialized disordered eating programs, and patient preferences. Often an interdisciplinary team involving nutritionist and educators, primary care physician, and mental health professionals offers the best support for patients with either bulimia or anorexia nervosa.[42,43,55–57]

ANOREXIA NERVOSA

HOSPITALIZATION   In patients with anorexia nervosa, the history, physical examination, and laboratory studies need to guide the decision about hospitalization as the initial site of treatment. About 50 percent of anorectic patients are hospitalized early in the course of their illness. Patients who have evidence of severe wasting (generally defined as 75 percent or less of expected body weight) or rapid weight loss, severe electrolyte imbalances, or cardiac abnormalities require inpatient care initially.[41] Severe or intractable purging, psychosis or high risk of suicide, and symptoms refractory to outpatient management are additional reasons for hospital management. Although used frequently in the past, tube feeding and parenteral nutrition are not recommended, unless there is a life-threatening situation, because of the needs of these patients to have some control over their lives.

Refeeding must proceed cautiously to avoid cardiac decompensation, especially if the patient is chronically malnourished or has not eaten for 7 to 10 days. Serum electrolytes should be measured and abnormalities corrected before refeeding. The traditional hospital-based refeeding regimen consists of a high-calorie diet with modified bed rest in the supportive, controlled environment of a psychiatric unit.[58] Patients are initially given 1200 to 1500 kcal/d with gradual increase (by 200 to 300 kcal/d every 3 to 5 days) to 3000 to 3600 kcal/d; the goal is a sustained increase of about 0.5 to 1.0 kg/wk. These high levels of intake are often necessary to achieve weight restoration. Serum chemistries should be monitored every 3 days for the first week of refeeding and weekly during the rest of the refeeding.[44] Patients should be carefully monitored for tachycardia or edema.

MANAGING MEDICAL COMPLICATIONS

Cardiac Complications. Discovery of a prolonged QT interval should lead to a search for and correction of any electrolyte abnormalities because a prolonged QT interval may increase the risk of ventricular tachycardia and sudden death. The use of tricyclic antidepressants is contraindicated.

Gastric Complications. Adjunctive treatment with prokinetic agents (cisapride, domperidone) may provide symptomatic relief from postprandial bloating. Alleviation of severe constipation may require stool softeners and bulk-forming agents.

Amenorrhea. Primary therapy for amenorrhea is directed at improving nutritional status. The decision to treat with hormones (usually oral contraceptives) must be individualized. Women with symptoms of estrogen deficiency, such as breast atrophy and dry skin, will likely benefit from treatment.[41]

Osteoporosis. Weight gain, restoration of gonadal function, calcium and vitamin D supplementation, and moderate but not excessive exercise are the components of managing this complication (Table 6-17). Indices of bone resorption are increased in patients with anorexia, and bisphosphonates may be useful, but their role has not been established.

Table 6-17

Goals and Strategies of Nutritional Care for Women With Anorexia Nervosa or Bulimia Nervosa

ANOREXIA NERVOSA	BULIMIA NERVOSA
• Increased energy intake to promote weight restoration; initially 800–1200 kcal/d gradually increased to achieve 0.5–1 kg/wk • Specific meal plan and dietary guidelines to promote normalization of intake • An approach to food choices, based on nutrient contributions rather than energy content • Formerly forbidden foods introduced with reassurance and sensitivity to fears of uncontrollable eating and weight gain • Adequate dietary calcium (1000–1500 mg/d) to permit improved bone mineralization as weight is restored • Low-dose daily multiple vitamin (including vitamin D, 400 IU/d) with minerals, especially if the patient is chronically ill • Avoidance of strategies to reduce energy intake and manage hunger or promote energy expenditure (such as excessive exercise)	• Establish a regular pattern of nutritionally balanced planned meals and snacks • Adequate but not excessive levels of energy intake, with the goal of weight maintenance • Adequate dietary fat and fiber intake, with the goal of promoting meal satiety • Avoidance of dieting behavior, excessive exercise, and associated strategies (such as overuse of caffeine-containing beverages) • Inclusion of formerly forbidden foods in the diet, with the goal of minimizing food avoidance, using behavioral strategies • Dietary record keeping and review to assess progress and plan strategy • Stimulus control strategies, with the goal of controlling exposures and high-risk situations • Weighing at scheduled intervals only

SOURCE: Adapted from Rock and Curran-Celentano.[58]

Because these medications will not correct the decrease in bone formation seen in patients with anorexia nervosa, they are unlikely to be fully effective.[59] Investigational agents that are anabolic to bone, such as parathyroid hormone, hold promise for higher efficacy. Estrogen therapy, usually in the form of oral contraceptives, cannot be universally recommended because it is relatively ineffective in preserving bone mass.[59]

Patients with osteoporosis should be counseled about their higher risk of fracture and instructed to avoid high-impact physical activities. Although these measures are important in improving osteopenia and osteoporosis, the problem is not corrected by calcium or hormone therapy alone and requires weight restoration; in fact, the problem may not be fully corrected despite full recovery.

NUTRITIONAL CARE   The goals and strategies of nutritional care for patients with anorexia nervosa managed as outpatients are listed in Table 6-17. Nutrition education should emphasize new approaches to food choices (e.g., focus on contribution of nutrients such as protein, vitamins, and minerals within foods) rather than following a specific diet and is often best accomplished in collaboration with a nutritionist. Adequate weight gain is the primary goal of treatment and is critical to reversing the adverse effects of this disorder. Again, rapid refeeding and rapid weight gain should be avoided because they may lead to gastric bloating, edema, and, in rare cases, CHF.

PSYCHIATRIC TREATMENT   Young patients with anorexia nervosa may respond best to family therapy.[57] Even if this is not possible, education of the family or partner is often useful in promoting acceptance of the patient and enlisting support for the planned treatment. Psychodynamic psychotherapy and concomitant use of behavioral strategies to control symptoms are cornerstones of therapy.[41] Although psychopharmacologic therapy is generally not effective in patients with anorexia, fluoxetine may be of benefit, particularly among patients who restrict their food intake.[60] Fluoxetine

may stabilize recovery for patients with anorexia who have attained 85 percent of their expected body weight.[41] Antidepressant medications may be considered when evidence suggests a significant mood disturbance or obsessive-compulsive disorder. Fluoxetine is the preferred agent, initiated at 10 to 20 mg/d. If obsessive-compulsive disorder is diagnosed, higher doses (e.g., 60 mg/d) should be used and can be reached for most patients over several weeks.[61]

BULIMIA NERVOSA

Cornerstones of treatment for women with bulimia include a trusting relationship with provider(s) and treatment based on a careful history of triggers for dysfunctional eating behaviors. Collaboration with the patient in assuming responsibility for healthy eating patterns is important along with support offered through therapy groups of patients with similar disorders. Education about healthy nutritional patterns may be useful for assisting women in interrupting their binge-purging patterns. Behavioral and psychological referral for insight and problem-solving is usually recommended.

HOSPITALIZATION   Management of patients with bulimia rarely requires hospitalization. It is reserved for patients who have life-threatening complications, such as heart failure or renal compromise associated with electrolyte disturbances, severe concurrent substance abuse, or evidence of suicide risk.[58] The nutritional goal for these patients is to maintain adequate weight by providing adequate intake, while medical problems are managed.

NUTRITIONAL CARE   For many women with bulimia, controlling the dysfunctional eating behaviors is often required before addressing weight management. Weight loss strategies, as discussed in the section on obesity, can then be used with obese women with bulimia. Goals and strategies of nutritional care for patients with managed bulimia nervosa are listed in Table 6-17. Dieting behavior is to be avoided. In a study of 75 patients with bulimia nervosa, subjective assessment of helpful components of treatment included encouragement to eat a balanced diet at regular intervals and to avoid binge foods.[62] Less helpful components were recording food intake and bingeing and purging episodes and making meal plans.

MANAGING DYSFUNCTIONAL EATING BEHAVIOR Because bingeing and purging are often viewed as behaviors initiated to gain control of one's life, decisions about therapy should be shared, rather than mandated, and bulimic patients should be self-monitors of their progress. The only exception to this principle is if there is life-threatening risk to health from the bulimia, which is rare.

Cognitive-behavioral therapy (CBT) is the most well-established treatment for bulimia. It consists of time-limited therapy that systematically addresses both the cognitive aspects of the disorder, such as preoccupation with weight and food, perfectionism and low self-esteem, and the dysfunctional eating behaviors.[41,43] Although CBT has been used effectively and appears to be more effective than medication,[63] both interpersonal therapy and pharmacologic therapy are also effective in patients with bulimia nervosa and binge-eating disorder.[41] Combination therapy with CBT and medication may be superior to either therapy alone.[44,64]

PSYCHIATRIC TREATMENT   Sometimes, antidepressant medications are helpful, but these should be used when there is a psychological diagnosis to support such therapy. Antidepressants from either the selective serotonin reuptake inhibitor or the tricyclic category are the drugs preferred for control of either depressive or obsessive symptoms.[65] Fluoxetine (60 mg/d) is the best studied and most easily tolerated medication effective in patients with bulimia nervosa. Women of normal or greater weight can usually be started on this dose at initiation of therapy or the medication can be increased from 20 to 60 mg over 1 to 2 weeks. Other medications effective for the treatment of bulimia nervosa are shown in Table 6-18. Desipramine (up

Table 6-18

Response of Bulimia Nervosa to Antidepressants

MEDICATION	EVIDENCE FOR EFFICACY
Tricyclics	
Desipramine	++++
Imipramine	++++
Amitriptyline	+
Serotonin reuptake inhibitors	
Fluoxetine	++++
Fluvoxamine	++
Paroxetine	++
Monoamine oxidase inhibitors	
Phenelzine	++++
Tranylcypromine	++
Atypical agents	
Bupropion	+++
Trazodone	+++

NOTES: Symbols: ++++, efficacy superior to placebo in at least two controlled studies; +++, efficacy superior to placebo in one controlled study; ++, significant efficacy in open-label studies; +, trend toward superior efficacy to placebo in a controlled study.
SOURCE: Reproduced with permission from Hudson et al.[65]

to 300 mg/d) and imipramine (up to 300 mg/d) are other first-line agents.[41]

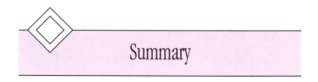

Summary

The best treatment for obesity and disordered eating patterns is prevention. This is becoming more difficult each year in a culture bombarded with high-fat foods and sedentary lifestyles and media images of the idealized thin body. The time to start preventive efforts related to healthy eating and exercise is in childhood. This does not necessarily mean competitive sports, but it does mean regular physical activity that continues throughout life. It does not mean rigid and restrictive diet plans, but emphasis on healthy eating patterns with food selections weighted toward the base of the food pyramid. In addition, children should be taught to eat only when hungry and to stop eating when full.

Appendix
Organizations

Take Off Pounds Sensibly
  (800) 932-8677
America Anorexia/Bulimia Association, Inc.
  293 Central Park West
  New York, NY 10021
  (212) 501-8531
National Association of American Anorexia Nervosa
  P.O. Box 7
  Highland Park, IL 60035
  (708) 831-3483
Anorexia Nervosa and Related Eating Disorders, Inc.
  P.O. Box 5102
  Eugene, OR 97405
  (503) 344-1144
Overeaters Anonymous
  P.O. Box 92870
  Los Angeles, CA 90009
  (213) 542-8363

References

1. National Heart, Lung and Blood Institute: *Clinical Guidelines on the Identification, Evaluation, and Treatment of Overweight and Obesity in Adults.* Bethesda, MD: National Institutes of Health; 1998 (www.nhlbi.nih.gov).

2. Anderson D, Wadden TA: Treating the obese patient: suggestions for primary care practice. *Arch Family Med* 8:156, 1999.

3. Launer LJ, Harris T, Rumpel C, et al: Body mass index, weight changes, and risk of mobility disability in middle-aged and older women. *JAMA* 271:1093, 1994.

4. Byers T: Body weight and mortality. *N Engl J Med* 333:723, 1995.

5. Harris T, Cook EF, Garrison R, et al: Body mass index and mortality among nonsmoking older persons. The Framingham Heart Study. *JAMA* 259:1520, 1988.

6. Lissner L, Odell PM, D'Agostino RB, et al: Variability of body weight and health outcomes in the Framingham population. *N Engl J Med* 324:1839, 1991.

7. Manson JE, Willett WC, Stampfer MJ, et al: Body weight and mortality among women. *N Engl J Med* 333:677, 1995.

8. Bray GA, Gray DS: Obesity; Part I. Pathogenesis. *West J Med* 149:429, 1988.

9. Kumanyika SK: Special issues regarding obesity in minority populations. *Ann Intern Med* 119:650, 1993.

10. Najjar MF, Kuczmarski RJ: Anthropometric data and prevalence of overweight for Hispanics: 1982–1984. In: *Vital and Health Statistics.* Series 11, No. 239. DHHS Publication No. (PHS) 89–1689. Washington, DC: U.S. Government Printing Office; March 1989.

11. Williamson DF, Pamuk E: The association between weight loss and increased longevity; a review of the evidence. *Ann Intern Med* 119:731, 1993.

12. Kuczmarski RJ, Flegal KM, Campbell SM, et al: Increasing prevalence of overweight among US adults: the National Health & Nutrition Examination Surveys, 1960–1991. *JAMA* 272:205, 1994.

13. Gortmaker SL, Must A, Perrin JM, et al: Social and economic consequences of overweight in adolescence and young adulthood. *N Engl J Med* 329:1008, 1993.

14. Kortt MA, Langley PC, Cox ER: A review of cost-of-illness studies on obesity. *Clin Ther* 20:722, 1998.

15. Gorsky RD, Pamuk E, Williamson DF, et al: The 25-year healthcare costs of women who remain overweight after 40 years of age. *Am J Prev Med* 12:388, 1996.

16. Andres R, Muller DC, Sorkin JD: Long-term effects of change in body weight on all-cause mortality. *Ann Intern Med* 119:737, 1993.

17. Colditz GA, Willett WC, Rotnitzky A, et al: Weight gain as a risk factor for clinical diabetes mellitus in women. *Ann Intern Med* 122:481, 1995.

18. Rhoades GG, Kagan A: The relation of coronary disease, stroke, and mortality to weight in youth and middle age. *Lancet* 1:493, 1983.

19. Galtier-Dereure F, Montpeyroux F, Boulot P, et al: Weight excess before pregnancy: complications and cost. *Int J Obesity Rel Metab Disord* 19:443, 1995.

20. Garfinkel L: Overweight and cancer. *Ann Intern Med* 103:1034, 1985.

21. Edwards LE, Dickes WF, Alton IR, et al: Pregnancy in the massively obese: course, outcome and obesity prognosis of the infant. *Am J Obstet Gynecol* 131:479, 1978.

22. National Research Council (U.S.) Committee on Diet and Health: *Diet and Health: Implications for Reducing Chronic Disease Risk.* Washington DC: National Academy Press; 1989;563.

23. Bender R, Trautner C, Spraul M, Berg M: Assessment of excess mortality in obesity. *Am J Epidemiol* 147:42, 1998.

24. *Healthy People 2000, Mid-Course Review.* Washington, DC: U.S. Department of Health and Human Services, 1995.

25. Rosenbaum M, Leibel RL, Hirsch J: Medical progress: obesity. *N Engl J Med* 337:396, 1997.

26. Stonkard AJ, Foch TT, Hrubec Z: A twin study of human obesity. *JAMA* 256:51, 1986.

27. Price RA, Cadoret RJ, Stonkard AJ, et al: Genetic contributions to human fatness: an adoption study. *Am J Psychiatry* 144:1003, 1987.

28. Bouchard C: Genetics of obesity: an update on molecular markers. *Int J Obesity* 19(suppl 3):S10, 1995.

29. Yanovski SZ: A practical approach to treatment of the obese patient. *Arch Fam Med* 2:309, 1993.

30. Institute of Medicine: Weighing the options: criteria for evaluating weight management programs. Washington, DC: Author; 1995;131.

31. Dietary Guidelines Advisory Committee, 1995: Report to the Secretary of Health and Human Services and the Secretary of Agriculture. Springfield, VA: U.S. Department of Agriculture, Agricultural Research Service. National Technical Information Service; 1995.

32. National Task Force on the Prevention and Treatment of Obesity: Long-term pharmacotherapy in the management of obesity. *JAMA* 276:1907, 1996.

33. Grubbs L: The critical role of exercise in weight control. *Nurse Pract* 18:20, 1993.

34. NIH Technology Assessment Conference Panel: Methods for voluntary weight loss and control. *Ann Intern Med* 119:764, 1993.

35. Federal Trade Commission, Food and Drug Administration, National Association of Attorneys General: *The Facts About Weight-Loss Products and Programs.* Washington, DC: Food and Drug Administration; 1992.

36. Bray GA: Use and abuse of appetite-suppressant drugs in the treatment of obesity. *Ann Intern Med* 119:707, 1993.

37. Doering P: Weight control products. In: *Handbook of Non-Prescription Drugs.* Washington, DC: American Pharmaceutical Association; 1996:423.

38. Kolankowski J: A risk-benefit assessment of anti-obesity drugs. *Drug Safety* 20:119, 1999.

39. McNeely W, Goa KL: Sibutramine: a review of its contribution to the management of obesity. *Drugs* 56:1093, 1998.

40. McNeely W, Benfield P: Orlistat. *Drugs* 56:241, 1998.

41. Becker A, Grinspoon SK, Klibanski A, Herzog DB: Eating disorders. *N Engl J Med* 340:1093, 1999.

42. Andolsek KM: Eating disorders. In: Rosenfeld JA (ed): *Women's Health in Primary Care.* Baltimore, MD: Williams & Wilkins; 1997.

43. McGilley BM, Pryor TL: Assessment and treatment of bulimia nervosa. *Am Fam Phys* 57:2743, 1998.

44. Woodside DB: A review of anorexia nervosa and bulimia nervosa. *Curr Probl Pediatr* 25:67, 1995.

45. Nielsen S, Moller-Madsen S, Isager T, et al: Standardized mortality in eating disorders—a quantitative summary of previously published and new evidence. *J Psychosom Res* 44:413, 1998.

46. Mehler PS, Gray MC, Schulte M: Medical complications of anorexia nervosa. *J Women's Health* 6:533, 1997.

47. Biller BMK, Saxe V, Herzog DB, et al: Mechanisms of osteoporosis in adult and adolescent women with anorexia nervosa. *J Clin Endocrinol Metab* 68:548, 1989.

48. Franko DL, Walton BE: Pregnancy and eating disorders: a review and clinical implications. *Int J Eat Disord* 13:41, 1993.

49. Palmer EP, Guay AT: Reversible myopathy secondary to abuse of ipecac in patients with major eating disorders. *N Engl J Med* 313:457, 1986.

50. Herzog DB, Nussbaum KM, Marmor AK: Comorbidity and outcome in eating disorders. *Psychiatr Clin North Am* 19:843, 1996.

51. Hsu LKG: Outcome of bulimia nervosa. In: Brownell KD, Fairburn CG (eds): *Eating Disorders and Obesity.* London: Guildford Press; 1995.

52. Gidwani GP, Rome ES: Eating disorders. *Clin Obstet Gynecol* 40:601, 1997.

53. Maloney MJ, McGuire J, Daniels SR, Speckler B: Dieting behavior and eating attitudes in children. *Pediatrics* 84:482, 1989.

54. American Psychiatric Association: *Diagnostic and Statistical Manual of Mental Disorders,* 4th ed. Washington DC: Author; 1994.

55. Jinks MJ, Garrison MW: Obesity and eating disorders. In: Herfindal ET, Gourley DR (eds): *Textbook of Therapeutics: Drug and Disease Management,* 6th ed. Baltimore, MD: Williams & Wilkins; 1996.

56. Yager J: Psychosocial treatments for eating disorders [review]. *Psychiatry* 57:153, 1994.

57. Russell GF, Szmukler GI, Dare C, et al: An evaluation of family therapy in anorexia nervosa and bulimia nervosa. *Arch Gen Psychiatry* 44:1047, 1987.

58. Rock CL, Curran-Celentano J: Nutritional management of eating disorders. *Psychiatr Clin North Am* 19:701, 1996.

59. Grinspoon S, Herzog D, Klibanski A: Mechanisms and treatment options for bone loss in anorexia nervosa. *Psychopharmacol Bull* 33:399, 1997.

60. Crow SJ, Mitchell JE: Rational therapy of eating disorders. *Drugs* 48:372, 1994.

61. Mayer LES, Walsh BT: The use of selective serotonin reuptake inhibitors in eating disorders. *J Clin Psychiatry* 59(suppl 15):28, 1998.

62. Gannon MA, Mitchell JE: Subjective evaluation of treatment methods by patients treated for bulimia. *J Am Diet Assoc* 86:520, 1986.

63. Mitchell JE, Pyle RL, Eckert ED, et al: A comparison study of antidepressants and structured intensive group psychotherapy in the treatment of bulimia nervosa. *Arch Gen Psychiatry* 47:149, 1990.

64. Walsh BT, Wilson GT, Loeb KL, et al: Medication and psychotherapy in the treatment of bulimia nervosa. *Am J Psychiatry* 154:523, 1997.

65. Hudson JI, Carter WP, Pope HG: Antidepressant treatment of binge-eating disorder: research findings and clinical guidelines. *J Clin Psychiatry* 57(suppl 8):73, 1996.

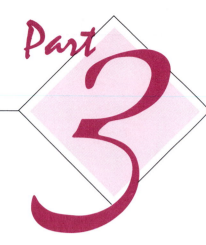

Women in Trouble

Valerie J. Gilchrist

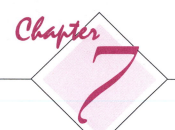

Chapter
7

Abuse of Women

Overview: Understanding Abuse of Women

Prevalence of Abuse

Almost 5 million women each year are violently victimized by men, especially by men who they know and with whom they have been intimate.[1] Of the 3/100,000 female homicides in the United States in 1997, almost 30 percent were committed by husbands or boyfriends.[2,3] Annually, 8/1000 women experience violent victimization by their current or former spouse or boyfriend[2] and an estimated 1 million women are stalked.[2]

These figures do not reveal the full effect of abuse primarily because of the limited scope of the types of abuse considered and lack of reporting. For example, in addition to physical violence, abuse of women includes emotional abuse, sexual harassment, prostitution, and pornography.[4] Statistics most often cited include only completed acts of violence reported to authorities. However, fewer than 1 in 10 rapes are reported to the police and less than 1 percent are ultimately resolved by arrest and conviction of the perpetrator.[5] Recurrent or threatened abuse may go unreported and abuse is highly underreported in certain vulnerable populations of women including adolescents, the homeless, ethnic minorities, women who are disabled, lesbians, and women in institutions.[4]

Consequences of Abuse

Abuse has a devastating effect on the health of women. Thirty percent of women treated in emer-gency rooms are suffering from injuries or symptoms related to abuse.[6] Even low level abuse is associated with increased physical and psychological symptoms and substance abuse.[7] The long-term consequences of abuse include mental health problems,[4,5] substance abuse,[8–10] increased use of medical services,[11,12] restricted activities and careers, and decreased self-efficacy of the victims.[4,5,13] There are also ramifications for friends and family members, especially children, including stress, fear, and loss of support. [5,14–16]

Common Features Across Types of Abuse

Several common features characterize physical and sexual assault, domestic violence, and harassment of women. First, each represents an exercise of power. Abusive acts are not ones of sexual desire, love, or normal relations but are ways of establishing control and power of one individual, usually male, over another individual, usually female. There is always coercion.[17] Feminists believe that all violent acts against women serve to control women in general.[4,13]

Second, although some groups of women are at higher risk of abuse (young women, students or women of low socioeconomic status [SES], unmarried women, and victims of childhood abuse),[5,17,18] every woman is vulnerable. Abuse crosses race, ethnicity, religion, age, SES, and professional barriers.[5,19] Adult survivors of child abuse are an especially vulnerable population to adult trauma and abuse. The very strategies they evoked to survive cloud their judgment. They have difficulty establishing boundaries, tend to idealize others, and self-denigrate, not trusting their own judgment. They are attuned to the wishes of others, almost unconsciously obey those in authority, tend to dissociate, and put themselves in dangerous situations.[5]

Third, most perpetrators are considered, by themselves and others, as "normal." Ninety percent of men who batter have no criminal record.[20] Studies on acquaintance rape show that perpetrators rarely have criminal records and most do not consider their actions a crime.[18] Abuse of women is supported by elements of our culture that normalize male sexual aggression and female compliance.[21–23] In this context, women are often blamed, by themselves and others, for the crimes perpetrated against them.[13,18,24] Women are seen as provoking men's abuse by their behavior, dress, or attitude. Even if a woman reports the abuse, she is assumed to have lied or exaggerated. Men are seen as exhibiting normal behavior ("men will be men") in acting on their sexual urges or jealousy or in creating what to women seems a hostile work environment.[4,5,18] Assumptions or myths about women that are used to justify abuse are listed in Table 7-1.

Finally, with the exception of care of physical injuries, it is the survivor alone who can determine her healing. Clinicians can only assist a woman, helping her identify normal and abnormal behaviors and reactions, acknowledging injustice, respecting confidentiality and autonomy, providing support, expanding options, and providing education.[5,22] Clinicians have often not been trained for this role and providing care for these woman requires them to step beyond the basic medical paradigm to confront their own personal feelings and social beliefs.[25–29] The clinician's discomfort may add to both the survivor's and clinician's denial of trauma. This potential lack of identification perpetuates violence and denies the survivor treatment.[5,22,26]

Recognition of Abuse

PUBLIC RECOGNITION

Public recognition of abuse of women in this country is less than three decades old. Historically women were considered men's property and rape was considered the fault of the woman.[30] Born of

Table 7-1

Assumptions or Myths that Perpetuate Abuse Against Women

RAPE MYTHS
She asked for it or she led me on She didn't really mean "no" Good women don't get raped She knew what she was getting in for (by going out alone)
SPOUSE ABUSE MYTHS
She asked for it by . . . being out late, not having dinner ready, etc. If you'd just do as I ask It's only because I love you It's the man's place to rule the house
HARASSMENT MYTHS
She asked for it by being so . . . (can substitute any behavior, but most commonly one that challenges the status quo) It was only a joke, you have no sense of humor She knew what she was getting in for (by taking this job) If she'd just be nice

the women's movement in the 1960s and 1970s, the first "speakout" on rape was in New York in 1971 and the First International Tribunal on Crimes against Women, which recognized the systematic rape of women in war for example, was held in Brussels in 1976.

UNITED STATES JUSTICE SYSTEM

Although the legal system has historically failed to acknowledge the abuse of women, changes have occurred over the past two decades.[30] California passed the first antistalking law in 1990, and in the last decade all states have recognized marital rape. Reforms in rape laws and in police investigation and enforcement have also taken place as summarized in Table 7-2.

Mandatory reporting of domestic violence is controversial because it may put the victim at increased risk and make the victim less likely to present for help.[26] Also although the use of restraining orders or mandated counseling have been helpful, enforcement is inadequate and women are at risk for murder despite the restraining order.[31] For example, women are five times more likely to be murdered by their partner during a separation than before the separation or after divorce.[32] Civil suits for abuse, although most common for sexual harassment, are increasingly an option for survivors of sexual assault and spouse abuse.

MEDICAL COMMUNITY

Clinicians have also frequently failed to recognize abuse of women. Even now, with domestic violence occurring as frequently as breast cancer and being potentially fatal, abuse is rarely inquired about as part of a routine medical exami-

Table 7-2

Legal Changes and Reforms

CHANGES IN THE LAWS CONCERNING SEXUAL ASSAULT AND RAPE
Sexual penetration broadened to include: Digital or object penetration not just penile penetration / Anal or oral penetration
Elimination of the need for physical signs of the victim's resistance as indication of lack of consent
Prohibition of reference to the victim's prior sexual history (rape shield laws)
CHANGES IN ENFORCEMENT PRACTICES
Specially trained police officers who are sensitive to victims' concerns and knowledgeable in investigating sexual assault and domestic violence exist in most communities
Restraining orders or mandatory counseling for domestic violence perpetrators are more frequently used by judges
In some states reporting of domestic violence is mandatory
In some communities removal of the perpetrators of domestic violence from the home is mandatory

nation.[10] Clinicians often have no training for this role and believe themselves powerless to effect change.[25–27] The health provider's discomfort may add to the survivor's and provider's denial of abuse.[5,26–28] Routine screening questions have been used in emergency room settings with some success.[33] Potential confounders resulting from abuse such as mental health problems, substance abuse, multiple somatic complaints, and patient denial make it imperative that clinicians ask about abuse even when it is not obvious.[4,11,34,35]

The single most important step that any health care professional can take is to ask every woman if she is being or has been abused or if she is afraid.[36,37] Questioning communicates to the patient that the problem is not trivial, shameful, or irrelevant. It conveys to all women the clinician's belief that it is important to talk about the problem of abuse.[18,19]

Prevention

PRIMARY

Primary prevention of abuse against women will only be achieved by challenging the roles of violence and patriarchy in society.[38,39] All individuals need to become aware of the destructive consequences of sexual stereotypes, rape myths, and pornography and to support and model nonviolent methods of conflict resolution.[40,41]

SECONDARY

Secondary prevention can be achieved by the interruption and elimination of intergenerational abuse of all kinds. Females need to be taught to recognize risk (e.g., distinguishing private parts of the body not to be touched by others, identifying dangerous situations) and practice self-defense (e.g., reporting inappropriate touching, avoiding dangerous situations, how to call for help).[18,42] Especially important is the recognition of a partner exercising control—directing dress, restricting friends, demeaning women, using intimidation, or being jealous. Recognition of the dangers associated with drugs or alcohol is also critical.[43]

TERTIARY

Tertiary prevention can be achieved by identifying victims and their abusers and helping them. This includes the education and training of medical and law enforcement personnel; specifically, medical providers and educators need to address issues of sexual and student harassment.[27] The Joint Commission on Accreditation of Healthcare Organizations requires policies for the identification and assessment of abuse victims and education of providers.[44] Community resources such as rape crisis centers and battered women's shelters are effective, but more are needed.[10,26,31,34] Court-ordered programs for male batterers have had some success in the reduction of battery.[45] Offenders need to be appropriately incarcerated.

SEXUAL ASSAULT

The most easily recognized form of abuse of women is sexual assault and/or rape. Sexual assault is an act of violence described by three defining characteristics: (1) the use of threat, physical force, intimidation, or deception; (2) sexual relations—the legal definitions vary from fondling to vaginal penetration; and (3) nonconsent or the inability to give consent for a sexual encounter.[18,46]

Prevalence

Thirteen to 25% of all women in the United States will experience a rape in their lifetime and the percentage is probably underestimated.[4] The difficulty in defining the incidence and prevalence of abuse of women is illustrated by rape statistics; prevalence rates reported in the literature vary by over 10-fold. The FBI Uniform Crime Reports (UCR) include those rapes reported to the police—70/100,000 women.[47] These tend to be underestimates for the following reasons. First, rapes are not reported because of the victim's fear of reprisal for self or others, shame, fear of the justice system, or because she does not define the act as rape (such as in marital rape).[8,24] Second, there may not be sufficient evidence to support a woman's report of rape. This is higher in rapes when the assailant is known to the victim, the victim has used alcohol or gone to the assailant's home, or if there has been a delay in reporting. Finally the UCR list only the most serious crime, so if there is both a rape and murder it is recorded as a murder.[18]

The second most often cited rape statistics come from the National Crime Survey. This is an annual telephone interview of randomly selected households organized by the Bureau of Justice Statistics. Since 1995, the survey has asked specifically about rape and found approximately double the rate of sexual assaults compared to the UCR.[8] A recent section of this, the National Women's Study, focused on women older than 18 years and found that 84 percent of rape victims did not report the offense to the police.[48]

Other population surveys reveal even higher prevalence rates. Koss, in a review of college student surveys, found that annually 10 percent described a rape, 17 percent an attempted rape, 26 percent unwanted sexual coercion, and 63 percent unwanted sexual contact.[49] A survey by the Crime Victim Research and Treatment Center of the Medical University of South Carolina concluded that over 12 million adult women had been rape victims, 61 percent before age 18 and 29 percent before age 11.[8] The most intensive survey was done by Diana Russell in which trained multilingual interviewers spoke with women older than 17 years in their homes. Even though in this survey the definition of rape was limited to vaginal penetration, 25 percent of women revealed a completed rape.[50]

Adolescent sexual assault is frequently unrecognized even though this group is at high risk for sexual assault (most of which are "date rapes").[51] The majority of teens younger than 15 years who engage in vaginal intercourse do so involuntarily.[52] Ten percent of undergraduate women report abuse in a dating relationship[18,51] and 25 percent report attempted or completed date rapes.[53,54] This underreporting may occur because adolescents lack experience with complex feelings or lack understanding about what is normal in a sexual relationship. Underreporting may also be exacerbated by less well-developed communication skills, reluctance to involve others as part of striving for autonomy, and having fewer resources such as money or transportation.[51,53]

Consequences

Physical Injuries

Five percent of victims of sexual assault have major nongenital injuries, 1 percent have genital injuries requiring surgery, and 0.1 percent have fatal injuries.[46] However, the majority of sexual assault victims (60 to 80 percent) do not have severe physical injuries but rather suffer from psychological trauma.[48]

Emotional Sequelae

Although every woman and situation differs, rape victims characteristically progress through stages described as the rape trauma syndrome. (Table 7-3). Initially there is acute disorganization that may last days to months. During this time, it is important for clinicians and counselors to educate the patient and her family about normal reactions to trauma, relieve guilt, and confirm and witness the survivor's experience of

Table 7-3
Rape Trauma Syndrome

ACUTE PHASE (DISORGANIZATION)

May be distraught or paradoxically detached and calm
All experience a triad of
    Haunting intrusive recollections
    Numbing constriction of feeling
    Heightened arousal
Also may experience any number of the following: shock, denial, disbelief, shame, fear, self-blame, feelings of helplessness and/or powerlessness, anger, mood swings, insomnia, headaches and muscle pain, anorexia, nausea, and abdominal pain

CHRONIC PHASE
Sexual dysfunction (25–40% at 1–6 y after the event) Depression (50% within the first 6 mo, 24% satisfying diagnostic criteria)[55] 22% attempt suicide; especially vulnerable for suicide are adolescents[102] Increased risk of substance abuse by a factor of 2.5[48]
CHARACTERISTICS OF RECOVERY[22]
Survivor has control over the memory of the traumatic event(s) rather than having them intrude into her life in the form of frightening dreams, flashbacks, or associations. Memory and affect are appropriately linked with, for example, sorrow, rather than dissociation. Memory and affect are tolerated and emotions do not overwhelm the survivor, as, for example, with paralyzing fear. Symptoms such as anxiety, depression, and sexual dysfunction have resolved or are tolerable. Survivor can relate to others with trust and attachment not isolation and detachment. Survivor has assigned some meaning to the trauma and to herself as a survivor.

trauma, allowing time for grieving. After the initial shock and disorganization, there may be denial, depression, psychosomatic complaints, and diffuse anger. Recovery is individual and characterized by such features as the ability to control memories.

tims.[55] In one study, 57 percent of women who were raped did not label their experience as rape.[17] In a study of adolescents, 71 percent of victims told only a friend.[40] Spousal rape is the most prevalent and least commonly reported.[50] Thus, all women should be asked about their exposure to violence.[35,56]

Identification

Recognition of sexual assault depends primarily on the type of assault. Stranger and gang rapes are often the most easily recognized because the victim is likely to suffer physical injury, be seen in the emergency room, and report the assault. However, even among women presenting for care to the emergency room following a rape, 26 percent did not identify themselves as assault vic-

Treatment

Prevention

Secondary prevention of sexual assault can be taught by reviewing the characteristics associated with assault. These are summarized in Table 7-4. However, there are no controlled trials of the effectiveness of such educational programs.

Table 7-4
Prevention of Sexual Assault

AVOIDANCE OF DATE RAPE
Examine feelings about sexual activity in general and in this relationship
Make communication as clear as possible
Avoid alcohol/drugs (excess is found in 33–50% of date rapes[18])
Avoid isolation
Prepare for own transportation
Avoid men who show jealousy or possessiveness, do not listen to your desires, demean women, use alcohol/drugs, threaten, or evoke guilt[17]
STRATEGIES IF AN ASSAULT IS THREATENED
Call for help
Run away
Resist but this is tempered by the presence of a weapon; self-defense reduced the chance of completed rape but increased injuries[6]
STRATEGIES IF ASSAULTED
Go to a friend—do not stay alone
Get medical attention
Report—whether or not you decide eventually to file charges
Get help and support—rape crisis center
Do not blame self[17]

Emergency Management

Most survivors of sexual assault report that they thought they were going to be killed. A survivor may appear distraught or may be calm, although there is likely to be acute psychological disorientation with either presentation.[18,46] She may be unable to give a complete history of the assault or the history may be disorganized. It is important that the clinician believe the victim, reassure her of her safety, and respect her autonomy by obtaining informed consent for the examination, procedures, or contact with others. With the victim's permission, the clinician should contact a rape crisis worker. Police are automatically contacted in the setting of assault, but the survivor decides if she wants to file criminal charges. When there is undisclosed assault, reporting is discussed individually between the health care provider and patient. The most important feature facilitating recovery is contact and support within 72 h.[18]

The emergency room treatment of the victim of sexual assault first and foremost involves assessment and management of the victim's injuries and prevention of sexually transmitted diseases and pregnancy (Table 7-5). Only secondarily, and with the patient's permission, should the clinician gather the information and samples necessary to support a criminal investigation. Most emergency rooms have rape or sexual assault kits that contain instructions for gathering materials to support legal charges.[18,46] Legal evidence collection must follow a "chain of evidence," which means that all samples have to be labeled and those samples kept under supervision. Although it is the survivor's decision to file charges, most clinicians attempt to gather evidence appropriately so this option remains open for the survivor.

HISTORY

Table 7-5 summarizes the history necessary from a survivor of sexual assault. The history directs the physical examination, sample collection, and risk assessment. It also provides information that will be necessary should the survivor choose to file criminal charges. However, it is critical to remember that the history is frequently partial and disorganized.[5]

PHYSICAL EXAMINATION

The purpose of the physical examination is to assess injuries to the survivor, as directed but not limited by the history, knowing that it is often incomplete. It is critical not to retraumatize the survivor at this time. Examination should be complete, starting with a general assessment, and then proceeding to the areas of trauma unless there is an obvious injury necessitating an initial intervention, such as vaginal bleeding (see Table 7-5).

GATHERING SAMPLES FOR LEGAL EVIDENCE

Semen samples, obtained using swabs moistened with saline for at least 60 sec before collection, may establish the time of ejaculation. On a wet preparation of a semen sample, motile sperm persist in the vagina for up to 8 h and in the cervical mucus for 2 to 3 days. Immotile sperm persist in the vagina and rectum for up to 24 h and in the cervical mucus for up to 7 days; the presence of a seminal plasma glycoprotein p30 indicates ejaculation within 48 h.[46] Soluble ABO antigens are found in saliva, semen, and vaginal secretions in 80% of the population and can help establish the identity of the perpetrator.[46]

LABORATORY TESTING AND PROCEDURES

Cultures for sexually transmitted diseases (STDs) and serum testing should be obtained as noted in Table 7-5. Vaginal colposcopic pictures may show lacerations. However, because laceration may also occur with volitional sexual activity, colposcopy is not always required evidence and the need for colposcopic investigation is controversial.[18,46]

TREATMENT

Table 7-5 summarizes the risks and recommended treatments for STDs in the setting of

Table 7-5
Emergency Treatment of Sexual Assault

1. History
   General medical history including illnesses, medications, allergies
   Gynecologic history
   History of the assault
   Date, time, location, number of assailants, and any descriptors offered of the assailant(s) such as race, age, and identifying characteristics
   Type of bodily and sexual contact—record specifics, need often to ask for details such as urination, defecation, oral or anal penetration
   Presence of weapons
2. Physical examination (gentle and slow with survivor's permission)
   Observations include emotional state of survivor, clothing and stains, ecchymoses, abrasions, lacerations, bites
   Observation and exploration of any lacerations, abrasions, areas of ecchymosis or edema or pain
   Start with the less traumatized areas unless necessary to attend to immediately (i.e., pain, bleeding)
   A general examination should be done as well as a detailed genital examination and a detailed examination of any area directed by the history (e.g., oral, anal)
3. Additional testing/gathering of samples
   Gather samples for legal evidence of
   Semen (will fluoresce under Wood's light)
   Clothing
   Hair/pubic hair combing
   Nail clipping
   Saliva sample
   Swabs of any open areas such as bites
   Vaginal aspirate or washings
   Oral, vaginal, and anal swabs for semen
   Photographs
   Oral, vaginal, and anal swabs for STDs (*Neisseria gonorrhea, Chlamydia, Trichomonas*)
   Serum samples for pregnancy testing, VDRL, hepatitis B, HIV, ABO type, drug screens
4. Treatment for and prevention of STDs or pregnancy
   Pregnancy risk: 2–5%[46]; 4.7%[48]; prophylaxis: oral contraceptive tablet with ethinyl estradiol 100 μg plus norgestrel 0.5 mg (2 tablets Ovral or 4 tablets of LoOvral taken within 72 h and repeated 12 h later or 0.75 mg of levonorgestrel taken at once and repeated in 12 h; the latter is not currently available in the United States[104]). Also available by prescription as a kit under the name Preven (see Chap. 2).
   STD risk: gonorrhea 6–12%, chlamydia 4–17%, syphilis 0.5–3%, HIV <1%; prophylaxis: azithromycin 1 g PO and metronidazole 2 g PO (or doxycycline 100 mg PO bid for 7 d and ceftriaxone 250 mg IM or spectinomycin 2 g IM, see Chap. 14)[46]
   Offer hepatitis B vaccination[46]
   Offer HIV prophylaxis with zidovudine and lamivudine with or without indinavir for 4 wk[105]
   Tetanus booster if necessary

sexual assault. The current recommendation is not only to offer STD and pregnancy prophylaxis but to include hepatitis B and HIV prophylaxis. Although the risk may be individualized by knowledge of the assailant's HIV status, often this is unknown and the traumatic nature of the event, especially for those who experienced anal penetration, puts the victim at risk.[46]

DECISION-MAKING

Most of the patient decision-making with sexual assault concerns disclosure. This is especially true with acquaintance rape. Filing criminal charges is the most public of disclosures. The longer the survivor waits to file criminal charges, the less likely the case is to be successfully litigated. However, even later filing of charges may be key to a survivor's recovery and establishing control over her life.[5,22] Decision-making also involves taking appropriate preventive measures, neither living in seclusion or denying risk settings, as the survivor rebuilds her life and struggles with the reestablishment of intimacy and trust.[22]

FOLLOW-UP

Most survivors will not clearly recall the emergency room visit and so it is important to give written instructions about what was done and what should be done in follow-up.[18,46] The first follow-up visit with the primary care provider is usually within 1 to 2 weeks, but over 50 percent of these women do not keep follow-up appointments.[18] It is important to have good communication between the emergency room clinician and the primary care provider so that patients are not lost to follow-up. Follow-up should include education, support, and patient advocacy. The results of tests drawn initially should be reviewed and a plan outlined for a redraw of samples (VDRL in 4 to 6 weeks and HIV in 3 to 6 months). Timing for completion of the hepatitis B vaccination series, if begun, should be reviewed.

Office Management

The office management of the victims of sexual assault is determined by the time at which the assault is recognized by the clinician. With a known sexual assault, Burgess and Holmstrom found that one-third of victims reported recovery within 1 year, another third stated that it took longer than 1 year, and one-quarter of women felt they had not recovered after 4 to 6 years.[57] Recovery appears to be dependent on the individual, her life stage, and the characteristics and context of the traumatic event. For example, stranger rape leaves the victim feeling like there is no way to prevent an attack, whereas acquaintance rape leaves the victim feeling like no one can be trusted.[13] Victims of date or marital rape show the greatest long-term effects with more depression and social phobias.[40,48,50] Individuals who have been previously victimized are especially vulnerable to a complex posttraumatic stress disorder (Table 7-6). Finally, although women's physical and psychological symptoms usually directly correlate with the severity of the violence experienced, even women exposed to low severity assaults (e.g., pushing, threats) experience an increase in physical and psychological health problems.[7] Recognition of the duration of symptoms and the effects on physical and mental health as well as interpersonal relationships can help the clinician provide needed support. Education of the family and the patient about normal recovery and such things as anniversary reactions is also key.[22]

A clinician may also be contacted by a patient after an assault before she goes to the emergency department. If the clinician has such a telephone contact with a victim, immediate safety and physical well-being should be assessed. She should be told not to brush her teeth, change her clothing, or shower, although in reality, many victims have already done so.[18] Most clinicians would recommend that the patient go to an emergency room for assessment and treatment and also to gather

Table 7-6

Posttraumatic Stress Disorder[103]*

Criterion A—exposure to and extreme trauma involving intense fear, helplessness, or horror
Criterion B—persistent reexperiencing the traumatic event (flashbacks, nightmares, etc.)
Criterion C—avoidance of stimuli associated with the event and a numbing of general responsiveness (avoiding places and people, emotional blunting, etc.)
Criterion D—persistent symptoms of increased arousal (exaggerated startle, poor concentration, outbursts, etc.)
Criterion E—symptoms for > 1 mo
Criterion F—distress or impairment in social, occupational, or other important areas of function

COMPLEX POSTTRAUMATIC STRESS DISORDER[5]

1. Subjection to totalitarian control for a prolonged period (months to years)
2. Alteration in affect (e.g., persistent dysphoria, self injury, etc.)
3. Alterations in consciousness (dissociation, depersonalization, amnesia, etc.)
4. Alterations in self-perception (helplessness, shame, guilt, self-blame, etc.)
5. Alterations in perception of the perpetrator (preoccupation, sense of being special, acceptance of perpetrator's belief system, etc.)
6. Alterations in relations with others (withdrawal, persistent distrust, etc.)
7. Alterations in systems of meaning (hopelessness and despair, etc.)

*Complete description of criteria in Chap 9.

legal evidence so that the option of filing criminal charges remains open to her.

Clinicians may also be contacted many days or weeks after an assault. Although evidence is unlikely to be obtained after several days, the victim needs to still be assessed and treatment given for STDs. Pregnancy prevention is only effective within 72 h. The patient may be offered 600 mg mifepristone followed by 400 μg misoprostol 2 days later if a pregnancy test is positive and it is within 50 days of the assault[58] (see Chap. 2).

Clinicians may also see women without realizing that they have been victims of a sexual assault. These women may have posttraumatic stress disorder or other problems as described previously, but often they have difficulty with pelvic exams occasionally to the point of having a flashback. All women should be asked about any experience of violence and violation.

DOMESTIC VIOLENCE

Prevalence

Domestic violence, an intimate partner's physical, emotional, or sexual abuse, effects up to one-half of women in the United States at some time in their lives.[10,34,36–38,56,59,60] Battery (an unlawful beating of another person or any threatening touch to her clothes or body) is the single greatest cause of injury to women.[36] As many as 35 percent of women who visit emergency departments are battered, and studies in these settings reveal a lifetime prevalence of 11 to 54 percent, depending on the definition of abuse and the reporting method used.[34,59]

One-third to one-half of women presenting to mental health centers have been battered.[36,39] Up to one in five women are battered during pregnancy, and this may become more frequent in the postpartum period.[34] Two surveys in family practice settings revealed current abuse in 25 percent to 48 percent of women, with a lifetime prevalence of 38.8 percent.[45,61] Annually, an estimated 10 million children witness wife battering.[2]

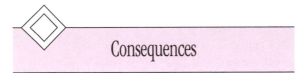

Consequences

Physical Injuries

Eight to 39 percent of battered women report receiving medical care[20] and 10 percent require hospital treatment. Most women, however, present for routine not emergency medical care, and most injuries do not require hospitalization.[10,36] Abused women have an increased rate of surgical procedures, pelvic pain, functional gastrointestinal problems, chronic headaches, and chronic pain problems in general.[10,36,39] Women who experience serious assault average almost double the number of days in bed due to illness compared with other women. Fear of abuse has also limited partner notification of HIV status.[62]

Abused women are twice as likely to delay seeking prenatal care, twice as likely to miscarry, and four times as likely to have a low birth weight infant. In addition, these infants are 40 percent more likely to die during the first year of life.[63] After battery, victims have demonstrated a ninefold increased risk for drug abuse, and the use of alcohol increased 16-fold.[39] There is concurrent use of alcohol and drugs during 25 percent to 80 percent of the battering episodes, and the presence of one should precipitate questions about the other.[34,38,39]

Emotional Sequelae

Batterers exercise control by using male privilege, threats and coercion, intimidation, minimizing, denying and blaming, isolating and emotionally abusing the victim, using the children, and controlling financial resources. These are enforced and reinforced by the threat or actuality of physical and sexual violence.

Survivors of chronic trauma universally experience depression, insomnia, nightmares, and psychosomatic complaints.[5] The diagnoses of borderline personality disorder and substance abuse are particularly common among abused women, although in a family practice center study, depression was the strongest indicator of domestic violence.[5,64] It is often these symptoms that are presented to clinicians. Judith Herman has proposed the diagnostic category of complex posttraumatic stress disorder[5] to apply to this constellation of symptoms (see Table 7-6). The associated depression may be so severe that up to one in six victims of abuse attempts suicide and up to 50 percent of suicide attempts among African American women are associated with domestic violence.[39]

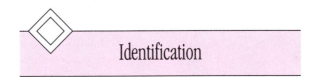

Identification

In unselected patients, clinicians identify only 1.5 to 8.5 percent of domestic violence victims.[28] Teenagers, elderly women, and never-married women are even less commonly identified.[64] Although various screening measures have been used in the emergency department[33,65] or outpatient / family medicine settings,[66–68] what seems most important is to incorporate some question about exposure to violence. It is critical for the clinician to breach the battered woman's isolation and to validate her view of reality.[5,19]

Battered women present with repeated, increasingly severe physical injuries, self-abuse, and psychosocial problems that include depression, drug or alcohol abuse, and suicide attempts. Battered women may lack money for or transportation to medical facilities, or they may be prevented by their abuser from seeking medical care. Once with a clinician, victims may withhold information because they feel ashamed, humiliated, that the injuries are not serious, or the abuse was deserved. A victim also may lie about the source of her injuries in an effort to protect her partner or her children or because she fears retribution for any disclosure or police involvement.[10]

Treatment

Prevention

Recognition of partner control is key to the avoidance of establishing a relationship in which abuse persists. Once domestic violence is established, trying to break the cycle of violence through victim education and the availability of community resources is likely to prevent further injury.[6]

Emergency Management

HISTORY

It is important for clinicians to remain nonjudgmental and relaxed because abused women are extremely sensitive to nonverbal cues.[10,36] The goal of history taking is not only to establish the presence of abuse but to assess the woman's immediate danger (Table 7-7). Clinicians may inadvertently cause additional emotional trauma by blaming her, diagnosing anxiety, depression, or substance abuse without realizing that these are a result of ongoing abuse. This oversight may result in both a delay in appropriate intervention or, if psychoactive drugs are given, increased risk of suicide.[25,26,28,39] The quality of medical care that a battered woman receives often determines if she will follow through with referrals to legal, social service, and health care agencies.[35]

PHYSICAL EXAMINATION

The battering injuries are often bilateral and only in areas covered by clothing. There may be contusions, lacerations, abrasions, pain without obvious tissue injury, evidence of injuries of different ages, and evidence of rape.

Table 7-7

Introductory Questions Concerning Spouse Abuse

1. General questions about relationships—How are things going at home?
2. Questions about conflict resolution—How do you and your partner resolve differences?
3. Questions about nonviolent but psychologically abusive acts—Are you insulted, threatened, or fearful or afraid of your partner?
4. Questions about the use of force such as grabbing or restraining, pushing, throwing objects (be specific about the type of objects thrown)—Have you ever been pushed or grabbed by your partner?
5. Questions about serious violence (forced sex, clubbing, beating, choking, and the use of weapons)—Have you ever been badly hurt or raped by your partner?
Negative responses to general questions do not preclude positive responses to specific questions.[10,36]

QUESTIONS TO ESTABLISH IMMEDIATE DANGER FOR SPOUSE ABUSE
6. Are you safe tonight?
7. Can you go home now?
8. Are your children safe?
9. Where is your partner (batterer) now?[10,36,61]

TREATMENT

The battered woman needs to develop a *safe plan* so she can escape quickly. It may save her life. A safe plan consists not only of consideration of where to flee but includes such things as a set of clothes packed for her and her children; an extra set of keys to home and car; evidence documenting the abuse, such as names and addresses of witnesses, pictures of injuries, and medical reports; cash, checkbook, and other valuables; legal documents such as birth certificates, social security cards, driver's license, insurance policies, protection orders, prescriptions; something meaningful for each child (blanket, toy, book); and a list of important telephone numbers and places to stay. If the children are old enough, she should talk to them about safety—how to call for help and where to go to keep themselves safe.[10,36]

Once recognized, the abuse also needs to be *documented* by the clinician.[45,61,64] The abused woman needs to know that her records are confidential unless she decides to use them. The clinician's documentation provides the history and evidence of abuse. Notes should be nonjudgmental, precise, and document the chronology. The chief complaint and a description of abusive events should be recorded in the patient's own words. A complete description should be included of any injuries with body diagrams, describing the type, number, size, location, age of the injuries, and the explanation offered of any injuries. Photographs should be taken before medical treatment if possible and should include a reference object and the face of the woman in at least one. All photographs should be dated and kept with the consent form.[28] The medical record should also include the results of diagnostic procedures, referrals, recommended follow-up, and a record of any contact with the abuser. Recording the badge number of the investigating officer, if the police are notified, is important.[10,36,44]

DECISION-MAKING

If the victim says she is in immediate danger, the clinician should believe her and begin to explore safer options. Isolation, power imbalance, and alternating abusive and kind behaviors predispose victims to the formation of strong emotional attachments to their abusers, explaining why battered women struggle to separate themselves emotionally from their abusers and often return after leaving.[5,35,69]

FOLLOW-UP

Regular follow-up for continued assessment of risk, documentation, and expanding options must be established. The battered woman may take civil actions, which include filing a protective order, injunction, or restraining order, or file criminal charges including prosecution for assault and battery, aggravated assault or battery, harassment, intimidation, or attempted murder. However, the legal response to domestic violence is less than optimal and the woman is likely to know whether the batterer will adhere to court orders.[10,36]

Office Management

Continued support, validation, risk assessment, and documentation comprise the clinician's "treatment" of domestic violence. Scheduled follow-up visits provide the victim with opportunities to acknowledge the validity of her experiences, the difficulties in her situation, and the chance to reassess her options. Clinicians need to review factors associated with increasing risk of violence (Table 7-8), review and expand options, and focus on the process of empowerment rather than the outcome of leaving.

RECOGNIZING THE CYCLE OF VIOLENCE

The cycle of violence, described by Walker,[60] consists of violence followed by a honeymoon phase of perpetrator remorse and apology, then a tension-building phase during which the victim is

Table 7-8

Features Associated with Increasing Risk of Assault with an Intimate

1. An increasing frequency of violence
2. Severe injuries
3. The presence of weapons*
4. Substance abuse*
5. Threats and overt forced sexual acts
6. Threats of suicide or homicide
7. Surveillance
8. Abuse of children, pets, other family members, or the destruction of treasured objects
9. Increased isolation*
10. Extreme jealousy and accusations of infidelity*
11. Failure of multiple support systems
12. Decreased or elimination of remorse expressed by the batterer[10]

*Characterize increasing risk for an acquaintance or date rape.

controlled, isolated, and systematically stripped of resources. Tension culminates in the violent phase and the cycle repeats with increasing frequency and severity.[5,60] In any captive setting, the methods of establishing control of another person are based on systematic repetitive psychological trauma.[5] This includes terror, isolation, enforced dependency, and, most elaborately in domestic violence, intermittent reward.[5] Victims disassociate, suppress thoughts, minimize, and deny to tolerate their reality.[5] Ongoing ego battering erodes the victim's self-image. She comes to believe that she is somehow to blame for the violence she suffers and that she is worthless, helpless, and incapable of survival without her abuser.[10,19,38,39]

Separation from an abusive partner is an ongoing process.[32,39,70] The abuser responds predictably when his partner leaves by first trying to locate her, apologizing, then threatening, then promising religion or counseling, and often embarrassing her in public or harassing her.[32] If she does not comply, she is at risk for significant injury. Women are at the greatest risk of being brutally beaten or killed when they leave their abuser.[37] Seventy-five percent of the calls to the police and 73 percent of the emergency room visits occur after separation.

RECOVERY

Women report going through stages of *"reclaiming self"* as they separate from their abusive partners.[70] They progress from initial denial, shame, humiliation, shock, and fear, through guilt, through staying in the relationship trying to minimize the abuse and hoping for improvement, to realization of the unavoidable abuse and the need to separate both emotionally and physically, to eventually establishing a safe and separate living situation and finally a new sense of themselves and their abuse history.[32,70]

EFFECT ON CHILDREN

The influence of domestic violence on children must also be considered. Parents often claim the children are unaware of the violence, but 40 to 80 percent of children have witnessed the violence and many others will hear the assault from another room or witness the results. Thirty to 40 percent of children are physically injured themselves.[16,71] Many consider spousal abuse to be, in and of itself, child abuse. Conversely, in 45 to 60 percent of child abuse cases, there is concurrent domestic violence.[63]

Treatment of domestic violence requires working in partnership with community agencies.[27,36] Many communities and states operate toll-free 24-h domestic violence hotlines. Other resources include the Domestic Violence Hotline (1-800-799-SAFE).

ELDER ABUSE

Elder abuse encompasses the following: *physical abuse*, including sexual abuse, is any act resulting in pain, injury, or disease; *neglect* can be either physical (such as the withholding of medical care) or psychological (such as forced isolation); *psychological abuse* includes acts that result in emotional distress such as harassment or intimidation; *financial exploitation* is the unauthorized use of funds, property, or resources; and the *violation of rights* is the failure to allow competent elders to make their own decisions or the denial of freedom of speech, personal property, and privacy.[72]

Prevalence

Estimates of the prevalence of elder abuse range from 1 to 5 percent of elderly women, depending on the definition and method of detection. Similar to other forms of violence, underreporting makes it difficult to determine the extent of the problem.[72] One study estimated that only 1 in 14 elder mistreatment cases is reported to a public agency.[73] Abuse of the elderly takes place in both the community and institutional settings. There are no reliable national data on the prevalence of abuse in institutional settings.[73]

Elder abuse was originally described as "granny bashing."[74] Most of the victims of elder abuse are women; however, it can occur across genders, socioeconomic, racial, or ethnic groups.[73] This reflects the fact that women make up the majority of the elderly, especially institutionalized elderly and also that women across all ages are more likely to be victims of abuse.[75] The institutionalized elderly are often dependent or demented, resulting in a loss of agency—acting for oneself—and allowing people to be more easily objectified.[76] The majority of caretakers of the elderly are also women. Feminists note that the societal assumption that females are naturally nurturing makes this abuse perhaps even more invisible.[76]

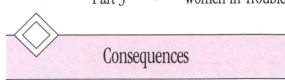

Consequences

Nearly 50 percent of incidents of elder abuse lead to physically apparent trauma.[75] There is not only the societal costs of medical care, institutional care, law enforcement, and adult protective services but there is the emotional pain and sometimes the perpetuation of intergenerational violence.

Identification

Elder abuse is rarely reported by either the victim or abuser; therefore, the key to the recognition of elder abuse is awareness and a high index of suspicion.[75] Elder abuse may be missed because of lack of clinician recognition of the signs of abuse in the elderly, ageism such that the problems of the elderly are thought of as inevitable and unmanageable, irregular medical visits, or the patient's inability to communicate. There may also be denial by the clinician, victim, or caretaker.[72] As in domestic violence, clinicians may avoid the time-consuming nature of such an investigation, feeling that they have inadequate training, or because they are frustrated, feeling they cannot effect a resolution.[73] It is important to ask patients directly about their living situation and relationships with others in the home and specifically about physical violence and neglect.

Risk Factors

Factors that increase disability and dependency put the elderly at risk for abuse (Table 7-9). Elder abuse may be intentional or nonintentional.[73] Risk factors, however, include not only those related to the needs and conditions of the elderly (e.g.,

Table 7-9
Risk Factors for Elder Abuse[72,75]

PATIENT FACTORS
Cognitive impairment/dementia
Increasing dependency
Incontinence
Psychological disorder
Alcohol or substance abuse
CAREGIVER FACTORS
Inexperience
Dementia
Burnout from a prolonged or burdensome caregiving role
Psychological disorder
Alcohol or substance abuse
Blaming or critical personality
Unrealistic expectations
Economic dependence on the elderly patient
SITUATIONAL FACTORS
Isolation
History of intergenerational conflict
Financial stress
Prior domestic violence, abuse or violence in the home
Overcrowding
Sudden changes in the patient's financial status/resources

cognitive impairment or incontinence) but also those of the caregiver (e.g., alcohol abuse or psychological disease).

The burden of caregiving may necessitate a rearrangement of work schedules or interference with other activities (e.g., hobbies) and family demands (care of children, activities with spouse). The care of a cognitively impaired relative is the most stressful and stress is greatest if the patient exhibits disruptive behaviors. Not uncommonly caregivers feel both physically and mentally exhausted. Thus "burnout" is not uncommon among caregivers. Depression has been found in 25 per-

cent of caregivers, and caregivers are more likely to use psychotropic medications than are peers who are not caregivers.[77] In one study of the rural elderly, a significantly higher percentage of individuals providing caregiving for a relative with dementia took more psychotropic medications and used nonprescription sleep aids than noncaregivers.[78]

In a community study, some risk factors for psychological and physical abuse were similar[79]; both were associated with an elder, usually female, living with a partner or other. In addition, verbal abuse was directed toward those in poor health, and having depressive symptoms was a risk factor for psychological abuse. In contrast, financial mistreatment was most often associated with being male, living alone, having depressive symptoms, and being partially dependent in instrumental activities. Alcohol abuse or psychological disease in the caretaker has been found in up to 35 percent of the identified cases of elder abuse.[75]

Institutional abuse is most often associated with increasing disability. Abuse may be perpetrated by a staff member, another patient, an intruder, or a visitor.[73] Fifty percent of the institutionalized elderly have some form of dementia.[73] Clinicians may be one of the few individuals who have regular contact with this vulnerable population and thus can notice and report abuse. This abuse may also include either failure to carry out a plan of care or unauthorized use of medication, restraints, or isolation.[73]

Treatment

Prevention

Primary prevention involves the social policies and cultural mores that prevent sexism and ageism. Secondary prevention such as identification of risk factors among the elderly and their caretakers may allow a clinician to intervene before abuse transpires. The most significant risk factor is a prior history of abuse. As the stress of the caregiver and the dependency of the elderly person rises, the risk of abuse increases.[75] Tertiary prevention consists of the recognition and treatment of abuse to prevent ongoing trauma.

Emergency Management

HISTORY

Up to one-third of victims specifically deny abuse.[75] Victims may be unable or fearful about reporting abuse. They may excuse their caretakers, blame themselves, or be fearful of abandonment. The clinician should be alert to similar features as found in domestic violence—a story that does not fit the injury, delay in seeking treatment, evasiveness exhibited by either the patient or caretaker, lack of concern by the caretaker, the patient who looks to the caretaker before answering questions, or the caretaker who answers for the patient and will not leave the patient alone.

The clinician should interview the patient without the caretaker present and attempt to get a picture of the patient's life. As much as possible, direct quotes should be used to document this history. As in the case of domestic violence, it is helpful to ask about relationships in general and any conflicts in particular. An inquiry into financial relationships may also be revealing. A history of abuse needs to include a description of the home environment; a detailed history of any trauma from both the victim and caretaker; inquiry into prior injuries, threats, emotional abuse; and any current or past denial or delay of food, shelter, clothing, or necessary services. Specific questions are found in Table 7-10, but no studies have reported the specificity or sensitivity of these or other questions to reveal elder abuse. A positive response to any of these questions should be followed up to determine the specific details of incidents, including the perpetrator and outcome.

Table 7-10

Screening Questions for Elderly Abuse or Neglect[73,75]

Has anyone at home ever hurt you?

Has anyone ever touched you without your consent?

Has anyone ever forced you to do something against your will?

Has anyone ever taken anything of yours without asking your permission?

Has anyone threatened you?

Have you ever signed any documents you didn't understand?

Are you afraid of anyone?

Has anyone ever failed to help you take care of yourself?

Have you ever been tied or locked in a room?

Have you ever had to wait long periods of time for food or medication?

Do you have enough money?

PHYSICAL EXAMINATION

In the setting of acute trauma, the physical examination will obviously focus on any overt trauma such as fractures, hematomas, burns, welts, and lacerations; more subtle signs of abuse are listed in Table 7-11. Presentation late in the stages of disease or repeated presentations for injury should also arouse a clinician's suspicion.[75] Somatic complaints, depression, withdrawal, agitation, or mental status changes may also indicate abuse. Part of the examination should also be the determination of competency.

LABORATORY TESTING AND PROCEDURES

Laboratory testing is directed by the history or physical examination. Simple tests including a complete blood count, electrolytes, albumin, renal function tests, and a urinalysis can document such things as dehydration or malnutrition. Serum levels of drugs may reveal either under- or overdosing of medication. X-rays to reveal old and new fractures may be indicated.

Table 7-11

Subtle Signs of Elder Abuse

Traumatic alopecia
Poor dental hygiene or oral trauma
Traction burns from dragging
Perineal trauma, rashes, or fecal impaction
Genital trauma or STDs
Decubitus ulcers
Bruises of various ages
Poor hygiene
Lack of clean clothing
Weight loss
Dehydration
Poor nutrition
Medication noncompliance
Missing eye glasses, hearing aids, dentures, or
   prostheses

TREATMENT

The first concern is always safety, and any person at immediate risk should be removed from the setting if agreeable. Adult protective services may need to be contacted to accomplish this if the person is incompetent or institutionalized.

As in the care of victims of domestic violence, documentation is critical. This must be comprehensive including findings, interpretations, investigations, recommendations, and follow-up. Photographs may be used as documentation, although informed consent with an impaired adult may be problematic.

DECISION-MAKING

If the victim is able to make a decision, options must be discussed with her. However, regardless of her desires, mandatory reporting of suspected abuse may be required. Health care providers risk being found negligent for not reporting suspected elder abuse. The difficulty surrounding mandatory reporting is the same as for domestic violence. Clinicians are caught between respecting the confidentiality and agency of a competent adult and the dictates of the law when victims may elect to stay in an abusive setting.[73,75] Also, there is wide variation in the state protective services, age of client eligibility, types and definitions of abuse, and reporting requirements.[80] Adult protective services or the state ombudsperson will provide clinicians with specific state and county information.

FOLLOW-UP

If the patient is a resident in a long-term care facility or if the patient is not competent, reporting to adult protective services is necessary.[72] There are also in most states, long-term care ombudsperson programs that can be contacted for institutionalized adults.[73] Adult protective service organizations exist in every state to protect the rights of vulnerable adults.[73] If the patient is competent, she must decide whether or not to accept voluntary agency help or file charges. The clinician must provide ongoing support in either case. If she is willing to explore the use of other services, such agencies often will provide financial management, homemaker services, and drug or alcohol rehabilitation.[75]

Office Management

The clinician's role is to provide ongoing support at regularly scheduled visits, document incidents, educate the patient about the ongoing nature and tendency for increasing severity of abuse over time, and expand her options.[75] Ongoing assessment should include safety, access to medical care and other services, competency, emotional status, health and functional status, and social and financial resources.[73]

As in the care of victims of domestic violence, a safe plan should be developed. The patient should receive information about the multiple community agencies and resources from social service workers to adult protective services or senior advocacy groups that are available to her.

Information about support services may also be made available to the caretaker although that must be balanced with keeping patient information confidential. It has been estimated that 20 percent of the chronically ill community-living elderly in the United States require at least minimal assistance with activities of daily living (ADL). Family caregivers provide three times as much elder care as do all nursing homes, hospitals, and other institutions combined; 72 percent of all days of care are provided by families. In addition, 80 percent of caregivers provide this care every day of the week.[77]

Primary care providers should periodically meet with the caregivers to assess their needs and concerns. Caregivers are usually women (daughter, daughter-in-law) or spouses. Nearly 4 of every 10 women will provide care for a disabled adult. Husbands are the oldest aged caregivers, with 42 percent being 75 years of age or older. Aggressive attention to and management of problems such as incontinence (see Chap. 12) and mobilization of

Table 7-12

Office Checklist for Elder Abuse

Social support
  Primary provider
  Attending at office visit
  Observed relationship/interactions
  Power of attorney—financial
  Power of attorney—medical
Social function
  Activities
Activities of daily living
  Transportation
  Shopping
  Finances
  Home making
  Meals
  Personal hygiene
Physical function
Mental function
  Competency assessment—Mini-Mental Status
  Affect

community resources (e.g., respite care, companion services, the Alzheimer's Disease Foundation, etc.) may improve the patient's and caregiver's quality of life and reduce the risk of abuse. The clinician, working as a team member, both within an office practice and within a community, will be much more effective than trying to make change alone.[73] It is often helpful to have a standard checklist for the use of all providers in a practice to assess abuse, especially over time[73] (see Table 7-12).

SEXUAL HARASSMENT

Definitions

SEXUAL HARASSMENT

Sexual harassment is a form of sexual discrimination forbidden by Title VII of the Civil Rights Act, 1964. The Equal Employment Opportunity Commission (EEOC) in 1980 issued specific guidelines on sexual harassment as follows:

Unwelcome sexual advances, requests for sexual favors, and other verbal or physical conduct of a sexual nature constitutes sexual harassment when (1) submission to such conduct is made either explicitly or implicitly a term or condition of an individual's employment, (2) submission to or rejection of such conduct by an individual is used as the basis for employment decisions affecting such individual, or (3) such conduct has the purpose or effect of unreasonably interfering with an individual's work performance or creating an intimidating, hostile or offensive work environment.[81,82]

The initial two parts of the definition are often referred to as quid pro quo harassment. Although the definition is clear and more easily identified by all parties, the hostile work environment is based on assessment by the victim, the severity and frequency of the behavior, and how it interferes with work performance.

Since the establishment of the EEOC guidelines, the following clarifications have emerged: (1) the victim as well as the harasser may be a woman or a man and the victim does not have to be of the opposite sex (1998 Supreme Court decision); (2) the harasser can be the victim's supervisor, an agent of the employer, a supervisor in another area, a co-worker, or a nonemployee; (3) the victim does not have to be the person harassed but could be anyone affected by the offensive conduct; (4) unlawful sexual harassment may occur without economic injury to or discharge of the victim; (5) the harasser's conduct must be unwelcome.[82]

STALKING

Stalking is a form of sexual harassment that is considered a type of sexual assault. Stalking is defined as a constellation of unwanted behaviors inflicted by one person (usually male) on another (usually female). Common behaviors include surveillance, multiple forms of communication, and specified or implied threats to the victim herself, her important others, or her property.[83]

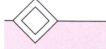

Prevalence

The prevalence of sexual harassment varies greatly based on the method of assessment and definition used. Surveys of sexual harassment reveal higher prevalence rates than formal reports. Surveys of female college students report a prevalence of 30 percent and for working women up to 70 percent.[17] The prevalence of sexual harassment of women during medical training varies from 7 to 60 percent, depending on the definition used in the study (e.g., sexual favors to sexual slurs).[84–88] In the first comprehensive survey of federal employees in 1980, the U.S. Merit Systems Protection Board Survey of over 10,000 women revealed that 62 percent

reported sexual harassment (such as sexual touching) and 20 percent reported actual or attempted rape. Forty-two percent had experienced sexual harassment within the past 2 years.[81,89] A repeat survey in 1987 found similar results.[81] MacKinnon estimates that 85 percent of women will experience sexual harassment at some time in their working lives.[90]

Consequences

Common responses to sexual harassment are a decrease in self-confidence and self-esteem, a sense of not being able to control one's own environment, anger, and stress symptoms (such as anxiety, depression, fear, helplessness).[17,81,89,91] Somatic symptoms most commonly include nausea, headaches, and chronic fatigue.[81,89,92,93] In an investigation of the type of harassment and its effect on either negative feelings about work or psychological symptoms, researchers found that harassment from superiors, quid pro quo harassment, work groups dominated by men, and increasing duration of harassment caused more psychological trauma.[94] Students experiencing harassment report trouble learning, become fearful and isolated, experience a loss of self-esteem, and more often drop out of school.[95]

The most common symptoms experienced by stalking victims are nightmares, appetite disturbances, anxiety, and depressed mood. In a study of 100 stalking victims, Pathe and Mullen found that flashbacks were reported by 55 women, 24 admitted to suicidal ruminations, and 37 fulfilled the criteria for posttraumatic stress disorder.[83]

Organizations experience lower productivity, lower employee moral, increased employee turnover, and diminished performance because of sexual harassment.[86] The EEOC records indicate that 15,618 charges of sexual harassment were filed in 1998. Of these, 87 percent were filed by women. Although only 20.9 percent required settlement (excluding litigation), this cost 43.3 million dollars.[82]

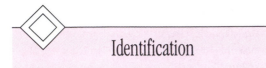

Identification

Gender Bias

Gender bias is differential treatment based on gender; it can be positive or negative. If negative, it is referred to as gender discrimination. Gender discrimination is a continuum of behavior that ranges from sexual remarks, jokes, teasing, questions; suggestive looks, gestures, and favoritism to pressure for dates, deliberate touching, leaning over, caressing, pressure for sexual favors, sexual letters, phone calls, written materials and pictures, and actual or attempted sexual assault.[96] Some forms of gender discrimination, although objectionable, are not illegal. The more subtle forms of gender discrimination, referred to as microinequities, are not illegal.[97] Examples of these include language that minimizes women, negative perceptions of women's abilities, treating women as invisible, or the exclusion of women from informal networks.

Sexual Harassment

There are gender differences in the perception of sexual harassment.[81] Women note a high incidence, identify with the victim, and recognize effects. Men tend to identify with the perpetrator and the intent and more often blame the victim. Men in the work environment are more likely to report finding overtures from women flattering; women find overtures from men insulting. In general, a hostile work environment is less about sexual exploitation and more about exclusion and harassing behavior that undermines an individual's competence. Behaviors such as these are only now being interpreted as harassment,

Table 7-13

Barriers to Reporting Sexual Harassment

1. A lack of an informal policy, which is favored by women[87]
2. Gender difference in the interpretation of behaviors
3. Harassing behaviors viewed as normative
4. Fear of victim blaming (you must have provoked it)
5. Fear of minimization or not being taken seriously (you overreacted)
6. Fear of being labeled as a troublemaker[86,87,89]
7. Fear of accusations of fabrication[88]

because they function to exclude women from certain tasks or positions in the workplace.[98]

Sexual harassment is rarely reported. Of those experiencing sexual harassment in one study, 11 percent reported to a higher authority and 2.5 percent initiated a formal complaint.[81] The barriers to reporting are both operational and social (Table 7-13). One-third of the federal employees who filed formal complaints reported that it made things worse.[81] Often women just want the behavior to stop without further investigation or retribution.

Treatment

Organizational Strategies

Organizations need to establish educational programs and policies to deal with sexual harassment. The educational programs must clearly outline definitions of sexual harassment and review the organization's policy. Policies need to establish mechanisms for both formal and informal reporting[99] (Table 7-14). The purpose of an informal report is often to solve the problem

Table 7-14

Components of a Sexual Harassment Policy

Definition of sexual harassment
Procedure for handling complaints including
   Differences between a formal and informal
    report
   Names and means to contact individuals to
    lodge a complaint
   Timelines
   An outline of
    How records will be kept
    How the complaint will be investigated
    How the alleged harasser will be
     approached
    How the outcomes will be monitored
   How grievance, disciplinary, and appeal
    committees will be structured
Sources for additional information such as
   the EEOC

rather than establish the harasser's guilt or innocence. It is confidential, future-focused, and resolved when the victim is satisfied. Adherence to any recommendations is voluntary.[81]

The purpose of a formal report is to establish the guilt or innocence of an accused harasser. It is focused on past behavior, and resolution is usually mandated by an appointed board and carries binding consequences. In a formal report, a standard written format is proscribed and confidentiality may not be maintained. A grievance committee screens and reviews complaints, usually within 60 to 90 days. The individual may be referred for mediation or to a disciplinary committee. If an appeal is made, this usually requires notice and a hearing. A complaint to the EEOC may be made in the setting of either a formal or informal report.[81]

Individual Decision-Making

Victims predictably go through stages of coping with harassment. Initially they question the offender's true intention. Next they blame themselves for the offender's behavior. Afterward they identify the behavior as abnormal and worry about whether they will be believed by others and whether there will be retaliation if they formally protest the behavior.[81]

Individuals first need to identify a behavior as sexual harassment. Women often ignore the behavior, hoping it will go away. It is important not to blame oneself or delay documentation. The victim should keep a record (diary) of incident(s). This should be factual and include the behavior, the effect on the victim, what was done to end the harassment, and any reports made. The victim should keep any evidence such as notes, talk with trusted co-worker(s), and get information from the institution on their policy. The individual may contact the appropriate individual or office in the work environment or use outside resources such as a lawyer, the EEOC, or organizations such as the National Organization for Women.

The victim may decide to contact the harasser. It is always helpful to speak up at the time of the harassment but that may not be possible. Contact may also be made through a third party or by letter. If a letter is used it is important to include facts, dates and description of incidents, effect, and future desired behaviors. It is necessary to keep a copy of the letter and make sure the harasser receives it.[17] The victim needs to be prepared for adverse consequences of reporting,[89] such as denial and accusations of exaggeration or outright fabrication, being treated as a "whistle blower," and having co-workers refuse to collaborate and blaming the victim.

Working with Survivors of Abuse

Understanding Posttraumatic Stress Sequelae

Traumatic events such as sexual assault, domestic violence, elder abuse, or sexual harassment produce long-lasting changes in physiologic arousal, emotion, cognition, and memory.[5] Initially victims of abuse are overwhelmed by symptoms of hyperarousal such as irritability, exaggerated startle, and sleep disorder. These will fade as safety is established. Intrusive symptoms including flashbacks during waking states and nightmares while sleeping then dominate. Eventual integration of these memories requires naming the event, verbalizing and connecting images, and finally linking these with emotion and feeling. As intrusive symptoms diminish, constrictive symptoms become evident. Constrictive symptoms not only include an "inability to feel" but an inability to actively plan and establish initiative.[5] Clinicians can use a number of pharmacologic and nonpharmacologic aids, at different stages, to help the survivor. These are summarized in Table 7-15.

Table 7-15

Treatment Options for Survivors of Abuse

> Medication
>   To reduce hyperarousal
>   To control depression
> Behavioral techniques to control intrusive
>   symptoms
>   Relaxation
>   Exercise
> Cognitive therapies to clarify and sort through
>   confused memories
>   Educate
>   Learn to plan
> Interpersonal therapy
>   Establish therapeutic alliances
> Group therapy
>   Initially structured groups focus on
>   education, risk appraisal, and self-care
>   Closed groups focus on recovering memories
>   Open groups focus on empowerment
> Social action
>   Establish connections
>   Engage social supports including legal
>   contacts

Stages of Recovery

The stages of recovery from psychological trauma are (1) establishing safety, (2) reconstructing the trauma story, and (3) restoring a connection between survivors and their community. The initial stage of *establishing safety* is critical, especially in the case of domestic violence; an example being the establishment of a safe plan. However, equally important is the therapeutic alliance between the clinician and survivor to control self-destructive behaviors such as eating disorders, substance abuse, or suicidal risk. *Reconstructing the trauma story* involves the witnessing by the clinician as the patient struggles to construct meaning from disorganized painful memories. Feelings of shame and doubt emerge; guilt is especially intense if the victim feels she has been complicit, and emotional control and the regulation of intimacy are fractured. The final stage of *restoring connection* is best established with the collective empowerment present in therapeutic groups. Initially structured, didactic, flexible groups focus on present self-care of survivors. In the second stage of recovery, homogeneous, closed, goal-directed, cohesive groups focus on remembering, mourning, and transforming traumatic memories so that they can be integrated into the survivor's life. Finally, future-oriented heterogeneous unstructured groups aid in the survivor's full integration.[5]

The Primary Care Clinician's Role

It is the role of the clinician to bear witness to a crime, support truth telling, and confront denial. Because the core experiences of psychological trauma are disempowerment and disconnection, recovery is based on empowerment and reconnection. Each survivor is the author of her own recovery. The clinician cannot direct this process but must support autonomy, acting as the survivor's assistant.[5] Clinicians may be emotionally overwhelmed and want to either professionally distance or attempt to rescue the survivor. Clinicians may also experience a heightened sense of vulnerability, grief, rage, and doubt. In addition, feelings about personal experiences may be rekindled. Up to 38 percent of clinicians report a history of personal or family violence.[100,101] Clinicians also need a support system and should be encouraged to consider co-management with a colleague or consultant.

References

1. Female Victims of Violent Crime, Bureau of Justice Statistics web site, 8/12/98 http://www.ojp.usdoj.gov/bjs/abstract/fvvc.htm.

2. Intimate partner violence fact sheet, National Center of Injury Prevention and Control, Center for Disease Control, 9/16/98 http:/www.cdc.gov/ncipc/dvp/ipvfacts.htm.

3. Homicide trends in the U.S., Bureau of Justice Statistics web site, 12/11/98 http://www.ojp.usdoj.gov/bjs/homicide/gender.htm.

4. Cromwell NA, Burgess AW (eds): *Understanding Violence Against Women*. Panel on Research on Violence Against Women, Committee on Law and Justice, Commission on Behavioral and Social Sciences and Education, National Research Council. Washington, DC: National Academy Press; 1996.

5. Herman JL: *Trauma and Recovery*. New York: Basic Books; 1992.

6. Centers for Disease Control and Prevention web http://www.cdc.gov/od/owh/whvio.htm.

7. McCauley J, Kern DE, Kolodner K, et al: The battering syndrome: prevalence and clinical characteristics of domestic violence in primary care internal medicine practices. *Ann of Intern Med* 123:737, 1995.

8. Schafran LH: Topics for our times: rape is a major public health issue. *Am J Public Health* 86:15, 1996.

9. McLeer SV: The role of the emergency physician in the prevention of domestic violence. *An Emerg Med* 16:1155, 1987.

10. Sassetti MR: Battered women. In: *Violence Education: Toward a Solution*. Kansas City, MO: Society of Teachers of Family Medicine; 1992;31.

11. Koss MP, Heslet L: Somatic consequences of violence against women. *Arch Fam Med* 1:53,1992.

12. Koss MP, Koss PG, Woodruff WJ: Deleterious effects of criminal victimization on women's health and medical utilization. *Arch Intern Med* 151:342,1991.

13. Gordon MT, Riger S: *The Female Fear*. New York: Free Press; 1989.

14. Strauss MA: Injury and frequency of assault and the "representative sample fallacy" in measuring wife beating and child abuse. In: *Physical Violence in American Families: Risk Factors and Adaptations to Violence in 8,145 Families*. New Brunswick, NJ: Transaction Publishers; 1990.

15. Wolfe DA, Korsch B: Witnessing domestic violence during childhood and adolescence: implications for pediatric practice. *Pediatrics* 94:594,1994.

16. Zuckerman B: Silent victims revisited: the special case of domestic violence. *Pediatrics* 96:511, 1995.

17. Hughes JO, Sandler BR: *In Case of Sexual Harassment: A Guide for Women Students*. Washington, DC: Association of American Colleges; 1986.

18. Dunn SFM, Gilchrist VJ: Sexual assault. *Prim Care* 20:359, 1993.

19. Burge SK: Violence against women as a health care issue. *Fam Med* 21:368, 1989.

20. Gilchrist VJ: Domestic violence. In: Taylor R (ed): *Fundamentals of Family Medicine*. New York: Springer-Verlag; 1996.

21. Lottes IL: Sexual socialization and attitudes toward rape. In: Burgess AW (ed): *Rape and Sexual Assault II*, Garland Reference Library of Social Science, vol 361. New York: Garland Publishing; 1988;193.

22. Koss MP, Harvey MR: *The Rape Victim: Clinical and Community Interventions*, 2nd ed. Newbury Park, CA: Sage; 1991.

23. Malamuth NM: Predictors of natualistic sexual aggression. *J Pers Soc Psychol* 50:953, 1986.

24. Madigan L, Gamble N: *The Second Rape*. New York: Lexington Books of Macmillan; 1991.

25. Bryant W, Panico S: Physician's legal responsibilities to victims of domestic violence. *NC Med J* 55:418, 1994.

26. Warshaw C: Domestic violence: changing theory, changing practice. *J Am Med Womens Assoc* 51:87, 1996.

27. Warshaw C: Intimate partner abuse: developing a framework for change in medical education. *Acad Med* 72(suppl):S26,1997.

28. Gremillion D, Evins G: Why don't doctors identify and refer victims of domestic violence? *NC Med J* 55:428, 1984.

29. McCauley J, Kern DE, Kolodner K, et al: Relation of low-severity violence to women's health. *J Gen Intern Med* 13:687, 1998.

30. Brownmiller S: *Against Our Will: Men, Women and Rape*. New York: Simon and Schuster; 1975.

31. Carden AD, Boehnlein T: Intervention with male batterers: continuous risk assessment. *The Ohio Psychologist* Sept 9, 1997.

32. Campbell A: Epidemic of women battering. *J Florida Med Assoc* 82:684, 1995.

33. Feldhaus KM, Koziol-McLain J, Amsbury HL, et al: Accuracy of 3 brief screening questions for detecting partner violence in the emergency department. *JAMA* 277:1357, 1997.

34. Wilt S, Olson S: Prevalence of domestic violence in the United States. *J Am Med Womens Assoc* 51:77, 1996.

35. Burge SK: How do you define abuse? *Arch Fam Med* 7:31, 1998.

36. American Medical Association: *Diagnostic and Treatment Guidelines on Domestic Violence.* Chicago: Authors; 1992.

37. Browne A: Violence against women by male partners. *Am Psychol* 48:1077, 1993.

38. Gelles RJ, Cornell CP: *Intimate Violence in Families,* 2nd ed. Newbury Park, CA: Sage; 1990.

39. Stark E, Flitcraft A: *Women at Risk: Domestic Violence and Women's Health.* Thousand Oaks, CA: Sage; 1996.

40. Warshaw R: *I Never Called It Rape: The MS Report on Recognizing , Fighting and Surviving Date and Acquaintance Rape.* New York: Harper & Row; 1988.

41. Rosenberg ML, Fenley MA, Johnson D, Short L: Bridging prevention and practice: public health and family violence. *Acad Med* 72(suppl):S13, 1997.

42. Hughes JO, Sandler BR: *Friends Raping Friends: It Could Happen to You.* Washington, DC: Association of American Colleges; 1987.

43. Gilchrist VJ, Carden A: Domestic violence. In: Taylor R (ed): *Fundamentals of Family Medicine,* 2nd ed. New York: Springer; 1999.

44. Hyman A: Domestic violence: legal issues for health care practitioners and institutions. *J Am Med Womens Assoc* 51:101, 1996.

45. Hamberger LK: Identifying and intervening with men who batter. In: *Violence Education: Toward a Solution.* Kansas City, MO: Society of Teachers of Family Medicine; 1992;55.

46. Hampton HL: Care of the woman who has been raped. *N Engl J Med* 332:234, 1998.

47. Uniform Crime Reports for the United States 1997. Federal Bureau of Investigation, US Department of Justice, Washington, DC.

48. Rape Fact Sheet, National Center of Injury Prevention and Control, Centers for Disease and Prevention Control and Prevention, 9/16/98, http:/www.cdc.gov/ncipc/fivpt/spotlite/rape.htm.

49. Koss MP: Detecting the scope of rape; a review of prevalence research methods. *Journal of Interpersonal Violence* 8:198,1993.

50. Russel DE: *Sexual Exploitation: Rape, Child Sexual Abuse, and Workplace Harassment.* Beverly Hills, CA: Sage; 1984.

51. Levy B (ed): *Dating Violence: Young Women in Danger.* Seattle: Seal Press; 1991.

52. Elders MJ: Adolescent pregnancy and sexual abuse. *JAMA* 280:648, 1998.

53. Sugarman DB, Hotaling GT: Dating violence: a review of contextual and risk factors. In: Levy B (ed): *Dating Violence: Young Women in Danger.* Seattle: Seal Press; 1991:100.

54. Koss M: Hidden rape: sexual aggression and victimization in a national sample in higher education. In: Burgess AW (ed): *Rape and Sexual Assualt II,* Garland Reference Library of Social Science, vol 361. New York: Garland Publishing; 1988;3.

55. Gise L, Paddison P: Rape, sexual abuse and its victim. *Psychiatr Clin North Am* 11:629, 1988.

56. Flitcraft A: Learning from the paradoxes of domestic violence. *JAMA* 277:1400, 1997.

57. Burgess AW, Holmstrom LL: Adaptive strategies and recovery from rape. *Am J Psychiatry* 136:1266, 1979.

58. Spitz IM, Bardin CW, Benton L, Robbins A: Early pregnancy termination with mifepristone and misoprostol in the United States. *N Engl J Med* 338:1241, 1998.

59. Abbott J, Johnson R, Koziol-McLain J, Lowenstein S: Domestic violence against women. *JAMA* 273:1763, 1995.

60. Walker LE: *The Battered Woman Syndrome.* New York: Springer; 1984.

61. Rath GD, Jarratt LG, Leonardson G: Rates of domestic violence against adult women by men partners. *J Am Board Fam Pract* 2:227, 1989.

62. Rothenberg K, Paskey S, Reuland M, Zimmerman S, North R: Domestic violence and partner notification: implications for treatment and counseling of women with HIV. *J Am Med Womens Assoc* 50:87, 1995.

63. Newberger EH, Barkam SE, Lieberman ES, et al: Abuse of pregnant women and adverse birth

outcome: current knowledge and implications for practice [commentary]. *JAMA* 267:2370, 1992.

64. Saunders DG, Hamberger K, Hovey M: Indicators of woman abuse based on a chart review at a family practice center. *Arch Fam Med* 2:537, 1993.

65. McFarlane J, Greenberg, L, Weltge A, et al: Identification of abuse in emergency departments: effectiveness of a two-question screening tool. *J Emerg Nurs* 21:391, 1995.

66. Pan HS, Ehrensaft MK, Heyman RE, et al: Evaluating domestic partner abuse in a family practice clinic. *Fam Med* 29:492, 1997.

67. Sherin KM, Sinacore JM, Li XQ, et al: HITS: a short domestic violence screening tool for use in a family practice setting. *Fam Med* 30:508, 1998.

68. Brown JB, Lent B, Brett PJ, et al: Development of the woman abuse screening tool for use in family practice. *Fam Med* 28:422, 1996.

69. Barnett OW, Laviolette AD: *It Could Happen to Anyone: Why Battered Woman Stay*. Beverly Hills, CA: Sage; 1993.

70. Merritt-Gray M, Wuest J: Counteracting abuse and breaking free: the process of leaving revealed through women's voices. *Health Care for Women International* 16:399, 1995.

71. Jaffe P, Wolfe DA, Wilson S: *Children of Battered Women*. Newbury Park, CA: Sage Publications; 1990.

72. Swagerty DL, Takahashi PY, Evans JM: Elderly mistreatment. *Am Fam Pract* 59:2804, 1999.

73. AMA Diagnostic and Treatment Guidelines on Elder Abuse. Chicago: Authors, 1992.

74. Burston GR: Granny-battering (letter). *BMJ* 3:592, 1975.

75. Costa AJ, Anetzberger G: Recognition and intervention for elder abuse. In: *Violence Issues for Health Care Educators and Providers*. Binghamton, NY: Haworth Maltreatment & Trauma Press; 1997.

76. Griffin G, Aitken L: Visibility blues: gender issues in elder abuse in institutional settings. *J Elder Abuse Negl* 199:1/2; 29, 1999.

77. Larry PP, Gondek K, Feinberg MV, et al: The family caregiver. *Elder Care News* (The Parke-Davis Center for the Education of the Elderly, University of Maryland, Baltimore.) 7:17, 1991.

78. Mort JR, Baspar PM, Juffer DI, Kovarna MB: Comparison of psychotropic agent use among rural elderly caregivers and noncaregivers. *Ann Pharmacother* 30:583, 1996.

79. Comijs HC, Smith JH, Pot AM, et al: Risk indicators of elder mistreatment in the community. *J Elder Abuse Negl* 9:67, 1998.

80. Goodrich CS: Results of a national survey of state protective services programs: assessing risk and defining victim outcomes. *J Elder Abuse Negl* 9:69, 1997.

81. Riger S: Gender dilemmas in sexual harassment policies and procedures. *Am Psychol* 46:497, 1991.

82. EEOC web site, http://www.eeoc.gov/facts/fs-sex.html 1/15/97, http://www.eeoc.gov/stats/hrass.html 1/14/99

83. Pathe M, Mullen PE: The impact of stalkers on their victims. *Br J Psychiatry* 170:12, 1997.

84. Komaromy M, Bindman AB, Haber RJ, et al: Sexual harassment in medical training. *New Engl J Med* 328:322, 1993.

85. Wolf TM, Randall HM, von Almen K, et al: Perceived mistreatment and attitude change by graduating medical students: a retrospective study. *Med Educ* 25:182, 1991.

86. Thorne S: Several medial schools have begun to tackle sexual harassment issue. *Can Med Assoc J* 147:1567, 1992.

87. Farley MM, Kozarsky P: Sexual harassment in medical training. *N Engl J Med* 329:661, 1993.

88. Vukovich C: The prevalence of sexual harassment among female family practice residents in the United States. *Violence Vict* 11:175, 1996.

89. Shrier DK: Sexual harassment and discrimination: impact on physical and mental health. *N J Med* 87:105, 1990.

90. MacKinnon CA: *Feminism Unmodified: Discourses on Life and Law*. Cambridge, MA: Harvard University Press; 1987.

91. MacKinnon CA: *Sexual Harassment of Working Women*. New Haven, CT: Yale University Press; 1979.

92. Stewart D, Abbey S, Meana M, Boydell KM: What makes women tired? A community sample. *J Womens Health* 7:69, 1998.

93. Goldenhar LM, Swanson NG, Hurrell JJ, et al: Stressors and adverse outcomes for female construction workers. *Journal of Occupational Health Psychology* 3:19, 1998.

94. Thacker RA, Gohmann SF: Emotional and psychological consequences of sexual harassment: a descriptive study. *J Psychol* 130:429, 1996.

95. U.S. Department of Education web site, http://www.ed.gov/offices/ocr/ocrshpam.html 8/27/97.

96. Lenhart SA, Evans CH: Sexual harassment and gender discrimination: a primer for women physicians. *J Am Med Women's Assoc* 46:77, 1991.

97. Nora LM: Sexual harassment in medical education: a review of the literature with comments from the law. *Acad Med* 71:S113, 1996.

98. Yoroshefsky E: More than sex: why the courts are missing the point. *MS* 8:56, 1998.

99. *AMA Guidelines for Establishing Sexual Harassment Prevention and Grievance Procedures.* Chicago: American Medical Association; 1989.

100. Sugg NK, Inui T: Primary care physicians' response to domestic violence: opening pandora's box. *JAMA* 267:3157, 1992.

101. Hendricks-Matthews MK: Ensuring students' well-being as they learn to support victims of violence. *Acad Med* 72:46, 1997.

102. Moscarello R: Psychological management of victims of sexual assault. *Can J Psychiatry* 35:25, 1990.

103. American Psychiatric Association: *Diagnostic and Statistical Manual of Mental Disorders,* 4th ed. Washington, DC: Author; 1994.

104. Anonymous: An emergency contraceptive kit. *Med Let Drug Ther* 40:102, 1998.

105. Pinkerton SD, Holtgrave DR, Bloom FR: Cost-effectiveness of post-exposure prophylaxis following sexual exposure to HIV. *AIDS* 12:1067, 1998.

Bertram Stoffelmayr
William C. Wadland
Sally K. Guthrie

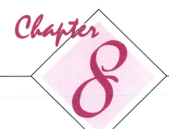

Chapter
8

Substance Abuse

Overview

The Concept of Dependence

This chapter addresses problems of abuse and dependence on alcohol, illegal drugs, and nicotine by women. Although there is controversy over potential linkages between these drugs and the persons who use and abuse them, one clinically relevant commonality among these drugs is that their consumption can lead to dependence.

The construct of dependence is basic to the modern diagnosis of substance abuse problems. Today, we speak of alcohol-dependent persons rather than alcoholics. Although the difference between these terms might appear insignificant, they refer to a different style of thinking about addiction. The term *dependence* denotes a continuum, from mild to severe, whereas terms such as *addict* and *alcoholic* separate individuals into discrete groups, namely, alcoholics and nonalcoholics.

The markers for dependence are the severity of withdrawal symptoms and the degree of tolerance to the drug. In the psychiatric classification, dependence is diagnosed if a patient meets more than three of the criteria listed in the *Diagnostic and Statistical Manual of Mental Disorders* (DSM) (Table 8-1).

Along with dependence, other terms are used to describe individuals' problems with drugs and alcohol. Among them are *substance abuse* and *harmful use*, referring to patterns of substance use that are characterized by "recurrent and significant adverse consequences due to the repeated use of substances." *Hazardous use* is defined as "an established pattern of use placing the user at greater risk of future damage to physical and mental health"; the use, however, has not resulted in significant medical or psychiatric consequences. As will be discussed later, these diagnostic categories have treatment implications.

Women and Drugs

It is men, and not women, who capture medical attention and resources in the area of substance abuse.[1,2] Because of the preponderance of men in treatment, most treatment outcome research only allows for conclusions about men. Treatment outcome studies that address these problems in woman can be counted on one hand.[3–5] In fact, the only issue that draws attention to women with substance abuse problems concerns whether or

Table 8-1

DSM-IV Criteria for Substance Abuse and Dependence

CRITERIA FOR SUBSTANCE ABUSE
A. A maladaptive pattern of substance use leading to clinically significant impairment or distress, as manifested by one (or more) of the following, occurring within a 12-month period: 1. Recurrent substance use resulting in a failure to fulfill major role obligation at work, school, or home (e.g., repeated absences or poor work performance related to substance use; substance-related absences, suspension, or expulsions from school; neglect of children or household) 2. Recurrent substance use in situations in which it is physically hazardous (e.g., driving an automobile or operating a machine when impaired by substance use) 3. Recurrent substance-related legal problems (e.g., arrests for substance-related disorderly conduct) 4. Continued substance use despite having persistent or recurrent social or interpersonal problems caused or exacerbated by the effects of the substance (e.g., arguments with spouse about consequences of intoxication, physical fights) B. The symptoms have never met the criteria for Substance Dependence for this class of substance
CRITERIA FOR SUBSTANCE DEPENDENCE

A maladaptive pattern of substance use, leading to clinically significant impairment or distress, as manifested by three (or more) of the following, occurring at any time in the same 12-month period:
 	
1. Tolerance, as defined by either of the following:
  a. A need for markedly increased amounts of the substance to achieve intoxification or desired effect
  b. Markedly diminished effect with continued use of the same amount of substance
2. Withdrawal, as manifested by either of the following:
  a. The characteristic withdrawal syndrome for the substance
  b. The same (or closely related) substance is taken to relieve or avoid withdrawal symptoms
3. The substance is often taken in larger amounts or over a longer period than was intended
4. There is a persistent desire or unsuccessful efforts to cut down or control substance use
5. A great deal of time is spent in activities necessary to obtain the substance (e.g., visiting multiple doctors or driving long distances), use the substance (e.g., chain-smoking), or recover from its effects
6. Important social, occupation, or recreational activities are given up or reduced because of substance use
7. The substance use is continued despite knowledge of having a persistent or recurrent physical or psychological problem that is likely to have been caused or exacerbated by the substance (e.g., current cocaine use despite recognition of cocaine-induced depression, or continued drinking despite recognition that an ulcer was made worse by alcohol consumption)

SOURCE: Reproduced with permission from *Diagnostic and Statistical Manual of Mental Disorders*, 4th ed. Washington, DC, American Psychiatric Association, 1994.

not women who use drugs while pregnant should be charged with child abuse.[6,7]

Research and the media are not alone in ignoring the plight of women with substance abuse problems. Professionals, including primary care physicians, identify a smaller proportion of women with substance abuse problems than men and are less likely to diagnose these difficulties in women.[8]

BARRIERS TO THE IDENTIFICATION AND REFERRAL OF WOMEN

Why this apparent inattention by professionals to the plight of substance abuse by women? One possible explanation involves the stigma traditionally attached to women with substance abuse problems. For example, one old prejudice is that alcohol use leads to promiscuity and that only "loose" women take drugs.[9–11] Therefore, if one were to ask a woman about alcohol and drug abuse, one would be accusing her of immorality. Further, despite the fact that women consult physicians more often than men, they are less likely than men to mention substance abuse as a problem.[8] It has been suggested that this is so because of the shame women attach to substance abuse and the fear of the consequences of admitting to substance abuse problems. For example, they might be accused of being ineffective mothers and be worried about losing their parental rights.

Another barrier to identification is that women who abuse substances frequently present with somatic complaints. Symptoms of fatigue, tiredness, changes in appetite, and increased anxiety may be the first presentation of substance abuse in women. Clinicians may focus on the somatic complaints or identify depression and not consider the possibility of associated substance abuse. In fact, clinicians may very well prescribe and add psychoactive medications that confound treatment and abuse.

Possibly the most important barrier to the identification of substance abuse problems by the clinician is that women's substance abuse problems are often embedded in complex psychological and social problems. These women report high levels of depression, anxiety, and sexual and physical abuse.[12,13] In one study, 67 percent of alcohol-abusing women reported sexual abuse in childhood, whereas only 28 percent of the control group reported similar abuse.[12] Up to 40 percent of women in treatment report having been abused sexually and physically during their lifetime and 25 percent during the last 12 months.[12–16]

RISK FACTORS FOR SUBSTANCE ABUSE

Disorganized family life and substance-abusing parents are important risk factors for the initiation of substance abuse.[17] Although some twin studies point to genetic influences on drinking, the degree of genetic predisposition for alcoholism is less clear in women than men, and the climate in the family of origin assumes more importance.

Women who present with substance abuse problems also report experiencing serious life stresses.[18] The effect of psychological and social problems may be most apparent among adolescents. Gomberg[19] lists the following risk factors for problem drinking in female adolescents:

1. Peer use of alcohol
2. Behavior problems and problems in school
3. Alienation and symptoms of stress/distress
4. Early experience of intoxication and early use of marijuana
5. Positive family history and/or dysfunctional family
6. Positive expectancies about alcohol

For women in their late adolescence and early twenties, risk factors for substance abuse include not being married, living with a substance-abusing partner, depression, being unemployed, single parenthood, atypical sexual practices, and early onset of smoking.[19] Although it is difficult to determine the degree to which these factors are risks or consequences, they do have implications for treatment.

BIOLOGIC RISKS

Women become more impaired than men after consumption of a similar quantity of alcohol. This may be explained by physiologic differences. A single dose of alcohol produces higher blood levels in women than in men[20] for two reasons:

1. The total body water content is smaller in women than men due to smaller body size and a higher ratio of fat to lean tissue in women.
2. Women possess a smaller amount of alcohol dehydrogenase in the gastric mucosa than men.[21]

Alcohol dehydrogenase is responsible for some of the first-pass metabolism of alcohol. Consequently, a larger portion of ingested alcohol is absorbed in women.

Physical differences between men and women also have an effect on the diagnosis of substance abuse. For example, screening tests may not be sensitive enough to detect problems in women because the threshold of abuse is lower for women due to body size and metabolic differences.[22]

Principal Diagnoses

Prevalence and Health Risks of Substance Abuse in Women

TOBACCO SMOKING

PREVALENCE The percentage of women who smoke has decreased over the last 30 years from 34 to 22 percent.[23] This decline, however, is considerably less than for men (52 to 28 percent). Adolescent girls have about the same rates of smoking as adolescent boys (36.4 percent of high school students are regular smokers).[24,25]

GENDER DIFFERENCES A number of studies have shown that women find it more difficult to quit smoking than men, especially in studies using nicotine replacement therapies.[26,27] Women appear to smoke less than men and for reasons not related to nicotine,[26] such as enhanced social pleasures and stimuli. Women smoke fewer cigarettes per day, and they smoke brands with lower nicotine yield and inhale less deeply than men. However, during smoking cessation, women seem to have more withdrawal symptoms such as craving, irritability, anxiety, excessive hunger, and tenseness than men.[27] More research is needed to understand these differences.

Although smoking overall is declining among Americans, most of the decrease is attributed to changes in male smoking activity. Due to the special barriers to smoking cessation and the prevalence differences between the sexes, women smokers may outnumber men over the next decade.

HEALTH CONSEQUENCES The health consequences of smoking for women are many. Lung cancer, which is directly associated with smoking activity, has become the most common form of cancer in women, surpassing breast cancer.[23] Smoking in women is also associated with other cancers (lung, oral, renal, and cervical), osteoporosis, chronic lung disease, vascular diseases (cardiac, cerebral, and peripheral), and embolic disease associated with the use of oral contraceptives. For pregnant women, smoking is associated with premature birth, lower-birth-weight infants, and spontaneous abortion.[28]

DRUG INTERACTIONS In addition to adversely affecting health and causing an addiction, nicotine in the form of a tobacco cigarette alters the metabolism of some commonly used medications. Tobacco cigarettes induce a component of the CYP450 enzyme system, specifically CYP1A2, which is responsible for the elimination of a large proportion of theophylline, caffeine, and clozapine. The enzyme induction is due to factors in the cigarette other than nicotine; therefore, when cigarette smoking is terminated, even with concomitant nicotine replacement, the induction of CYP1A2 subsides over time. Patients who are stabilized on a particular theophylline dose will experience a decrease in drug clearance and an increase in theophylline concentration over time.[29] This could result in toxicity if the dose is not monitored. Similarly, toxicity might be seen with clozapine, an antipsychotic agent that can cause seizures at elevated blood concentrations.

ALCOHOL USE

PREVALENCE AND RISK FACTORS Studies estimate that there are 15.1 million alcohol-abusing or alcohol-dependent persons in the United States; approximately 4.6 million (nearly one-third) are women.[30] Risk factors for alcohol use and abuse among women include age, marital status, and race. Younger women (age 18 to 34) report more drinking-related problems than older women (older than age 35), yet actual alcohol dependence is higher among middle-aged women (age 35 to 49).[31] Women who have never been married or who are divorced or separated are more likely to drink heavily and to have alcohol-related health problems than are women who are married or widowed. This may be related to role identity and density, because women who have multiple roles, such as work and parenting, have lower rates of alcohol-related health problems than women with fewer defined roles.[32] Physicians should be aware of changing risk factors for substance abuse across the life span[19] (see Appendix A).

Surveys of racial and ethnic groups show that black women (46 percent) are more likely to abstain from alcohol than white women (34 percent).[33] Despite this, equal proportions of black and white women are heavy drinkers.[30,34] Hispanic women are infrequent users of alcohol.[30,34]

GENDER DIFFERENCES   There are gender differences in alcohol use and abuse. Generally, women consume less alcohol than men and have fewer health-related problems and dependence symptoms than men. However, the heaviest consumers of alcohol among women have more alcohol-related health problems than men.[32,35] Women tend to develop alcoholism at a later age than men, but rapidly develop symptoms at the onset (i.e., they "telescope" into the illness). This rapid onset of alcoholism is more common if primary depression is present concurrently.[36] Social relationships also appear to influence women's drinking patterns; women often have the same drinking patterns as their husband, siblings, and close friends.[30,35]

HEALTH CONSEQUENCES   The health risks of heavy alcohol use appear to be greater for women than men.[37] Women who are heavy alcohol users have death rates 50 to 100 percent higher than men who are heavy alcohol users,[37] with greater proportions of suicides, alcohol-related accidents, circulatory disorders, and cirrhosis of the liver. Depression is four times more frequent among women with alcohol dependence than among men with alcohol dependence (19 versus 5 percent).[36] Evidence also indicates that alcohol has more detrimental effects on the liver for women than men.[38] Excess alcohol use is also associated with menstrual disorders, infertility, and early menopause.[39]

ILLICIT DRUG USE

PREVALENCE AND RISK FACTORS   In 1996, 29.9 percent of U.S. women, 12 years of age and older, reported having used illicit drugs at least once in their life.[40] Over 30 million women reported having used marijuana at least once and more than 4.7 million women had used an illicit drug at least once in the month preceding the survey, with 603,000 using cocaine, 241,000 using crack cocaine, and 547,000 using hallucinogens. In 1996, 56,000 women reported use of a needle to inject drugs. Nearly 1.2 million women, aged 12 and older, had taken prescription drugs (sedatives, tranquilizers, or analgesics) for nonmedicinal purposes in the preceding month.[40]

Experiencing abuse is a major risk factor for substance abuse among women. Over 70 percent of women who abuse drugs report histories of physical and sexual abuse. Adolescent females, who are vulnerable to substance abuse, often have a history of victimization, sexual and physical abuse, family exposure to substance abuse, dysfunctional family life, poor self-esteem, poor school performance, and early sexual activity.[19]

HEALTH CONSEQUENCES   Cocaine use, especially in the form of crack or intravenous cocaine, can lead to severe medical problems such as hypertension, myocardial infarction, hyperthermia, and stroke. In pregnant users, cocaine is associated with a higher rate of abruptio placenta. Cocaine can also lead to paranoia, psychosis, and violent acts, all of which impair a woman's functioning. Cocaine is highly reinforcing and those who routinely abuse it will go to great lengths to acquire more of the drug.

Substance abuse also places women at high risk of comorbid illness and infection. Women who abuse substances or who are in treatment for substance abuse are more anxious and depressed than men.[41–43] Bulimia is more common among women who abuse alcohol and drugs.[36] Drug-addicted women are also at higher risk for infections, HIV, and poorly controlled chronic conditions such as hypertension, diabetes, and cardiovascular disease.

POLYSUBSTANCE ABUSE

Polysubstance abuse or linkage patterns exist between smoking, alcohol, illicit drug use, and prescribed psychoactive medications in women.[44]

Higher rates of smoking occur among female alcoholics and illicit drug users. The prevalence of smoking among female alcoholics and illicit drug users is over 60 percent, or twice to three times the general prevalence rate of smoking. Multiple drug abuse patterns are typical, especially when psychiatric symptoms or comorbidities exist.[43]

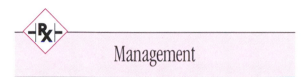

Management

Substance Abuse Counseling

Primary care clinicians have an important role in the prevention and treatment of substance abuse problems and they provide the most effective smoking cessation interventions. Recent research[45,46] also demonstrates that brief intervention delivered by primary care physicians to patients with alcohol problems resulted in a significant reduction in alcohol consumption.

Given these findings, why then do primary care clinicians address substance abuse problems less often than they might? Some physicians might feel that asking patients, in particular women, about substance abuse is accusing them of immorality. More important, however, is that physicians are unaware of their effectiveness, are uncertain about how to address substance abuse, and possibly have experienced failure. Their advice has not always been heeded. Even patients with serious health problems did not stop smoking and some, despite the fact their lives were disintegrating, kept on drinking.

Although acknowledging how discouraging it is to fail, it would be helpful if physicians were to keep in mind the following two points when evaluating their own effectiveness as agents of behavior change. First, even the most effective clinician will only influence a proportion of patients. The correct evaluative question is, "What proportion of smokers in my practice did I influence?" and not "Was I able to help Ms. Jones?" This is a difficult challenge because the usual unit for medical intervention is the individual. Second, change is not an all or nothing proposition, but an ongoing process. Physicians are successful if they help patients in this process. For example, a patient who has never questioned her drinking, even if her consumption of alcohol is a great hazard to her and her family, will not stop drinking just because she is told to, but can be helped, in the first instance, to view her drinking realistically. Only later, after acknowledging that her drinking is excessive, will she reduce it or accept treatment.

APPROACHES TO SUBSTANCE ABUSE COUNSELING

In recent years the work of substance abuse treatment specialists has undergone changes relevant to primary medical care. Previously, it was thought that the most important task in counseling patients who had problems with substance abuse was to "break down denial" through confrontation. Two lines of research have challenged traditional approaches, pointing to the ineffectiveness of confrontation and proposing different styles of interacting with patients.

STAGES OF CHANGE   Research on the stages of change indicates that communication with patients should be tailored to the patient's stage of change (Tables 8-2 and 8-3).[47,48] For example, patients who never thought about stopping smoking will not give up cigarettes simply on the physician's advice. Similarly, patients who do not consider the amount of alcohol they consume excessive are not likely to cut back. Therefore, the goal of an initial consultation with a patient who is in precontemplation will be to raise problem awareness. The conversations between the physician and a patient who acknowledges a substance abuse problem will deal with different issues. Here, the physician will offer concrete help, will talk with the patient about ways to change the problematic behavior, and, if indicated, arrange a referral to a specialist.

Stages of change assessments are specific to the problem under discussion, for example, smoking, drinking more than four drinks a day, using cocaine, and so on. To determine a patient's

Table 8-2

Interview Approaches that Account for the Patient's Readiness for Behavioral Change

SIGNS OF READINESS	INTERVIEW APPROACHES
Precontemplation	• Express concern about the patient and substance abuse
	• State nonjudgmentally that substance use is a problem
	• Agree to disagree about the severity of the problem
	• Consider a trial of abstinence to clarify the issue
	• Suggest bringing a family member to an appointment
	• Explore the patient's perception of a substance use problem
	• Emphasize the importance of seeing the patient again
Contemplation	• Elicit positive and negative aspects of substance use
	• Ask about positive and negative aspects of past periods of abstinence
	• Summarize the patient's comments on substance use and abstinence
	• Make explicit discrepancies between values and actions
	• Consider a trial of abstinence
Determination	• Acknowledge the significance of the decision to seek treatment
	• Support self-efficacy
	• Affirm patient's ability to successfully seek treatment
	• Help the patient decide on appropriate, achievable action
	• Caution that the road ahead is tough but very important
	• Explain that relapse should not disrupt the patient-provider relationship
Action	• Be a source of encouragement and support
	• Acknowledge the uncomfortable aspects of withdrawal
	• Reinforce the importance of remaining in recovery
Maintenance	• Anticipate difficulties as a means of relapse prevention
	• Recognize the patient's struggle
	• Support the patient's resolve
	• Reiterate that relapse should not disrupt the medical care relationship
Relapse	• Explore what can be learned from the relapse
	• Express concern and even disappointment about the relapse
	• Emphasize the positive aspect of the effort to seek care
	• Support the patient's self-efficacy so that recovery seems achievable

readiness to change and to assign her a stage of change, the provider will have to explore: (1) if the patient has any awareness of the problem, (2) if she plans to do anything about the problem, (3) if she is ready to take action within the next 6 months, (4) if she will do something about it during the next 30 days, (5) if she is already working on the problem, or (6) if she has already coped with the problem but is at risk of relapse. Patients who have no awareness that they have a problem are said to be in "precontemplation"; those who acknowledge a problem, are aware of drinking too much, or that they should stop smoking or using illegal drugs but do not have a plan to do so are in "contemplation." Patients who plan to act on their problem within the next 30 days are in "preparation," and those who are already doing something about it are in "action." Velicer and Prochaska[49] published algorithms to determine a patient's stage of change (Table 8-4).

Communication strategies appropriate for the different stages of change are presented in Table 8-2.

Table 8-3

The Longitudinal Brief Intervention

	PATIENT STAGE	PHYSICIAN INTERVENTION	FREQUENCY OF FOLLOW-UP
Precontemplation	No conception of a problem and no plans to change.	Agree to disagree about presence of chemical dependence. Briefly bring up your concern periodically in future. Reassess for a change in readiness.	Follow-up visits as needed for other primary care problems or health maintenance.
Contemplation	Perception that there probably is a problem but ambivalent about change.	Present evidence of dysfunction and disability from the screening and assessment questionnaires, as well as the laboratory and toxicology testing. Be sure to use SOAPE to avoid a confrontation.	Schedule follow-up visits as needed for other primary care problems or health maintenance.
Determination	Awareness that a problem definitely exists and something must be done about it.	Problem solve with patient about what forms of action she/he might take.	Frequent visits, perhaps every 2–4 wk for a month or more.
Action	Ready for the initiation of behavior change.	Provide strong encouragement and support; assist with referral as needed; encourage family participation; consider pharmacotherapy; collaborate and consult with treatment program staff.	Weekly to every other week.
Maintenance	Incorporation of behavior changes into daily routine.	Encourage success; discuss difficulties and problems; encourage compliance with outpatient counseling (aftercare and self-help meetings); reassess pharmacotherapy; monitor for relapse signs; routine toxicology testing; and GGT testing if indicated.	Initially monthly, then decreasing in frequency as appropriate.
Relapse	Reversion back to contemplation or precontemplation with continued substance abuse.	Voice continued optimism; encourage return to determination, action, and maintenance; aid continued treatment and recovery attempts by patient or family members.	Frequently at first, then plan according to the new stage of patient readiness.

ABBREVIATIONS: GGT, γ-glutamyltransferase; SOAPE, subjective, objective, assessment, plan, evaluation.

Table 8-4

Smoking Algorithm

Are you currently a smoker?
1. Yes, I currently smoke.
2. No, I quit within the last 6 months.
   (ACTION STAGE)
3. No, I quit more than 6 months ago.
   (MAINTENANCE STAGE)
4. No, I have never smoked. **(NONSMOKER)**
For smokers only:
In the last year, how many times have you quit
   smoking for at least 24 h?
For smokers only:
Are you seriously thinking of quitting smoking?
   • Yes, within the next 30 days.
     (PREPARATION STAGE if they have one
     24-h quit attempt in the past year—refer to
     previous question)
     (CONTEMPLATION STAGE if they have
     zero 24-h quit attempts in the past year—
     refer to previous question)
   • Yes, within the next 6 months.
     (CONTEMPLATION STAGE)
   • No, not thinking of quitting.
     (PRECONTEMPLATION STAGE)

SOURCE: Reproduced with permission from Velicer WF, Prochaska JO.[49]

The goal of the communication is to help patients to move from one stage to the next. The impact of framing communication according to the stages of change model has been evaluated in numerous studies.[49,50] Stage-matched interventions achieve higher behavior change rates (such as smoking cessation or reduction of alcohol use) than interventions that focus only on the action of modifying drug-taking behavior. Possibly even more important is that patients are helped to move from stage to stage. Patients who are in precontemplation during their first contact with the provider can be helped to move to contemplation and ultimately to preparation and action. The criteria for success of behavior change counseling is not only changing habits but also progressing along the continuum of stages of change.

MOTIVATIONAL INTERVIEWING Motivational interviewing is the approach to patients arising from the realization that confrontation, long advocated as a major tool for treating substance abusers, does not usually result in the desired behavior change, but rather in the patient's anger and rejection of advice.[51] The alternatives suggested are that the counselor, in this case the clinician, be nonconfrontational and assist the patient in making her own decisions.[52–56]

The principles of motivational interviewing are (1) express empathy, (2) develop discrepancy, (3) avoid argumentation, (4) roll with resistance, and (5) support self-efficacy (Table 8-5). The similarity between motivational interviewing and

Table 8-5

Five General Principles of Motivational Interviewing

1. **Express empathy:**
   • Acceptance facilitates change.
   • Skillful reflective listening is fundamental.
   • Ambivalence is normal.
2. **Develop discrepancy:**
   • Awareness of consequences is important.
   • A discrepancy between present behavior and important goals will motivate change.
   • The client should present the arguments for change.
3. **Avoid argumentation:**
   • Arguments are counterproductive.
   • Defending breeds defensiveness.
   • Resistance is a signal to change strategies.
   • Labeling is unnecessary.
4. **Roll with resistance:**
   • Momentum can be used to good advantage.
   • Perceptions can be shifted.
   • New perspectives are invited but not imposed.
   • The client is a valuable resource in finding solutions to problems.
5. **Support self-efficacy:**
   • Belief in the possibility of change is an important motivator.
   • The client is responsible for choosing and carrying out personal change.
   • There is hope in the range of alternative approaches available.

patient-centered interviewing, a style of interviewing familiar to most physicians, is apparent. Rolling with resistance, although consistent with patient-centered interviewing, is rarely discussed specifically in interviewing textbooks.[57] This principle is meant to suggest that talking to a patient is not like combat; it is not the clinician's task to impose his or her will on the patients, but to acknowledge reluctance and ambivalence as natural and understandable.

A General Model of Intervening with Substance Abuse Problems in Primary Care

The Agency for Health Care Policy and Research (AHCPR) guidelines for smoking intervention in primary care[58] and the Physicians' Guide to Helping Patients with Alcohol Problems[59] point to a common strategy for dealing with substance abuse in primary care. This four-step process includes: (1) all patients should be asked; (2) patients who use should be assessed; (3) if the assessment points to problems, the patient should be advised about appropriate actions; and (4) the patient's progress should be monitored (Table 8-6). Some find it useful to divide the third step, advising, into two steps: advising on the appropriate action and assisting patients to engage in such action (Table 8-7).

DIAGNOSING SUBSTANCE ABUSE

The first step in identifying substance abuse problems is "asking." This step should be integrated into regular clinical work and is separate from assessing. Asking, in this schema, is finding

Table 8-6

Agency for Health Care Policy and Research Guidelines

Brief Advice for ALL Smokers
- **ASK** all patients at each visit if they smoke.
- **ADVISE** every smoker to quit.
- **IDENTIFY** which smokers are ready to quit.
- **ASSIST** in their quit attempt.
- **ARRANGE** a follow-up call or meeting.

Table 8-7

Steps for Screening and Brief Intervention

Step 1	**Ask about alcohol use:**
	a. Inquire about the patient's alcohol consumption.
	b. Use the CAGE questionnaire.
Step 2	**Assess for alcohol problems:**
	a. Alcohol-related medical problems.
	b. Alcohol-related behavioral problems.
	c. Alcohol dependence.
Step 3	**Advise appropriate action:**
	a. If alcohol dependence is suspected:
	1. Advise him or her to abstain.
	2. Refer the patient to a specialist.
	b. If the patient is at risk for or evidences alcohol problems:
	1. Advise him or her to cut down.
	2. Set a drinking goal.
Step 4	**Monitor the patient's progress.**

out whether the patient uses a given drug. Assessing is determining whether or not the drug use is problematic. Alternatives to the physician asking are computerized health risks or lifestyle assessments. The instrument developed by Skinner, for example, includes questions about tobacco, alcohol, and illicit drug use.[60,61] This computerized lifestyle assessment provides immediate feedback, which can become the basis of the provider's discussion with the patient. Evidence also suggests that patients may respond more openly and honestly to self-administered questionnaires than to direct questioning by a clinician.

ASKING All patients should be asked about drug and alcohol use. Examples of appropriate questions are:

- *Tobacco*: Do you smoke cigarettes? Do you use tobacco products? Do you smoke or chew tobacco?
- *Alcohol*: Do you drink alcohol, including beer, wine, or distilled spirits?

- *Illicit drugs*: Have you ever used recreational drugs (such as marijuana or cocaine) other than alcohol and cigarettes?

How often should patients be asked? The AHCPR Guidelines suggest that patients be asked about the use of tobacco products every time they are seen in primary medical care. Although this recommendation may be excessive for patients who are seen regularly in a medical setting, patients should be asked about alcohol and illicit drugs at least annually at health maintenance visits. Also, annual reviews of prescribed drugs will provide clues to inappropriate use of these medications.

Clues to the Diagnosis of Substance Abuse.   Patients usually do not come to the physician with a complaint of substance abuse, but rather with other complaints ranging from depression and sexual

Table 8-8

Common Symptoms and Physical and Laboratory Findings Suggestive of Substance Abuse

SYMPTOMS	
Fatigue (1–5)*	History of late-term abruption (2)
Insomnia (1–5)	Frequent respiratory infections (1,5)
Anxiety spells (1–5)	Frequent absences from work/school (2–5)
Somatic complaints out of proportion to physical findings (1–5)	Frequent trauma/accidental injuries (2–5)
Blackout spells (4)	Depression (2–4)
Poor school and work performance (1–5)	Atypical chest pain (2)
Weight loss (1–5)	Rhinorrhea/sinusitis (1,2,5)
Low energy (1–5)	Chronic cough (1,2,5)
Irregular menses (2–4)	Gastrointestinal complaints (4)
Frequent spontaneous abortions (1–5)	Sexual dysfunction (2–4)

PHYSICAL FINDINGS	
Staining of fingers and teeth (1)	Black sputum (2)
Jaundice (4)	Labile hypertension (2–4)
Needle tracks (2,3)	Mild tremor (4)
Nasal irritation and bleeding (2)	Odor of alcohol (4)
Tachycardia and mild hypertension (2,4)	Conjunctival irritation (5)
Hepatomegaly (4)	Perfume/mouthwash use to mask alcohol odor (4)
Expiratory wheezing (1,5)	Pupillary dilatation (5)
Decreased peak flow rate (1,5)	Pupillary constriction (3)
Easy bruising (4)	Osteoporosis (1,4)
Hemangiomata (4)	

LABORATORY FINDINGS/DIAGNOSTIC TESTS	
Elevated liver function tests (GGT, AST, ALT) (4)	Worsening peak flow (1,5)
Increased mean corpuscular volume (4)	Drug screens positive (2–5)
Carbohydrate-deficient transferrin (4)	Low blood glucose (4)
Hemoccult positive (4)	Cardiac arrhythmias (2)

*Smoking (1); cocaine (2); heroin (3); alcohol (4); marijuana (5).
ABBREVIATIONS: ALT, alanine aminotransferase; AST, aspartate transaminase; GGT, γ-glutamyltransferase.

dysfunction to atypical chest pain and gastrointestinal complaints. Common symptoms, physical findings, and laboratory studies related to alcohol use and other substances are listed in Table 8-8.

The clinician may need to look for clusters of symptoms and findings, due to multiple drug use and abuse. Abnormal laboratory study results may be transient, due to timing and degree of exposure.

Table 8-9
Assessing Levels of Disease Severity

	PSYCHOLOGICAL DEPENDENCE	**ORGAN SYSTEM DAMAGE**	**PSYCHOSOCIAL MORBIDITY**
Mild	One or more of the following: • Inability to stop • Insomnia • Anxiety AUDIT (Questions 1–3)* Combined score > 5: • Frequency (1) • Average # of drinks (2) • Six or more drinks (3)	One of the following: • High normal GGT • Memory loss • Physical injury • Bloodshot eyes • Depression • Sexual dysfunction • High blood pressure • Gastritis/ulcers • Headaches • Osteoporosis	One of the following: CAGE:† • Cut down (C) • Annoyed (A) • Guilty (G) AUDIT: • Failed expectations (5) • Remorse (7) • Memory loss (8) • Injured self or others (9) • Concern expressed by others (10)
Moderate	Any of the above mild symptoms with one or more of the following: • Hand tremor • "Eye opener" • Diaphoresis • BAL > 100 mg/dL • Positive urine toxicology	Two or three of the following: • Elevated GGT • Memory loss • Injury/broken bones • Elevated MCV • Elevated liver function profile • Depression • Sexual dysfunction • High blood pressure • Gastritis/ulcers • Headaches • Osteoporosis	Two of the following: CAGE: • Cut down (C) • Annoyed (A) • Guilty (G) AUDIT: • Failed expectations (5) • Remorse (7) • Memory loss (8) • Injured self or others (9) • Concern expressed by others (10)
aSevere	Any of the above mild or moderate symptoms with one or more of the following: • Hallucinations • Seizures • Delirium tremens • BAL > 200 mg/dL • Prolonged positive toxicology	Four or more of the following: • Elevated GGT • Memory loss • Injury/broken bones • Elevated MCV • Elevated liver function profile • Depression • Sexual dysfunction • High blood pressure • Gastritis/ulcers • Headaches • Osteoporosis • Hepatomegaly • Elevated prothrombin time	Positive on three or more of the following: CAGE: • Cut down (C) • Annoyed (A) • Guilty (G) AUDIT: • Failed expectations (5) • Remorse (7) • Memory loss (8) • Injured self or others (9) • Concern expressed by others (10)

*For AUDIT questionnaire see Appendix B.
†For CAGE questionnaire see Table 8-11.
ABBREVIATIONS: BAL, blood alcohol level; GGT, γ-glutamyltransferase; MCV, mean corpuscular volume.

ASSESSMENT   Patients who admit to using (or in the case of illicit drugs, of having used drugs) or who present with other indications of drug use on physical examination or laboratory testing should be assessed further. Most primary care providers are concerned about assessments that would facilitate treatment decisions rather than provide a formal diagnosis. Two factors that are most helpful in tailoring treatment are problem severity and stage of change.

Problem Severity.   To assess problem severity (Table 8-9), it is useful to rely on established instruments with known sensitivity and specificity.

Tobacco   Fagerstrom developed a scale for assessing the level of dependence on nicotine (Table 8-10). This scale is a good example of an instrument for the assessment of dependence. In smoking, however, dependence correlates highly with consumption (e.g., the more cigarettes a person smokes, the more dependent they are). It is debatable whether or not there are nondependent smokers, but persons who smoke less than five cigarettes a day rarely enroll in treatment.

Alcohol   Best known for the identification of alcohol problems is the CAGE (Table 8-11). If at least two questions are answered positively, further

Table 8-10

Mini-Fagerstrom Nicotine Tolerance Questionnaire

Values for each answer are coded immediately behind the answer. Total > 7 assumes addiction.
1. On the average, how many cigarettes do you smoke per day?
   0–10 cigs/day = 0
   11–20 cigs/day = 1
   21–30 cigs/day = 2
   ≥31 cigs/day = 3
2. Do you smoke more frequently in the first hours of the morning than during the rest of the day?
   Yes = 1
   No = 0
3. How soon after you wake up do you have your first cigarette? (in min)
   0–5 = 3
   6–30 = 2
   31–60 = 1
   >60 = 0
4. Which cigarette of the day would you hate to give up most?
   First in the morning = 1
   Any other = 0
5. Do you find it difficult to refrain from smoking when you are in places where it is forbidden, like in church, at the library, or in a movie theater?
   Yes = 1
   No = 0
6. Do you find it difficult to refrain from smoking when drinking coffee?
   Yes = 1
   No = 0
7. Do you find it difficult to refrain from smoking when drinking alcohol?
   Yes = 1
   No = 0
8. Do you smoke if you are so ill that you are in bed most of the day?
   Yes = 1
   No = 0

Source: Adapted from Fagerstrom KO: Measuring degree of physical dependence on tobacco smoking with reference to individualization of treatment. *Addictive Behavior* 3:235, 1998.

Table 8-11

CAGE Questionnaire

1. Have you ever felt you should cut down on your drinking?
2. Have people ever annoyed you by criticizing your drinking?
3. Have you ever felt bad or guilty about your drinking?
4. Have you ever had a drink first thing in the morning to steady your nerves or to get rid of a hangover (eye opener)?

SOURCE: Adapted from Ewing JA: Detecting alcoholism: the CAGE questionnaire. *JAMA* 252:1905, 1984.

assessment with respect to the amount of alcohol consumed, situations of use, and potential health consequences is indicated. In recent years, variations of the CAGE have been published, most notably the TWEAK (Table 8-12). The MAST (Michigan Alcohol Screening Test) and its variations are among other instruments that have been used to assess alcohol use.[62]

Screening may be accomplished most simply, however, using the following two questions

suggested by Brown et al.[63] Either question answered positively is a good indicator for the presence of substance abuse problems.

1. In the last year, have you ever drank or used drugs more than you meant to?
2. Have you felt you wanted or needed to cut down on your drinking or drug use in the last year?

Other Forms of Substance Abuse   CAGE-AID (Table 8-13) can be used to assess the presence of problems of drug abuse other than alcohol abuse. Specific drugs to inquire about are marijuana (hashish, pot, grass), amphetamines (stimulants, uppers, speed), barbiturates (sedatives, downers, sleeping pills, Seconal, quaaludes), tranquilizers (Valium, Librium), cocaine (coke, crack), heroin, opiates (codeine, Demerol, morphine, methadone, Darvon, opium), and psychedelics (LSD, Mescaline, peyote, psilocybin, DMT, PCP).

If problematic substance use is suggested by the screening interviews, then further examination with instruments such as the AUDIT[64,65] (see Appendix B) or the DAST[66] is indicated. Should assessment at this stage indicate substance abuse problems, then a history of substance abuse problems should be taken and medical problems that might be the consequence of substance abuse should be explored (Table 8-8).

Table 8-12

TWEAK Test

T	Tolerance: How many drinks can you hold?
W	Have close friends or relatives worried or complained about your drinking in the past year?
E	Eye opener: Do you sometimes take a drink in the morning when you first get up?
A	Amnesia: Has a friend or family member ever told you about things you said or did while you were drinking that you could not remember?
K(C)	Do you sometimes feel the need to cut down on your drinking?

SOURCE: Adapted from Russell M: New assessment tools for risk-drinking during pregnancy: T-ACE, TWEAK, and others. *Alc Health and Research World* 18:55, 1994.

Table 8-13

CAGE-AID

1. Have you ever felt you ought to cut down on your drinking or drug use?
2. Have people annoyed you by criticizing your drinking or drug use?
3. Have you ever felt bad or guilty about your drinking or drug use?
4. Have you ever had a drink or used drugs first thing in the morning to steady your nerves or get rid of a hangover (eye opener)?

SOURCE: Reproduced with permission from Brown RL, Rounds LA: Conjoint screening questionnaire for alcohol and drug abuse. *Wis Med J* 94:135–140, 1995.

MANAGING SUBSTANCE ABUSE

ADVISE/ASSIST Primary care providers face a choice: they can either give righteous, firm but ineffective, advice or work with patients to help them make reasonable decisions leading to important, albeit small, steps toward dealing with substance abuse. Just telling someone what to do, often justified as an act of moral courage, is an established practice not only in medicine but in many walks of life including education and politics. However, in this situation such advice is ineffective partially because it is difficult for patients to quickly change long-established habits. A provider who decides to assist the patient has two options: (1) to work with her within the practice using a brief office intervention, or (2) to refer her to a substance abuse specialist or a specialized substance abuse treatment program.

In deciding which strategy to follow, the provider should be guided by the patient's readiness to change, the severity of the substance abuse problem, and concomitant psychiatric, medical, and social problems. The patient's degree of readiness will become apparent through the patient's answers to questions like "Do you think you have a problem with drinking?" and "Have you ever thought about cutting back?" When evaluating the severity of the substance abuse problem, both degrees of dependence and acute intoxication will be considered. Concomitant problems enter the decision-making process because they might be too severe to allow the primary care physician the alternative of office-based intervention.

Brief Office Intervention. Brief advice or minimal intervention is at times discussed as if it were a discrete stand-alone model of behavior change. The overlap between brief advice and the general approach to patient counseling described in this section is apparent.[64,67] Brief advice is, in effect, an extension of assist and advise in the general model and will, in appropriate cases, also include pharmacologic support. Brief advice is the appropriate intervention for patients with positive but low scores on any of the screening instruments (CAGE, AUDIT, and DAST) and for all cigarette smokers. Those interested in learning more about brief advice should consult volume NR 24, Treatment Improvement Protocol (TIP Series).[68]

The components of a brief intervention are:

1. Giving feedback about screening results, impairment, and risks while clarifying the findings
2. Informing patients about safe consumption limits and offering advice about change
3. Assessing patient's readiness to change
4. Negotiating goals and strategies for change
5. Arranging for follow-up treatment

Giving Feedback   To give feedback, clinicians tell the patient that they believe that the patient has a problem by reporting and interpreting findings, while conversing with the patient in a nonadversarial, nonconfrontational manner. Examples of what clinicians might say can be found in Appendix C. It is important to remember that the patient cannot be made to accept advice, but a patient's ability to process the information given will increase if the patient is encouraged to verbalize feelings about the advice and the reasons for rejecting advice.

Informing Patients   The goal of informing patients about safe consumption limits and offering advice about change is to engage the patient in problem-solving. To be effective givers of advice, providers should maintain communication styles conforming to the principles of motivational interviewing. Clinicians should be clear and firm about their opinion, but statements of opinion need to be followed by exploration of the readiness for change and negotiations.

There is some disagreement about how to advise patients who use illegal drugs. When talking about alcohol, clinicians are encouraged to discuss safe drinking. In contrast, when talking about illegal drugs, it is suggested that clinicians advise only total abstinence, even though this approach may be less effective than simply encouraging a decrease in consumption. Few patients will be ready to stop using drugs altogether, but many others will be at the stage where they can control consumption.

Assessing Readiness to Change   Only some patients will opt immediately for action. They, for example, will stop smoking. Frequently, the task of the clinician will be helping patients move from one stage to the next. Examples of provider interventions linked to stages of change are shown in Tables 8-2 and 8-3 and questions for determining the stage of readiness can be found in Table 8-4.

Negotiating   The result of the negotiation will be a decision. Decisions might range from a willingness to come back to discuss the problem with the clinician to a plan to enter substance abuse treatment. The decision that the clinician and patient arrive at must be the patient's.

Referral.   Referral to a substance abuse specialist or a substance abuse treatment program is indicated for patients who have been judged to be too highly dependent to be able to respond to brief intervention and for patients at different levels of dependence with severe concomitant social, psychological, medical, and financial problems. Although some patients are ordered into treatment by the judicial system, the primary care provider's success in completing a referral depends on the patient's readiness to accept the referral. A patient's readiness is influenced by the clinician's skill in counseling.

Type of Referral   Usually, primary care providers have few or no choices about clinicians and institutions to whom to refer and no influence on the treatment the patient receives. Financial matters are primary; the patient's medical insurance or financial means determine the route of referral. Only if a patient has insurance or private funds can a referral to private substance abuse treatment specialist or treatment program be contemplated. Many patients suffering from substance abuse problems are without resources for private care.[69] For them, admission to publicly funded programs is the only option. Fortunately, public and private programs cannot be differentiated with regard to their effectiveness in helping patients.

Choices are limited even if funds are available. The number of substance abuse specialists, particularly physicians and psychiatrists, is small, and it is difficult to differentiate specialists by the approach that they take to treatment. In addition, the list of treatment alternatives actually refers to the setting in which treatment is given rather than to different therapies. The reason for this is that assignment of patients is primarily to programs and not to a particular form of therapy; most programs follow the same treatment model shaped by the 12-step movement (Table 8-14).

In the public treatment network, patients are often evaluated by a central assessment organization before they are assigned to a program. The task of these organizations is to determine the level of care needed by each patient. In many states the ASAM criteria (American Society of Addiction Medicine Patient Placement Criteria for the Treatment of Psychoactive Substance-Related Disorders)[70] guide the decision-making. Although the ASAM criteria mention 10 different levels or types of care, only 4 alternatives are available in most jurisdictions: detoxification, outpatient, intensive outpatient, and long-term residential. Also, only some places have methadone maintenance, drug-free outpatient, and specialized programs for subpopulations such as women, adolescents, and patients with a dual diagnosis of substance abuse and other psychiatric disorders.

Hospitalization is rarely used today and is only indicated if patients' psychiatric or medical problems are severe enough to lead to hospitalization even without a substance abuse disorder. Although the ASAM criteria for the assignment of patients to different levels of care are complex, many substance abuse professionals base their decision to admit their patients to residential programs primarily on the severity of social problems. For example, homelessness is a common indicator for admission to residential programs.

MONITORING PATIENT PROGRESS   Follow-up and monitoring are essential components for any substance abuse intervention. Follow-up in primary medical care has two functions. In the context of brief advice, it is an essential part of "treatment." Through repeated follow-up visits, primary care providers will check compliance with the treatment plan negotiated and provide encouragement.

Table 8-14

The Twelve Steps of Alcoholics Anonymous

1. We admitted we were powerless over alcohol and that our lives had become unmanageable.
2. Came to believe that a Power greater than ourselves could restore us to sanity.
3. Made a decision to turn our will and our lives over to the care of God as we understood Him.
4. Made a searching and fearless moral inventory of ourselves.
5. Admitted to God, to ourselves, and to another human being the exact nature of our wrongs.
6. Were entirely ready to have God remove all these defects of character.
7. Humbly asked Him to remove our shortcomings.
8. Made a list of all persons we had harmed, and became willing to make amends to them all.
9. Made direct amends to such people wherever possible, except when to do so would injure them or others.
10. Continued to take personal inventory and when we were wrong promptly admitted it.
11. Sought through prayer and meditation to improve our conscious contact with God as we understood Him, praying only for knowledge of His will for us and the power to carry that out.
12. Having had a spiritual awakening as the result of these steps, we tried to carry this message to alcoholics, and to practice these principles in all our affairs.

The frequency of follow-up visits will depend on the severity of the substance abuse problem. As a general rule, however, there should be one follow-up visit shortly after the initial visit during which the treatment plan was negotiated. The purpose of this follow-up visit is to help patients stick to their treatment plan. The visit therefore ought to occur after the patient has an opportunity to put the plan into action. For example, in smoking cessation, where patients in the action stage will agree on a stop smoking date, it is helpful for patients to be seen the day after the stop smoking date. On the other hand, if the patient developed a plan that called for the reduction of the number of drinks during a week, then the follow-up visit ought to occur after the patient had a chance to practice the new style of drinking for at least a week.

Even after referral of patients to treatment programs, it will often be the primary care clinician who will provide medical care even while the patient is in active substance abuse treatment. Primary care providers will work with the patient for long periods of time, and they often know when relapse has occurred and additional treatment is needed. Patients value the primary care provider's encouragement, and they may be the only one who knows about the patient's ongoing struggle with substance abuse. Given the intractability of substance abuse problems, the issue of substance abuse should be a frequently discussed topic.

Has the Primary Care Provider Made the Best Referral?

The simplest and most discouraging answer is that there is no way to know. Research on substance abuse treatment, which might provide guidance, has had little influence on the field. Fortunately, what seems to matter most is for a patient to be treated and to stay in treatment for a long time.[71,72] The actual nature of treatment, in particular the type of program to which one is referred, is of secondary importance.

The practice of assigning patients to different levels of care, however, is not supported by research.[73,74] Not only is there no evidence that patients who were correctly placed according to ASAM criteria did better than those randomly assigned to different levels of care, there is also no convincing evidence that residential programs are superior to outpatient care.[75,76] Recent studies, however, note higher retention rates in residential programs. In addition, although patients who are maintained in outpatient programs achieve the same improvements as those in residential programs, a larger proportion of residential patients complete treatment.[77] One additional issue of importance is the program "attraction rate," that is, the percentage of those in need of treatment who are willing to enter a given treatment program. It is possible that the attraction rate for outpatient programs is higher than that of residential programs. If this is the case, then outpatient treatment could have a greater impact on the problem of substance abuse.

Pharmacologic Treatments

The indication for detoxification for any abused drug is that the drug is having an adverse effect on physical health or is interfering with the individual's ability to perform social, job, school, or parenting functions. Virtually any drug that is abused (marijuana, alcohol, cocaine, or heroin) can interfere with these functions. Although smoking may not directly interfere with functioning, the health risks to a woman, her children, and those around her dictate that smoking cessation at least be attempted.

Although the drugs listed above can all cause significant problems with health or functioning, not all drugs cause a severe enough withdrawal syndrome on acute discontinuation to warrant medical treatment. For example, marijuana abuse can cause impairment of functioning but it causes little in the way of physical dependence; consequently, a severe withdrawal reaction is not seen when marijuana is abruptly discontinued. Even in

very heavy users of marijuana (up to 20 joints per day), withdrawal consists only of irritability and transient insomnia.

Cocaine withdrawal consists primarily of fatigue, lethargy, increased appetite, anhedonia, and a persistent craving for more cocaine. These physical symptoms, however, are not severe enough to warrant medical treatment. The major problem with cocaine is that women using it tend to relapse readily. Unfortunately, no medical treatments have been shown to reliably decrease the craving for cocaine.

The pharmacologic treatments discussed below focus on abused substances that cause severe withdrawal syndromes or health problems that can be at least somewhat effectively treated by pharmacologic interventions. These withdrawal syndromes and their management are outlined in Table 8-15.

ETHANOL DETOXIFICATION

It can be assumed that alcohol tolerance is present when any woman ingests more than 8 oz of absolute (100 percent) alcohol per day (about 1 pint of hard liquor daily; Table 8-16).[78] This is not to imply that this is the minimum amount of daily alcohol needed to create dependence, and less alcohol intake may be associated with dependence, especially if other drugs are also being taken.[79]

Alcohol withdrawal severity occurs along a continuum, with many persons only experiencing mild withdrawal symptoms such as tremor, headache, nausea, irritability, and insomnia. However, at the other end of the spectrum, severe symptoms may occur and possibly lead to seizures or delirium tremens. Up to 5 percent of those withdrawing from alcohol use experience delirium tremens. It is difficult to predict who will suffer the most severe withdrawal syndrome; the majority of individuals withdrawing from alcohol can be treated as outpatients.

HOSPITALIZATION   Some specialized populations should always be hospitalized for treatment, such

Table 8-15

Withdrawal Symptoms and Their Treatment

SUBSTANCE	WITHDRAWAL SYMPTOMS		TREATMENT
Alcohol	Onset within 6–48 h		Nonpharmacologic if syndrome is mild, benzodiazepines for moderate to severe symptoms
	Mild:	restlessness, tachycardia, irritability, hypertension, anorexia, insomnia, tremor	Vitamins and fluids
	Moderate:	nausea, nightmares, vomiting, impaired concentration, sweating, increased hypertension, tachycardia	
	Severe:	increased tremulousness, agitation, increased sweating, delirium, hallucinations, delusions, grand mal seizures	
Opioids	Heroin:	onset within 6–8 h; duration 5–7 d	Methadone
	Methadone:	onset within 36–72 h; duration 2–3 wk	Clonidine (Catapres)
			Phenobarbital
	Opioid withdrawal symptoms in adults:		Paregoric
	Mild:	anxiety, drug craving, restlessness, muscle and joint aches, lower back pain, tension, mild insomnia, lethargy, diaphoresis, mydriasis	
	Moderate:	chills with flushing, diaphoresis, rhinorrhea, lacrimation, anorexia, back pain, piloerection, tachycardia, mild increase in blood pressure, yawning, nausea, stomach cramps	
	Severe:	diarrhea, vomiting, tremors, tachycardia (>100 beats/min), increased respirations, severe stomach cramps, kicking movements, low-grade temperature elevation	
	Opioid withdrawal symptoms in neonates:		
	Onset within 72 h (heroin; longer with methadone)		
	Symptoms include: irritability, hypertonia, hyperreflexia, abnormal suck, poor feeding, seizures, diarrhea, vomiting, tachypnea, sneezing		
Tobacco	Onset within 24 h		Nicotine gum
	Symptoms include: dysphoria, insomnia, irritability, frustration, anger, anxiety, difficulty concentrating, restlessness, decreased heart rate, increased appetite, weight gain		Nicotine patch
			Nicotine nasal spray
			Nicotine oral inhaler
			Bupropion (Zyban)

Table 8-16

Amounts of Alcoholic Beverages Equivalent to 1 Drink
(12 g or 0.5 oz absolute ethanol)

- 1 "shot" (1.5 oz) of hard liquor (80 proof, 40% alcohol)
- 1 glass (5 oz) of wine (11–12% alcohol)
- 1 bottle or can (12 oz) beer (4–5% alcohol)
- 1 wine cooler (12 oz) (5% alcohol)

as those who are medically unstable or are pregnant. The Center for Substance Abuse Treatment (CSAT) has developed guidelines recommending that any pregnant woman undergoing alcohol withdrawal be treated as an inpatient, even if the withdrawal syndrome does not appear to be very severe. The treatment team should include collaboration with an experienced obstetric provider, and fetal well-being should be monitored throughout withdrawal (fetal heart tones, sonograms, or nonstress test).

VITAMINS Although all individuals undergoing alcohol withdrawal may not require pharmacologic treatment, thiamine (100 mg) should be given to all patients because thiamine is deficient in 30 to 80 percent of alcohol abusers. Administration of thiamine can prevent the Wernicke-Korsakoff syndrome (classically presenting as ophthalmoplegia, ataxia, and global confusion). Treatment of this syndrome requires immediate administration of 50 mg thiamine, either intravenously or intramuscularly, with continued administration daily until the patient is tolerating a normal diet.

Heavy alcohol consumption may also lead to depletion of other water-soluble vitamins, so administration of a multivitamin containing B vitamins, vitamin C, and folic acid is advised.

BENZODIAZEPINES In patients in whom pharmacologic treatment is necessary, the standard treatment is benzodiazepines (Table 8-17). Although the benzodiazepines are considerably safer than their precursors (barbiturates), they are not without hazards. Benzodiazepines can result in sedation if their use is not carefully monitored. They may also cause respiratory depression, although it is rarely problematic except in those with preexisting pulmonary disease or obstructive sleep apnea syndrome.

Although there have been concerns about birth defects, in particular cleft palate, associated with the use of benzodiazepines during pregnancy, the data supporting this connection or any other teratogenic effect are weak.[80] The risk to the fetus from severe alcohol withdrawal is likely to outweigh the potential risk of benzodiazepine-induced teratogenicity.

In the last trimester of pregnancy, an effort should be made to taper the benzodiazepine before delivery because when high doses of benzodiazepines are taken by the woman, her infant is likely to show sedation and to undergo benzodiazepine withdrawal postpartum. In the case of benzodiazepine intoxication, the neonate may display a "floppy," lethargic appearance and have difficulty breathing. Usually benzodiazepine withdrawal, consisting of hyperreflexia, tremor, and hypertonia, resolves spontaneously.

ETHANOL DETERRENTS

Alcohol deterrents are drugs that can be used to curtail alcohol ingestion. Some of these agents (aversive agents) cause a distressful reaction when alcohol is taken following their ingestion and others are used to reduce craving and decrease the pleasurable effects of alcohol. An excellent review on the pharmacologic treatment of alcohol dependence has recently been published and provides a more detailed review of current and experimental agents.[79]

AVERSIVE AGENTS This class of drugs includes disulfiram (Antabuse®), calcium carbamide, and metronidazole (Flagyl®). Of these, only disulfiram has an approval from the Food and Drug Administration (FDA) for use as an aid to maintain sobriety from alcohol.

Table 8-17

Benzodiazepine Dosing Options in Acute Alcohol Withdrawal

DRUG	REGIMEN (ORAL UNLESS OTHERWISE STATED)	
Chlordiazepoxide (Librium®)	Day 1	100 mg q6h
	Day 2	100 mg q8h
	Day 3	100 mg q12h
	Day 4	100 mg hs
OR		
	Day 1	50 mg q8h + 50 mg prn X 1
	Day 2	50 mg q8h
	Day 3	25 mg q8h
	Day 4	25 mg bid
Clorazepate (Tranxene®)	Day 1	30 mg initially, followed by 15 mg bid
	Day 2	15 mg tid
	Day 3	15 mg bid
	Day 4	7.5 mg tid
	Day 5	7.5 mg bid
Diazepam (Valium®)	Day 1	10 mg tid
	Day 2	10 mg, 5 mg, 10 mg
	Day 3	5 mg tid
	Day 4	5 mg bid
OR		
	Day 1	20 mg initially, followed by 20 mg q2h until reaction controlled, then drug d/c'd
Lorazepam (Ativan®)	Day 1	2 mg q8h + 2 mg prn X 1
	Day 2	2 mg q8h
	Day 3	1 mg q8h
	Day 4	1 mg bid
OR		
	Day 1	5 mg IM
	Day 2	Average daily oral dose of 2 or 3 mg continued as long as needed

Disulfiram. Disulfiram inhibits acetaldehyde dehydrogenase, the enzyme responsible for eliminating acetaldehyde from the body. Most ethanol is metabolized by alcohol dehydrogenase to acetaldehyde, which is then metabolized, by acetaldehyde dehydrogenase, to acetate and carbon dioxide. Normally acetaldehyde is easily cleared from the body, but when it accumulates, it causes a series of unpleasant symptoms including vasodilation, diaphoresis, tachycardia, elevated blood pressure, headache, and nausea. Not only is this reaction uncomfortable, but it has been fatal, especially in those who are medically unstable.[81]

Efficacy In general, the success of disulfiram in maintaining abstinence has not been impressive. Two randomized clinical trials have compared disulfiram to placebo.[82,83] One trial found a slight increase in abstinence at 6 months, whereas the other found no significant differences in the number of patients remaining abstinent, the time to first drink, or number of drinking days over 12 months among three groups who received placebo, a 1-mg daily disulfiram dose (subtherapeutic), and the usual 250-mg daily disulfiram dose. Although statistical significance was not achieved, the group taking the 250-mg daily dose of disulfiram drank 49 ± 8.4 days (mean $\pm$ standard deviation), and those taking placebo drank 86.5 ± 13.6 days. If disulfiram is ordered by the court as a condition of parole, compliance appears to be much better than in a random sample of alcohol abusers who are not as motivated.

Dose and Regimen   Although the recommended dose of disulfiram is 250 mg daily, this might not be the most appropriate dose in all individuals because the metabolism of disulfiram varies. The activity of disulfiram depends on one of its metabolites, diethylthiocarbamate, which is generated to varying degrees in different individuals. Another metabolite generated by the biotransformation of disulfiram is carbon disulfide, which produces centrilobular hepatic necrosis in animal experiments. It may be that the hepatotoxicity seen in humans is related to this metabolite.

Side Effects   Disulfiram itself has also been associated with some rather severe side effects. Sedation, dizziness, and headache are common side effects, especially at the beginning of treatment. Nausea, vomiting, hypotension, dry mouth, and blurred vision are less commonly seen, as well as urticarial, acneiform, or allergic dermatitis type skin rashes. Hepatotoxicity and peripheral neuropathy have been rarely reported. The incidence of peripheral neuropathy may be disproportionately high in women.[84] The hepatic reactions usually occur within 60 days, the peripheral neuropathy usually within 2 to 3 months, and skin reactions usually within the first 3 weeks of disulfiram treatment. Such side effects tend to be dose related; consequently, daily doses greater than 250 mg are discouraged.

Use in Pregnancy   There is little information on the use of disulfiram in pregnancy. There are several case reports of teratogenicity (limb reductions and cleft palate), but there are not enough data to conclusively determine whether disulfiram actually causes these reported abnormalities.[85] Although these case reports are neither numerous nor conclusive, it would be prudent to avoid disulfiram during pregnancy.

Drug Interactions   In addition to inhibiting acetaldehyde dehydrogenase, disulfiram also inhibits some of the cytochrome P450 metabolic enzymes, altering the biotransformation of a variety of drugs (Table 8-18). In particular, the increase in warfarin effect and an increase in phenytoin blood concentrations seen after addition of disulfiram could be quite problematic. Additionally, because polysubstance abuse is fairly common, it should be noted that chronic disulfiram use results in higher cocaine concentrations following intranasal cocaine administration.

Metronidazole causes a similar type of reaction with alcohol, but it has never been used as a deterrent for drinking alcohol. One effort was made to determine if combined treatment with disulfiram and metronidazole would be more effective than disulfiram alone, and the combination caused an unacceptable (20 percent) level of psychosis.

OPIOID ANTAGONISTS   Although many drugs, including lithium and serotonin reuptake inhibitors, have been used for reduction of alcohol craving, only naltrexone (ReVia®) has substantial data to support its use for this indication.

Naltrexone.   The use of naltrexone to treat alcohol abuse is a relatively new phenomenon. Naltrexone was developed for use as an aid in the maintenance of sobriety in heroin addicts, but it was never widely accepted for this indication because unlike methadone, it does not replace heroin, but only blocks its pharmacologic effects.

Efficacy   When naltrexone is given to heavy alcohol drinkers, both the overall number of drinks

Table 8-18

Drug Interactions for Drugs Used in the Treatment of Drug Dependence and Withdrawal

DRUG	INTERACTING DRUG	TYPE OF INTERACTION AND APPROPRIATE ACTION
Clonidine	Amitriptyline, imipramine, desipramine, (also likely with nortriptyline, doxepin, protriptyline, and trimipramine)	Decrease in clonidine antihypertensive effect (unknown if this interaction would interfere with detoxification effects); monitor closely, the dose may need to be increased.
	Cyclosporine	Clonidine may cause an increase in cyclosporine levels; monitor cyclosporine blood levels.
Disulfiram	Benzodiazepines (including: alprazolam, chlordiazepoxide, diazepam, flurazepam, halazepam, prazepam, triazolam)	Disulfiram decreases the metabolism; may see increased pharmacologic effect; might have to decrease benzodiazepine dose.
	Cocaine	Disulfiram decreases the clearance of cocaine from the body; may see increased cocaine effects.
	Isoniazid	The addition of disulfiram to isoniazid has resulted in changes in affect and behavior and decreased coordination; avoid the combination if possible; if they must be given concomitantly, monitor closely.
	Phenytoin	Phenytoin blood levels increase, possibly associated with toxicity; phenytoin dose may need to be decreased, monitor phenytoin blood levels.
	Theophylline	Increased theophylline blood concentration; may need to decrease theophylline dose, monitor theophylline blood levels.
	Warfarin	Increased warfarin effect has been noted when disulfiram is added; monitor PT/INR, may need to decrease warfarin dose.
Methadone	Many anticonvulsants (phenytoin, phenobarbital, carbamazepine, primidone)	Dose of methadone may have to be increased to prevent the development of withdrawal symptoms.
	Rifampin	When added to methadone an increase in methadone clearance is seen; dose of methadone may have to be increased to prevent the development of withdrawal symptoms.
(Possible inter-action)	*Tricyclic antidepressants, phenothiazines, metroprolol, timolol, codeine, dextromethorphan, tramadol*	*Methadone might decrease clearance of these drugs; monitor and change dose if necessary.*
Tobacco smoke	Caffeine, theophylline, tricyclic antidepressants, propranolol	Smoking tobacco increases the metabolism of these drugs, if smoking is discontinued the dose of these drugs may need to be decreased.

ABBREVIATIONS: INR, International Normalized Ratio; PT, prothrombin time.

consumed per drinking episode and the number of drinking episodes decrease. Although naltrexone decreases alcohol intake, this does not necessarily result in abstinence. A prospective follow-up study was conducted after the completion of a 12-week course of naltrexone or placebo.[86] During the follow-up, no drug therapy was administered and all subjects were monitored for the next 6 months. During the active drug phase, the naltrexone group showed a greater abstinence rate, but by 2 months following the active drug trial, the group that had received naltrexone no longer maintained a higher abstinence rate than those who had received placebo. The researchers concluded that naltrexone was able to help promote abstinence when it was taken, but this effect did not last beyond 2 months after the drug was discontinued. Evidently, breaking the "habit" of drinking for this short period of time was not enough to bring about continued abstinence after discontinuation of the drug.

Dose and Regimen   For the treatment of alcoholism, naltrexone is given in a dose of 50 mg/d. The manufacturer recommends treatment duration of up to 12 weeks; however, it has been used for a longer duration in the treatment of opioid addiction. Although most of the studies have used a 12-week treatment period, longer treatment is probably indicated, assuming careful monitoring for side effects, especially increases in liver function tests (LFTs).

Side Effects   Naltrexone is generally well tolerated, and it is remarkably free of any reported drug interactions. Side effects found in an open study of alcohol abusers included nausea (10 percent), headache (7 percent), dizziness (4 percent), nervousness (4 percent), and fatigue (4 percent). The most severe adverse effect has been hepatotoxicity, but this was reported primarily when naltrexone was used in doses up to 300 mg/d to treat obesity. When the recommended dose of 50 mg/d is used, hepatotoxicity is not likely. In one study, LFTs actually improved during naltrexone treatment, probably as a function of abstinence from alcohol.[87]

Because naltrexone is an opioid antagonist, it is contraindicated if there is known opioid use due to the likelihood of opioid withdrawal. If there is a suspicion of opioid use, a urine screen for opioids or a naloxone (Narcan®) challenge could be used to determine whether naltrexone should be used.

Use in Pregnancy   Naltrexone has a category C listing for use in pregnancy. When given in huge doses (approximately 140 times the human dose), embryocidal effects were noted in rats and rabbits. There are no data in humans. Although naltrexone would not generally be used in a pregnant woman, a risk/benefit decision would be necessary. If the alcohol abuse is heavy enough to result in fetal alcohol syndrome, then naltrexone therapy might be worth the risk.

HEROIN DETOXIFICATION

Heroin, or diacetylmorphine hydrochloride, is two to four times more potent than morphine as an analgesic and also more euphorigenic. Much of its action is a consequence of rapid deacetylation to monoacetyl morphine (MAM) and morphine. Withdrawal from heroin begins about 8 h or less after the previous dose and symptoms increase in severity over the next 2 days, with peak withdrawal occurring within the first 48 h. Opioid withdrawal is uncomfortable, resembling a case of influenza, but is rarely life-threatening. The withdrawal syndrome is described in Table 8-15.

OPIOID AGONISTS   Several different methods are used for heroin detoxification. One strategy involves opioid replacement with another opioid agonist such as methadone or L-α-acetyl methadyl (LAAM).

Agents.   Methadone is commonly used because it has relatively high oral bioavailability, so it can be given orally, and it has a more prolonged effect than morphine or heroin, up to 48 h. Methadone also has a slower onset of effect, so it is not associated with the "rush" seen when heroin is injected and rapidly enters the brain. Withdrawal from methadone is similar to withdrawal from heroin except that symptoms of withdrawal are less intense and do not occur for up to 3 days after the last dose. Withdrawal from methadone reaches a peak at about 6 days and lasts for 2 to 3 weeks.

L-α-Acetyl methadyl (LAAM) is also an opioid agonist, but it displays a more prolonged elimination half-life than methadone and can be administered every other day, instead of daily. It is recommended for use in maintenance programs rather than for acute withdrawal, due to slow onset of effect (8 to 12 h). Withdrawal from LAAM is also similar to withdrawal from methadone except that the onset is later and its duration is longer due to the fact that LAAM is eliminated from the body more slowly than methadone.

Efficacy.   Follow-up studies have shown that about 20 to 30 percent of heroin users who have been detoxified are still abstinent at 1.5 to 2.7 years after detoxification. Philosophies regarding whether heroin addicts should be maintained on methadone or should undergo detoxification and achieve complete opioid abstinence differ. Although not many studies have compared detoxification programs of different length, the most frequently quoted study[88] reported more treatment dropouts and more urine samples positive for opioids in a group of addicts treated in a 21-day program in comparison to an 84-day program. Some clinicians have argued that detoxification is neither desirable nor appropriate for all opioid addicts.[89,90] An example is the HIV-infected opioid addict for whom relapse poses additional risks to public health as well as to the individual.

Dose and Regimen.   When the amount of heroin used daily can be estimated, methadone can be substituted at a rate of 1 mg methadone per 2 mg heroin. The usual methadone dose for heroin detoxification ranges from 30 to 60 mg daily. However, in a recent randomized trial, higher doses (80 to 100 mg daily) were more effective in decreasing illicit opioid use during detoxification, although the higher doses were not associated with increased retention in the study.[91]

Methadone detoxification regimens range in duration from 7 to 180 days. When methadone is administered for the treatment of heroin abuse for longer than 180 days, it is considered maintenance treatment. Methadone maintenance programs must have both FDA and state authority approval. There are also federal guidelines governing methadone detoxification. Physicians not affiliated with methadone detoxification clinics can administer opioids for the purpose of relieving acute withdrawal symptoms for a period not to exceed 3 days. According to guidelines from the Drug Enforcement Agency (DEA), administration of methadone for detoxification for longer than 3 days requires a special license. Additionally, methadone cannot be given as a take-home medication; patients must take methadone in the presence of and under the direct observation of the physician.

Side Effects.   Side effects caused by methadone are similar to those resulting from other opioid agonists. These most commonly include sedation, lightheadedness, miosis, nausea and vomiting, decreased libido, urinary hesitancy, and constipation. With an increase in dose, respiratory and circulatory depressions are seen. Allergic reactions, especially skin rash, are also seen.

Use in Pregnancy.   Most experts agree that methadone maintenance is the most appropriate management for pregnant opiate abusers because detoxification may cause intrauterine fetal death. Controlled methadone dosage is preferred to unknown doses of drugs that are obtained on the street, and with licit methadone the mother and fetus are not at risk from possible contaminants found in street drugs. However, the appropriate dose of methadone to use for pregnant women is unknown. The recommendation (CSAT) is to administer an initial oral methadone dose of 10 to 40 mg, with an additional dose of 5 to 10 mg within 3 to 4 h if signs of withdrawal persist. This can be repeated if necessary. The total required methadone dose over the first day is assumed to be the necessary 24-h dose, but daily doses may be adjusted by 5 to 10 mg/d as needed. As the pregnancy progresses, the maternal volume of distribution increases and the clearance of most drugs also increases, resulting in the necessity for a dosage increase. Some evidence also indicates that women who enter a methadone program early in their pregnancy tend to show greater compliance, in the form of fewer urine samples indicating use of heroin or cocaine.

Neonatal opioid withdrawal symptoms can be severe and possibly fatal if untreated. A withdrawal syndrome occurs in approximately 60 to 80 percent of infants whose mothers used heroin. Symptoms usually develop within 72 h postpartum with heroin or within a week with methadone. The withdrawal symptoms are similar to, but more severe, than those seen in adults (see Table 8-15). Additionally, the infant usually feeds poorly, and seizures may occur in up to 3 percent of heroin or 7 percent of methadone withdrawals. Neonatal opioid withdrawal is treated with either paregoric or phenobarbital (see Table 8-15).

Drug Interactions. Methadone interacts with many anticonvulsant medications. When these medications are added to a methadone regimen, they may precipitate a withdrawal reaction because they induce the enzymatic biotransformation of methadone. Alternatively, if these medications are discontinued in a patient receiving methadone, the methadone clearance will slowly decrease, possibly necessitating a decrease in methadone dose at some point. Additionally, methadone is a moderately potent inhibitor of cytochrome P450 isoenzyme CYP2D6, which is important for the metabolism of a variety of drugs (see Table 8-18). Theoretically, methadone would be likely to decrease the metabolism of these drugs leading to increased levels, but this has not yet been studied.

OPIOID ANTAGONISTS　Another strategy for treating heroin dependence is to block the euphoria caused by heroin with an opioid antagonist, such as naltrexone. Naltrexone blocks the opioid receptors, thereby preventing the effects of an opioid agonist as long as it remains in the body. This sounds like an excellent solution (similar to disulfiram without

the unpleasant reaction); however, in practice it is rarely effective except in populations of highly motivated opioid addicts, such as physicians or other professionals who have much to lose if they cannot remain abstinent. The two largest double-blind, placebo-controlled studies conducted using naltrexone to treat heroin addicts were plagued with study dropouts; less than 20 percent of subjects completed either trial. Although naltrexone use was associated with a decreased use of opioids in those who remained in the study, use of other drugs (barbiturates or amphetamines) did not decrease.[92] In general, the drug was not well accepted by the addict population because it possesses no opioid agonist effects, and many complained they felt dysphoric while taking it. It is probable that most individuals addicted to heroin will not comply with a naltrexone regimen.

α-ADRENERGIC AGONISTS　Another strategy for heroin detoxification is the use of the α-adrenergic agonist clonidine. Many opioid withdrawal symptoms are probably a result of hyperarousal of the norepinephrine system in the central nervous system. A drug that dampens this system, such as clonidine, should be effective in alleviating many of the symptoms of opioid withdrawal. Unlike methadone, clonidine is not a strictly regulated drug so it is easier for clinicians not affiliated with methadone treatment facilities to use this agent for detoxification.

Early investigations by Gold et al.[93] reported that, because patients experienced no euphoria, clonidine would be unlikely to be abused or diverted to the street. Unfortunately, this has not proved to be the case. In one study, 33 percent of pregnant women who abused opioids and were attending a methadone clinic tested positive for clonidine by urinalysis, but many did not report taking the medication when asked.[94] Most of these women were also abusing cocaine or intravenous opioids as well as receiving methadone. Self-reported reasons for using clonidine (sometimes in much higher than the recommended doses for withdrawal) included reduction of withdrawal symptoms or potentiation of methadone effects or as an anxiolytic.

Efficacy. At least five placebo-controlled, double-blind studies of clonidine use in opioid withdrawal have been published.[93,95–98] In all studies, clonidine significantly decreased many withdrawal symptoms including chills, rhinorrhea, lacrimation, stomach cramps, and diaphoresis. Although clonidine often causes sedation, it does not alleviate the muscle aches, insomnia, or drug craving seen during withdrawal. The effects on withdrawal are usually evident within 2 h of clonidine administration.

Dose and Regimen. A sample dosing protocol used for the treatment of opioid withdrawal is to begin with 0.005 mg/kg body weight as a test dose. Patients showing a positive response are then treated with 0.017 mg/kg body weight in divided doses, adjusted to avoid hypotension and oversedation. Heroin withdrawal is most often treated with 7 days of clonidine, whereas methadone withdrawal may require 10 days or longer. The dose should then be reduced by 50 percent for 3 more days and then discontinued.

Side Effects. When used to treat opioid withdrawal, clonidine has most commonly caused the adverse effects of sedation, dizziness, and hypotension.

Use in Pregnancy. Clonidine is a pregnancy category C drug. The unsupervised use of clonidine in doses that exceed either therapeutic doses or the usual length of treatment of withdrawal is especially worrisome in pregnant women because abrupt withdrawal during chronic use could result in rebound hypertension, headache, tachycardia, and anxiety. These effects could adversely affect the fetus as well as the mother.

SMOKING CESSATION

Several methods can be used to promote smoking cessation. Simply discontinuing smoking works for some, but relapse is, unfortunately, common. Experiencing nicotine withdrawal is one of the reasons for relapse. Symptoms of nicotine withdrawal include dysphoric mood, insomnia, irritability, anxiety, difficulty concentrating, restlessness, bradycardia, and increased appetite and weight gain. Although the physiologic effects of withdrawal are unpleasant, one of the major reasons women relapse is the weight gain associated with smoking cessation. This issue is important also to men, but it is a much more potent psychological issue in women.[99,100] More women than men admit to using smoking as a means of maintaining their weight within a desirable range. Although the average weight gain with smoking cessation is about 3 to 5 kg, women tend to gain more weight than men and some may gain in excess of 13 kg.

Unfortunately, other than warning women that they will likely gain weight when they quit smoking and urging them to watch their caloric intake and engage in regular exercise, there is no mechanism to prevent the weight gain. It is wise to avoid trying to diet at the same time as attempting to quit smoking because failure to control weight might doom both the diet and the smoking cessation. Dieting should be put off until after smoking cessation when the patient may be more reasonably certain that she can remain free from cigarette smoking when undergoing the stress of dieting.

NICOTINE REPLACEMENT Rather than abruptly ceasing the intake of nicotine, nicotine replacement is a commonly used method to promote smoking cessation. Nicotine for this purpose can be administered by four different routes: chewing gum, transdermal patches, nasal inhalers, and oral inhalers (Table 8-19). All of these products can provide adequate nicotine concentrations within a range that will prevent withdrawal symptoms, but they differ with regard to rate of absorption and peak nicotine blood level achieved. Theoretically, the oral inhalation and nasal spray should provide a more rapid elevation and a higher peak concentration of nicotine. It is hypothesized that the rapid achievement of a peak nicotine concentration similar to that provided by smoking a cigarette will deliver a nicotine boost, which is more likely to satisfy the craving for a cigarette. However, neither the nasal spray nor the oral inhaler consistently provides a similar rapid maximum nicotine concentration to that achieved when a cigarette is

Table 8-19

Nicotine Replacement Products

Dosage Form	Product	Preparation
Buccal—Chewing gum	Nicorette*	2 mg
	Nicorette DS*	4 mg
Topical—Patch	Nicotrol*	15 mg/16 h (24.9 mg/30 cm²)
	Habitrol	7 mg/24 h (17.5 mg/10 cm²)
	NicoDermCQ—Step 3*	7 mg/24 h (36 mg/7 cm²)
	Prostep	11 mg/24 h (15 mg/3.5 cm²)
	Habitrol	14 mg/24 h (35 mg/20 cm²)
	NicoDermCQ—Step 2*	14 mg/24 h (78 mg/15 cm²)
	Habitrol	21 mg/24 h (52.5 mg/30 cm²)
	NicoDermCQ—Step 1*	21 mg/24 h (114 mg/22 cm²)
	Prostep	22 mg/24 h (30 mg/7 cm²)
Nasal spray	NicotrolNS	0.5 mg/metered spray
Oral inhaler	Nicotrol Inhaler	4 mg/plastic cartridge

*Available as nonprescription product.

smoked. After the administration of the nasal spray, the peak concentration is achieved within 5 to 15 min. The peak concentration after a single dose of spray (1 mg, 1 spray in each nostril) of 2 to 17 ng/mL is variable, although 17 ng/mL is similar to peak venous blood levels following a cigarette. When the oral inhaler is used, peak concentrations of 3 to 6 ng/mL are usually reached within 15 min. A proportion of the nicotine spray is probably swallowed, and when the oral inhaler is used the majority of nicotine is deposited in the oral cavity. In both cases, the rate and extent of absorption are decreased because oral or buccal absorption of nicotine is slower than absorption via the lungs.

When the gum is chewed, the rate of nicotine release depends on many variables, including the rate, intensity, and duration of chewing. Although levels are variable when the gum is used, peak nicotine concentrations are not comparable to those achieved following cigarette smoking. Following transdermal use, relatively low peak concentrations are reached more slowly, at approximately 8 h.

Efficacy. The cessation rates for the first few months for all these products range from 20 to 40 percent. The 1-year abstinence rates are rarely greater than 10 to 15 percent. Although these rates are not impressive, they are approximately twice those seen when placebo is administered in clinical comparison studies.

Dose and Regimen. The recommended regimens for withdrawal using these replacement systems vary depending on the manufacturer, but are well described in the package inserts. Anyone smoking more than half a pack of cigarettes per day should probably receive the high-dose patches, with tapering over time based on individual tolerance. The higher-dose patches are generally associated with fewer withdrawal symptoms. Replacement doses should be individualized. Those smoking more than a pack of cigarettes per day may require a replacement dose of 33 to 35 mg/d; those smoking more than 2 packs per day may require a transdermal dose in the range of 44 mg/d.[101] Because transdermal patches in this dosage range are not currently available in the United States, multiple patches of smaller doses may be used simultaneously to alleviate withdrawal symptoms in heavier smokers.

Lower-dose patches are then recommended to wean off of nicotine. However, weaning should be individualized. Some might use the spray, gum, or inhaler to supplement the low steady-state nicotine levels produced by the patch (i.e., to provide a nicotine boost when a cigarette is craved). Most manufacturers recommend a step-down approach lasting 10 to 12 weeks, which may be of insufficient duration for many smokers. Although biologic withdrawal from nicotine is achieved with this regimen, the risk of relapse is still present. It would be reasonable to continue nicotine replacement beyond 10 or 12 weeks if the patient desires. There is no reason that the discontinuation of nicotine replacement should be rushed to meet a schedule because, in most cases, continuing nicotine replacement is less of a health risk than smoking (if relapse should occur).

Side Effects.   In 20 to 40 percent of patients, the gum, nasal spray, and oral inhalers cause symptoms of gastrointestinal upset including diarrhea, nausea, or heartburn. Initially, cardiovascular disease was a concern, but nicotine replacement appears to cause less strain on the cardiovascular system than cigarette smoking. However, it is still a good idea to monitor response to nicotine replacement therapy in those with underlying cardiovascular disease.

The nicotine patches are associated with localized skin irritation, but the gastrointestinal effects are not seen with this dosage form. Rotation of sites should be used each time a patch is placed. The nasal spray is often irritating to the nose and throat, resulting in sneezing or coughing. Although the irritation may abate over time, some patients find these side effects intolerable. The oral inhaler may be irritating to the lungs, so it should be avoided in those with severe bronchospastic disease.

Replacement therapies can be helpful for some individuals, but they are not without potential hazards. Patients need to be informed that the combination of smoking cigarettes and using nicotine replacement treatment could result in an overdose. The simultaneous placement of multiple nicotine transdermal patches has been used as a means of attempting suicide, usually in combination with other prescription or nonprescription drugs. The

symptoms seen on overdose include lethargy, dizziness, vomiting, hyper- or hypotension, and possibly seizures. Accidental poisoning in children and pets has also been reported, often resulting from children playing with discarded transdermal patches that still contain relatively large amounts of residual nicotine even after a 16- to 24-h application to skin. Patients should be advised to carefully dispose of patches after use.

Use in Pregnancy.   Because smoking is associated with complications during pregnancy and an increased risk of perinatal death, many women want to discontinue smoking when they become pregnant. Smoking adversely affects the fetus, causing decreased birth weight as well as changes in the walls of the umbilical artery and vein and in the placenta. Nicotine causes increases in maternal blood pressure and heart rate and also elevates fetal heart rate. These effects appear to be related to nicotine blood levels, so if replacement achieves a similarly high nicotine concentration, then these effects will also be seen during nicotine replacement treatment. The FDA has acknowledged that nicotine replacement products are associated with risks during pregnancy, and the nicotine spray, inhaler, and patches are placed in pregnancy category D. The risk of these products during pregnancy is likely worth the benefits if the woman is able to cease smoking altogether using replacement treatment, which will be tapered.

Drug Interactions.   Although nicotine is not associated with any documented drug interactions, cigarette smoking increases the metabolism of many drugs. Health care providers need to be aware that the doses of some drugs will probably have to be decreased following cessation of cigarette smoking (see Table 8-18).

BUPROPION   Bupropion when used as an aid to quit smoking is marketed under the name Zyban; when used as an antidepressant it is marketed under the name Wellbutrin. Bupropion is helpful in decreasing the craving for cigarettes in smokers.

Efficacy.   Following a 7-week bupropion or placebo treatment, efficacy was dose related, with the greatest abstinence effect seen in the group receiving 300 mg/d (44.2 percent), significant effects (38.6 percent) seen in the 150-mg/d group, and some effect (28.8 percent) seen in the 100-mg/d group of patients. Only 19.0 percent of patients randomized to the placebo group were abstinent at 7 weeks. After discontinuing bupropion, the 1-year abstinence rates were still significantly higher for the group who had received 300 mg/d (23.1 percent) compared with the placebo group (12.4 percent). Additionally, bupropion has the advantage of not being associated with weight gain; however, this only lasts as long as the drug is actually being given. Once bupropion is discontinued, the usual weight gain seen in abstinent smokers is likely to occur.

In a recently published study, it was found that the combination of a nicotine patch and bupropion (300 mg/d) was more effective than either placebo or the nicotine patch alone.[102] The drug treatment period lasted 7 weeks, then abstinence rates were monitored at 12 months. At 1 year, 35.5 percent of the combination group, 30.3 percent of the bupropion alone group, 16.4 percent of the nicotine patch alone group, and 15.6 percent of the placebo group still abstained from smoking. Discontinuation rates due to adverse effects were similar in the bupropion (11.9 percent) and the combination (11.4 percent) groups.

Dose and Regimen.   The most commonly used smoking cessation dose is 150 mg of the sustained-release product twice a day. Because bupropion can be associated with activating effects, it is wise to begin with 150 mg/d and increase to 150 mg twice-daily after 3 days or more.

Side Effects.   Although bupropion is relatively safe, it does cause some side effects. The most common side effects are tremor, insomnia, restlessness, dizziness, and dry mouth. It can also cause seizures in a dose-dependent manner. Consequently, it is important to ascertain whether a patient desiring to take Zyban for smoking cessation is already taking Wellbutrin as an antidepressant. Additionally, bupropion is contraindicated

in patients with either preexisting seizure disorders or eating disorders because of an increased risk of seizures in these populations.

Use in Pregnancy.   In animal studies, bupropion has not shown any teratogenic effects, but no data are available from human studies (pregnancy category B). Although it is always best to avoid the use of drugs during pregnancy, it should be remembered that tobacco has some deleterious effects on the fetus. After being informed about the risks of treatment with bupropion versus the risks associated with continued smoking, most women should be given the opportunity to make the choice themselves.

Appendix A
Risk Factors for Alcohol and/or Drug Misuse by Women

RISK FACTORS FOR ADOLESCENTS AND YOUNG WOMEN

First, the risk factors for adolescents and young women need not all be present to be concerned, but the more of these risk factors that are present, the greater the likelihood of development of substance abuse problems. These risk factors are:

- A family history positive for substance abuse.
- Dysfunctional, disruptive, often chaotic early family life in the family of origin. Vulnerable young women often report early life unhappiness, depression, and feelings of deprivation.
- School-related problems, including low achievement, drive, and expectations, and trouble with school authorities. Young women with substance abuse problems also manifest lesser school achievement than their age peers and so come into the job market with fewer skills and are employed at relatively lower status jobs than their age peers.
- Positive expectancies about alcohol and drugs. Evidence suggests that positive expectancies about alcohol/drugs are strong predictors of adolescent drinking.

- Peer pressure and participation in social groups in which use of alcohol and/or drugs is facilitated both by encouragement and availability.
- Early experience with alcohol intoxication, marijuana use; early sexual experience.
- Behavior problems: e.g., difficulties in impulse control, shoplifting, vandalism, temper tantrums, etc. These include antisocial aggressive behavior and rejection of authority.

RISK FACTORS FOR ADULT AND MIDDLE-AGED WOMEN

Risk factors specific to adult and middle-aged women include:

- A family history positive for substance abuse.
- Marital status: there is greater likelihood of heavy drinking among single women, divorced/separated women, and those who are in cohabiting relationships. Married women are less likely to develop heavy drinking problems although a spouse's heavy drinking may be a factor for young and middle-aged women.
- Participation in a social group where there is heavy drinking. Although this is more likely to be a mixed gender group, there are social groups of women who facilitate each others' drinking.
- Gynecologic/obstetric problems are sometimes antecedent to high-risk drinking. In a study of alcoholic women in treatment, compared with a matched nonalcoholic control group, the problem drinking women reported significantly more miscarriage and hysterectomy; whether those preceded or followed heavy drinking is not clear.
- Depression is reported as antecedent to problem drinking among a large proportion of women problem drinkers. Other antecedent symptomatic behaviors include eating disorders, phobias, panic states, and anxiety attacks.
- Use and abuse of prescribed psychoactive drugs may precede, accompany, or follow problematic drinking.
- Among middle-aged women (45 to 60), difficulty in redefining one's role—marital, occupational, maternal—may create conditions for the development of problem drinking. Although the loss of youth produces, in most women, adaptations of one sort or another, this adjustment in role is difficult for some middle-aged women.

RISK FACTORS FOR ELDERLY WOMEN

Risk factors for elderly women include:

- Although problem drinking of long duration can occur in elderly women, more recent onset is more frequent among female older drinkers than among male elderly problem drinkers. When they present for treatment, they come with a shorter duration of alcohol-related problems than do men.
- Marital disruption is present among elderly women problem drinkers more than it is among men. The disruption often takes the form of widowhood rather than divorce or separation. Widowhood and its accompanying sense of loss and depression appear to be an antecedent.
- Work situation: for those women who have been employed outside the home most of their adult lives, retirement from the workforce may act as antecedent to problematic use of alcohol. This is probably because, for those women, most of their social networks have been within the workplace.
- Throughout their lives, women have been bigger users of prescribed psychoactive drugs than men. There may, in fact, be more elderly women with psychoactive drug misuse than those manifesting misuse of alcohol. Elderly women problem drinkers report more dependence on such drugs than elderly male problem drinkers.
- Depression associated with aging or losses may clearly act as antecedent.
- Among elderly women alcohol abusers, there are frequent reports of drinking with the spouse or a significant other. This may well be, again, the transmission of problem drinking from male to female.

Appendix B
The AUDIT Questionnaire

Circle the number that comes closest to the patient's answer.

1. How often do you have a drink containing alcohol?
   - (0) Never
   - (1) Monthly or less
   - (2) Two to four times a month
   - (3) Two to three times a week
   - (4) Four or more times a week

2. How many drinks containing alcohol do you have on a typical day when you are drinking? [Code number of standard drinks.*]
   - (0) 1 or 2
   - (1) 3 or 4
   - (2) 5 or 6
   - (3) 7 to 9
   - (4) 10 or more

3. How often do you have six or more drinks on one occasion?
   - (0) Never
   - (1) Monthly or less
   - (2) Two to four times a month
   - (3) Two to three times a week
   - (4) Four or more times a week

4. How often during the last year have you found that you were not able to stop drinking once you had started?
   - (0) Never
   - (1) Monthly or less
   - (2) Two to four times a month
   - (3) Two to three times a week
   - (4) Four or more times a week

5. How often during the last year have you failed to do what was normally expected from you because of drinking?
   - (0) Never
   - (1) Monthly or less
   - (2) Two to four times a month
   - (3) Two to three times a week
   - (4) Four or more times a week

6. How often during the last year have you needed a drink first thing in the morning to get yourself going after a heavy drinking session?
   - (0) Never
   - (1) Monthly or less
   - (2) Two to four times a month
   - (3) Two to three times a week
   - (4) Four or more times a week

7. How often during the last year have you had a feeling of guilt or remorse after drinking?
   - (0) Never
   - (1) Monthly or less
   - (2) Two to four times a month
   - (3) Two to three times a week
   - (4) Four or more times a week

8. How often during the last year have you been unable to remember what happened the night before because you had been drinking?
   - (0) Never
   - (1) Monthly or less
   - (2) Two to four times a month
   - (3) Two to three times a week
   - (4) Four or more times a week

9. Have you or someone else been injured as a result of your drinking?
   - (0) No
   - (2) Yes, but not in the last year
   - (4) Yes, during the last year

10. Has a relative or friend or doctor or other health worker been concerned about your drinking or suggested you cut down?
   - (0) Never
   - (1) Monthly or less
   - (2) Two to four times a month
   - (3) Two to three times a week
   - (4) Four or more times a week

Record sum of individual items here._____

The minimum score (for nondrinkers) is 0 and the maximum possible score is 40. A score of 8 or more indicates a strong likelihood of hazardous or harmful alcohol consumption.

*In determining the response categories it has been assumed that one drink contains 10 g alcohol. In countries where the alcohol content of a standard drink differs by more than 25 percent from 10 g, the response category should be modified accordingly.
SOURCE: Reproduced with permission from Saunders JB, Aasland OG, Babor TF, Unreal N: Development of the Alcohol Use Disorders Identification Test (AUDIT): WHO collaborative project on early detection of persons with harmful alcohol consumption. *Addiction* 88:791, 1993.

Appendix C
Critical Components of Brief Interventions

1. Give feedback about screening results, impairment, and risks while clarifying the findings.

   The following are some sample scripts:

   • "I notice from your answers to the CAGE questionnaire that your drinking has caused you some concern. You also state that you are consuming a six-pack every afternoon. Can you tell me more specifically what your concerns are?"

   • "I'm concerned about your GGT levels. These indicate you may be drinking heavily, and this could be causing you some liver damage. Just how much and how often are you drinking?"

   • "Your urine screen shows the presence of cocaine (or heroin or cannabis). Could you tell me about your drug use?"

   • Your responses to our screening questionnaire and my physical examination indicate that you have some symptoms of alcohol dependence. I noticed that you have a slight tremor in your hand, and you're reporting insomnia and occasional morning drinking as well as substantial drinking overall. Has this been a concern of yours too?"

   • "I'm concerned about how your alcohol use is affecting your pregnancy. Your baby could suffer severe abnormalities as a direct result of your drinking."

   • "I'm concerned that your alcohol use is related to many of the problems that we've been talking about."

   • "At this level of consumption, you are at increased risk for some health problems as well as accidents."

   • "You've said that you've been smoking pot for the past several years. You know about the trouble you could get into legally, but I'm concerned about your health."

2. Inform the patient about safe consumption limits and offer advice about change.

   The following are some sample scripts:

   • "Your blood pressure is high and your abdominal pain may be caused by gastritis or an ulcer.

Until we can investigate further, I'd like you to stop drinking for at least 6 weeks to let your stomach heal. Do you think you can do this?"

   • "Since I'm going to prescribe some pain medication for your shoulder that interacts with alcohol, I don't want you to drink for the next several weeks. I'm also concerned that your regular consumption habits seem to be above safe levels for women. When you are finished with the medication, I suggest that you cut down to no more than one drink a day, especially since you're also complaining about occasional insomnia. Let's talk more about this when you come back in 2 weeks."

   • "Thank you for being honest with me about your marijuana use. One concern of mine is your asthma, because marijuana smoke does affect your lungs. Why don't we work on a plan to help you quit."

   • "In reviewing your responses to our screening questionnaire, I notice that you are drinking a lot of beer on weekends. You don't seem to be having any direct problems as a result, but I'm concerned that driving while intoxicated is not safe and you have a young family to consider. I'd like you to read this pamphlet and talk more about this when you come back next month to get your allergy shot. I hope you will think seriously about cutting back on the beer before you do have some problems."

   • "You say you've been taking 'speed' to stay awake during your second job, and I'm worried that you're developing a dependence on amphetamines. Let's talk about other, healthier ways to get you through your night job."

3. Assess the patient's readiness to change.

4. Negotiate goals and strategies for change.

   The following are some sample scripts:

   • "Based on what we've been discussing, would you be willing to change your drinking habits (or drug use)?"

   • "Can we set a specific date to reduce your alcohol use? Could you cut back, beginning this week?"

- "Since you agreed to cut back on your drinking, you may find that this booklet offers some helpful advice about how to go about it."
- "Would you be willing to see a counselor to discuss your drug use further? Think of this referral as comparable to sending you to a cardiologist for a heart problem."

References

1. Califano JA: Crime and punishment—and treatment, too. *Washington Post*, p. C-7, February 8, 1998.
2. Youssef NA: Help urged for inmate addicts, most prisoners linked to drug, alcohol use. *Chicago Tribune*, p. 1–20, January 9, 1998.
3. Dahlgren L, Willander A: Are special treatment facilities for female alcoholics needed? A controlled 2-year follow-up study from a specialized female unit (EWA) versus a mixed male/female treatment facility. *Alcohol Clin Exp Res* 13:499, 1989.
4. Roberts AC, Nishimoto RH: Predicting treatment retention of women dependent on cocaine. *Am J Drug Alcohol Abuse* 22:313, 1996.
5. Jarvis TJ: Implications of gender for alcohol treatment research: a quantitative and qualitative review. *Br J Addict* 87:1249, 1992.
6. Trafford A: Should women who use drugs while pregnant be locked up? *Washington Post*, p.WH-6. August 18, 1998.
7. Herbert B: Pregnancy and addiction. *New York Times* p. A-31. June 11, 1998.
8. Chang G, Behr H, Goetz MA, Hiley A, Bigby J: Women and alcohol abuse in primary care. Identification and intervention. *Am J Addict* 6:183, 1997.
9. Blume SB: Sexuality and stigma: the alcoholic woman. *Alcohol Health Res World* 15:139, 1991.
10. Kumpfer KL: Treatment programs for drug abusing women. *Future Child* 1:50, 1991.
11. Sandmaier M: *The Invisible Alcoholics: Women and Alcohol*, 2nd ed. New York: McGraw-Hill; 1992.
12. Windle M, Windle RC, Scheidt DM, Miller GB: Physical and sexual abuse and associated mental disorders among alcoholic inpatients. *Am J Psychiatry* 152:1322 , 1995.
13. Liebschutz JM, Mulvey KP, Samet JH: Victimization among substance-abusing women. Worse health outcomes. *Arch Intern Med* 157:1093, 1997.
14. Hill S: Personality characteristics of sisters and spouses of male alcoholics. *Alcohol Clin Exp Res* 17:733, 1993.
15. Miller BA, Downs WR, Gondoli DM, et al: The role of childhood sexual abuse in the development of alcoholism in women. *Violence Victims* 2:157, 1987.
16. Miller BA, Downs WR, Testa M: Interrelations between victimization experiences and women alcohol/drug use. *J Stud Alcohol* 11(suppl):109, 1993.
17. Zucker RA, Fitzgerald HE: Early developmental factors and risk for alcohol problems. *Alcohol Health Res World* 15:18, 1991.
18. Finkelstein N, Derman L: Single parent women: what's a mother to do? In: Roth P (ed): *Alcohol and Drugs Are Women's Issues*. New York: Scarecrow Press; 1991:78.
19. Gomberg ESL: Social predictors of women's alcohol and drug use: implications for prevention and treatment. In: Graham AW, Schultz TK (eds): *Principles of Addiction Medicine*, 2nd ed. Chevy Chase, MD: American Society of Addiction Medicine Inc; 1998. 1191–1198.
20. Jones BM, Jones MK: Women and alcohol; intoxication, metabolism, and the menstrual cycle. In: Greenblatt M, Schuckit MA (eds): *Alcohol Problems in Women and Children*. New York: Grune & Stratton; 1976:103.
21. Frezza M, di Padova C, Pozzato G, et al: High blood alcohol levels in women. The role of decreased gastric alcohol dehydrogenase activity and first-pass metabolism (published errata appear in *N Engl J Med* 322:1540, 1990 and 323:553, 1990 [see comments]). *N Engl J Med* 322:95, 1990.
22. Smith AR: Alcoholism and gender: patterns of diagnosis and response. *Journal of Drug Issues* 16:407, 1986.
23. National Center on Addiction and Substance Abuse (CASA) at Columbia University: *Under the Rug: Substance Abuse and the Mature Woman*. New York: CASA; 1998.
24. Gritz ER: *Which Women Smoke and Why?* Washington, DC: U.S. Department of Health and Human Services; 1987.
25. Recer P: Teen smokers who quit may be too late. *Lansing State Journal* 1, April 7, 1999.
26. Perkins KA: Sex differences in nicotine versus non-nicotine reinforcement as determinants of tobacco smoking. *Experimental and Clinical Psychopharmacology* 4:166, 1996.
27. Hatsukami D, Skoog K, Allen S, Bliss R; et al: Gender and the effects of different doses of nicotine gum on tobacco withdrawal symptoms. *Exper Clin Psychopharmacol* 3:163, 1995.

28. Department of Health and Human Services: Reducing the health consequences of smoking: 25 years of progress. A report of the Surgeon General. Publication no. DHHS (CDC) 89-8411. Rockville, MD: Department of Health and Human Services; 1989.

29. Lee BL, Benowitz NL, Jacob P, 3rd: Cigarette abstinence, nicotine gum, and theophylline disposition. *Ann Intern Med* 106:553, 1987.

30. Williams GD, et al: Population projections using DSM-III criteria: alcohol abuse and dependence, 1990–2000. *Alcohol Health Res World* 13:366, 1989.

31. Williams GD, Stinson FS, Parker DA: Demographic trends, alcohol abuse and alcoholism, 1985–1995. *Alcohol Health Res World* 11:80, 1987.

32. Wilsnack RW, Wilsnack SC, Klassen AD: Women's drinking and drinking problems: patterns from a 1981 national survey. *Am J Public Health* 74:1231, 1984.

33. Herd D: Drinking by black and white women: results from a national survey. *Social Problems* 35:493, 1988.

34. Gilbert J: Alcohol consumption patterns in immigrant and later generation Mexican American women. *Hispanic Journal of Behavioral Sciences* 9:299, 1987.

35. Malin H, Coakley J, Kaelber C, et al: *An Epidemiologic Perspective on Alcohol Use and Abuse in the United States*. In: Alcohol consumption and related problems. Alcohol and Health Monograph; 1. National Institute on Alcohol Abuse and Alcoholism. Washington, DC: U.S. Government Printing Office; 1982. Pub No. ADM 82-1190 DHHS, 99–153.

36. Blume SB: Understanding addictive disorders in women. In: Graham AW, Schultz TK (eds): *Principles of Addiction Medicine,* 2nd ed. Chevy Chase, MD: American Society of Addiction Medicine, Inc; 1998; 1173–1190.

37. Hill SY: *Biological Consequences of Alcoholism and Alcohol-Related Problems Among Women*. Alcohol and Health Monograph; 4. National Institute on Alcohol Abuse and Alcoholism. Washington, DC: US Government Print Office; 1982.

38. Saunders JB, Davis M, Williams R: Do women develop alcoholic liver disease more readily than men? *BMJ* 282:1140, 1981.

39. Mello NK: *Drug Use and Premenstrual Dysphoria*. NIDA Research Monograph. Rockville, MD: National Institute on Drug Abuse; 1986;65:31.

40. National Household Survey on Drug Abuse (NHSDA): *Survey.* Substance Abuse and Mental Health Services Administration. 1996.

41. Gomberg ESL: Alcoholic women in treatment: new research. *Substance Abuse* 12:6, 1991.

42. Griffin ML, Weiss RL, Mirin SM, Lange U: A comparison of male and female cocaine abusers. *Arch Gen Psychiatry* 46:122, 1989.

43. Helzer JF, Pryzbeck RT: The co-occurrence of alcoholism with other psychiatric disorders in the general population and its impact on treatment. *J Stud Alcohol* 49:219, 1988.

44. El Guebaly Nady: Alcohol and polysubstance abuse among women. *Can J Psychiatry* 40:73, 1995.

45. Fleming MF, Barry KL, Manwell LB, Johnson K, London R: Brief physician advice for problem alcohol drinkers. A randomized controlled trial in community-based primary care practices [see comments]. *JAMA* 277:1039, 1997.

46. Wilk AI, Jensen NM, Havighurst TC: Meta-analysis of randomized control trials addressing brief interventions in heavy alcohol drinkers. *J Gen Intern Med* 12:274, 1997.

47. Prochaska JO, DiClemente CC, Norcross JC: In search of how people change: applications to addictive behaviors. *Am Psychol* 47:1102, 1992.

48. Carmin CN: Addicted woman: when your patient can't stop drinking, smoking, shopping, eating. *International Journal of Fertility and Women's Medicine* 43:179, 1998.

49. Velicer WF, Prochaska JO: An expert system intervention for smoking cessation. *Patient Education and Counseling* 36:119, 1999.

50. Perz CA, DiClemente CC, Carbonari JP: Doing the right thing at the right time? The interaction of stages and processes of change in successful smoking cessation. *Health Psychol* 15:462, 1996.

51. Miller WR, Rollnick S: *Motivational Interviewing: Preparing People to Change Addictive Behavior.* New York: Guilford Press; 1991.

52. Colby SM, Monti PM, Barnett NP, et al: Brief motivational interviewing in a hospital setting for adolescent smoking: a preliminary study. *J Consult Clin Psychol* 66:574, 1998.

53. Bombardier CH, Rimmele CT: Motivational interviewing to prevent alcohol abuse after traumatic brain injury: a case series. *Rehabilitation Psychology* 44:52, 1999.

54. Handmaker NS, Miller WR, Manicke M: Findings of a pilot study of motivational interviewing with pregnant drinkers. *J Stud Alcohol* 60:285, 1999.

55. Lawendowski LA: A motivational intervention for adolescent smokers. *Prevent Med* 27:A39, 1998.

56. Trigwell P, Grant PJ, House A: Motivation and glycemic control in diabetes mellitus. *J Psychosom Res* 43:307, 1997.

57. Smith RC: *The Patient's Story: Integrated Patient-Doctor Interviewing*. New York: Little, Brown; 1996.

58. The Smoking Cessation Clinical Practice Guideline Panel and Staff: The Agency for Health Care Policy and Research: smoking cessation clinical practice guideline. *JAMA* 275:1270, 1996.

59. National Institute on Alcohol Abuse and Alcoholism: National Institutes of Health; NIH Pub. No. 95-3769; 1995.

60. Skinner H, Allen B: Does the computer make a difference? Computerized versus face-to-face versus self-report assessment of alcohol, drug, and tobacco use. *J Consult Clin Psychol* 51:267, 1983.

61. Skinner H, Palmer W, McIntosh M, Sanchez-Craig M: *Computerized Lifestyle Assessment in Family Practice: Early Intervention for Alcohol Problems*. Toronto: Addiction Research Foundation; 1985.

62. Selzer ML: The Michigan Alcoholism Screening Test: the quest for a new diagnostic instrument. *Am J Psychiatry* 127:1653, 1971.

63. Brown RL, Leonard T, Saunders LA, Papasouliotis O: A two-item screening test for alcohol and other drug problems [see comments]. *J Fam Pract* 44:151, 1997.

64. Babor TF: Brief intervention strategies for harmful drinkers: new directions for medical education. *J Can Med Assoc* 143:1070, 1990.

65. Volk RJ, Steinbauer JR, Cantor SB, Holzer CE, 3rd: The Alcohol Use Disorders Identification Test (AUDIT) as a screen for at-risk drinking in primary care patients of different racial/ethnic backgrounds. *Addiction* 92:197, 1997.

66. Levy M, Spino M: Neonatal withdrawal syndrome: associated drugs and pharmacologic management. *Pharmacotherapy* 13:202, 1993.

67. Miller WR: Techniques to modify hazardous drinking patterns. *Recent Dev Alcohol* 5:425, 1987.

68. Sullivan E, Fleming M: *Treatment Improvements Protocol (TIP) Series; 24*. Rockville, MD: Substance Abuse and Mental Health Services Administration; 1997.

69. Finkelstein N: Treatment issues for alcohol- and drug-dependent pregnant and parenting women. *Health Soc Work* 19:7, 1994.

70. Mee-Lee D, Shulman G, Gartner L: *Patient Placement Criteria for the Treatment of Substance-Related Disorders*, 2nd ed. Chevy Chase, MD: American Society of Addiction Medicine; ASAM PPC-2.

71. Hubbard RL, Marsden ME, Rachel JV, Harwood HJ, Cavanaugh ER, Ginzburg HM: *Drug Abuse Treatment: A National Study of Effectiveness*. Chapel Hill, NC: University of North Carolina Press; 1989.

72. Miller WR, Hester RK: The effectiveness of alcoholism treatment methods: what research reveals. In: Miller WR, Heather N (eds): *Treating Addictive Behaviors: Process of Change*. New York: Plenum Press; 1986.

73. Alterman AI, McLellan AT, O'Brien CP, et al: Effectiveness and costs of inpatient versus day and hospital cocaine rehabilitation. *J Nerv Men Dis* 182:157, 1994.

74. Miller WR, Hester RK: Inpatient alcoholism treatment: who benefits? *Am Psychol* 41:794, 1986.

75. McKay JR, Cacciola JS, McLellan AT, Alterman AI, Wirtz PW: An initial evaluation of the psychosocial dimensions of the American Society of Addiction Medicine criteria for inpatient versus intensive outpatient substance abuse rehabilitation. *J Stud Alcohol* 58:239, 1997.

76. McKay JR, Alterman AI, McLellan AT, et al: Treatment goals, continuity of care, and outcome in a day hospital substance abuse rehabilitation program. *Am J Psychiatry* 151:254, 1994.

77. McLellan AT, Alterman AI, Metzger DS, et al: Similarity of outcome predictors across opiate, cocaine, and alcohol treatments: role of treatment services. *J Consult Clin Psychol* 62:1141, 1994.

78. Jessup M, Green JR: Treatment of the pregnant alcohol-dependent woman. *J Psychoactive Drugs* 19:193, 1987.

79. Swift RM: Drug therapy for alcohol dependence. *N Engl J Med* 340:1482, 1999.

80. Bergman U, Rosa FW, Baum C, et al: Effects of exposure to benzodiazepine during fetal life. *Lancet* 340:694, 1992.

81. Jacobsen E: Deaths of alcoholic patients treated with disulfiram. *Q J Stud Alcohol* 13:16, 1952.

82. Fuller RK, Roth HP: Disulfiram for the treatment of alcoholism: an evaluation of 128 men. *Ann Intern Med* 90:901, 1979.

83. Fuller RK, Branchley L, Brightwell DR, et al: Disulfiram in the treatment of alcoholism: a Veterans Administration cooperative study. *JAMA* 256:1449, 1986.

84. Frisoni GB, Di Monda V: Disulfiram neuropathy: a review (1971–1988) and report of a case. *Alcohol Alcohol* 24:429, 1989.

85. Reitnauer PJ, Callanan NP, Farber RA, Aylsworth AS: Prenatal exposure to disulfiram implicated in the cause of malformations in discordant monozygotic twins. *Teratology* 56:358, 1997.

86. O'Malley SS, Jaffee AJ, Chang G, et al: Six month follow-up of naltrexone and psychotherapy for alcohol dependence. *Arch Gen Psychiatry* 53:217, 1996.

87. Volpicelli JR, Alterman AI, Hayashida M, O'Brien CP: Naltrexone in the treatment of alcohol dependence. *Arch Gen Psychiatry* 49:876, 1992.

88. Senay EC, Dorus W, Showalter CV: Short-term detoxification with methadone. *Ann N Y Acad Sci* 362:203, 1981.

89. Resnick R: Methadone detoxification from illicit opiates and methadone maintenance. In: Cooper JR, Altman F, Brown BS, Czechowicz D (eds): *National Institute of Drug Abuse Research Monograph*. Washington, DC: U.S. Government Printing Office; 1983; 160.

90. Sorensen JL, Batki SL, Good P, Wilkinson K: Methadone maintenance program for AIDS-affected opiate addicts. *J Subst Abuse Treat* 6:87, 1989.

91. Strain EC, Begelow GE, Liebson IA, Stitzer ML: Moderate- vs. high-dose methadone in the treatment of opioid dependence: a randomized trial. *JAMA* 281:1000, 1999.

92. Bradford HA, Kaim SC, Ling W: A summary of the phase II clinical studies of the narcotic antagonist, naltrexone. In: Schecter AJ (ed): *Drug Dependence and Alcoholism*. New York: Plenum Press; 1981:981.

93. Gold MS, Pottash AC, Sweeney DR, Kelber HD: Opiate withdrawal using clonidine. *JAMA* 243:343, 1980.

94. Anderson F, Paluzzi P, Lee J, et al: Illicit use of clonidine in opiate-abusing pregnant women. *Obstet Gynecol* 90:790, 1997.

95. Gold MS, Redmond DE, Kleber HD: Clonidine blocks acute opiate-withdrawal symptoms. *Lancet* 2:599, 1978.

96. Gold MS, Redmond DE, Kleber HD: Noradrenergic hyperactivity in opiate withdrawal supported by clonidine reversal of opiate withdrawal. *Am J Psychiatry* 136:100, 1979.

97. Gold MS, Pottash ALC, Sweeney DR, et al: Efficacy of clonidine in opiate withdrawal: a study of thirty patients. *Drug Alcohol Depend* 6:201, 1980.

98. Washtkon AM, Resnick RB: Clonidine for opiate detoxification: outpatient clinical trials. *Am J Psychiatry* 137:1121, 1980.

99. French SA, Jeffery RW, Pirie PL, McBride CM: Do weight concerns hinder smoking cessation efforts? *Addict Behav* 17:219, 1992.

100. Camp DE, Klesges RC, Relyea G: The relationship between body weight concerns and adolescent smoking. *Health Psychol* 12:24, 1993.

101. Dale LC, Hurt RD, Offord KP, Lawson GM, Croghan IT, Schroeder DR: High-dose nicotine patch therapy. Percentage of replacement and smoking cessation [see comments]. *JAMA* 274:1353, 1995.

102. Jorenby DE, Leischow SJ, Nides MA, et al: A controlled trial of sustained-release bupropion, a nicotine patch, or both for smoking cessation. *N Engl J Med* 340:685, 1999.

Jonathan G. A. Henry

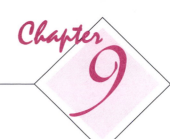

Depression and Anxiety

Overview

Psychiatric conditions have lagged far behind the more "mainstream" medical conditions in both recognition and treatment. Their effect on people's lives, however, can be devastating and far-reaching. The human costs of depression and anxiety disorders include not just the suffering of the individual but also the effect on the lives of the people around them. Interpersonal stress can manifest itself in work dysfunction and marital and family disruption. Divorce and all of its consequences are possible outcomes. The economic costs of these conditions are high indeed. Some $40 billion per year is lost in both direct and indirect costs for depression alone.

Unfortunately, the diagnosis of depression and anxiety can be difficult, even elusive, and psychiatric diagnosis remains more art than science. The clinician remains the de facto diagnostic instrument because of the paucity of technology available to play a confirmatory role in the diagnostic process. Blood and neuroimaging tests are useful primarily to exclude or confirm the presence of coexisting processes. Because symptoms such as mild insomnia, irritability, loss of pleasure, and negative

thinking patterns are so subjective, they are often missed and may not even be mentioned during visits to a clinician's office. This is especially true of anxiety disorders. Thus, a high level of suspicion should be maintained when evaluating symptoms that might indicate a mood or anxiety disorder.

Fortunately, ever-improving methods of treatment are available. Seven different classes of antidepressant medications are now available. Psychotherapies have also advanced, now with well-established efficacy of cognitive-behavioral treatments and interpersonal therapy, in addition to the more traditional psychotherapies. However, management of patients with depression or anxiety continues to present a therapeutic challenge. Treatment refractoriness and comorbidity along with the sheer breadth of depression and anxiety symptoms call for the constant need to tailor treatment plans to the broad needs of the patient.

Principal Diagnoses

Because depression and anxiety were so poorly understood and often went unrecognized in the past, patients with these conditions were left with the feeling that their symptoms were "all in their head" or just represented some poorly defined "stress." Patients experienced an increased sense of guilt that their symptoms were somehow of their own making. This approach to diagnosis would often leave patients more demoralized than when they first came to the clinician's office. Prepared now with a more complete understanding of the phenomenology of these disorders, clinicians can be much more precise in their diagnosis. Patients can be educated about the biochemical basis for their symptoms, although care should be taken to avoid creating the impression that the condition will resolve with simple pharmacologic manipulation. Powerful sociocultural forces are often a part of the expression of depression and anxiety, especially for women, and the most effective treatment strategies usually include pharmacotherapy and psychotherapies.

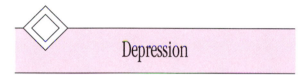

Depression

Epidemiology

The incidence of major depression in women is substantially higher than that in men. In the 1980s, the National Institutes of Mental Health (NIMH) Epidemiologic Catchment Area (ECA) Program conducted a study of depression in five major cities in the United States.[1] The 1-month prevalence of major depression across all adult age groups was 2.6 to 3.9 percent in women and 1.2 to 2.2 percent for men. The lifetime risk of major depression has been reported as 20 to 26 percent in women and 8 to 12 percent in men. These figures were recently confirmed in the National Comorbidity Survey,[2] the first community study using more recently operationalized criteria from the *Diagnostic and Statistical Manual of Mental Disorders-III-R* (DSM-III-R).

Many differences in the incidence, presentation, and course of depression appear to exist between women and men (Table 9-1).[3] The dif-ference between men and women in the incidence of major depression first begins to appear during adolescence; one study showed that by ages 14 to 16, over 13 percent of girls had suffered depression, compared to 2.7 percent of boys.[4] The age of onset may be earlier and the association with stressful life events and a number of medical and psychiatric conditions is greater.[3] Atypical symptoms such as hypersomnia, hyperphagia, and weight gain are experienced more often among women than men. In addition, the course and self-reported severity of an episode of depression appears to be different for women in that the episode may be of longer duration and greater severity, with more frequent recurrence.

In the elderly, the increased relative risk of depression and depressive symptoms among women versus men continues, although the diagnosis of major depression in the elderly is made less often. Depressive symptoms in the elderly often fall into an area of less specific and sometimes confusing nomenclature. The terms that are used to describe this kind of depression are "minor depression," "subsyndromal depression," dysthymia, or depression NOS (not otherwise specified).

Etiology

Throughout their life span, it is clear that biologic, psychosocial, and cultural factors all play interrelated roles in predisposing adolescent girls and women to depression and anxiety. These factors are listed in Table 9-2.

BIOLOGIC CONSIDERATIONS

RELATIONSHIP TO FEMALE HORMONES The connection between depressive symptoms and female sex hormones has been extensively investigated. Supporting evidence includes the increase in incidence of depression with the onset of puberty,[5] the development of depressive symptoms during the postpartum period,[6] and the link between depressive symptoms and the menstrual cycle, specifically the late luteal phase.[7] In addition, women who have

Table 9-1

Depression in Women Compared with Men

PARAMETERS	DIFFERENCES IN WOMEN COMPARED WITH MEN
Lifetime prevalence rate	20% (10% in men)
Age of onset	May be earlier
Duration of episodes	May be longer
Course of illness	May more often be recurrent
Seasonal effect on mood	Greater
Association with stressful life events	More frequent
Atypical symptoms of depression (e.g.,hypersomnia, hyperphagia)	Experienced more often
Severity of depression	May be greater if self-rated by the patient
Guilt feelings	May be experienced more often
Suicidal behavior	Suicide attempted more often but much less often successfully
Association of anxiety disorders, especially panic and phobic symptoms	Greater
Association of eating disorders	Greater
Association of alcoholism or substance use disorder	Usually less
Association of thyroid disease	Greater
Association of migraine headache	Greater
Association of antisocial, narcissistic, and obsessive-compulsive personalities	Less
Effect of exogenous and endogenous gonadal steroids on mood	Greater

SOURCE: Reproduced with permission from Bahatia SC, Bahatia SK: Depression in women: diagnostic and treatment considerations. *Am Fam Physician* 60:225, 1999.

previously established depression often note an increase in depressive symptoms or their intensity during the premenstrual period.[7] Finally, depressive symptoms *can* occur during the use of oral contraceptives, but the relationship between depression and the use of combined oral contraceptives is controversial. Depressive symptoms can occur with use of progestin-only contraceptives.

The biochemical synthesis, metabolism, and turnover of the putative neurotransmitters thought to be germane to depression (serotonin, norepinephrine, and dopamine) are known to be affected by estrogen.[8] The biogenic amine theory holds that it is underactivity in serotonin and norepinephrine transmission that leads to depression, whereas overactivity can lead to mania. The synaptic effects of antidepressants on these neurotransmitters has led to significant success in treating depression.

BIOCHEMICAL MARKERS OF DEPRESSION   To date, finding biochemical markers with clinical utility has been elusive. In research settings, measurement of the urinary metabolites of norepinephrine, 3-methoxy-4-hydroxyphenylglycol and 3-methoxy-4-hydroxymandelic acid; the cerebrospinal fluid (CSF) metabolite of dopamine, homovanillic acid; and the CSF metabolite of serotonin, 5-hydroxyindoleacetic acid (5-HIAA), appear to have a role in depression, but they have not proven helpful in clinical settings. Research findings have corroborated the theoretical

Table 9-2
Risk Factors for Depression in Women

BIOLOGIC FACTORS
Sex Hormones
Puberty
Postpartum period
Menopause (rapid cycling in those with bipolar depression)
Oral contraceptives
Medroxyprogesterone acetate
Thyroid hormones (hypothyroidism)
Melatonin

PSYCHOSOCIAL FACTORS
Adolescent developmental tasks
Maintcnance of self-esteem
Maintenance of sense of control
Adjustment to emerging sexuality and physical changes
Management of emerging sense of identity
Adulthood tasks
Family planning
Marriage/partnering
Decisions about parenthood
Family responsibilities
Occupation and career

OTHER FACTORS
Age
Low socioeconomic status
Marital status
Stressful life events
Divorce
Death of family member
Loss of parent before age 10
Domestic violence
Abortion
Miscarriage
Caretaking roles
Childhood abuse
Family history of mood disorders
Previous history of mood disorders
Physical illness

prediction of the biogenic amine theory that these metabolites of norepinephrine, serotonin, and dopamine all are present in reduced concentrations in both urine and CSF. However, these findings are not reliable enough to be clinically useful.

NEUROENDOCRINE CONSIDERATIONS   The role of the hypothalamic-pituitary-adrenal axis has also been thoroughly studied; hypersecretion of cortisol, as documented by 24-h urinary corticoid output or serum cortisol levels, and failure of a response of cortisol to the dexamethasone suppression test (DST) has been demonstrated in depressed patients. The DST was initially developed to measure the observed hypercortisolemia that has been repeatedly found in depressed patients. However, the DST is relatively nonspecific and, as a result, has limited clinical utility. Factors that can confound DST interpretation include acute illness, dementia, weight loss, smoking, alcohol use, and medications that accelerate dexamethasone metabolism.

Another neuroendocrine system of clinical significance is the hypothalamic-pituitary-thyroid axis. Thyroid disorders are more common in women, and both hypothyroidism and hyperthyroidism can precipitate depression.[9] The symptoms of hypothyroidism tend to be more subtle and can easily be overlooked, especially in older women. Conversely, some depressed patients, especially those with bipolar disorder, can develop mild or subclinical hypothyroidism. These conditions can be detected through an elevated thyroid-stimulating hormone (TSH) level and often by the presence of antimicrosomal thyroid or antithyroglobulin antibodies. Treatment can result in resolution of the depression. The mechanisms by which thyroid hormones mediate mood symptoms are complex. They regulate biologic cycles and neurotransmitter and receptor functions. Thyroid dysfunction has been shown to induce abnormal fluctuations in norepinephrine and serotonin systems involved in mood control.

Melatonin, a hormone of the pineal gland, has also been shown to play a biochemical role in depression.[10] It is synthesized from serotonin and is under the regulatory effects of norepinephrine.

The hormone is secreted by the pineal gland during the night, but secretion is stopped by exposure to sunlight during the day. Seasonal affective disorder (SAD), a specific subtype of depression, is believed to result from delayed circadian rhythms and abnormalities in melatonin secretion. SAD is more common in women (80 percent of all patients diagnosed with SAD), and light therapy has been effective.[11] No data are available to demonstrate the efficacy of melatonin in the treatment of depression.

PSYCHOSOCIAL CONSIDERATIONS

Extreme caution must be used in ascribing gender differences in mood and anxiety disorders to sex hormones alone. Sociocultural influences affect boys and girls as well as men and women, and it seems certain that they play a critical role in the development of depression and anxiety. The work of Carol Gilligan and others has been enlightening in identifying the tasks facing girls growing up in our culture.[12,13] In preadolescence, the self-esteem of boys and girls appears equal, but with the onset of adolescence, girls show a predisposition to a loss of self-esteem and a belief that they can no longer influence the course of events in their lives. At the same time, boys become increasingly aggressive, in part due to increasing testosterone levels. Girls may react to this aggressiveness with interpersonal withdrawal, because a large proportion of self-esteem in girls is based on relationships. Boys, in distinction, usually have their self-esteem tied to a sense of achievement in work, activities, and sports.

PHYSICAL CHANGES   The physical changes in girls' bodies also play a role in the development of mood and anxiety disorders. Preadolescent girls are unencumbered with concerns about menstruation, birth control, pregnancy, and the effect of these concerns on their life choices. Intrapsychic conflict can occur, however, with girls' changing bodies and the implications of these changes. This transition into womanhood coincides with an increase not only in depression and anxiety but also in eating disorders, substance abuse, and educational difficulties ranging from poorer grades to outright academic failure. Western cultural norms, and particularly American culture, reinforce problems with self-esteem and body image, plaguing girls incessantly with messages from magazines, books, television shows, movies, and popular music.

FAMILY OF ORIGIN A girl's family may complicate the difficulty she has in understanding herself sexually. The attitudes of parents serve as a template on which the girl's own identity starts to grow and develop. Both the female role models in a girl's life and the way in which the men and boys in her life react to women in general are of significant consequence to her sense of emerging self.

CHALLENGES OF ADULTHOOD Adulthood presents similar challenges for women. Balancing roles of career and motherhood in adulthood can be extremely stressful. The issues of birth control, marriage, parenthood, and family affect women in fundamentally different ways than men. Women still take primary responsibility for contraception, and once pregnant, they confront an enormous array of physical changes. The changes that attend pregnancy in terms of their relationship with their mate and their work life provide additional challenges. Developing effective strategies of compromise and balance in their life becomes of paramount importance in achieving and maintaining emotional equilibrium. The costs of achieving this equilibrium, unfortunately, can be high. Lack of life satisfaction and interpersonal conflict with significant people in their lives are common. A paternally oriented work and cultural environment may provide little understanding or empathy for the difficult processes women confront. In marriage, an unenlightened and unresponsive spouse may have great difficulty in adequately responding to the issues women face on a daily basis, leading to marital conflict and sometimes divorce.

As life progresses, women continue to confront different psychological challenges. As a consequence of greater involvement in child-rearing and family cohesiveness, they may suffer a sense of loss as their children grow and leave home.

Menopause and all of its attendant features must be addressed and managed. In late adulthood, increasing physical frailty and the potential loss of a life partner accompanies a longer life span.

OTHER RISK FACTORS FOR DEPRESSION

A number of other factors play a role in the development of major depression and other mood disorders (see Table 9-2). Age is one of them. Although there is virtually no age at which depression can not appear, major depression in women is at its highest prevalence between the ages of 18 and 44, with the average time of onset of about 25 years of age.[14] In older people, the prevalence of the diagnosis of major depression declines, although clinically significant symptoms of depression that fall short of the total syndrome of major depression (i.e., minor depression or depression NOS) are still common. Race does not appear to be a factor in the prevalence of depression. Several studies have demonstrated that lower socioeconomic status is positively correlated with the development of depressive symptoms.[15,16]

MARITAL STATUS Marital status is a risk factor for both major and minor depression.[17] Although married women have higher rates of depression than single women, some studies show that happily married women have lower rates of depression than single women.[18] Stressful life events that are associated with marital status (e.g., death, divorce, domestic violence, sexual abuse, abortion, and miscarriage) also increase the risk of depression. Many women find themselves in caretaker roles, and assuming this role is a risk factor for the development of depression.[19] Women caring for demented spouses or parents are at higher risk for depression.[20] Mothers of children with attention deficit-hyperactivity disorder also have more symptoms of depression.[21]

FAMILY HISTORY AND EXPERIENCES Family history and childhood experience are also risk factors for depression. There is an increased risk of depression among first-degree relatives of individuals with depression[22]; however, environmental factors likely contribute to this risk as well. Genetic transmission is more clearly established in bipolar disorder.[22] There is an increased risk of both bipolar disorder and major depression in first-degree relatives of persons with bipolar disorder. Among childhood influences, parental loss before the onset of adolescence clearly contributes to risk, as do major life events such as divorce and separation.[23] Subtle influences, such as parental neglect, are more difficult to quantify in terms of their ability to affect the development of depression.

Previous episodes of depression are a risk factor for future episodes, and increased vigilance is necessary in monitoring patients with a history of depression.[24] Fifty percent of people with a first episode of depression experience a second episode of depression within 5 years.[24] Two previous episodes confer an 80 to 90 percent risk of subsequent depressive episodes.[24]

PSYCHOSOCIAL STRESSORS   Psychosocial stressors, both acute and chronic, often presage the development of depression. Obvious life-changing events such as marriage, divorce, birth, and death can have a role in the development of depression. More chronic stressors, however, such as interpersonal problems, finances, and chronic illness also predispose to the development of depression.[25] One life event of special importance to women, menopause, by itself does not give rise to an increased risk of depression; however, among women suffering from insomnia or excessive hot flashes, there is an increased risk of depression.[26] Another life-changing event in women is the postpartum period. Up to 10 percent of women following delivery will develop major depression within 6 months.[27] Miscarriage and abortion also pose an increased risk for depression.

SOCIAL SUPPORT   The presence or absence of social supports can influence the development and course of depression. This may be especially important in women for whom psychological needs correlate with their sense of interpersonal connectedness. The presence of a functioning social network with family, friends, co-workers, and others can be both a source of strength and a source of stress (see Chap. 10). The degree of community cohesiveness is also an important factor. Data from the NIMH ECA studies show that the risk of depression is double for women living in a rural versus an urban area.[16] This factor was shown to be independent of socioeconomic status. Unemployment also confers an increased risk, with more depressive symptoms reported in people unemployed at least 6 months in the past 5 years.[16]

PHYSICAL ILLNESS   Finally, serious physical illness, especially in the elderly, increases the risk of depression.[28] Depression can affect up to 50 percent of hospitalized patients, especially those with serious or life-threatening illnesses, such as stroke, trauma, myocardial infarction, and cancer.[28] Some illnesses that disproportionately affect women are also known to increase the risk of depression. These illnesses include thyroid disease, multiple sclerosis, and systemic lupus erythematosus. Medications may also cause depression (Table 9-3). Among the most common medications specifically known to cause depression are β-blockers, corticosteroids, and most importantly in the case of women, progestin-containing contraceptives.

Diagnosis

As our knowledge about depression continues to expand, it is becoming increasingly important to develop a careful and thorough approach to diagnosis. A comprehensive history is necessary to identify various medical causes of depression, any contribution of substance abuse, and a history of psychiatric comorbidities, such as anxiety, psychosis, or personality disorders, because each of these factors can have a major bearing on treatment decisions. It is also no longer sufficient, indeed, if it ever was, to simply diagnose the *syndrome* of depression. It is now also important to make an effort to understand what *subtype* of

Table 9-3

Medications that Cause Depression

Antihypertensives	Antibiotics
α-Methyldopa (Aldomet)	Sulfonamides
Reserpine (Serpasil)	Ethambutol (Myambutol)
Propranolol (Inderal)	Psychotropic medications
Guanethidine (Ismelin)	Antipsychotics
Clonidine (Catapres)	Benzodiazepines
Thiazide diuretics	Illicit drugs
Steroids	Cocaine
Adrenocorticotropic hormone	Amphetamines
Glucocorticoids	Miscellaneous
Anabolic steroids	Digitalis
Oral contraceptives	Levodopa (Sinemet)
Progestins (medroxyprogesterone acetate	Cyclosporin (Sandimmune)
[Provera, Depo-Provera], levonorgestrel	Disulfiram (Antabuse)
[Norplant], norgestrel [Ovrette])	Baclofen (Lioresal)
Gastrointestinal medications	
Cimetidine (Tagamet)	
Ranitidine (Zantac)	
Metoclopramide (Reglan)	

depression the patient may have because this distinction can have a direct bearing on treatment decisions. Finally, it is **always** necessary to conduct a careful assessment of the risk of suicide, including ongoing monitoring of suicide risk, given the inherent risk of suicide that depression can pose.

CRITERIA

The use of psychiatric epidemiologic data led to the establishment of diagnostic criteria for depression. These criteria continue to be refined and are published in the *Diagnostic and Statistical Manual of Mental Disorders* of the American Psychiatric Association (DSM-IV).[24] The current diagnostic criteria for depressive illnesses are shown in Tables 9-4, 9-5, and 9-6. Despite the use of these criteria, the determination of the "clinical significance" of behavioral or psychological syndromes causing either "distress" or "disability" is more art than science. Distinguishing between sig-

nificant psychopathology and normal variants is no easy task, even for experienced clinicians.

The presence of depressed mood is one of the two core criteria for the diagnosis of depression. Depressed mood, however, can mean different things to different people and may be described as anguish, anxiety, irritability, or mournfulness. In addition, depression may have a somatic presentation. Common somatic expressions of depression include headache, epigastric pain, and chest discomfort. Depression manifesting as somatic symptoms is more commonly seen in the elderly and in people who have difficulty describing feelings and physical sensations.[29] Somatoform manifestations of depression appear to disproportionately affect women.[24]

Loss of interest, or anhedonia, is a symptom that it is also critical to explore; it is the other core criterion for the diagnosis of depression. The easiest way to demonstrate anhedonia is to identify the loss of previously pleasurable pastimes. This loss

Table 9-4

DSM-IV Criteria for Major Depression

A. Presence of at least one Major Depression Episode

  Five or more of the following symptoms have been present during the same 2-week period and represent a change from previous functioning; at least one of the symptoms is either (1) depressed mood or (2) loss of interest or pleasure.

  (1) Depressed mood most of the day, nearly every day

  (2) Markedly diminished interest or pleasure in all, or almost all, activities most of the day, nearly every day

  (3) Significant weight loss when not dieting or weight gain, or decrease or increase in appetite nearly every day

  (4) Insomnia or hypersomnia nearly every day

  (5) Psychomotor agitation or retardation nearly every day

  (6) Fatigue or loss of energy nearly every day

  (7) Feelings of worthlessness or excessive or inappropriate guilt nearly every day

  (8) Diminished ability to think or concentrate, or indecisiveness, nearly every day

  (9) Recurrent thoughts of death (not just fear of dying), recurrent suicidal ideation without a specific plan, or a suicide attempt or a specific plan for committing suicide

  • The symptoms do not meet the criteria for a Mixed Episode.

  • The symptoms cause clinically significant distress or impairment in social, occupational, or other important areas of functioning.

  • The symptoms are not due to the direct physiological effects of a substance or a general medical condition.

  • The symptoms are not better accounted for by bereavement.

B. The major depressive episode is not better accounted for by Schizoaffective Disorder and is not superimposed on Schizophrenia, Schizophreniform Disorder, Delusional Disorder, or Psychotic Disorder Not Otherwise Specified

C. There has never been a Manic Episode, a Mixed Episode, or a Hypomanic Episode.

SOURCE: Reproduced with permission from *Diagnostic and Statistical Manual of Mental Disorders*, 4th ed. Washington, DC, American Psychiatric Association, 1994.

can be so severe that the patient exhibits no enjoyment of friends, family, or career.

SCREENING FOR DEPRESSION

Using a screening instrument for depression in primary care settings can provide a ready way to identify whether depressive symptoms are present and, consequently, require further attention. A number of instruments have been used over the years, including the Beck,[30] Carroll,[31] Center for Epidemiologic Studies,[32] and Zung[33] scales. These scales are straightforward to use and can be scored by office staff within minutes. The Hamilton Depression Scale[34] is the one most frequently used in research settings and by psychiatrists, but its use requires some training and an interview is required. The Carroll Scale has the advantage of most closely resembling the Hamilton Depression Scale, but can be self-administered (Table 9-7). A scoring system has been developed for the Carroll Scale, with 0 to 11 points indicating no or minimal depression, 12 to 18 points indicating mild depression, 19 to 25 points indicating moderate depression, and 26 or more points indicating severe depression. However, there is no clear cutoff point for where depression does or does not exist, and the clinician is still left with deciding when further inquiry into the nature of symptoms identified on these scales is necessary.

Table 9-5

DSM-IV Criteria for Dysthymic Disorder

A. Depressed mood for most of the day, for more days than not, as indicated either by subjective account or observation by others, for at least 2 years.

B. Presence, while depressed, of two or more of the following:
   (1) Poor appetite or overeating
   (2) Insomnia or hypersomnia
   (3) Low energy or fatigue
   (4) Low self-esteem
   (5) Poor concentration or difficulty making decisions
   (6) Feelings of hopelessness

C. During the 2-year period of the disturbance, the person has never been without the symptoms in Criteria A and B for more than 2 months at a time.

D. No Major Depressive Episode has been present during the first 2 years of the disturbance; i.e., the disturbance is not better accounted for by chronic Major Depressive Disorder, or Major Depressive Disorder, In Partial Remission.

E. There has never been a Manic Episode, a Mixed Episode, or a Hypomanic Episode, and criteria have never been meet for Cyclothymic Disorder.

F. The disturbance does not occur exclusively during the course of a chronic Psychotic Disorder, such as Schizophrenia or Delusional Disorder.

G. The symptoms are not due to the direct physiological effects of a substance or a general medical condition.

H. The symptoms cause clinically significant distress or impairment in social, occupational, or other important areas of functioning.

SOURCE: Reproduced with permission from *Diagnostic and Statistical Manual of Mental Disorders*, 4th ed. Washington, DC, American Psychiatric Association, 1994.

SUBTYPES OF DEPRESSION

One of the newer trends in conceptualizing depression is the further subclassification of the disorder. The primary interest in subtyping depression is to optimize treatment approaches.

DYSTHYMIA Dysthymia is characterized by a chronically depressed mood that occurs most of the day, for more days than not, for at least 2 years (see Table 9-5).[24] Accompanying symptoms include poor appetite or overeating, insomnia or hypersomnia, low energy or fatigue, low self-esteem, poor concentration or inability to make decisions, and feelings of hopelessness. This symptom profile is a subset of the symptoms of major depression and underscores the current thinking in psychiatry that there is likely a *spectrum* of

depressive symptoms. Some authors also use the term *minor depression*, denoting a set of symptoms that does not quite merit a diagnosis of major depression. This terminology is in need of further study; in particular, the implications for treatment are not clear. In the past, dysthymia was considered to be more treatment resistant than major depression, but this assertion is now in doubt.[35]

ATYPICAL DEPRESSION Atypical depression is actually the most common form of depression seen among outpatients. The symptoms of depression that characterize this subtype include mood reactivity (i.e., the capacity to be cheered up temporarily by positive interactions or events), hypersomnia (increased sleepiness), "leaden paralysis" (severe fatigue), hyperphagia (increased eating), and rejection sensitivity (an increased sensitivity to

Table 9-6

DSM-IV Criteria for Bipolar Disorder

A. Presence of Manic Episode (see criteria below) and no past Major Depressive Episodes
  • A distinct period of abnormally and persistently elevated, expansive, or irritable mood, lasting at least 1 week.
  • During the period of mood disturbance, three or more of the following symptoms have persisted (four, if the mood is only irritable) and have been present to a significant degree:
  (1) Inflated self-esteem or grandiosity
  (2) Decreased need for sleep
  (3) More talkative than usual or pressure to keep talking
  (4) Flight of ideas or subjective experience that thoughts are racing
  (5) Distractibility
  (6) Increase in goal-directed activity or psychomotor agitation
  (7) Excessive involvement in pleasurable activities that have a high potential for painful consequences
  • The symptoms do not meet criteria for a Mixed Episode.
  • The mood disturbance is sufficiently severe to cause marked impairment in occupational functioning or in usual social activities or relationships with others, or to necessitate hospitalization to prevent harm to self or others, or there are psychotic features.
  • The symptoms are not due to the direct physiologic effects of a substance or a general medical condition.
B. The Manic Episode is not better accounted for by Schizoaffective Disorder and is not superimposed on Schizophrenia, Schizophreniform Disorder, Delusional Disorder, or Psychotic Disorder Not Otherwise Specified.

SOURCE: Reproduced with permission from *Diagnostic and Statistical Manual of Mental Disorders*, 4th ed. Washington, DC, American Psychiatric Association, 1994.

interpersonal rejection and conflict). Patients with atypical depression tend to have an earlier age at onset of their first depressive episode, and women seem to be more often affected by this type than men.[36] The episodes appear to be of shorter duration than those of melancholic depression, but more frequent. Patients with coexisting obsessive-compulsive, avoidant, and passive-aggressive personalities are more prone to this type of depression.[37] The importance of recognizing this particular subtype is that monoamine oxidase inhibitors (MAOIs) have the greatest efficacy in treatment.[38] Tricyclic antidepressants (TCAs) are less effective.[43] Selective serotonin reuptake inhibitors (SSRIs) are also effective treatments and may be considered as first-line therapy because of their high safety and low risk of side effects.[39]

ANXIOUS DEPRESSION Anxiety and depression are often considered to be two separate entities; however, it is now clear that there is significant overlap of these disorders. In fact, the *majority* of patients diagnosed with *either* a depressive or anxiety disorder will actually have both conditions. The anxiety disorders that are more likely to coexist with major depression are panic disorder, social phobia, obsessive-compulsive disorder, posttraumatic stress disorder, and generalized anxiety disorder. When significant coexisting anxiety is identified, care must be directed toward its treatment as well. In the cases of panic disorder, social phobia, and obsessive-compulsive disorders, for example, the recommendation to seek cognitive-behavioral treatments to a patient would be of great importance.

Table 9-7
Carroll Depression Self-Rating Scale

Patient's Name _____	Date _____

Answer the following questions in terms of how you have felt in the *last few days*; circle your answers and please do not leave any questions unanswered. Please do not write any comments on this form.

1.	I feel just as energetic as always	Yes	No
2.	I am losing weight	Yes	No
3.	I have dropped many of my interests and activities	Yes	No
4.	Since my illness I have completely lost interest in sex	Yes	No
5.	I am especially concerned about how my body is functioning	Yes	No
6.	It must be obvious that I am disturbed and agitated	Yes	No
7.	I am still able to carry on doing the work I am supposed to do	Yes	No
8.	I can concentrate easily when reading the papers	Yes	No
9.	Getting to sleep takes me more than half an hour	Yes	No
10.	I am restless and fidgety	Yes	No
11.	I wake up much earler than I need to in the morning	Yes	No
12.	Dying is the best solution for me	Yes	No
13.	I have a lot of trouble with dizzy and faint feelings	Yes	No
14.	I am being punished for something bad in my past	Yes	No
15.	My sexual interest is the same as before I got sick	Yes	No
16.	I am miserable or often feel like crying	Yes	No
17.	I often wish I were dead	Yes	No
18.	I am having trouble with indigestion	Yes	No
19.	I wake up often in the middle of the night	Yes	No
20.	I feel worthless and ashamed about myself	Yes	No
21.	I am so slowed down that I need help with bathing and dressing	Yes	No
22.	I take longer than usual to fall asleep at night	Yes	No
23.	Much of the time I am very afraid but don't know the reason	Yes	No
24.	Things which I regret about my life are bothering me	Yes	No
25.	I get pleasure and satisfaction from what I do	Yes	No
26.	All I need is a good rest to be perfectly well again	Yes	No
27.	My sleep is restless and disturbed	Yes	No
28.	My mind is as fast and alert as always	Yes	No
29.	I feel that life is still worth living	Yes	No
30.	My voice is dull and lifeless	Yes	No
31.	I feel irritable or jittery	Yes	No
32.	I feel in good spirits	Yes	No
33.	My heart sometimes beats faster than usual	Yes	No
34.	I think my case is hopeless	Yes	No
35.	I wake up before my usual time in the morning	Yes	No
36.	I still enjoy my meals as much as usual	Yes	No
37.	I have to keep pacing around most of the time	Yes	No
38.	I am terrified and near panic	Yes	No

(Continued Overleaf.)

Table 9-7

Carroll Depression Self-Rating Scale *(Continued.)*

Patient's Name _____	Date _____	
39. My body is bad and rotten inside	Yes	No
40. I got sick because of the bad weather we have been having	Yes	No
41. My hands shake so much that people can easily notice	Yes	No
42. I still like to go out and meet people	Yes	No
43. I think I appear calm on the outside	Yes	No
44. I think I am as good a person as anybody else	Yes	No
45. My trouble is the result of some serious internal disease	Yes	No
46. I have been thinking about trying to kill myself	Yes	No
47. I get hardly anything done lately	Yes	No
48. There is only misery in the future for me	Yes	No
49. I worry a lot about my bodily symptoms	Yes	No
50. I have to force myself to eat even a little	Yes	No
51. I am exhausted much of the time	Yes	No
52. I can tell that I have lost a lot of weight	Yes	No

SOURCE: Reproduced with permission from Carroll et al.[31]

BIPOLAR DEPRESSION To help distinguish unipolar from bipolar depression, it is helpful to recognize the different symptomatology of these disorders (see Table 9-6). Patients with unipolar depression are more physically and mentally active and have complaints of somatic and sleep disturbances as well as anxiety and anger. Bipolar patients tend, in contrast, to be more quietly withdrawn, with psychomotor slowing and hypersomnia.[40] They also tend to have fewer signs and symptoms of anxiety, fewer physical complaints, and less reported anger. Bipolar patients are also less likely to identify and complain of depression and are, as a result, at increased risk for undertreatment and suicide.[41] Although bipolar disorder has the same incidence in both men and women, so-called "rapid-cycling" (at least four episodes of a mood disturbance in the previous 12 months meeting the criteria for a major depressive, manic, mixed, or hypomanic episode) more commonly affects women. Menopause is a risk factor for developing rapid cycling; sex hormone influences likely play a role.

The recognition of bipolar depression is of critical importance because treating this subtype of depression with an antidepressant without the coadministration of a mood stabilizer (e.g., lithium) can lead to a manic episode.[42] Table 9-6 lists the criteria for diagnosis. Manic episodes can be difficult enough to treat in their own right, but are especially difficult to treat when they are precipitated by an antidepressant. The treatment of bipolar depression is somewhat complicated, in that a number of different types of approaches are possible, including the use of lithium, anticonvulsants, antidepressants, atypical antipsychotics, and electroconvulsive therapy.

DEPRESSION WITH ANGER ATTACKS This newly identified subtype is characterized by sudden episodes of anger accompanied by symptoms of autonomic activation, such as tachycardia, sweating, flushing, and tightness of the chest.[43] Depressed patients affected this way experience these attacks as uncharacteristic of themselves and inappropriate to the situations in which they occur. About one-third of depressed patients will present with such attacks; coexisting anxiety and somatic symptoms are relatively common. This subtype appears to have a predilection for affecting patients with avoidant, dependent, borderline, narcissistic, and antisocial personality disorders. Anger attacks improve with antidepressant treatment, although there is insufficient evidence to indicate a differential response to different types of antidepressants.

SEASONAL AFFECTIVE DISORDER This subtype of depression is characterized by the onset and remission of major depressive episodes at recurrent and distinct, regular times of the year. It is greater at higher latitudes, in younger people, and in women.[24] The symptom profile of SAD consists of increased appetite, carbohydrate craving, weight gain, and hypersomnia. Treatment for SAD includes full-spectrum bright light at an intensity of 10,000 lux for 30 min, preferably administered in the morning.[44] However, light is often not sufficient for treating SAD because nearly two-thirds of patients also require supplemental treatment with antidepressants.[45]

PSYCHOTIC DEPRESSION The diagnosis of psychotic depression requires the presence of hallucinations or delusions in the presence of depressive symptoms. These psychotic symptoms can be either "mood-congruent," such as delusions of guilt or deserved punishment, or "mood-incongruent," such as persecutory delusions and delusions of thought insertion (the belief that someone or something is inserting thoughts into one's mind) or thought broadcasting (the belief that other people can hear one's thoughts as if they were being broadcast). Psychotic depression is present in about 15 percent of patients with major depression and is more common in bipolar depression than unipolar depression.[46] This subtype of depression, compared to all the other subtypes, is the most dangerous, because it is the one most frequently associated with suicide. It does ***not*** respond to antidepressant therapy alone; antipsychotics are necessary in combination with antidepressant therapy, and electroconvulsive therapy is frequently needed.[46]

DEPRESSION IN PREGNANCY

Pregnancy does not confer any protection against depression; it appears that there is no significant difference in the prevalence of depression when comparing pregnant with nonpregnant women.[47] Risk factors for depression during pregnancy include a prior history of depression, ambivalent or negative attitudes about being pregnant, limited or absent social and family support, living alone, having a higher number of children, the presence of significant marital conflict, and a younger age.[48] The evidence is conflicting about the course of depression during pregnancy, with some studies showing general improvement as pregnancy progresses and other studies suggesting the opposite. However, the presence of depression during pregnancy raises the specter of higher risk for prematurity and lower Apgar scores for the infant and mood instability in the mother.[49]

Treatment with medication should be considered for pregnant women if the symptoms of depression are moderate to severe or if they persist into the second trimester. Despite the desire of most women and their physicians to avoid medication in the first trimester, if a patient has a history of recurrent moderate to severe depression with multiple failed attempts at antidepressant discontinuation, maintaining antidepressant treatment during conception attempts and pregnancy is preferable. Antidepressant medication is usually well tolerated during pregnancy. Further information on treatment is discussed below.

POSTPARTUM DEPRESSION

Postpartum depression affects 5 to 20 percent of women. True postpartum depression must be distinguished from a milder form of depression, sometimes referred to as the "postpartum blues." This milder form of depression is characterized by typical depressive symptoms (e.g., depressed mood, loss of energy, loss of appetite, and decreased libido) accompanied by feelings of being overwhelmed and interpersonally sensitive to the feelings and comments of others. This condition can affect up 85 percent of women in the first week after the infant's birth. To be distinguished from nonpregnancy depression, postpartum depression must begin within 6 months of giving birth. Among women who have experienced postpartum depression previously, the risk increases up to 50 to 60 percent.[50] Other factors that increase the risk of this type of depression include marital conflict, the emotional state of the father, stressful life events, ambivalent or negative feelings regarding the pregnancy and child, and the temperament of the child.[51] Hormonal influences are thought to provide the biologic substrate for the subsequent development of depression; rapidly falling levels of estrogen are thought to contribute.[52] Less well known is the potential contribution of thyroid dysfunction in the postpartum period. Hypothyroidism is more common in the first 6 months after giving birth, and the rates of thyroid dysfunction can be as high as 9 percent after pregnancy compared to 3 to 4 percent in the population at large.[53]

Assessing the Risk of Suicide

Suicide merits special mention because up to 15 percent of untreated or inadequately treated patients with depression will commit suicide.[54] Suicide is a major public health issue in the United States, representing the ninth leading cause of death in the country overall. In people under 45 years of age, suicide is the *fifth* most common cause of death, more common than homicide and only slightly less frequent than coronary heart disease. Women are more likely than men to attempt suicide, usually choosing drug overdose as the preferred method.[55] Men, however, choose more lethal methods and, as a result, men are four times more likely to die than women.[55]

The risk of suicide for an individual must be aggressively defined during the patient evaluation through skillful and detailed questioning, while being mindful that patients will often find thoughts of suicide to be the most distressing and painful. Figure 9-1 presents an algorithm that may be used for assessing the risk of suicide. Inquiry should include assessment of associated demographic risk factors, psychosocial stressors, comorbid anxiety or agitation symptoms, and substance abuse.

Pharmacologic Treatment

PHARMACOLOGIC AGENTS

The pharmacology of treating depression has become significantly more complicated. There are now three identified neurotransmitter receptor systems (norepinephrine, dopamine, and serotonin) and seven distinct mechanisms of action. Medication options are listed in Table 9-8. In considering initial medication treatment, side-effect profiles and potential drug interactions should be considered (Table 9-9).

MONOAMINE OXIDASE INHIBITORS   The MAOIs are the oldest class of antidepressants. MAOIs act by increasing the neurotransmission of serotonin, dopamine, and norepinephrine by inhibiting their metabolism in the synapse. In general, the MAOIs have unsurpassed efficacy in the treatment of depression, comparable to that observed with the TCAs.[56] They are especially effective in depression complicated by anxiety and in atypical depression.

Dosing Regimens.   The usual dosing range for MAOIs is listed in Table 9-8.

Adverse Effects.   The chief drawback to the use of MAOIs is the potential tyramine reaction. This reaction, characterized by headache and acute hypertension, is precipitated by tyramine acting as a false transmitter and displacing norepinephrine from presynaptic storage granules. As a result, large amounts of dietary tyramine can cause a hypertensive crisis by displacing large amounts of norepinephrine into the circulation. Tyramine is found in a number of foods, such as aged cheeses and soy sauce. Some drugs with sympathomimetic activity, such as diet medications, ephedrine, and phenylephrine, can also provoke a hypertensive crisis because their metabolism will also be impaired by the presence of an MAOI.

Another potential danger of using MAOIs is the emergence of the *serotonin syndrome*. Although this syndrome can also appear with the use of SSRIs, it is potentially deadly in the case of the

Figure 9-1

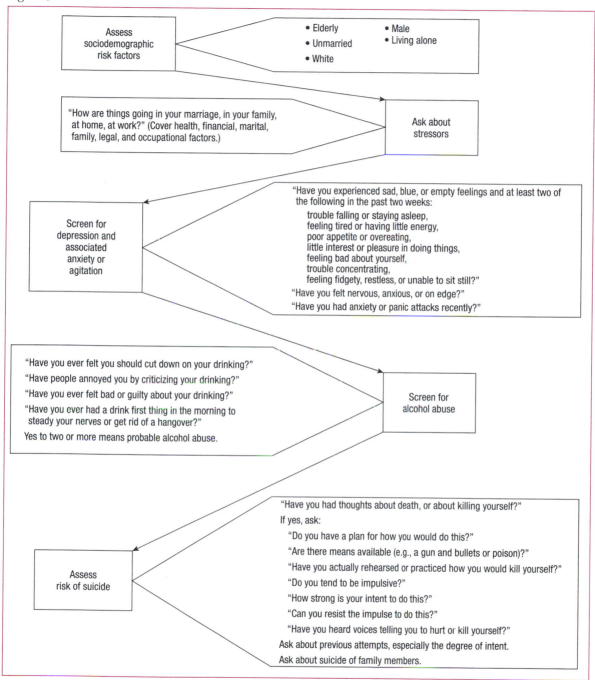

Algorithm for assessing the risk of suicide. *(Reproduced with permission from RM Hirschfeld, JM Russell: Assessment and treatment of suicidal patients. N Engl J Med 337:910–915, 1997.)*

Table 9-8

Antidepressants and Anxiolytics

GENERIC NAME	BRAND NAME	USUAL ADULT DAILY DOSAGE (mg)	SIDE-EFFECT PROFILE FOR DRUG CLASS	COST*
MONOAMINE OXIDASE INHIBITORS				$$
phenelzine	Nardil (C)†	45–90	Orthostatic hypotension	
tranylcypromine	Parnate (C)	30–60	Insomnia, restlessness	
			Peripheral edema	
			Drowsiness	
			Increased appetite	
			Weight gain	
			Sexual dysfunction	
TRICYCLICS (MOST AVAILABLE AS GENERIC AGENTS)				$–$$
amitriptyline	Elavil (D)	50–150	Dry mouth	
clomipramine	Anafranil (C)	75–250	Blurred vision	($$$)
desipramine	Norpramin (C)	50–300	Constipation	
doxepin	Sinequan (C)	75–150	Urinary retention	
imipramine	Tofranil (D)	150–200	Drowsiness	
nortriptyline	Pamelor (D)	75–150	Orthostatic hypotension	($$$)
			Dizziness	
			Increased appetite, weight gain	
			Sexual dysfunction	
			Confusion (especially for elderly)	
SELECTIVE SEROTONIN REUPTAKE INHIBITORS				$$$–$$$$
citalopram	Celexa (C)	20–40	Agitation	
fluoxetine	Prozac (C)	20–40	Anxiety	
fluvoxamine	Luvox (C)	100–300	Insomnia	
paroxetine	Paxil (C)	20–50	Sexual dysfunction	
sertraline	Zoloft (C)	50–200	Confusion	
			Dizziness	
			Sedation	
			Nausea	
			Gastrointestinal distress/diarrhea	
			Headache	
			Restlessness	
			Increased sweating	
ATYPICAL AGENTS				$$–$$$$
venlafaxine	Effexor (C)	75–225	Nausea, decreased appetite	
			Sexual dysfunction, visual disturbance	
			Abnormal dreams	
			Sweating	
			Agitation, anxiety	
			Taste perversion	
			Insomnia, hypertension, headache	

Table 9-8

Antidepressants and Anxiolytics *(Continued.)*

GENERIC NAME	BRAND NAME	USUAL ADULT DAILY DOSAGE (mg)	SIDE-EFFECT PROFILE FOR DRUG CLASS	COST*
	ATYPICAL AGENTS			$$–$$$$
nefazodone	Serzone (C)	300–600	Sedation, weakness Dizziness, dry mouth Blurred vision Nausea Constipation	
mirtazapine	Remeron (C)	15–45	Sedation, weight gain	
bupropion	Wellbutrin (B)	300–450	Anxiety, agitation, insomnia Nausea, poor appetite, weight loss Dizziness, sweating, dry mouth	
maprotiline	Ludiomil (B)	100–225	Sedation, dry mouth Constipation	
trazodone	Desyrel (C)	150–400	Sedation, orthostatic hypotension, dizziness Dry mouth Headache Nausea, vomiting, unpleasant taste	
	ANXIOLYTICS			$–$$
alprazolam	Xanax	0.75–1.5	Drowsiness Dizziness, ataxia	
chlordiazepoxide	Librium	15–100	Slurred speech Headache	
clonazepam	Klonopin	0.5–6	Gastrointestinal distress	
clorazepate	Tranxene	15–60	Euphoria Weakness	
diazepam	Valium	4–40	Depression	
halazepam	Paxipam	60–160		
lorazepam	Ativan	2–6		
oxazepam	Serax	30–120		
buspirone	Buspar	30–60	Dizziness, lightheadedness $$$–$$$$ Headache Nausea Weakness Restlessness Drowsiness Muscle pain or stiffness	

*Relative cost per drug class, based on Red Book. $, inexpensive (<$25); $$, moderately expensive ($26–60); $$$, expensive ($61–125); $$$$, very expensive (>$125).
†Food and Drug Administration drug rating for drugs in pregnancy: B, no evidence of risk to fetus; C, risk to fetus cannot be ruled out; D, evidence of risk to fetus.

MAOIs. The syndrome is characterized by lethargy, restlessness, confusion, flushing, diaphoresis, tremor, and myoclonic jerking. In its full expression, the syndrome can progress to hyperthermia, hypertonicity, myoclonus, and death. The deadliest interaction that can produce the serotonin syndrome is the combination of a MAOI and meperidine (Demerol). Thus, patients taking an MAOI must never be given meperidine. It is advisable for patients taking MAOIs to wear a Medic Alert bracelet indicating that they cannot be given meperidine. If a patient is in need of a narcotic analgesic, it is safe to use codeine or morphine.

Common Side Effects.   Other potential side effects of MAOIs are listed in Table 9-8. The most common side effects are orthostatic hypotension and insomnia.

TRICYCLIC ANTIDEPRESSANTS   These medications act as both serotonin and norepinephrine reuptake inhibitors. Their actions at three other receptors result in anticholinergic-antimuscarinic effects (e.g., side effects of dry mouth, blurred vision, and constipation), α_1-receptor antagonism (e.g., potential for hypotension), and antihistamine effects (e.g., possible drowsiness). The varying intensity of the medication effects at these receptors provides a differential side-effect profile for these agents. These medications also inhibit sodium channels conferring a risk of cardiac arrhythmias, particularly in the case of overdose.

A major benefit of use of the TCAs is the availability of accurate and clinically usable serum plasma levels to monitor therapy. Plasma levels of nortriptyline, desipramine, and imipramine can all be followed to optimize dosing. Monitoring drug levels is also helpful if a patient has not responded to what should be a therapeutic dose, if the patient is at higher risk of drug side effects because of age or medical illness, if the patient requires rapid increases in medication because of high risk of suicide, if compliance is in question, to document the optimal therapeutic level for a patient, and to monitor potential drug interactions when TCAs are given with medication known to

increase blood concentration (e.g., cimetidine, SSRIs).

Dosing Regimens.   The starting dose for nortriptyline is usually 25 mg/d and can be increased to 75 mg/d over 7 to 14 days, depending on the patient's response and the emergence of side effects. The maximum dose of nortriptyline should not exceed 150 mg/d. Starting doses for most of these medications is 25 mg with gradual increases to the therapeutic ranges shown in Table 9-8. The therapeutic range for imipramine is calculated as the sum of the concentration of both imipramine itself and its metabolite, desipramine. The total concentration of both imipramine and desipramine should be 200 to 250 ng/mg. In the case of using desipramine alone, the concentration should not exceed 125 ng/mL. For clomipramine (Anafranil), a TCA with additional effectiveness in the treatment of obsessive-compulsive disorder, the maximum dose should not exceed 250 mg/d to avoid the risk of seizures encountered at higher doses.

Adverse Effects and Common Side Effects.   The major adverse effect is the risk of cardiac arrhythmias, particularly in the case of overdose. These medications also commonly cause dry mouth, blurred vision, and sedation (see Table 9-8).

SELECTIVE SEROTONIN REUPTAKE INHIBITORS   Five SSRIs are now available commercially in the United States: fluoxetine (Prozac), sertraline (Zoloft), paroxetine (Paxil), fluvoxamine (Luvox), and citalopram (Celexa). The mechanism of action is complex and includes inhibition of serotonin neurotransmission. These medications have a wide spectrum of psychiatric application, including depression, obsessive-compulsive disorder, panic disorder, and bulimia. In treating depression, the onset of action is generally within 3 to 8 weeks. Transient symptom worsening may be noted early in the course of treatment for patients with anxiety. There is some sense that SSRIs are not as efficacious in treating *melancholic* depression as TCAs and MAOIs.

Dosing Regimens. The usual treatment doses of the SSRIs are listed in Table 9-8. It is important to begin with small doses and gradually increase the medication to the levels indicated in Table 9-8 over several weeks to minimize side effects.

Adverse Effects. Sexual dysfunction, generally defined as decreased sexual interest and inhibited orgasm, is often the most troublesome side effect associated with the use of these medications. The incidence of this adverse effect is high, generally estimated at 40 to 50 percent.[57] It is thought to be mediated through both central and spinal serotonin effects as well as effects on dopamine pathways.

Many methods have evolved to address SSRI-mediated sexual dysfunction (Table 9-10). Using agents with a shorter half-life and withholding the pills for 1 to 2 days before anticipated sexual activity are initial management strategies. Counteractive medications may also be used. For example, one strategy is to increase dopamine concentrations by adding bupropion (Wellbutrin), amantadine (Symmetrel), methylphenidate (Ritalin), or pramipexole (Mirapex) to the regimen.[58] Another option is to increase norepinephrine activity through the use of yohimbine (Yocon).[59] Inhibition of serotonin via cyproheptadine (Periactin) or buspirone (Buspar) is another approach that has been used.[60] Ginkgo biloba and ginseng have some demonstrated efficacy, but their mechanisms of action are unknown.[61] It may be necessary to use a different antidepressant altogether. Good alternatives to consider are bupropion (Wellbutrin), nefazodone (Serzone), and mirtazapine (Remeron). It is also possible that one SSRI will not induce the same sexual dysfunction as another, and switching SSRIs may be a successful strategy.

Common Side Effects. Early observations suggested that weight loss was associated with the use of SSRIs through serotonin-mediated effects on the brainstem and hypothalamus. However, long-term weight gain is observed in 1 to 50 percent of patients.[62] The mechanism of weight gain is not well understood, but it may be mediated through a serotonin receptor subtype, 5-HT2C. Most often, the effect is a loss of a sense of satiety as opposed to a reduction in metabolism. It is important to counsel patients at the time of beginning a trial of an SSRI about possible weight gain and to monitor their food consumption and exercise. Other side effects are listed in Table 9-8.

Discontinuation Syndrome. A discontinuation syndrome is sometimes observed when a patient stops using an SSRI.[63] The discontinuation syndrome is characterized by flulike symptoms including fatigue, dizziness, chills, sweating, lightheadedness, anxiety, and incoordination. Abrupt discontinuation of the medication is most likely to provoke this problem, but even tapering the medication will sometimes trigger the syndrome. The reported frequency of the syndrome varies widely, with rates of 5 to 80 percent quoted in the literature.[64] Short half-life agents (sertraline, paroxetine, fluvoxamine, and venlafaxine) are more prone to this problem than fluoxetine. Symptoms are usually not severe, though, and generally remit within 3 weeks. Tapering the dose over 3 to 4 weeks before stopping a short-acting agent will decrease the likelihood of provoking the discontinuation syndrome. The cause of this adverse effect is unclear, but some posit that the symptoms represent hyposerotonergic tone in the central nervous system (CNS) or remodulation of other neurotransmitter systems in the setting of hyposerotonergic tone.[65]

Drug-Drug Interactions. Much has been written about the potential drug-drug interactions of the SSRIs (see Table 9-9). These agents can be significant enzyme inhibitors of the P_{450} system of hepatic metabolism. A number of drug interactions with the potential for clinical significance exist (see Table 9-9). Of particular concern, however, is the combination of SSRIs with other agents that may elevate serotonin levels because a lethal hyperserotonergic state can develop. Patients should be asked about concomitant use of alternative therapies that affect serotonin, such as St. John's wort, before prescribing SSRIs. TCAs

Table 9-9

Potential Drug Interactions with Antidepressants

Drug Class	Effect	Action
Monoamine Oxidase Inhibitors (MAOIs)		
Tricyclic antidepressants	Hyperpyretic crisis, seizures, death	Avoid use of TCA concurrently or within 2 wk of MAOI therapy
Selective serotonin reuptake inhibitors (citaloprim, fluoxetine, fluvoxamine, paroxetinc, sertraline, nefazodone, venlafaxine)	Serotonin syndrome (e.g., CNS irritability, increased muscle tone, shivering, myoclonus, altered consciousness)	Do not use concurrently. Allow at least 1 wk after nefazodone or venlafaxine; at least 2 wk after citaloprim, fluvoxamine, or paroxetine; and at least 5 wk after fluoxetine before starting MAOI therapy. After stopping an MAOI allow at least 2 wk before starting any SSRI.
Bupropion	Risk of bupropion toxicity	Avoid concurrent use or use of bupropion within 14 d of use of an MAOI.
Anorexiants (e.g., phentermine, mazindol, diethylpropion, amphetamines)	Increased pharmacologic effect of anorexiants (hypertensive crisis, seizures, hyperpyrexia)	Avoid concurrent use or use of anorexiants for several weeks after MAOI therapy is discontinued.
Sulfonylureas (e.g., glipizide, glyburide, tolbutamide, chlorpropamide, tolazamide, acetohexamide)	Enhanced hypoglycemic effect	Adjust doses of sulfonylureas if necessary.
Insulin	Enhanced hypoglycemic effect	Adjust doses of insulin if necessary.
Sympathomimetics (e.g., pseudoephedrine, phenylpropanolamine, ephedrine, phenylephrine)	Hypertensive crisis, high fever, severe headache	Avoid concurrent use.
Levodopa	Hypertensive reaction	Avoid concurrent use.
Meperidine	Agitation, seizures, fever, apnea, coma, death	Avoid concurrent use.
Sumatriptan	Risk of sumatriptan toxicity	Avoid use of sumatriptan concurrently or within 2 wk of MAOI therapy.
Tricyclic Antidepressants (TCA)		
Carbamazepine	Increased carbamazepine serum levels and toxicity and decreased TCA serum levels	Monitor levels of both agents; watch for toxicity or loss of therapeutic effect.
Cimetidine	Increased TCA serum levels	Monitor patient status and/or levels of TCA; adjust dose if necessary.
Clonidine	Loss of blood pressure control; hypertensive reaction	Avoid concurrent use.
Sympathomimetics (e.g., pseudoephedrine, phenylpropanolamine, ephedrine, phenylephrine)	Hypertensive reaction, arrhythmia	Avoid concurrent use or adjust dose of sympathomimetic.
Selective serotonin reuptake inhibitors (see below)	Increased TCA serum levels and possible toxicity	Monitor patient status and/or levels of TCA; adjust dose if necessary.
Quinolones (grepafloxacin, sparfloxacin)	Risk of cardiac arrhythmia, including torsades de pointes	Use alternative quinolone.
Guanethidine	Hypertensive reaction	Monitor blood pressure; use alternative antihypertensive.
MAOI	See above	
Rifampin, rifabutin	Decreased TCA serum levels; loss of therapeutic effect	Monitor patient status and/or levels of TCA; adjust dose if necessary.

Table 9-9

Potential Drug Interactions with Antidepressants *(Continued.)*

Drug Class	Effect	Action
Tricyclic Antidepressants (TCA)		
Valproic acid, valproate sodium	Increased TCA serum levels and possible toxicity	Monitor patient status and/or levels of TCA; adjust dose if necessary.
Selective Serotonin Reuptake Inhibitors (SSRIs)		
Sympathomimetics (e.g., pseudoephedrine, phenyl-propanolamine, ephedrine, phenylephrine)	Risk of serotonin syndrome (see above)	Avoid concurrent use or monitor for CNS effects.
Clozapine	Increased serum clozapine levels and possible toxicity	Monitor patient status and/or levels of clozapine; adjust dose if necessary.
Cyproheptadine	Decreased therapeutic effect of SSRI	Avoid concurrent use.
MAOI (includes selegiline)	See above	
Tricyclic antidepressants	See above	
Hydantoins (e.g., phenytoin)	Increased serum hydantoin levels and possible toxicity	Monitor patient status and/or levels of hydantoin; adjust dose if necessary.
Phenothiazines	Increased plasma phenothiazine level and possible toxicity	Monitor patient status and/or levels of phenothiazine; adjust dose if necessary.
Astemizole (with fluvoxamine and nefazodone; not with paroxetine or sertraline)	Risk of cardiac arrhythmia, including torsades de pointes	Avoid concurrent use; use alternative antihistamine.
Tacrine (with fluvoxamine; not with fluoxetine)	Increased plasma tacrine level and possible toxicity	Avoid concurrent use; use alternative SSRI.
Carbamazepine (with fluoxetine; possibly with fluvoxamine)	Increased carbamazepine serum levels and toxicity	Monitor patient status and/or levels of carbamazepine; adjust dose if necessary.
Atypical Antidepressants		
Bupropion		
Carbamazepine	Decreased bupropion serum levels; loss of therapeutic effect	Monitor patient status: adjust bupropion dose if necessary.
MAOI	See above	
Ritonavir	Increased bupropion serum levels; and possible toxicity	Avoid concurrent use.
Nefazodone (See also MAOI–SSRI and SSRI–Astemizole above)		
Cisapride	Increased plasma cisapride level and possible toxicity	Avoid concurrent use.
Venlafaxine		
MAOI (including selegiline)	See MAOI–SSRI above	

Source: Compiled from Drug Interactions Facts (Level 1 and 2 drug interactions); Facts and Comparison, St. Louis; 1999.

Table 9-10

Management of Antidepressant-Induced Sexual Dysfunction

Optimization strategies
    Manipulate current treatment
        Wait for tolerance
        Reduce dose
        Introduce drug holidays
Antidote strategies
    Add another drug
        Serotonin (5-hydroxytryptamine) antagonists
            Cyproheptadine
            Methysergide
            Nefazodone
            Mirtazapine
            Mianserin
        Dopamine agonists
            Amantadine
            Amphetamine
            Methylphenidate
            Pramipexole
        Other agents
            Yohimbine
            Bupropion
            Buspirone
            Bethanechol
            Ginkgo biloba extract
Substitution strategies
    Bupropion
    Nefazodone
    Mirtazapine
    St. John's wort

SOURCE: Adapted from Delgado PL, McGahuey CA, Moreno FA, et al: Treatment strategies for depression and sexual dysfunction. *J Clin Psychiatry* Monograph 17:1, 15, 1999.

and SSRIs are occasionally used together, but SSRIs are capable of significantly increasing TCA levels. Frequent use of plasma levels of TCAs may be indicated in these situations.

OTHER NEW AGENTS

Bupropion (Wellbutrin). This antidepressant affects both norepinephrine and dopamine neuro-transmission, leaving the serotonin system un-affected. It is unique in its mechanism of action. It has also been shown to be effective in treating attention deficit disorder and in helping people with smoking cessation. The dosage range and side effects are listed in Table 9-8. Of note is that bupropion causes no sexual dysfunction or weight gain.[66] It can cause seizures with overdose.[67]

Venlafaxine (Effexor). This antidepressant has reuptake blockade properties that are dose dependent. At lower doses, it blocks serotonin reuptake, but at higher doses it also blocks norepinephrine; at maximal doses, it blocks dopamine reuptake, too. It has a very short half-life, making it the most likely antidepressant medication to provoke a discontinuation syndrome. As a result, it is very important to remember to taper venlafaxine slowly when stopping the drug. The most common side effect is nausea, but this problem is minimized if the medication is taken with food. Other side effects are listed in Table 9-8. Increased blood pressure, a novel side effect for antidepressants, is seen generally only in older men. Venlafaxine has demonstrated some effectiveness in treating resistant depression, which is a distinguishing characteristic.[68]

Nefazodone (Serzone). Nefazodone is a specific 5-HT2 reuptake blocker. It is also a weak norepinephrine uptake inhibitor. It has several clinically significant drug interactions (see Table 9-9). Unlike a structurally related compound, trazodone (Desyrel), it does not cause priapism because it has no significant α_2 effects. Nefazodone also enjoys the distinction of preserving sleep architecture better than any other antidepressant. For this reason, both nefazodone and trazodone are often used in lower doses to promote sleep.

Mirtazapine (Remeron). Mirtazapine has the unique profile of antagonizing 5-HT2, 5-HT3, and α_2-receptors. This combination of effects results in the therapeutic effect being mediated through the 5-HT1 receptor. At low doses, mirtazapine has significant antihistaminic effects; as a consequence,

Figure 9-2

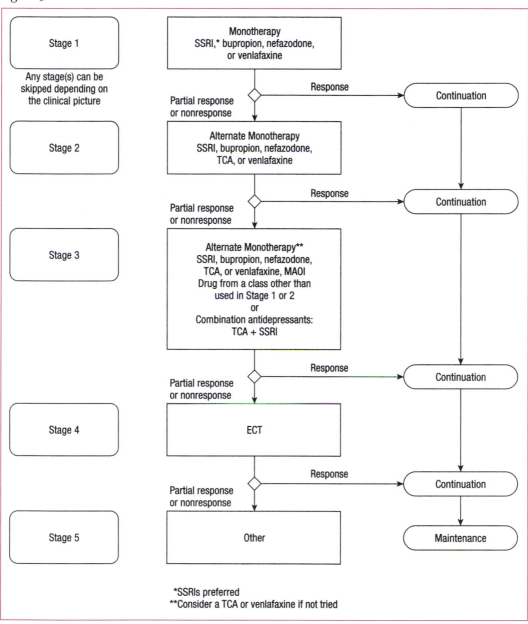

Algorithm for choosing an antidepressant. ECT, electroconvulsive therapy; MAOI, monoamine oxidase inhibitor; SSRI, selective serotonin reuptake inhibitor; TCA, tricyclic antidepressant. Drug trade names: bupropion, Wellbutrin; citalopram, Celexa; mirtazapine, Remeron; nefazodone, Serzone; venlafaxine, Effexor. *(Reproduced with permission from M Crimson et al: J Clin Psychiatry 60:142, Copyright 1999.)*

it is quite sedating in the 7.5- to 15.0-mg range. Typical side effects include increased appetite and weight gain, but no sexual dysfunction. It is sometimes used in combination with SSRIs to reduce the nausea and sexual side effects associated with these drugs.

SELECTION OF AN INITIAL ANTIDEPRESSANT

Figure 9-2 presents an algorithm for selection of an initial antidepressant developed by the Texas Medication Algorithm Project.[69] It can be used as a guide to assist clinicians in making therapeutic choices and changes when patients fail to respond to initial therapy.

INITIAL SELECTION   The initial treatment is usually monotherapy (single agent) with an SSRI. These medications are highly effective, safe and well tolerated, and dose titration is rarely necessary. If sexual side effects are a concern, initial treatment with bupropion or venlafaxine should be considered.

RESPONSE TO TREATMENT   When a patient fails to completely respond to an adequate trial of a single agent (generally defined as using an agent at a therapeutic dose for at least 8 weeks), many options can be tried. With an SSRI as the initial agent, switching to another SSRI is now accepted practice because these agents differ enough from each other that they cannot be thought of as interchangeable (step 2 of algorithm). Using combination and augmentation strategies is another frequently used option (step 3 of algorithm).

The subject of combination and augmentation strategies is a complex one, and older approaches to augmentation are coming under further scrutiny. Simple and safe augmentation can be accomplished through the use of bupropion. Another agent that is often used is methylphenidate (Ritalin). One time-honored approach to augmentation has been to use lithium or thyroid supplementation. The benefit of lithium augmentation has been documented; doses of lithium are similar to those used to treat bipolar disorder. After the addition of lithium, benefit is often seen within a few days

(up to 6 weeks). Early response is a predictor of a good outcome. Thyroid is usually used as triiodothyronine (Cytomel) in a dose of 25 µg/d. Consultation with a psychiatrist should be considered for patients who reach stage 4 with only a partial response or no response to treatment.

Especially important in perimenopausal and postmenopausal women is the use of estrogen. Some studies indicate that antidepressants are more effective in women during this time if estrogen is prescribed concurrently.[70] However, it is clear that estrogen by itself is insufficient to treat significant depressive symptoms.

ANTIDEPRESSANT USE IN PREGNANCY AND THE POSTPARTUM PERIOD

Generally, antidepressants are well tolerated in pregnancy, and careful assessment of the risk of significant untreated psychiatric illness (e.g., poor maternal nutrition, suicide) must be weighed against the potential risk of teratogenicity. As a guiding principle, the use of medication in pregnancy should be correlated with the severity of mental illness. It is not unreasonable to maximize nonpharmacologic approaches in women with mild to moderate depression with a single episode of depression beginning in the first trimester. Likewise, women who are taking medication for their first episode of depression, with only mild or moderate symptoms, can be considered for tapering their medication when they become pregnant or if they wish to try to conceive. Medication is indicated, however, if the symptoms of depression are moderate to severe of if they persist into the second trimester.

Despite the desire of most women and their health care providers to avoid medication in the first trimester, if a woman has a history of recurrent moderate to severe depression with multiple failed attempts at antidepressant discontinuation, maintaining antidepressant treatment during conception attempts and pregnancy is preferable. The research to date would indicate that bupropion, maprotiline, fluoxetine, sertraline, paroxetine, or desipramine are probably safe to use. Only bupropion and maprotiline, however, are rated as Pregnancy Category B (no evidence of risk to fetus). In a study of 228 pregnant women treated with fluoxetine during the first trimester of pregnancy, investigators found no increase in teratogenicity, but did report perinatal neurobehavioral effects.[71] Other investigators, however, found no effect on the neurobehavioral development of preschool children exposed in utero to either TCAs or fluoxetine.[72]

It is especially important to monitor the affective state of women with a history of depression after delivery because up to 25 percent of these patients will develop a postpartum depression. Given the inherent stresses of new parenthood, increased vigilance for this possibility is required. There are no differences in the treatment of women in the postpartum period from the treatment of women at other times, unless the woman is breast-feeding. For these mothers, antidepressants that have no adverse effects on breast-fed infants may be considered for use. These include amitriptyline, clomipramine, imipramine, desipramine, nortriptyline, bupropion, and sertraline.

Nonpharmacologic Treatment

PSYCHOTHERAPY

Despite the rapid expansion of pharmacologic treatments for depression, it is important not to forget the place and the effectiveness of psychotherapy. In a review of the recommendations of the Depression Guideline Panel of the Agency for Health Care Policy and Research, time-limited depression-targeted psychotherapies were as effective as antidepressant pharmacotherapy.[73] The therapies showing the most consistent effectiveness are cognitive behavioral therapy and interpersonal psychotherapy. Cognitive behavioral therapy is a type of therapy targeting maladaptive thoughts or "cognitions" underlying depression or anxiety through the use of a focused, generally time-limited, problem-solving approach. Interpersonal therapy is a type of therapy that focuses on improving current interpersonal skills through a number of techniques that include reassurance, clarification

of feeling states, and improving interpersonal communication. Brief psychodynamic therapy and group therapy have also shown benefit in treating depression. The former is a psychoanalytically oriented type of therapy that uses at least some examination of early life or childhood experiences through a variety of techniques including free association and the latter refers to therapies that involve applying therapeutic techniques to a group of people rather than an individual.

Substantial controversy still exists as to whether psychotherapy or medication should be the initial intervention and patient preference should play a significant role in this decision. Ample research data indicate that psychotherapy is equally effective as antidepressants in treating mild to moderate depression, although there is less information supporting psychotherapy as a first-line treatment for more severe forms of depression. Other data suggest that combined antidepressant therapy and psychotherapy may produce the best outcomes.

COMPLEMENTARY THERAPIES

There clearly has been an increased interest in alternative medicine over the past several years, and some of these therapies have been effective in the treatment of depression. Some of the best data support the "prescription" of exercise to depressed patients. The antidepressant effect of exercise is observed with all types of regular exercise and is independent of gender or age. Some data suggest that the antidepressant effect of exercise may be on a par with psychotherapy.

Another popular complementary therapy is St. John's wort (Hypericum perforatum). The usual dose of hypericum is 300 mg tid. Experience in this country is still limited, however, and there is a general clinical sense that hypericum is useful primarily in depressions of mild intensity. St. John's wort should not be used by patients taking SSRIs because both agents increase serotonin levels, placing patients at risk for serotonin syndrome.

A variety of other therapies have been put forth as effective in treating depression. Examples are aromatherapy, dance and movement therapy, homeopathy, hypnotherapy, massage therapy, acupuncture, music therapy, and relaxation therapy. Of these, however, supportive data are available only for acupuncture, massage, and relaxation. There are no controlled research trials regarding the relative efficacy of these other forms of therapy.

DIET

Recent information suggests a link between the amount and type of dietary fat and psychiatric illness. There has long been puzzlement over why depression occurs at such different rates in different societies, and diet may be one reason. Dietary fat may be important in mental health because of its role in supporting normal brain function. The cell membrane at neuron synapses is composed almost entirely of essential fatty acids. Speculation has centered on omega-3 polyunsaturated fatty acids in particular. These fatty acids are found in especially high concentrations in fish oils, and rates of major depression are markedly different depending on how much fish is consumed. In Japan, for example, people consume over 140 lb of fish per person per year, and the rate of depression in Japan is just 0.12 percent! In Germany, people eat a little over 20 lb of fish per person per year and have a depression rate of 5 percent. These low rates of depression are in stark contrast to those in the United States.

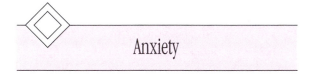

Anxiety

Introduction

Anxiety disorders are the most common of all psychiatric conditions, and they are disproportionately common in women. Although up to 25 percent of Americans may have a diagnosable anxiety disorder during their lifetime, over 30 percent of women will at some time in their life develop an anxiety disorder. In addition to being more common, anxiety disorders can be just as disabling as depression, and the acute sense of subjective discomfort is often worse with anxiety symptoms. In some studies, up to 7 percent of people with one common anxiety disorder, panic disorder, will eventually commit suicide.

MEDICAL CONDITIONS THAT CAN MIMIC ANXIETY

Because of the number of somatic symptoms that are a part of anxiety syndromes, nonpsychiatrists are often the first medical professionals consulted by patients suffering from these symptoms. Medical conditions that can mimic anxiety include a number of cardiac conditions, ischemic heart disease, and arrhythmias. Conversely, up to 20 percent of people referred to a cardiologist for the first time will actually have an anxiety disorder, especially panic disorder. Pulmonary conditions can likewise simulate anxiety. Chronic obstructive pulmonary disease, pulmonary embolism, and asthma can all cause the sense of dyspnea that is a frequent feature of anxiety. Gastrointestinal symptoms such as abdominal discomfort, cramping, and diarrhea can all be easily confused with anxiety. Other medical conditions such as hyperthyroidism, hypoglycemia, menopause, premenstrual syndrome, pheochromocytoma, transient ischemic attacks, vitamin deficiencies, and various drugs including caffeine, alcohol, bronchodilators, amphetamines, corticosteroids, and illicit drugs may produce symptoms identical to those occurring in anxiety disorders.

COEXISTING PSYCHIATRIC DISORDERS

As difficult as it can be to separate medical conditions and anxiety disorders, and indeed the two often coexist, the same is true of psychiatric disorders. The anxiety disorders themselves are not always easy to discern from each other (e.g., panic disorder and social phobia) and often coexist with other subtypes of psychiatric disorders. Anxiety can be a comorbid or complicating feature of psychotic, substance abuse, somatoform, sexual, personality, and especially mood disorders. Depression also commonly coexists with anxiety. The presence of significant anxiety symptoms not only complicates the treatment of depression, but it also signifies a more chronic and treatment-resistant course. Independent identification of anxiety symptoms is important because separate and effective treatments are available.

COEXISTING SUBSTANCE ABUSE

It is not uncommon for patients to resort to the use of alcohol or illicit substances to self-medicate anxiety symptoms. Alcohol is particularly treacherous because it can effectively ameliorate anxiety symptoms acutely, but it can aggravate them through complicating depression and inhibiting normal sleep. Withdrawal symptoms, when present, can provoke anxiety and lead to more alcohol consumption to reduce the discomfort associated with them. Unfortunately, some of the medications used to treat anxiety can themselves be problematic in that they can be abused. Barbiturates and benzodiazepines are the worst offenders in this regard.

To diagnose anxiety disorders, a high index of suspicion must be maintained by the clinician along with an open approach, using open-ended questions, careful listening, and observation. Given the increasing time constraints faced by clinicians, this task may appear daunting. Nevertheless, it is important to be successful in discerning and diagnosing these conditions, so that unnecessary, fruitless, and expensive workups for somatic symptoms of anxiety can be avoided. Effective treatment cannot begin until an accurate diagnosis is made.

Types of Anxiety Disorders

PANIC DISORDER

Of all the anxiety disorders, panic disorder is the best known. The definition of panic disorder consists of the recurrence of unexpected panic attacks, discrete periods of intense anxiety or fear, accompanied by at least four of the symptoms listed in Table 9-11. In addition, there must be a period of at least 1 month after at least one attack where there is persistent concern about having additional attacks, worry about the implications of the attack or its consequences, or a significant change in behavior related to the attacks. Furthermore, it must be determined that the panic attacks are not due to the effects of a substance, a medical condition, or another mental disorder. Panic disorder may or may not be complicated by agoraphobia. *Agoraphobia* is anxiety or fear about being in places or situations from which escape might be difficult or in which help may not be available in the event of having a panic attack.

The overall lifetime incidence of panic disorder is 3.5 percent in the United States; among women, the incidence is about 5 percent.[74] One-year prevalence rates are 1 to 2 percent. About one-third to one-half of patients with panic disorder also have agoraphobia.[24] Age of onset is generally between adolescence and the midthirties, although it can begin in childhood and, rarely, after age 45. The usual course is chronic, but symptom intensity can wax and wane with time. With treatment, about one-third of patients can achieve remission of their symptoms for long periods of time, one-third achieve some improvement in their symptoms, and the remaining third have chronic symptoms that sometimes get worse. Although a genetic factor is involved in the development of panic disorder, at least half of the patients do not have an affected first-degree relative.

There are no significant differences between men and women in panic symptoms noted at the onset of the disorder, in symptom severity, or in remission rates (about 40 percent).[74] The clinical course of the disorder, however, appears different. Women are more likely to have panic disorder with agoraphobia (85 versus 75 percent).[24] In contrast, men are more likely to have uncomplicated panic disorder (25 versus 15 percent).[74] In addition, of those who achieve remission, 25 percent of women and 15 percent of men reexperienced symptoms within 6 months. Also, recurrence of panic symptoms remains higher among women (82 versus 51 percent).[74]

Table 9-11

DSM-IV Criteria for Panic Disorder

A. Both (1) and (2):
  (1) Recurrent unexpected Panic Attacks
      A discrete period of intense fear or discomfort, in which four or more of the following symptoms developed abruptly and reached a peak within 10 min:
      a. Palpitations, pounding heart, or accelerated heart rate
      b. Sweating
      c. Trembling or shaking
      d. Sensations of shortness of breath or smothering
      e. Feeling of choking
      f. Chest pain or discomfort
      g. Nausea or abdominal distress
      h. Feeling dizzy, unsteady, lightheaded, or faint
      i. Derealization (feelings of unreality) or depersonalization (being detached from oneself)
      j. Fear of losing control or going crazy
      k. Fear of dying
      l. Paresthesias
      m. Chills or hot flushes
  (2) At least one of the attacks has been followed by 1 month or more of one or more of the following:
      a. Persistent concern about having additional attacks
      b. Worry about the implications of the attack or its consequences (e.g., losing control, having a heart attack, "going crazy")
      c. A significant change in behavior related to the attacks
B. The Panic Attacks are not due to the direct physiologic effects of a substance or a general medical condition.
C. The Panic Attacks are not better accounted for by another mental disorder, such as Social Phobia, Specific Phobia, Obsessive-Compulsive Disorder, Posttraumatic Stress Disorder, or Separation Anxiety Disorder.

SOURCE: Reproduced with permission from *Diagnostic and Statistical Manual of Mental Disorders*, 4th ed. Washington, DC, American Psychiatric Association, 1994.

SOCIAL PHOBIA

According to DSM-IV, the core definition of social phobia is a marked and persistent fear of social or performance situations in which embarrassment may occur (Table 9-12). Exposure to the feared social situation almost invariably provokes anxiety that can mimic a panic attack. One potentially distinguishing feature of the anxiety of social phobia is the presence of blushing during the episode. Other associated features include the recognition by the patient that the fear is excessive or unreasonable, the avoidance of feared social or performance situations, and the impaired occupational or social functioning that results.

The most common symptom is fear of public speaking.[24] Other performance fears such as eating, drinking, or writing in public or using a public restroom are less common.

Social phobia is estimated to occur in 3 to 13 percent of individuals (lifetime prevalence). As with panic disorder, women appear to be more frequently affected than men. Symptom onset typically occurs in adolescence. There appears to be an increased incidence of social phobia in first-degree relatives of those with the disorder. Stressful or humiliating childhood experiences can predispose to the development of this disorder. At other times, the onset can be more insidious. The duration of the disorder is generally thought to be lifelong.

Table 9-12

DSM-IV Criteria for Social Phobia

A. A marked and persistent fear of one or more social or performance situations in which the person is exposed to unfamiliar people or to possible scrutiny by other. The individual fears that he or she will act in a way that will be humiliating or embarrassing.

B. Exposure to the feared social situation almost invariably provokes anxiety, which may take the form of a situationally bound or situationally predisposed Panic Attack.

C. The person recognized that the fear is excessive or unreasonable.

D. The feared social or performance situations are avoided or else are endured with intense anxiety or distress.

E. The avoidance, anxious anticipation, or distress in the feared social or performance situations interferes significantly with the person's normal routine, occupational (or academic) functioning, or social activities or relationships, or there is marked distress about having the phobia.

F. The fear or avoidance is not due to the direct physiologic effects of a substance or a general medical condition and is not better accounted for by another mental disorder.

G. If a general medical condition or another mental disorder is present, the fear in Criterion A is unrelated to it, e.g., the fear is not of stuttering, trembling in Parkinson's disease, or exhibiting abnormal eating behavior in anorexia nervosa or bulimia nervosa.

SOURCE: Reproduced with permission from *Diagnostic and Statistical Manual of Mental Disorders*, 4th ed. Washington, DC, American Psychiatric Association, 1994.

POSTTRAUMATIC STRESS DISORDER

The diagnosis of posttraumatic stress disorder, according to the DSM-IV, is listed in Table 9-13. Although this diagnosis is often considered in the context of exposure to such situations as war or large-scale natural disasters, it can also apply to physical or sexual abuse, which is more common for women and children. Because abuse is often surrounded by shame and secrecy, the possibility of this diagnosis as an explanation for anxiety symptoms may be easily overlooked.

When considering the prevalence of posttraumatic stress disorder, it is useful to divide the population into an "at-large" group and an "at-risk" group. In the general population (the at-large group), posttraumatic stress disorder affects between 1 and 14 percent of all people. However, in groups of people who have been exposed to a severe traumatic event (the at-risk group), the potential prevalence rate rises to 58 percent.

Three personal characteristics are noted to be pertinent in *both* genders: preexisting anxiety disorder or major depressive disorder, a family history of anxiety disorder, and early separation from parents.[75] The severity and course of the disorder can be quite variable. Different symptom clusters can dominate the clinical presentation at different times. The symptoms can disappear spontaneously without treatment, or they can persist indefinitely. Various factors, such as the nature of the traumatic event itself (e.g., severity, duration, or temporal proximity), the presence or absence of social supports, childhood experiences, personality variables, and preexisting mental illness, can influence the course of the disorder.

Consistent with both of the major epidemiologic psychiatric studies, the ECA survey and the National Comorbidity Study, Breslau et al. found that the lifetime prevalence rate of posttraumatic stress disorder in women is about double that observed in men.[75] Interestingly, these prevalence rates are consistent in the face of approximately equal numbers of traumatic events in the lives of men and women. The widest difference in prevalence rates occurred in childhood age groups; girls experiencing traumatic events developed posttraumatic stress disorder significantly more frequently than boys, but after the age of 15, the prevalence rates became

Table 9-13

DSM-IV Criteria for Posttraumatic Stress Disorder

A. The person has been exposed to a traumatic event in which both of the following were present:
  (1) The person experienced, witnessed, or was confronted with an event or events that involved actual or threatened death or serious injury, or a threat to the physical integrity of self or others.
  (2) The person's response involved intense fear, helplessness, or horror.
B. The traumatic event is persistently reexperienced in one or more of the following ways:
  (1) Recurrent and intrusive distressing recollections of the event, including images, thoughts, or perceptions
  (2) Recurrent distressing dreams of the event
  (3) Acting or feeling as if the traumatic event were recurring
  (4) Intense psychological distress at exposure to internal or external cues that symbolize or resemble an aspect of the traumatic event
  (5) Physiologic reactivity on exposure to internal or external cues that symbolize or resemble an aspect of the traumatic event
C. Persistent avoidance of stimuli associated with the trauma and numbing of general responsiveness (not present before the trauma), as indicated by three or more of the following:
  (1) Efforts to avoid thoughts, feelings, or conversations associated with the trauma
  (2) Efforts to avoid activities, places, or people that arouse recollections of the trauma
  (3) Inability to recall an important aspect of the trauma
  (4) Markedly diminished interest or participation in significant activities
  (5) Feeling of detachment or estrangement from others
  (6) Restricted range of affect
  (7) Sense of a foreshortened future
D. Persistent symptoms of increased arousal (not present before the trauma), as indicated by two or more of the following:
  (1) Difficulty falling or staying asleep
  (2) Irritability or outbursts of anger
  (3) Difficulty concentrating
  (4) Hypervigilance
  (5) Exaggerated startle response
E. Duration of the disturbance (symptoms in Criteria B, C, and D) is more than 1 month.
F. The disturbance causes clinically significant distress or impairment in social, occupational, or other important areas of functioning.

SOURCE: Reproduced with permission from *Diagnostic and Statistical Manual of Mental Disorders*, 4th ed. Washington, DC, American Psychiatric Association, 1994.

similar. It is not clear, however, why this discrepancy in prevalence rates in childhood exists.

GENERALIZED ANXIETY DISORDER

The chief feature of generalized anxiety disorder, according to the DSM-IV, is excessive worry or anxiety more days than not about a number of events or activities, and the person so affected finds it difficult to control the worry (Table 9-14). A number of accompanying symptoms (e.g., restlessness, easy fatigue, insomnia, and irritability) are also necessary to make the diagnosis. The 1-year prevalence rate is about 3 percent and the lifetime rate is 5 percent.[28] Women are affected more frequently than men by a ratio of about 3:2. Generalized anxiety disorder frequently coexists with other anxiety and depressive disorders, such as panic disorder and dysthymia. The usual course of the disorder is chronic with waxing and waning symptoms.

OBSESSIVE-COMPULSIVE DISORDER

The diagnosis of this anxiety disorder depends on the presence of obsessions and compulsions (Table 9-15). Obsessions are recurring and persistent ideas, thoughts, images, or impulses that are experienced by the patient as intrusive and that cause marked anxiety or distress. The most common obsessions are about contamination, repeated doubts, a need to have things in a particular order, aggressive or horrific impulses, and sexual images. Compulsions are repetitive behaviors that are intended to reduce anxiety or distress. The most common compulsions are washing and cleaning, counting, checking, requesting or demanding assurances, repeating actions, and ordering. Patients with this disorder recognize that the obsessions or compulsions are either excessive or unreasonable. They also experience these symptoms with significant distress. Although there is no gender difference in prevalence or incidence rates, women tend to be afflicted later in life, with the onset most frequently in their twenties. Stress predictably worsens symptoms, although the overall course is generally waxing and waning. Once thought to be rare, obsessive-compulsive disorder is actually relatively common, affecting 2 to 3 percent of the population over their lifetimes; the 1-year prevalence rate is estimated to be 1 to 2 percent. Patients do not often volunteer the presence of these symptoms, and a high degree of suspicion must be maintained, coupled with direct questions during the interview to elicit an accurate history.

Treatment

PHARAMACOLOGIC APPROACHES

ANTIDEPRESSANTS As if to underscore the neurochemical and pathophysiologic overlap between anxiety and depressive disorders, antidepressant agents are also the mainstay of pharmacologic treatment of anxiety. The main classes of antidepressants (i.e., MAOIs, TCAs, and SSRIs) all have proven efficacy in the treatment of anxiety (see Table 9-8). Nearly all of the newer antidepressants (e.g., Effexor, Serzone, and Remeron) also have

Table 9-14

DSM-IV Criteria for Generalized Anxiety Disorder

A. Excessive anxiety and worry (apprehensive expectation), occurring more days than not for at least 6 months, about a number of events or activities such as work or school performance.

B. The person finds it difficult to control the worry.

C. The anxiety and worry are associated with three or more of the following six symptoms (with at least some symptoms present for more days than not for the past 6 months).
   (1) Restlessness or feeling keyed up or on edge
   (2) Being easily fatigued
   (3) Difficulty concentrating or mind going blank
   (4) Irritability
   (5) Muscle tension
   (6) Sleep disturbance

D. The anxiety, worry, or physical symptoms cause clinically significant distress or impairment in social, occupational, or other important areas of functioning.

E. The disturbance is not due to the direct physiologic effects of a substance or a general medical condition and does not occur exclusively during a Mood Disorder, a Psychotic Disorder, or a Pervasive Developmental Disorder.

SOURCE: Reproduced with permission from *Diagnostic and Statistical Manual of Mental Disorders*, 4th ed. Washington, DC, American Psychiatric Association, 1994.

Table 9-15

DSM-IV Criteria for Obsessive-Compulsive Disorder

A. Either obsession or compulsions:

Obsessions as defined by (1), (2), (3), or (4):

(1) Recurrent and persistent thoughts, impulses, or images that are experienced, at some time during the disturbance, as intrusive and inappropriate and that cause marked anxiety or distress.

(2) The thoughts, impulses, or images are not simply excessive worries about real-life problems.

(3) The person attempts to ignore or suppress such thoughts, impulses, or images, or to neutralize them with some other thought or action.

(4) The person recognizes that the obsessional thoughts, impulses, or images are a product of his or her own mind (not imposed from without as in thought insertions).

Compulsions as defined by (1) and (2):

(1) Repetitive behaviors (e.g., handwashing, ordering, checking) or mental acts (e.g., praying, counting, repeating words silently) that the person feels driven to perform in response to an obsession, or according to rules that must be applied rigidly.

(2) The behaviors or mental acts are aimed at preventing or reducing distress or preventing some dreaded event or situation; however, these behaviors or mental acts either are not connected in a realistic way with what they are designed to neutralize or prevent or are clearly excessive.

B. At some point during the course of the disorder, the person has recognized that the obsessions or compulsions are excessive or unreasonable.

C. The obsessions or compulsions cause marked distress, are time consuming (take > 1 h a day), or significantly interfere with the person's normal routine, occupational (or academic) functioning, or usual social activities or relationships.

D. The disturbance is not due to the direct physiologic effects of a substance or a general medical condition.

SOURCE: Reproduced with permission from *Diagnostic and Statistical Manual of Mental Disorders*, 4th ed. Washington, DC, American Psychiatric Association, 1994.

antianxiety properties. Wellbutrin is the single exception to this rule.

Selective Serotonin Reuptake Inhibitors. The SSRIs have demonstrated efficacy in treating most anxiety disorders, including panic disorder (with or without agoraphobia), posttraumatic stress disorder, social phobia, obsessive-compulsive disorder, and generalized anxiety disorder. One caveat in using SSRIs in patients with anxiety disorders is that smaller *starting* doses are generally better tolerated than the usual starting doses. Suggested initial doses are: fluoxetine (Prozac), 5 to 10 mg/d; sertraline (Zoloft), 25 to 50 mg/d; paroxetine (Paxil), 10 mg/d; fluvoxamine (Luvox), 25 mg/d; and citalopram (Celexa), 10 to 20 mg/d. An irony in treating anxiety disorders, however, is that it is not uncommon to eventually use *higher*

doses than antidepressant doses to control anxiety symptoms.

Tricyclic Antidepressants. The TCAs were the mainstay of therapy for anxiety disorders for many years until the advent of SSRIs. More research is available about the use of imipramine (Tofranil) in panic disorder than any other antidepressant, and it was long considered to be the gold standard for treating panic. These agents have largely been supplanted by the SSRIs because of the better safety and side-effect profiles of SSRIs. When used, TCAs are also initiated at low doses. In the case of imipramine, a starting dose of 10 mg/d is appropriate. This class of antidepressants is effective especially in patients with panic disorder but is also useful in those with generalized anxiety disorder and posttraumatic stress disorder.

Monoamine Oxidase Inhibitors. The MAOIs also have a role in the treatment in anxiety disorders. In fact, they are still without peer in the treatment of social phobia,[76] although SSRIs have some efficacy in this disorder as well. Unlike other antidepressants, however, these agents are rarely associated with any initial exacerbation of anxiety when beginning treatment. In addition to social phobia, they are useful in treating panic disorder and posttraumatic stress disorder. While the concern about hypertensive crisis is justified, these agents are probably underused in treating anxiety just as they are underused in depression.

Other Agents. The atypical antidepressants Effexor and Serzone both have shown effectiveness as well.[77,78] As is the case with the SSRIs, lower starting doses are likely to be better tolerated by the anxious patient. With Effexor, begin with 18.75 mg bid, and with Serzone, the starting dose is 50 mg bid. Remeron has shown some efficacy with anxiety, but experience is limited to date.

ANXIOLYTIC AGENTS

Benzodiazepines. Benzodiazepines have an important but limited role in the treatment of anxiety disorders. The use of the benzodiazepines is associated with both tolerance and withdrawal symptoms. Because of these problems, benzodiazepines should *not* be considered first-line agents in the treatment of anxiety disorders. Their use is best reserved for acute situations, especially panic attacks. In clinical practice, SSRIs are used to provide prophylaxis against chronic anxiety; the benzodiazepines are used in an adjunctive role. Chronic use of benzodiazepines is discouraged, especially in the elderly and in patients with any significant history of substance abuse.

Virtually all of the benzodiazepines are equally effective in treating anxiety disorders when used in equipotent doses (see Table 9-8). The higher-potency agents, alprazolam (Xanax) and clonazepam (Klonopin), are used more frequently for the treatment of panic disorder, although diazepam (Valium), too, has a long history of proven effectiveness. For the most part, selection of these agents depends on the best match of pharmacokinetic properties to the clinical situation. In treating an acute panic attack, for example, use of an agent with a rapid onset of action (e.g., lorazepam, clorazepate) would be preferable to an agent with a slower onset.

Benzodiazepines can adversely affect gait and balance in the elderly, resulting in a higher incidence of falls. Another concern is the depression that can be caused or aggravated by chronic and especially high-dose use of benzodiazepines. However, benzodiazepines can be especially useful, in moderate doses, in the early phases of treating an anxiety disorder, as the clinician and patient wait for the onset of action of the antidepressant.

Buspirone. Buspirone (Buspar), a nonbenzodiazepine anxiolytic, is another agent with proven efficacy in the treatment of anxiety disorders, although its usefulness is limited to generalized anxiety disorder.[79] Advantages of buspirone include the absence of tolerance and withdrawal symptoms. However, it has a long onset of action and full effects may take as long as 4 to 8 weeks to achieve. Buspirone has gained the reputation of not being particularly effective, but this inaccurate perception is likely related to its slow onset of effect as well as inadequate dosing. Doses of 30 to 60 mg/d are necessary in most patients to achieve beneficial clinical effects. For patients who are being treated with benzodiazepines chronically, it is helpful to add buspirone and gradually decrease and taper the benzodiazepine dose in an effort to wean these agents. Buspirone occupies an especially useful niche in the treatment of generalized anxiety disorder in the elderly and in patients with a significant history of substance abuse.

Other Agents. Other pharmacologic agents that have been used adjunctively in the treatment of anxiety include β-adrenergic blockers and anticonvulsants. The β-adrenergic blockers decrease autonomic arousal and can be useful for the somatic symptoms of panic and generalized anxiety disorder, but not as primary treatment. They can be especially helpful in social phobia of the performance anxiety subtype.[80] Somewhat surprisingly, anticonvulsants can have efficacy in the adjunctive treatment of anxiety. Both valproate (Depakote) and gabapentin (Neurontin) are used for the treatment of panic disorder, and gabapentin has been successfully used in treating social phobia.[81]

TREATMENT DURING PREGNANCY AND POSTPARTUM
Many benzodiazepines are known to cross the placenta; information is not available for all agents. These agents should be avoided in the first trimester because diazepam and clordiazepoxide have been reported to increase the risk of congenital malformation, and other agents may also increase risk. The use of benzodiazepines during the last weeks of pregnancy may cause neonatal CNS depression. Maternal administration just before or during labor may also cause neonatal flaccidity. In addition, chronic use of these medications during pregnancy may cause withdrawal symptoms in the infant after delivery.

In contrast, buspirone (Pregnancy Category B) is not known to have any adverse effects on pregnancy or labor and delivery. Information on antidepressant use in pregnancy can be found in the previous section of this chapter on depression in pregnancy.

A number of benzodiazepines are known to be excreted in breast milk, and it is expected that all of these agents would appear in breast milk. There is a possibility of pharmacologic effects in nursing infants (e.g., sedation, lethargy, poor feeding, weight loss). Neonates metabolize benzodiazepines more slowly than adults, and accumulation of drug is possible. Potential adverse effects to the infant are a concern especially if exposure is prolonged or in the case of high maternal doses. No problems in humans have been documented with buspirone use during lactation; it is not known, however, whether this agent is excreted in human milk.

NONPHARMACOLOGIC TREATMENTS

As in depression, nonpharmacologic treatments are also helpful. It is wise to use a comprehensive treatment strategy in treating anxiety disorders, with pharmacologic interventions accounting for only one dimension of available treatments. Various types of psychotherapy and especially cognitive-behavioral therapy can be highly effective. Graded exposure to the anxiety-producing circumstances is a core component of this type of therapy. Other components include the correction of cognitive misperceptions, breathing retraining, and muscle relaxation. Improvement in anxiety symptoms is reported to be better sustained when patients engage in cognitive-behavioral treatment, as compared to use of only pharmacologic treatment.[82]

Using relaxation techniques, engaging in regular exercise, and avoiding stimulants such as caffeine, diet pills, and decongestants are also important. It is also necessary to address the potential complication of substance abuse in these patients (see Chap. 8). Finally, combined pharmacologic and psychotherapeutic interventions appear to hold the most promise in sustaining remission of symptoms.

Summary

Anxiety and depressive disorders are complex, important conditions with significant and often underestimated morbidity and mortality. The causes of these conditions are many and varied, and it is crucial to search for all of the components of the etiologies of depression and anxiety. A significant pitfall in clinical practice is to not allot sufficient time to explore the subtleties involved in eliciting an accurate and complete history. All too often, histories of abuse, substance abuse, and psychological conflict or family history are missed, to the detriment of effective treatment. It is not easy in this age of managed care and shrinking appointment times to give these conditions the time needed for both diagnosis and treatment, but it is nevertheless critical to do so. It is also crucial to be ever mindful that these conditions do not easily resolve with pharmacologic interventions alone. The construction of a comprehensive treatment plan is mandatory and needs to consider all forms of therapy that might be helpful. Most patients can be successfully managed by a primary care provider. It is incumbent on that provider to consider all of the etiologic and treatment factors pertinent to the individual patient.

References

1. Shapiro A, Skinner EA, Kessler LG, et al: Utilization of health and mental health services:three Epidemiologic Catchment Area sites. *Arch Gen Psychiatry* 41:971, 1984.

2. Kessler RC, McGonagle KA, Zhao S, et al: Lifetime and 12-month prevalence of DSM-III-R psychiatric disorders in the United States:results from the National Comorbidity Survey. *Arch Gen Psychiatry* 51:8, 1994.

3. Bhatia SC, Bhatia SK: Depression in women: diagnostic and treatment considerations. *Am Fam Physician* 60:225, 1999.

4. Kornstein SG, Schatzberg AF, Yonkers KA, et al: Gender differences in presentation of chronic major depression. *Psychopharmacol Bull* 31:711, 1996.

5. Fava M, Abraham M, Alpert J, et al: Gender differences in Axis I comorbidity among depressed outpatients. *J Affect Disord* 38:129,1996.

6. Gotlib LA, Whiffen VE, Mount JH, et al: Prevalence and demographic characteristics associated with depression in pregnancy and the postpartum. *J Consult Clin Psychol* 57:260, 1989.

7. Endicott J: The menstrual cycle and mood disorders. *J Affect Disord* 29:193, 1993.

8. DeBattista C, Smith DL, Schatzberg A: Modulation of monoamine neurotransmitters by estrogen: clinical implications. In: Leibenluft E (ed): *Gender Differences in Mood and Anxiety Disorders.* Washington, DC: American Psychiatric Press; 1999.

9. Joffe RT, Levitt AJ: The thyroid and depression. In: Joffe RT, Levitt AJ (eds): *The Thyroid Axis and Psychiatric Illness.* Washington, DC: American Psychiatric Press; 1993;195.

10. Wirz-Justice A: Biological rhythms in mood disorders. In: Bloom FE, Kupfer DJ (eds): *Psychopharmacology: The Fourth Generation of Progress.* New York: Raven Press; 1995.

11. Hellekson C: Phenomenology of seasonal affective disorder: an Alaskan perspective. In: Rosenthal NE, Blehar MC (eds): *Seasonal Affective Disorders and Phototherapy.* New York: Guilford, 1989.

12. Gilligan C: *In a Different Voice.* Cambridge MA: Harvard University Press; 1982.

13. Pipher M: *Reviving Ophelia.* New York: Ballantine Books; 1994.

14. Kessler R, McGonagle K, Swartz M, et al: Sex and depression in the National Comorbidity Survey: I. lifetime prevalence, chronicity, and recurrence. *J Affect Disord* 29:85, 1993.

15. Blazer DG, George LK, Landerman R, et al: Psychiatric disorders: a rural/urban comparison. *Arch Gen Psychiatry* 42:651, 1985.

16. Regier DA, Boyd JH, Rae DS, et al: One-month prevalence of mental disorders in the US: based on five epidemiologic catchment area (ECA) sites. *Arch Gen Psychiatry* 45:977, 1988.

17. Lehtinen V, Joukamaa M: Epidemiology of depression: prevalence, risk factors and treatment situation. *Acta Psychiatr Scand* 89(suppl):7, 1994.

18. Morano HE: Debunking the marriage myth: it works for women too. *New York Times* August 4, 1998.

19. Kessler RC, McLeod JD: Sex differences in vulnerability to undesirable life events. *American Social Review* 49:620, 1984.

20. Rosenthal CJ, Sulman J, Marshall VX: Depressive symptoms in family caregivers of long-stay patients. *Gerontologist* 33:249, 1993.

21. McCormick LH: Depression in mothers of children with attention deficit hyperactivity disorder. *Fam Med* 27:176, 1995.

22. Tsuang MT, Faraone SV: The inheritance of mood disorders. In: Hall LL (ed): *Genetics and Mental Illness: Evolving Issues for Research and Society.* New York: Plenum Press; 1996;79.

23. Angold A: Child and adolescent depression: parts I and II. *Br J Psychiatry* 152:601, 1988.

24. American Psychiatric Association: *Diagnostic and Statistical Manual of Mental Disorders,* 4th ed. Washington, DC: Author; 1994;341.

25. Brems C: Women and depression: a comprehensive analysis. In: Beckham EE, Leber WR (eds): *Handbook of Depression,* 2nd ed. New York: Guilford; 1995;539.

26. Yonkers KA, Austin LS: Mood disorders: women and affective disorders. *Primary Psychiatry* 3:27, 1996.

27. Warner R, Appleby L, Whitton A, et al: Demographic and obstetric risk factors for postnatal psychiatric morbidity. *Br J Psychiatry* 168:607, 1996.

28. Koenig HG, Meador KG, Cohen HJ, et al: Self-rated depression scales and screening for major depression in the older hospitalized patient with medical illness. *J Am Geriatr Soc* 36:699, 1988.

29. Kramer-Ginsberg E, Greenwald B, Aisen P, et al: Hypochondriasis in the elderly depressed. *J Am Geriatr Soc* 35:507, 1989.

30. Beck AT, Ward C, Mendelson M, et al: An inventory for measuring depression. *Arch Gen Psychiatry* 4:561, 1961.

31. Carroll BJ, Fineberg M, Smouse PE, et al: The Carroll rating scale for depression: development, reliability, and validation. *Br J Psychiatry* 138:194, 1981.

32. Fischer J, Corcoran K: *Measures for Clinical Practice: A Source Book,* vol 2, 2nd ed. New York: Maxwell MacMillan; 1994:114.

33. Zung WW: A self-rating depression scale. *Arch Gen Psychiatry* 12:63, 1965.

34. Hamilton M: A rating scale for depression. *J Neurol Neurosurg Psychiatry* 23:51, 1960.

35. Harrison WM, Stewart JW: Pharmacotherapy of dysthymia. *Psychiatric Annals* 23:638, 1993.

36. Asnis GM, McGinn LK, Sanderson WC: Atypical depression: clinical aspects and noradrenergic function. *Am J Psychiatry* 152:31, 1995.

37. Nierenberg AA, Alpert JE, Pava J: Course and treatment of atypical depression. *J Clin Psychiatry* 59 (suppl 18):5, 1998.

38. Liebowitz M, Quitkin F, Stewart J, et al: Antidepressant specificity in atypical depression. *Arch Gen Psychiatry* 45:129, 1988

39. Pande AC, Birkett M, Fechner-Bates S, et al: Fluoxetine versus phenelzine in atypical depression. *Biol Psychiatry* 40:1017, 1996.

40. Winokur G: Manic-depressive disease (bipolar): is it autonomous? *Psychopathology* 28(suppl 1):51, 1995.

41. McElroy SL, Keck PE, Pope HG, et al: Clinical and research implications of the diagnosis of dysphoric or mixed mania or hypomania. *Am J Psychiatry* 149:1633, 1992.

42. Wehr TA, Goodwin FK: Can antidepressants cause mania and worsen the course of affective illness? *Am J Psychiatry* 144:1403, 1987.

43. Fava M, Anderson K, Rosenbaum JF: "Anger attacks": possible variants of panic and depressive disorders. *Am J Psychiatry* 147:867, 1990.

44. Lam R, Kripke D, Gillin J: Phototherapy for depressive disorders: a review. *Can J Psychiatry* 34:140, 1989.

45. Schwartz PJ, Brown C, Wehr TA, et al: Winter seasonal affective disorder: a follow-up study of the first 59 patients of the National Institute of mental Health Seasonal Studies Program. *Am J Psychiatry* 153:1028, 1996.

46. Dubovsky SL, Thomas M: Psychotic depression: advances in conceptualization and treatment. *Hospital and Community Psychiatry* 43:1189, 1992.

47. Miller LJ: Psychiatric disorders during pregnancy. In: Steward DE, Stotland NL (eds): *Psychological Aspects of Women's Health Care. The Interface Between Psychiatry and Obstetrics and Gynecology.* Washington, DC: American Psychiatric Press; 1993;55.

48. O'Hara MW: Social support, life events and depression during pregnancy and the puerperium. *Arch Gen Psychiatry* 43:569, 1986.

49. Steer RA, Scholl TO, Hediger ML, et al: Self-reported depression and negative pregnancy outcomes. *J Clin Epidemiol* 45:1093, 1992.

50. Garvey MJ, Tuason VB, Lumry AD, et al: Occurrence of depression in the postpartum state. *J Affect Disord* 5:97, 1983.

51. Martin CJ, Brown GW, Goldberg DP, et al: Psychosocial stress and puerperal depression. *J Affect Disord* 16:283, 1989.

52. Sichel D, Cohen L: Oestrogen and the prevention of severe postnatal mental illness. *Neuropsychopharmacology* 10:904S, 1994.

53. Harris B, Othman S, Davies JA, et al: Association between postpartum thyroid dysfunction and thyroid antibodies and depression. *BMJ* 305:152, 1992.

54. Asnis GM, Friedman TA, Sanderson WC, et al: Suicidal behaviors in adult psychiatric outpatients: I. Description and prevalence. *Am J Psychiatry* 150:108, 1993.

55. Petronis KR, Samuels JF, Moscicki EK, et al: An epidemiologic investigation of potential risk factors for suicide attempts. *Soc Psychiatry Psychiatr Epidemiol* 25:193, 1990.

56. Thase ME, Mallinger AG, McKnight D, et al: Treatment of imipramine-resistant recurrent depression: IV. A double-blind crossover study of tranylcypromine for anergic bipolar depression. *Am J Psychiatry* 149:195, 1992.

57. Segraves RT: Antidepressant-induced sexual dysfunction. *J Clin Psychiatry* 59(suppl 4):48, 1998.

58. Gitlin MJ: Treatment of sexual side effects with dopaminergic agents (letter). *J Clin Psychiatry* 56:124, 1995.

59. Jacobsen FM: Fluoxetine-induced sexual dysfunction and an open trial of yohimbine. *J Clin Psychiatry* 53:119, 1992.

60. Aizenberg D, Zemishlany Z, Weizman A: Cyproheptadine treatment of sexual dysfunction induced by serotonin reuptake inhibitors. *Clin Neuropharmacol* 18:320, 1995.

61. Cohen A J, Bartlik G: Ginkgo biloba for antidepressant-induced sexual dysfunction. *J Sex Marital Ther* 24:139, 1993.

62. Sussman N, Ginsberg D: Weight gain associated with SSRIs. *Primary Psychiatry* 5:28, 1998.

63. Coupland NJ, Bell CJ, Potokar JP: Serotonin reuptake inhibitor withdrawal. *J Clin Psychopharmacol* 16:356, 1996.

64. Black DW, Wesner R, Gabel J: The abrupt discontinuation of fluvoxamine in patients with panic disorder. *J Clin Psychiatry* 54:146, 1993.

65. Schatzberg AF, Haddad P, Kaplan E, et al: Possible biological mechanisms of the serotonin reuptake inhibitor discontinuation syndrome. *J Clin Psychiatry* 58(suppl 7):23, 1997.

66. Haarto-Truax N, Stern WC, Miller LL, et al: Effects of bupropion on body weight. *J Clin Psychiatry* 44(sec2):183, 1983.

67. Settle EC: Bupropion sustained release: side-effect profile. *J Clin Psychiatry* 59 (suppl 4):32, 1998.

68. Kelsey JE: Dose-response relationship with venlafaxine. *J Clin Psychopharmacol* 16(3 suppl 2):21S, 1996.

69. Crismon M, Triredi M, Pigott TA, et al: The Texas Medication Algorithm Project: report of the Texas Consensus Conference Panel on Medication Treatment of Major Depressive Disorder. *J Clin Psychiatry* 60:142, 1999.

70. Schneider LS, Small GW, Hamilton SH, et al: Estrogen replacement and response to fluoxetine in a multicenter geriatric depression trial (Fluoxetine Collaborative Study Group). *Am J Geriatr Psychiatry* 5:97, 1997.

71. Cohen LS, Rosenbaum JF: Psychotropic drug use during pregnancy: weighing the risks. *J Clin Psychiatry* 59(suppl 2):18, 1998.

72. Nulman I, Rovet J, Stewart DE, et al: Neurodevelopment of children exposed in utero to antidepressant drugs. *N Engl J Med* 336:258, 1997.

73. Clinical Practice Guideline #5. *Depression in Primary Care: Vol 1. Detection and Diagnosis.* Agency for Health Care Policy and Research, Publication No. 93-0550. Rockville, MD: U.S. Department of Health and Human Services; 1993, April.

74. Yonkers KA, Zlotnick C, Allsworth J, et al: Is the course of panic disorder the same in women and men? *Am J Psychiatry* 155:596, 1998.

75. Breslau N, Davis GC, Andreski P, et al: Sex differences in posttraumatic stress disorder. *Arch Gen Psychiatry* 54:1044,1997.

76. Liebowitz MR, Schneier F, Campeas R, et al: Phenelzine vs atenolol in social phobia: a placebo-controlled comparison. *Arch Gen Psychiatry* 49: 290, 1992.

77. Geracioti TD: Venlafaxine treatment of panic disorder: a case series. *J Clin Psychiatry* 56:408, 1995.

78. DeMartinis NA, Schweizer E, Rickels K: An open-label trial of nefazodone in high comorbidity panic disorder. *J Clin Psychiatry* 57:245, 1996.

79. Rickels K, Schweizer E, Csanalosi I, et al: Long-term treatment of anxiety and risk of withdrawal: prospective comparison of clorazepate and buspirone. *Arch Gen Psychiatry* 45:444, 1988.

80. Hartley LR, Ungapen S, Davie I, et al: The effect of beta adrenergic blocking drugs on speakers' performance and memory. *Br J Psychiatry* 142:512, 1983.

81. Ballenger JC, Davidson JR, Lecrubier Y, et al: Consensus statement on panic disorder from the International Consensus Group on Depression and Anxiety. *J Clin Psychiatry* 59(suppl 8):47, 1998.

82. Clark DM, Salkovskis PM, Hackmann A, et al: A comparison of cognitive therapy, applied relaxation therapy and imipramine in the treatment of panic disorder. *Br J Psychiatry* 164:759, 1994.

Jenny Speice
Audrey Farley
Susan McDaniel

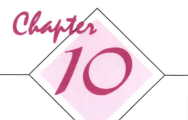

Relational Problems

Yolanda is a 43-year-old married woman with three children, two living at home. She presents at the office to follow up after an emergency room visit 6 days ago. Her symptoms in the emergency room were chest pain, shortness of breath, palpitations, a "funny feeling" in the back of her head, and dizziness. Her blood pressure in the emergency room was 205/106. She came to the office wondering if she is seriously ill; her blood pressure in the office is usually 120/80. Further questioning has revealed that her husband of 20 years is starting a new business and is less available to her emotionally and physically. This is especially stressful because her youngest son has been diagnosed with attention deficit-hyperactivity disorder and requires much energy and attention, both at home and at school.

Jean Baker Miller, a leading scholar on women and relationships, states that "women stay with, build on, and develop in a context of connections with others."[1] Women's most meaningful and significant relationships are with their partners, their parents, their children, and their friends. Within these relationships, women experience emotional intensity and opportunities for growth; these include the joys of connection and the pains of loss, abandonment, or abuse. As the case example above suggests, a key component of providing health care for women is the recognition of the importance of these relationships and their associated implications for women's health. It was virtually impossible to understand Yolanda and her health problems without understanding her connections to her husband and her son.

Most clinicians agree in theory that some psychosocial and relational information is useful with all patients. However, with increased time pressure and the push for shorter health care visits, it can be challenging to attend to all relevant aspects of a woman's biopsychosocial health in one brief encounter. In fact, if one is aware that a patient has a very complex and painful psychosocial history, it may seem less complicated to "stay clear" of opening up the

proverbial Pandora's box. In some ways it may appear easier to deal with the chief complaint and move on to the next examination room. However, in the context of continuity in the clinician-patient relationship, the assessment of a woman's relational health is a critical aspect of her care that is likely to enhance care over time. We propose that assessment of, and intervention to improve, a woman's relational health will lead to improved overall health status and better outcomes for the patient, as well as a more satisfying clinician-patient relationship.

As with any health or illness assessment, the relational context must always be considered within the larger sociocultural context. A woman's decisions about relationships are heavily influenced by gender roles, racial/ethnic identity, socioeconomic status, affectual and sexual orientation, geographical region, and community setting (urban, rural, suburban); what a woman reports to the clinician may be influenced by the sociocultural and power dynamics of the medical encounter. To conduct an accurate relational assessment, clinicians must remain aware of their own relationship experiences and expectations (with parents, partners, siblings, children, and close friends) and prevent the unwanted imposition of one's own values on patients and their families.

Research on Relationships and Health

For each patient who arrives for an appointment, a network of relationships has influenced her beliefs, values, and behaviors about her health. Some may enhance her health and others may be detrimental to her health. Studies have demonstrated links between patients' relationships with family members and their recovery from medical crises, management of chronic disease, and the prevention of illness.[2,3] Studies have also shown linkages between women's overall health and their relationships. For example, women in better health report fewer concerns about their roles as wives, mothers, and employees compared to less healthy women.[4]

Social Support

The literature on social support generally suggests that people who perceive that they have higher positive social support have better health, whereas people who perceive themselves as isolated are at increased risk for health problems.[5–7] For example, higher social support during pregnancy has been demonstrated to improve labor and delivery and postpartum outcomes for the mother and child, and lower social support appears to be associated with increased heart disease and mortality for bereaved widows.[8,9]

Partner Support

The importance of partner support is noted in a study by Ross et al.[10] In this study, employed women who experienced child care difficulties without the support of their husbands reported increased distress. In general, married couples are at an advantage compared to their unmarried counterparts.[11] However, negative aspects of the marital relationship, such as a wife's perception of conflict or hostility, are directly associated with reported symptoms of chronic fatigue and immune dysfunction syndrome[12] and negative immunologic changes.[13] The literature also identifies complexities in women's relationships with their husbands, and some scholars suggest that social support has less of a positive effect on women's health than on men's health because of the differences in emotional and instrumental support needs and contributions of women and men.[4,14] In addition, women report more relationship stressors than men,[14] and O'Leary and Helgeson[4] suggest that these relational stressors as well as financial difficulties may interfere with health care compliance.

Family and Work

Data about the impact of children on maternal health is mixed. Some studies suggest that parenthood may not improve health because of the depletion of economic and emotional resources from the marital couple and may actually increase psychological distress including maternal depression.[10] Women's health is clearly influenced by socioeconomic status,[15] and, although the balance of work and family benefits some women, others find that the pressures and strain result in psychosocial distress and increased physical symptoms.[16]

Abusive Relationships

Women who have experienced childhood or adult sexual abuse or other victimization report more medical complaints.[17,18] In particular, these women report more respiratory, gastrointestinal, musculoskeletal, neurologic, and gynecologic symptoms[19,21] than patients without abuse histories. These issues are discussed in greater detail in Chap. 7.

Women's relational and physical health are closely linked, but more research is needed to understand these complex interactions and the results of interventions aimed at reducing women's relational distress. In addition, more information is needed about the influence of relationships on health for lesbian women, racial/ethnic minority women, and poor women. Much of the research to date has focused on white, heterosexual, middle-class women. Several authors have proposed conceptual models and related research support for understanding women's relationships, family relationships, and health. These resources are listed at the end of the chapter.

Relational Health Assessment

Women's lives are increasingly more complex; time pressure while juggling multiple demands can be emotionally and physically draining. For women with chronic medical or mental conditions, relational distress may exacerbate symptoms or create barriers to adherence with treatment regimens.

These added stressors are against the background of the continual family transitions that shift relationships, bringing possibilities for forming new relationships and re-creating old ones—partnering and marriage, childbirth, parenting adolescents and launching young adults, caregiving for parents, and other life events.[21] Even the healthiest of families experience difficulties adjusting to the new ways of relating with each other during these transitions.

Many women turn to their primary health care clinicians to seek relief for overt psychosocial distress or for somatic complaints related to unsuccessful coping mechanisms. Health care professionals should understand the significance of relationships and life transitions to the health of patients. Although time pressures make it difficult to fully assess the complexities within a patient's family relationships, this information is critical in caring for women. A woman's relationships may sustain her through new diagnoses and illness recurrences and encourage her to be more vigilant in preventive health care behaviors. The health of these relationships sometimes "holds the key" to unlocking the mysteries of challenging or frustrating patients, patients with multiple vague somatic complaints that can never be adequately treated, and patients whose pain never seems to go away.

Gathering Relational Health Information in the Office

INITIAL ENCOUNTER

The usual informal greetings to patients and their family members often prompt the sharing of important psychosocial information. "How are you doing with the kids?" is all the invitation some patients need to start a lengthy explanation of the daily struggles or satisfactions they are experiencing. However, others may respond with a brief response, "fine" or "okay." Unless the patient reveals more through vocal tone, facial expression, or other nonverbal cues, the distress behind her short answer may go unexplored.

Many clinicians develop a repertoire of relationally-oriented questions to weave into their greeting at the beginning of visits or during the physical examination. (It is best not to wait until the close of the visit to avoid an "oh, by the way, my partner left me" bombshell.) Some of these questions might include "How are things at home?" or "Who else knows about your pain (or presenting complaint today) and what does he or she think might be the cause?" or "Who helps you deal with your illness?" or "Last visit you mentioned you were having problems with (significant relationship). Are things better or worse now?" To obtain a more specific response, a scaling question may provide more information: "On a scale of 1 to 10, how are things in your relationship with your partner right now?"[22–24] When relational problems are an issue, a graph for these numbers or brief note in the chart serves as a cue for follow-up on future visits to determine improvement or deterioration for the patient or family and to decide when intervention might be helpful. Additional questions are recommended in Appendix A.

SCREENING TOOLS

Some clinicians find it helpful to use established screening tools. Two that have been developed for family-oriented clinicians are the Family APGAR (an assessment of family satisfaction/functioning) and the GARF or Global Assessment of Relational Functioning (a tool to assess the domains of problem-solving, organization, and emotional climate). More information is included in Appendix B. All clinicians should routinely screen for domestic violence (see Chap. 7).

Some clinicians who think about a patient in the context of her relationships argue that screening tools are no substitute for good clinical interviewing skills, a high index of suspicion, and a brief overview of the patient's significant relationships. One method for organizing a patient's relationship network is the genogram.[25]

GENOGRAMS

A genogram is a useful framework to quickly gather relevant information regarding family members, emotional relationships, and significant family events (e.g., births, deaths, marriages, abuse).[25] It is surprisingly common to find previously unrecorded information regarding death of children, siblings, or parents; history of sexual abuse; family history of alcoholism; or children living somewhere other than with parents all in the few minutes it takes to sketch a genogram with a patient. Genograms frequently shed new light on a patient's insomnia, fatigue, headaches, body aches, or other complaints that are present despite a normal physical examination.

The genogram consists of symbols indicating female/male and lines indicating types and quality of relationships. For example, a genogram as in Fig. 10-1 would demonstrate that Olivia was previously married to a man who physically abused her and her son; her current household includes her second husband whom she married in 1990, her son

from the previous marriage, and her two daughters with her current husband. From this genogram, a clinician would be aware of the patient's potential concerns or risks for breast cancer and alcoholism; also, the clinician would inquire about any abuse in her current relationship due to Olivia's past abusive marriage. This genogram took 2 min but produced critical information that may not have come up in a biomedical focused history.

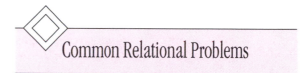

Common Relational Problems

Although each problem that a woman might experience in her significant relationships is unique to the circumstances of the particular patient, there

Figure 10-1

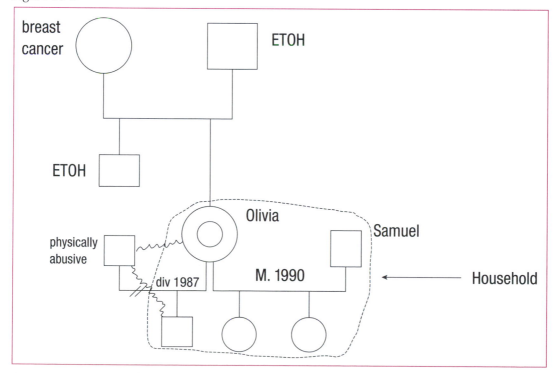

Genogram.

are a few common challenges that women often experience in their relationships with their parents, partners, and children. We summarize these common problems as well as more serious problems that may require crisis intervention or longer-term treatment.

Problems with Parents

Many patients experience strong positive connections with their parents in adulthood. Others find these relationships to be full of conflict or avoidance. Sometimes adult relationships with parents go smoothly until a parent's health crisis or family event.

CONFLICT

Katherine is a 46-year-old divorced woman who presents for routine gynecologic care. She has a history of migraine headaches. She has had increasingly severe headaches over the past few weeks. Further questioning reveals that, in the next month, she plans to travel to her home state to spend several weeks with her parents in preparation of their 50th wedding anniversary. In the presence of her parents, she always feels inadequate and criticized. Her nurse practitioner points out the likely relationship between her anxiety about the upcoming trip and her worsening migraines. A discussion ensues about her options including shortening the duration of the trip, taking a friend or another family member, and planning for conflict and relaxation techniques. Migraine abortive treatment and prophylaxis is discussed.

Similar to Katherine, many patients present with an interplay of biomedical complaints and relational stressors. In this case, her nurse practitioner routinely inquires about relational health and becomes aware of the possible links between Katherine's upcoming trip and exacerbated headaches. With this information, the nurse practitioner can help the patient to prepare for the family visit while attending to the biomedical treatment.

Relatively healthy families strive to balance the needs for separation and connectedness. At times this becomes a challenge when a woman is "sandwiched" between caring for her parents and her children.

CAREGIVING

Ida is scheduled for a mole removal; however, at the start of the visit, she requests time to talk about stressful caregiving issues instead. She is a 37-year-old woman who is one of three children of divorced parents. Ida is married and has two young children. Her siblings are pressuring her to have their father move in with her so she can take care of him. Her father has debilitating arthritis and chronic heart disease. Ida is very concerned about the demands that this would put on her personally and on her marriage and children. She has multiple chronic medical problems and a history of depression. However, she feels guilty for not taking care of her father because she feels that she is the one who relates best with him. Ida seemed to benefit from a 15-min discussion about balancing her own health and emotional and family needs with those of her father. She decided to convene a family meeting with her siblings and father to discuss how each member would contribute to their father's care.

Caregiving is often stressful. One family member may feel overburdened with caregiving tasks. Ida needed support from the health care professional to make decisions, to rally other caregiving resources and respite services, and to deal with the complicated emotional reactions of caring for an ailing parent.

DEATH OF A PARENT

Lenore is a 67-year-old married woman who assumed the primary caregiver role for her mother 3 years ago, after her mother's stroke.

Her mother died 16 months ago and Lenore presents frequently to her internist with concerns about her rising blood pressure and "pressure in her head." Her husband is worried about her chronic fatigue and irritability and her increasing complaints of headaches, back pain, and stomach trouble. She is wondering if there is a pill that she can take to give her more energy. When asked about her daily functioning, Lenore responds that she hasn't had much focus since her mother died and wonders how others find the strength to go on after the loss of a parent. She agrees to a referral for counseling and over the course of the next several months demonstrates improved mood and energy level as well as a reduction in physician visits and somatic complaints. In counseling, Lenore is able to create some rituals to memorialize her mother's life and decides to volunteer at a bereavement group at her church to help others who have recently experienced a loss.

When a parent dies, an adult child may experience a complex range of emotional reactions from intense sadness and grief, and feeling abandoned as an "orphan," to relief (and perhaps guilt) from the burden of caregiving demands. Many patients with acute grief reactions can find support in their family relationships, religious communities, or friendship circles. For most, it takes a full year of experiencing holidays, birthdays, anniversaries, and other celebrations without the loved one to feel some lessening of the grief. Others get "stuck" in the bereavement process and require more intensive psychotherapeutic treatment and occasionally psychotropic medication.

ABUSE AND NEGLECT

Ellen is a 37-year-old woman who has been married and divorced three times and has a history of unsatisfying relationships with men. She faithfully attends her annual gynecologic examination and is eager to talk about how she can change her patterns with men. Each year, however, it seems that she hasn't made

any progress toward positive change. Occasionally she mentions a strained relationship with her alcoholic father, because of his emotional distance and the verbal abuse that occurred during her childhood. At her most recent appointment, she tearfully remarked that her father was recently diagnosed with end-stage liver disease; she surprised herself by being so emotional at the news. This experience provided the needed impetus for her to accept a referral for psychotherapy to address the childhood pain and its connections with her current relationship patterns.

Sometimes the pain from a history of childhood abuse or neglect, or growing up in an alcoholic family, has so seriously impaired a relationship with one's parent that even geographical distance or years apart does not heal the emotional scars. These patients and families often require intensive psychotherapy to address and heal old wounds.

Several questions can provide an opening to discuss a patient's relationships with her parents. Answers to these questions may suggest satisfying relationships or point to underlying conflict or dissatisfaction that may benefit from supportive counseling, a referral for brief therapy, or intensive psychotherapy. Assessing sibling relationships may also be important because they are often part of the fabric of the patient's relationship to her parents. Questions that can be used to assess a patient's relationship with her parents are listed in Appendix A.

Problems with Partners

A relationship with a spouse or partner can be the most intimate and secure relationship in a woman's life. Others find their marital or committed relationship to be a source of ongoing strain and tension, with serious physical and emotional health consequences. Even the healthiest of partner relationships experience ups and downs and challenges to the commitment once made. With the current high divorce rate, some question the wisdom of attempting a committed relationship; others, by choice or circumstance, remain single.

People in healthy partnerships are able to communicate directly with each other, share power and decision-making, resolve conflicts, negotiate roles and responsibilities, and maintain a satisfying sexual relationship. The individuals respect each other and maintain a good balance of personal autonomy and connection with one another. In the face of family, work, or health stressors, the couple is able to adjust and adapt to new demands without significant impairment to the relationship or either individual.

Those who experience more difficulties in couple relationships struggle with conflict about power, decisions, roles, and responsibilities and have less satisfaction about most aspects of the relationship including sex. Sometimes these tensions are not overt and surface during a family, work, or health crisis. Women in these relationships often struggle with a low sense of self-esteem and lack of autonomy; they may experience somatic distress, depression, and anxiety.

CONFLICT

Gloria is a 78-year-old married woman who made an appointment for follow-up after a health fair screening. The test results were normal. She brings up an additional concern about leg cramps at night. When it appears that the visit is nearly over, she asks if she may take her Buspar more often than prescribed. On further questioning, she pours out her story of frustration. Her husband is in poor health and she finds him demanding and manipulative, using his health as a reason for her to be available to him at all times. She needs time for herself, "room to breathe," but feels guilty that she wants to leave him occasionally. Gloria is reluctant to ask her husband to go to marital counseling. She agrees to regular visits with her nurse practitioner for supportive counseling. Over the next 4 months it becomes clear that Gloria is concerned about repeating caregiving patterns that she witnessed in her parents' relationship. She begins to talk more openly with her husband about her concerns and invites him to attend several appointments with her nurse practitioner.

In Gloria's case, the marital dissatisfaction was able to be addressed over time with primary care counseling and a few couples' sessions with her husband. For other women, the relationship is more acutely strained and requires more urgent and intensive treatment with particular attention to safety issues, as in the case of Camille.

ABUSE

Camille is a 24-year-old married woman with two young toddlers who presents with headaches and tension in her neck and complains about her "nerves." Further direct questioning reveals that when she and her husband get into arguments, particularly after he's been drinking, he occasionally becomes physically threatening and has struck her in the past. She recently received a positive pregnancy test result. She wanted to continue the pregnancy but was unable to tell her husband because he was clear that he didn't want any more "noise" around the house and had been verbally abusive about her weight gain with her other two pregnancies. Recognizing the increased risk for abuse, her physician informs Camille of community resources for counseling and support to help her with determining her desires and plans. Also, her physician helps Camille brainstorm ways to tell her husband about the pregnancy and addresses possible safety plans, if needed.

Some couple relationships are seriously impaired by chronic unresolved marital conflict, alcohol or other substance abuse, or physical, verbal, sexual, or emotional abuse. Women in these relationships need assistance in seeking safety, support for decisions about staying in the relationship, and a long-term consistent, nonjudgmental presence by a caring clinician. Change in these abusive relationships often happens slowly. Many women in these situations are reluctant to seek psychotherapeutic services because of fears of disclosure, feelings of shame or self-blame, or ambivalence about the relationship, and the plan for making such a referral needs to be long-term and involve close collaboration with the psychotherapist. (See Chap. 7 for additional information.)

INFIDELITY

Emily is a 42-year-old woman who has been living with her partner, Abby, for 14 years. She was seen over the course of several months for complaints including weight gain, headaches, anxiety, and low-level depression. Her home situation recently became stressful because she and Abby had taken in a housemate and this has resulted in increasing conflict. Abby tended to side with the housemate and accused Emily of being too defensive and angry. At her next visit, Emily discloses that her suspicions about Abby and this housemate having an affair proved true when she found them in bed together. Emily was devastated and uncertain about the future of the relationship. She accepts a referral for psychotherapy and eventually Abby joined her for several sessions of couples therapy. They decide to end the relationship. Emily's depression and anxiety decrease over the next 8 months.

When women experience a crisis such as a partner's infidelity, the connections between the acute stressors and somatic complaints are often obvious for these patients. Some are willing to seek brief psychotherapy to address the crisis situation and are able to repair the damage to the relationship or make a decision to separate, and the somatic complaints are lessened or resolved.

Several questions (listed in Appendix A) can provide an opening to discuss and assess a patient's relationships with her spouse or partner. For patients who have been married or previously in a committed relationship, these questions may help determine patterns or unresolved concerns from former relationships.

Problems with Children

Parenting is one of the most significant and demanding of all life roles. Parents experience a roller coaster ride of immense joy, intense fear, outbursts of anger, and a mixture of pride and disappointment throughout their children's lives. With a majority of women working outside the home, balancing the pressures of work and family life and maintaining enough stamina for the boundless energy of children can be a daunting task. Parents rely on a repertoire of skills that they learned from their own parents and other parental models they have admired, trying to avoid those they disdained. Even so, much of the work of parenting is "feeling one's way" through what seems like uncharted territory.

In most families, women are responsible for the majority of daily parental tasks. Although some parents create more equitable role sharing, in general, mothers are more likely to attend a school meeting or a doctor's visit or to adjust a work schedule to be home with a sick child than fathers. Because of this, they may experience role strain and suffer from emotional distress, fatigue, and other somatic symptoms.

As children age, parents face new challenges. A child's first day at school, first overnight stay away from home, and leaving for summer camp can be transitions that provoke anxiety for parents of young children. When preadolescence appears on the horizon, parents hope that they have prepared their children for exposure to peer pressure, drugs, and sexual experiences. Parents anxiously await the return of their children from dates, driving the family car, and parties with friends. In healthy families, parents and children build strong relationships of support and caring while maintaining firm, clear guidelines and instilling important values for themselves and others. These families enter transitional experiences with a history of consistent love and nurturance and the ability to be flexible in adapting to new phases. These parents encourage children to explore and learn autonomy with the certainty of remaining securely connected to their family. When the inevitable conflicts arise around schoolwork, friends, clothing, or other preferences, parents and children who have healthy relationships can navigate these differences without serious long-term consequences.

CONFLICT

Shavonne is a 41-year-old married woman with three teenagers. She has always been involved with her children, paying attention to their friends and activities. She home-schooled her youngest daughter, concerned about the crowd that she was a part of at school. One day she called her family physician in great distress because her daughter Lakisha's menses was late and she just found out that Lakisha was sexually active. Her alarm brought out reactions that surprised her and she needed help dealing with the situation. A 20-min counseling session with mother and daughter opened communication between them and resulted in birth control pills for Lakisha, who was not pregnant.

Most parents at some time seek the support of a trusted friend, clergy person, or physician for advice or guidance during particularly challenging times. As with Shavonne and Lakisha, sometimes a primary care clinician offers a neutral territory and careful facilitation to help parents and children navigate through transitional conflicts.

ACUTE CRISES

Margareta is a 50-year-old married woman who presents with chest pain. After a thorough review of systems, physical examination, and electrocardiogram, there is no clear biomedical diagnosis for her pain. Further questioning reveals that her 16-year-old daughter ran away from home with a boyfriend, to Mexico, 2 weeks earlier, and Margareta hasn't heard anything from her since.

Her nurse practitioner helps Margareta with the local youth emergency services and offers more frequent visits, which Margareta declines. The nurse practitioner also contacts the school counselor, with Margareta's permission, to help assess the crisis situation. One month later, Margareta reports that her daughter has returned. She has had no further chest pain.

Occasionally a child or adolescent's acting-out behaviors push the limits of parental and social tolerance. Early teen pregnancy, truancy, failure or dropping out of school, running away, drug abuse, stealing, or assault or other criminal behaviors can be indicators that the individual child, the parents, and the family may require professional help to resolve the crisis and underlying concerns. At times, an acute crisis triggers somatic complaints that remit when the situation is resolved.

ABUSE AND NEGLECT

Rachel, a 19-year-old single mother of three, is seen for HIV/STD testing. She brought her infant daughter to the appointment with her because she did not have child care. In an attempt to quiet her crying daughter in the exam room, she shook her roughly. On questioning about her discipline strategies at home, Rachel admits that sometimes she "loses it" and has, on occasion, been forceful with her children to "teach them a lesson." Her two older children are often sent to stay with her mother to "get a break." Rachel describes being beaten with a belt as a child but denies "abusing" her own children. She reports that her current boyfriend occasionally hits them too hard when he's been drinking and that this has sometimes scared her. She said that a child protective worker visited her home a few weeks ago, but she hasn't heard anything since. She agrees that she may benefit from in-home services to learn other ways of disciplining her children and prevent having them placed outside the home. Her physician refers Rachel and her children to a family therapist who practices in the same office. An appointment is scheduled for the next day, and the physician briefly joins the therapy session to initiate collaboration between all parties.

Some parents struggle with a lack of emotional or physical resources to provide for their children. They are too overwhelmed with their own alcohol or other substance abuse, or emotional instability, to meet their children's needs in a consistent way. Some parents need the support of extended family and community resources to care for their children through foster care or in-home services that monitor safety and ensure protection of children. These families require intensive mental health intervention as well.

Several questions can provide an opening to discuss and assess a patient's relationships with her children (see Appendix A). The answers to these questions may reveal a need for additional parenting skills, support from her partner, or self-care skills to manage the multiple demands in her life. They may also reveal more serious concerns requiring collaboration with mental health, school, and legal professionals. It is important to involve the patient's partner in the assessment of child concerns. It is best to invite the partner to the visit to ask the questions with both present. If that is not possible, ask the patient how her partner might answer the questions.

Treatment

Once an assessment reveals that a patient is experiencing relational distress, the clinician must determine whether the appropriate intervention is within his or her skill level and practice time constraints, or whether a referral for family, couple, or individual psychotherapy is needed. In addition to relational distress, occasionally patients suffer from severe mental illness and intensive psychiatric care is indicated. A skilled mental health colleague can assist with the evaluation and referral process.

Psychotropic medications, when appropriate, can be a useful adjunct to supportive counseling or psychotherapy (see Chap. 9). Treatment decisions can be facilitated by identifying what the patient has tried in the past to resolve the conflict and whether it was helpful or not in reducing her distress.

Empathic Listening/Supportive Counseling in the Office

Kimberly is a 36-year-old married woman who experienced a miscarriage several years ago before transferring care. She and her husband are now considering another pregnancy. Her husband is discouraging another attempt because of how hard the miscarriage was on Kimberly last time. She acknowledges the concerns but is determined to try again. This issue is creating significant tension for this couple who otherwise have been able to work through other conflicts. Kimberly and her husband agree to come for several appointments to discuss the medical and relational aspects of this situation. After four visits, Kimberly and her husband state that they better understand each other's concerns and agree they both are ready to attempt another pregnancy.

Many physicians, nurse practitioners, and other health care clinicians manage patients' relational problems with supportive counseling during routine appointments.[26,27] Several common relational disorders appropriate for primary care counseling are presented in Table 10-1. Clinicians need a general overview of the relationship patterns, strengths, and challenges to provide brief primary care counseling for these relational problems. Assessment and intervention can occur during routine visits conducted over a period of weeks or months, depending on the acuity of the situation.

Components of a thorough assessment and areas to assess related to the family process are listed in Table 10-2. Good indicators for primary care counseling include a motivated couple or family with a history of a good relationship, a spe-

Table 10-1

Relational Disorders Commonly Seen
in Primary Care Counseling

- Adjustment to the diagnosis of a new illness
- Adjustment to a change in functioning or prognosis in a chronic illness (such as entering the terminal phase)
- Adjustment to caregiving for a parent
- New onset of child behavior problems
- New onset of marital problems
- New onset of problems with an aging parent
- New onset of workplace problems
- Uncomplicated grief reactions

SOURCE: Adapted from McDaniel SH, DeGruy FV: Relational disorders in primary care medicine. In Kaslow F (ed): *Handbook on Relational Disorders.* New York: Wiley; 1996;132.[27]

Table 10-2

Relational Assessment for the Primary Care Clinician

Components of a thorough relational assessment:

1. Information about the presenting problem (a detailed description, and what seems to make the problem better or worse)
2. Roles that each person plays with regard to this situation
3. Solutions that the patient/family have already attempted
4. Patient and family strengths
5. Support resources that the patient/family can access
6. The family process of communication and problem solving

Areas to assess related to the family process:

1. Do family members seem overinvolved or too detached?
2. Do family members talk directly with each other or focus on another person?
3. Are there unresolved issues from the past that seem to get in the way?
4. What are the important development/life cycle tasks for the family right now?

SOURCE: Adapted from McDaniel SH, Campbell TL, Seaburn DB: *Family-Oriented Primary Care: A Manual for Medical Providers.* New York: Springer-Verlag; 1990.[26]

cific situational problem of recent onset, and a clinician with appropriate time and skill.[26] Family therapists are good resources for consultation and referral for more intensive treatment.

It is common for clinicians to feel reluctant to invite family members for medical visits or primary care counseling due to time constraints or worry about the complexity of their complaints. Clinicians who routinely involve family members in new patient visits, maternity care, delivery of new diagnoses, or preparing for the death of a loved one have often developed the skills necessary for establishing rapport with family members, inviting multiple perspectives, and sharing information with more than one person in the room. These basic skills form the foundation for primary care couples or family counseling that allow a clinician to facilitate communication, reduce emotional reactivity among family members, and work toward conflict resolution.

Any counseling relationship should begin with a clear agreement as to the number (four to six), length (25 to 45 min), and frequency (weekly, monthly, etc.) of visits, as well as a plan for the changes that are desired and a specified way to evaluate progress.[26] McDaniel et al.[26] give the following recommendations for building strong alliances with couples/family members: (1) do not

talk about a person who is not present; (2) establish rapport with each person present; (3) validate each person's perception as important to him or her; and (4) do not agree to keep harmful secrets. Hahn[28] states that a key component of working with families is "empathic witnessing," which is accomplished by acknowledging that you have listened to their stories, seen what they cope with, and are impressed with their resilience, despite the challenges.

Sometimes, relational problems that are initially treated with primary care counseling are not resolved or require additional intensive psychotherapy beyond what the primary care clinician can offer. A referral to a family therapist is appropriate for these cases. Relational problems that are more severe or involve multiple family problems may benefit from an immediate referral to a family therapist or other mental health specialist who is trained to deal with the specific concerns (Table 10-3).

Referral for Family Therapy

Billie Jo is a 43-year-old woman with complaints of anorexia, weight loss, fatigue, decreased libido, and sleep problems. Her periods have been irregular over the past year and she complains of recent pelvic pain. She denies any current stressors. The nurse practitioner performs a workup to rule out occult malignancy, including a complete physical, mammogram, and laboratory tests. At this first visit, her nurse practitioner also mentions the possibility of depression. At Billie Jo's second visit, she is told about her normal test results. On repeat questioning about life stressors, she mentions concerns about her 13-year-old daughter's "reckless" behavior and fears that her daughter is drinking alcohol, sexually active, and "hanging" with the wrong crowd. Billie Jo said her husband downplays her worries, saying that Billie Jo is overreacting and their daughter is just "being a teenager." When asked about her own teenage years, Billie Jo tearfully and hesitantly

Table 10-3

Relational Disorders Commonly Referred from a Primary Care Provider to a Mental Health Specialist

- Sexual or physical abuse
- Homicidal ideation
- Moderate to severe marital and sexual problems
- Multiproblem family situations
- Families coping with serious mental illness
- Substance abuse
- Psychosis

Source: Reprinted from McDaniel SH, DeGruy FV: Relational disorders in primary care medicine. In: Kaslow F (ed). *Handbook on Relational Disorders*. New York: Wiley; 1996;132.[27]

discloses that she had been gang raped but hadn't told anyone about this until now. After several weekly sessions with her primary care physician, this patient accepts a referral for individual psychotherapy to deal with the rape trauma. Despite initial reluctance, Billie Jo and her husband eventually start family sessions with the therapist to address the transition to adolescence and to respond to their daughter's acting-out behaviors.

Making a successful referral to a mental health specialist is an art form. It requires understanding what motivates the patient and the family and communicating confidence in the therapist. A few important guidelines follow here and in Table 10-4. For additional recommendations, consult *Family-Oriented Primary Care: A Manual for Medical Providers.*[26]

After identifying the need for referral, select a family-oriented therapist who is communicative and collaborative in treating the patient or family. Then, discuss with the mental health specialist the patient's individual and relational concerns, your consultation question(s), and the history of caring for the patient. Because mental health professionals often have different practice styles than their medical and nursing colleagues, discuss the expectations that each of you have for communication, treatment decisions, and disclosure of information to all parties. Some relationally trained therapists are willing to come to a medical visit to facilitate the introduction and transition of care for patients or family members who are reluctant to see a therapist.

If the patient requests a referral to a mental health clinician, encourage the patient's initiative and state your interest in collaborating with the treating mental health specialist to provide the best integrated care. Also encourage the family members to become involved in the treatment as appropriate; support the patient's abilities to incorporate her family members and close friends if you do not have a direct relationship with them.

For patients who are hesitant or resistant to seeing a mental health therapist, continue to discuss the importance of the treatment as well as any barriers to following through on the referral. Some-

Table 10-4

The Do's and Don'ts of Referral to Mental Health Specialists

A. The Do's
  1. Clarify the consultation or referral question.
  2. Refer to someone you know and trust whenever possible.
  3. Consult with the intended therapist as early as possible.
  4. Work to maximize the patient's motivation to use the referral in a productive way:
     a. Use the patient's language.
     b. Refer for "evaluation," "consultation," or "counseling."
     c. Refer to the specialist as a "counselor" or an "expert on helping people with problems such as yours."
  5. Elicit family support for the referral.
  6. Have the patient call the therapist for an appointment before he or she leaves your office.
  7. Join the therapist for the first session for those patients who are difficult and need your support to accept the referral.
  8. Make explicit the frequency and kind of communication you want from the therapist.
  9. Negotiate and clarify what you will work on with the patient, what the therapist will work on, and how you will work together.
  10. When a patient strongly resists a referral:
     a. Take a longer view of the problems. Some difficult referrals take 1–2 y to accomplish.
     b. Wait for a crisis to occur, when referral is typically easier.
  11. Support the treatment with the mental health specialist.
     a. Communicate regularly with the therapist.
     b. Let the patient know you and the therapist are a team.
  12. Follow up with the patient after making the referral.
     a. Set up an appointment soon after the counseling begins to support treatment and reassure the patient of your interest.
     b. Set up an appointment with the patient soon after counseling ends to debrief and provide continuity.
B. The Don'ts
  1. Don't assume the mental health specialist has a similar working style to that of a primary care physician. Work to get to know the differences between yourself and a therapist you respect. By recognizing differences, the ground for efficient collaboration will be established.
  2. Don't wait until the last minute to refer a difficult patient or family. Therapists refer to this as a "dump" and feel it takes a very long time to bring the patient back to a place where treatment can be successful. Contact the therapist fairly early in the process, even for an informal consultation.
  3. Don't use medical or psychiatric diagnoses with patients when making the referral. Although patients may benefit from knowing their diagnosis, the language of the patient and the family is much more descriptive and understandable to them.
  4. Don't refer to a "family therapist" for "family therapy." Unfortunately, most patients hear these labels as conferring blame or inadequacy on their family. Exceptions to this principle are those problems patients themselves label "marital" or "family" problems.
  5. When patients strongly resist a referral, don't battle with them. Maintain your recommendation, monitor their functioning for deterioration, and just wait.
  6. Don't allow the patient to pit you against the therapist.
     a. Encourage the patient to talk directly to the therapist about any complaints he or she has about the treatment.
     b. Encourage the patient to attend several sessions and "give it a fair try."
     c. Tell the therapist the patient is reporting difficulty.
     d. When treatment is stuck or ineffective, ask the therapist for his or her assessment. Consider consultation, termination, or referral to another mental health specialist.
  7. Don't continue using a therapist who generally does not provide adequate feedback or effective treatment.

Source: Reprinted from McDaniel SH, Campbell TL, Seaburn DB: *Family-Oriented Primary Care: A Manual for Medical Providers.* New York: Springer-Verlag; 1990.[26]

times, patients and families wait for a crisis situation to force them into treatment. Other times, with the gentle and consistent reminders from a trusted physician, nurse, or other clinician, patients and family members are able to consider a referral. When possible, schedule to attend the first session for patients who are very challenging and may need the reassurance of your physical presence to facilitate their beginning treatment with a mental health specialist.[4]

Monitoring Progress

Patients benefit from ongoing attention to their relational concerns.[2,3,26] If common relational problems are not resolved with the use of brief supportive counseling, revisit the assessment and treatment plan; consider referral to an outside mental health specialist if appropriate. For more serious relationship problems, as with any patients receiving care from consulting or collaborating specialists, continue to monitor the treatment and encourage compliance with the therapist's recommendations. Support the patient and her family in the management of crises by scheduling regular visits. In some cases, the progress toward relational health is very slow and the primary care clinician functions as a consistent, supportive presence over many years and many episodes of relational distress. Patients appreciate a clinician who will "be with them" even if progress seems slow or crises persist. It is essential that patients not feel "abandoned" when struggling with relationship concerns, particularly when referred to a mental health colleague. Continue to schedule routine visits to reassure the patient of your support and tell the patient that you will collaborate closely with her psychotherapist.

Future Directions

The importance of women's relationships as a part of their overall health is increasingly recognized and health care practices are responding with re-

sources for support and treatment. Some primary care offices offer on-site mental health services, including couple and family therapy. A few include women's support groups and multifamily groups for coping with chronic conditions. Psychoeducation seminars for improving women's overall health often focus on the multiple stresses, including relationship demands, in women's lives. Targeted interventions aimed at improving women's relationships and outcome measures to demonstrate their effectiveness are much needed. Anecdotal reports suggest that patients and their family members and clinicians report satisfaction about the availability of on-site integrated clinical services.

Appendix A
Key Questions

GENERAL QUESTIONS/NEW PATIENT VISIT

How is life at home?
Possible follow-up questions:
   Who lives with you?
   Who do you turn to for support during
      difficult times?
Tell me about your relationship with your
   husband/partner.
Possible follow-up questions:
   How long have you been together?
   How is his/her health?
   Are there any concerns that you have about
      this relationship?
   How do the two of you make decisions/
      resolve conflicts?
   How satisfying is your sexual relationship?
   In what ways does he/she support you?
   Has he/she ever hit, kicked, or punched you?
   What stresses do you experience in this
      relationship (financial, sexual, role-sharing,
      emotional distress, substance use, infidelity,
      separation, etc.)?
[Have you been previously married or in a long-
   term relationship with a committed partner? If
   yes, repeat above questions re: previous
   husband/partner.]

Tell me about your relationship with your parents.

Possible follow-up questions:

Are they living/deceased?

How is their health?

How far away do they live from you?

How often do you see them?

Do you provide any caregiving for them?

In what ways do they support you?

How was your life growing up?

Was there any violence or abuse as a child? (If yes—is there any violence now?)

What stresses do you experience in this relationship (financial, caregiving, conflict, emotional distress, substance use, etc.)?

How do your siblings respond to the situation?

Do you have children? If yes,

Tell me about your relationship with your children.

Possible follow-up questions:

How old are they?

How is their health?

Do any of your children have serious medical or mental illness?

Have you experienced pregnancy loss or the death of a child?

What difficulties do you have in parenting them?

Do they have any problems at home, school, or with the law?

What support do you have in parenting them?

How do you talk with them about life's challenges and opportunities (sex, drugs, etc.)?

Is there any violence involving your children?

What stresses do you experience with your children (financial, acting-out, school problems, teen pregnancy, substance use, etc.)?

Other times to integrate a relational assessment/approach:

Patient Receiving a New Diagnosis

Who will you tell about this new diagnosis?

What do you think his/her reactions will be?

What involvement or support do you expect from your partner/parents/children?

What difficulties do you anticipate for you and for them?

How can we best involve them in your care?

Patient Managing a Chronic Condition

Who else knows about your illness?

Are there people close to you (parents/partner/children) that you have chosen not to tell? Why?

Who helps you maintain your treatment regimen?

In what ways can your spouse/partner, parents/siblings, or children be more helpful?

What difficulties are they having adjusting to your _____ ?

How can we best involve them in your care?

Appendix B
Screening Tools

THE FAMILY APGAR

This is a brief 5-item self-report measure to obtain a patient's perceptions of current family relationships. The focus is on "satisfaction" with family functioning in the areas of: emotional support and expression, communicating, problem-solving, acknowledging the patient's ideas for family activities/decisions, as well as shared time together. The scores range from 0–10, with 10 representing a family member's perception that the family is functioning very well.

SOURCE: Smilkstein G: The family APGAR: a proposal for a family function test and its use by physicians. *J Fam Pract* 6:1231, 1978.

THE GLOBAL ASSESSMENT OF RELATIONAL FUNCTIONING (GARF)

This assessment tool combines the dimensions of problem-solving, organization, and emotional climate. The ratings range from 1–100, with the highest category (81–99) indicating that the relationships meet the affective and instrumental needs of the members in a satisfactory way, both by the patient's report and by observation. Traditionally family therapists and other clinicians use the scale to assess relational functioning initially and report changes over time in response to interventions.

SOURCE: Yingling LC, Miller WE, McDonald A, et al: *GARF Assessment Sourcebook: Using the DSM-IV Global Assessment of Relational Functioning.*

DOMESTIC VIOLENCE

All clinicians should routinely screen for relational violence. Recommended resources can be found in Chap. 7.

References

1. Miller JB: *Toward a New Psychology of Women.* Boston: Beacon Press; 1976.
2. Campbell TL: Family's impact on health: a critical review. *Family Systems Medicine* 4:135, 1986.
3. Doherty WJ, Campbell TL: *Families and Health.* Newbury Park, CA: Sage; 1988.
4. O'Leary A, Helgeson VS: Psychosocial factors and women's health: integrating mind, heart, and body. In: Gallant SJ, Puryear Keita G, Royak-Schaler R (eds): *Health Care for Women.* Washington, DC: American Psychiatric Association; 1997.
5. Berkman LF: The role of social relations in health promotion. *Psychosom Med* 57:245, 1995.
6. Callaghan P, Morrissey J: Social support and health: a review. *J Adv Nurs* 18:203, 1993.
7. House JS, Robbins C, Metzner HL: The association of social relationships and activities with mortality: prospective evidence from the Tecumseh community health study. *Am J Epidemiol* 116:123, 1982.
8. Collins NL, Dunkel-Schetter C, Lobel M, et al: Social support in pregnancy: psychosocial correlates of birth outcomes and postpartum depression. *J Pers Soc Psychol* 65:1243, 1993.
9. Brezinka V, Kittel F: Psychosocial factors of coronary heart disease in women: a review. *Soc Sci Med* 42:1351, 1995.
10. Ross CE , Mirowsky J, Goldsteen K: The impact of the family on health: the decade in review. *Journal of Marriage and the Family* 52:1059, 1990.
11. Burman B, Margolin G: Analysis of the association between marital relationships and health problems: an interactional perspective. *Psychol Bull* 112:39, 1992.
12. Goodwin SS: The marital relationship and health in women with chronic fatigue and immune dys-function syndrome: views of wives and husbands. *Nurs Res* 46:138, 1997.
13. Kiecolt JK, Malarkey WB, Chee M, et al: Negative behavior during marital conflict is associated with immunological down-regulation. *Psychosom Med* 55:395, 1993.
14. Shumaker SA, Hill, DR: Gender differences in social support and physical health. *Health Psychol* 10:102, 1991.
15. Adler NE, Coriell M: Socioeconomic status and women's health. In: Gallant SJ, Puryear Keita G, Royak-Schaler R (eds): *Health Care for Women.* Washington, DC: American Psychiatric Association; 1997.
16. Marshall NL: Combining work and family. In: Gallant SJ, Puryear Keita G, Royak-Schaler R (eds): *Health Care for Women.* Washington, DC: American Psychiatric Association; 1997.
17. Thomas S: Psychosocial correlates of women's health in middle adulthood. *Issues in Mental Health Nursing* 16:285, 1995.
18. Drossman DA, Leserman J, Nachman G, et al: Sexual and physical abuse in women with functional or organic gastrointestinal disorders. *Ann Intern Med* 113:828, 1990.
19. Plichta SB, Abraham C: Violence and gynecologic health in women under 50 years old. *Am J Obstet Gynecol* 174:903, 1996.
20. Lechner ME, Vogel ME, Garcia-Shelton LM, et al: Self-reported medical problems of adult female survivors of sexual abuse. *J Fam Pract* 36:633, 1993.
21. Carter B, McGoldrick M (eds): *The Changing Family Life Cycle: A Framework for Family Therapy*, 2nd ed. New York: Gardner; 1988.
22. deShazer S: *Keys to Solutions in Brief Therapy.* New York: Norton; 1985.
23. deShazer S: *Clues: Investigating Solutions in Brief Therapy.* New York: Norton, 1988.
24. Giorlando ME, Schilling RJ: On becoming a solution-focused physician: The MED-STAT Acronym. *Families, Systems & Health* 15:361, 1997.
25. McGoldrick M, Gerson R, Shellenberger J: *Genograms : Assessment and Intervention,* 2nd ed. New York: Norton, 1999.
26. McDaniel SH, Campbell TL, Seaburn DB: *Family Oriented Primary Care: A Manual for Medical Providers.* New York:, Springer-Verlag; 1990.
28. McDaniel SH, DeGruy FV: Relational disorders in primary care medicine. In: Kaslow F (ed): *Handbook on Relational Disorders.* New York: Wiley; 1996.

29. Hahn SR: Working with special populations: families. In: Feldman MD, Christensen JF (eds): *Behavioral Medicine in Primary Care: A Practical Guide*. Stamford, CT: Appleton & Lange; 1997.

Additional Resources

Women's Experiences

Baker Miller J, Pierce Stiver I: *The Healing Connection: How Women Form Relationships in Therapy and in Life*. Boston: Beacon Press; 1997.

Candid LM: *Medicine and the Family: A Feminist Perspective*. New York: Basic Books; 1995.

Gallant S, Puryear Keita G, Royak-Schaler R (eds): *Health Care for Women*. Washington, DC: American Psychiatric Association; 1997.

Jordan JV: *Women's Growth in Diversity*. New York: Guilford; 1997.

Family-Oriented Health Care

Families, Systems, & Health: The Journal of Collaborative Healthcare. www.FSH.org

McDaniel SH, Campbell TL, Seaburn DB: *Family-Oriented Primary Care: A Manual for Medical Providers*. New York: Springer-Verlag; 1990.

McDaniel SH, Hepworth J, Doherty W: *Medical Family Therapy: A Biopsychosocial Aproach to Families with Health Problems*. New York: Basic Books; 1992.

McDaniel SH, Hepworth J, Doherty W: *The Shared Experience of Illness: Stories of Patients, Families and Their Therapists*. New York: Basic Books; 1996.

Intimacy and Health

Ornish D: *Love & Survival: The Scientific Basis for the Healing Power of Intimacy*. New York: Harper-Collins; 1998.

Spiegel D: *Living Beyond Limits: New Hope and Help for Facing Life-Threatening Illness*. New York: Times Books; 1993.

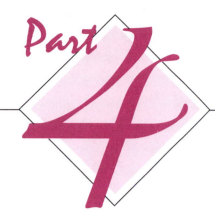

Gynecologic Concerns

Judith A. Suess
Claudia Holzman

Vulvar and Vaginal Disease

Overview

Women's Concerns

Vaginal and vulvar symptoms are among the most common health concerns of women of all ages and ethnic backgrounds. Women are often taught, implicitly as well as explicitly, that the vagina is intrinsically unclean while simultaneously it is the focus of female sexuality. Advertisements for "feminine" products, such as douches and scented panty liners that promise to eliminate unpleasant odors or to "clean" a dirty vagina, only reinforce these perceptions. Many women assume that any discharge is pathologic and needs to be treated.

Health messages about feminine hygiene products are constantly changing, and as a result, products widely used and recommended by previous generations of women are now implicated as potential health hazards. For example, today's women are reading reports that ordinary talcum powder may increase the risk of ovarian cancer,[1] that douching may lead to upper genital tract infections,[2] that tampon use may cause toxic shock syndrome,[3] and that tampons and panty liners may cause irritation or localized allergic reactions if deodorant or scents have been added.

Women are also confronted with the availability, without prescription, of antifungal vaginal products. This can be seen as empowering, enabling women to bypass the (at times) cumbersome medical system and self-treat vulvovaginal candidiasis (VVC). However, misdiagnosing another condition as VVC can have important consequences, especially in pregnancy. Therefore, women, as well as health care providers, have a concern about when it is appropriate to self-diagnose and self-treat VVC.

Vaginal conditions can have far-reaching physical and psychological effects. If dyspareunia is present, women's sexual relationships are adversely affected. In addition, the social stigmata of the classic sexually transmitted diseases (STDs) can carry over to any pathologic condition of the genital tract, leaving women feeling guilty or ashamed.

Pregnant women diagnosed with abnormal vaginal conditions are left wondering how this will affect the course of the pregnancy and the health of the fetus. Lesbian women wonder if information on vaginal conditions applies to lesbian relationships, given the paucity of studies that includes this population.

Prevalence and Morbidity

It is estimated that over one million physician office visits per year in the United States are motivated by concerns about vaginal symptoms.[4] The three most common vaginal conditions are bacterial vaginosis (BV), VVC, and trichomoniasis. Other reproductive tract infections are discussed in Chap. 14. Studies in the United States report that BV is present in 10 to 25 percent of women who attend gynecologic clinics and in more than 50 percent of women who attend STD clinics.[5–7] It has been estimated that 75 percent of women will experience at least one VVC infection during their childbearing years and that about half of these women will have at least one recurrence.[8] However, estimates of VVC incidence have been based mainly on self-reported history of physician diagnosis. This relies on the participant's memory, as well as the accuracy of physician diagnosis—often made without benefit of microscopy or culture.[9] The prevalence of trichomonas is about 13 percent, although there is considerable variation in prevalence among subgroups of women.[10]

These common vaginal conditions were once regarded as problems confined to the lower genital tract, as mainly a nuisance due to discomfort and symptomatology, and as having little effect on larger health concerns. More recently, BV has been linked to asymptomatic endometritis,[11] pelvic inflammatory disease (PID),[12] and ectopic pregnancies.[13] Both BV and trichomoniasis have been associated with an increased risk of acquiring HIV from infected partners at the time of vaginal intercourse[14,15] and with preterm birth.[10,16]

An increasing proportion of VVC is caused by *Candida* species other than *Candida albicans,* many of which are resistant to traditional antifungal treatment. At the same time, several topical antifungal preparations have been made available as nonprescription products. Self-treatment, although a very worthy modality, may result in ineffective treatment of resistant fungi, inadequate treatment of recurrent VVC (RVVC), or nontreatment for more serious gynecologic entities such as PID or cystitis. The latter may result in significant morbidity, especially during pregnancy.

Normal Physiology

The amount and character of normal vaginal secretions will vary depending on many factors. These include hormonal and fluid status, pregnancy, and medication use. Most of the liquid portion of vaginal secretions consists of mucus from the cervix. A very small amount of moisture is contributed by endometrial fluid, exudates from accessory glands such as Skene's and Bartholin's glands, and from vaginal transudate. Exfoliated squamous cells from the vaginal mucosa give a white to off-white color and provide some increase in consistency. Women produce, on the average, about 1.5 g of vaginal fluid per day. Secretions are not usually noticeable at the introitus and the discharge is flocculent, that is, nonhomogeneous. At the time of ovulation, the discharge is of higher viscosity and is often greater in quantity. Normal secretions have no odor; the pH is 3.5 to 4.5.

The squamous epithelium of the vagina is highly sensitive to estrogen, which induces a mature glycogen-containing epithelial lining. Glycogen is broken down into various organic acids by the action of local enzymes and bacteria. Lactobacilli predominate in this milieu and contribute to the low vaginal pH by producing lactic acid. Some *Lactobacillus* species also produce hydrogen peroxide (H_2O_2), which inhibits the growth of many organisms. Thus, a competitive inhibition is established, which serves to control pathogens.[17]

A wide range of aerobic and anaerobic bacteria may normally be found in the vagina at concentrations of 10^{8-9} col/mL. The most common organisms are lactobacilli, diptheroids, streptococci, and staphylococci. *C. albicans* is present in small numbers in 20 percent of women. Because the vagina is a potential space, not an open tube, a ratio of 5:1 anaerobic/aerobic bacteria is normal.[18] For a detailed analysis and description of vaginal secretions and flora, see the article by Huggins and Preti.[19]

Hormonal changes can result in a marked change in vaginal ecology. Whenever the absolute or relative concentration of estrogen decreases (such as with lactation, oral contraceptive use, or menopause), there is a corresponding decrease in glycogen. With menopause, the lack of estrogen results in thin vaginal epithelium and cells that are lacking in glycogen. This contributes to a reduction in lactic acid production and an increase in pH. The change in the environment can result in the overgrowth of nonacidophilic coliforms and the disappearance of lactobacilli.

Principal Diagnoses

Diagnosis in the Setting of an Office Visit

HISTORY

It is useful to begin with an open-ended approach to the history, which will often elicit information that might otherwise be missed, and then follow with symptom-related inquiry and relevant history (Table 11-1).

With a new patient, it is important to also obtain a sexual history including any new sexual partners, number of current or lifetime partners, sexual practices, sexual orientation, safety of sexual practices, contraceptive methods, use of new spermicidal agents or condoms, symptoms in partner(s), and the last time of vaginal intercourse (may increase vaginal pH). Note the estrogenic status of the patient (i.e., premenarchal, childbearing age, pregnant, perimenopausal, menopausal) and the use of

Table 11-1

Obtaining an Adequate History

  I.   Begin with open-ended questions about the purpose of the visit

 II.   Symptom-related inquiry and relevant history
- Pain: location (external versus internal), intensity, any radiation, associated aggravating or alleviating factors, description (burning, sharp, etc.)
- Dysuria (internal versus external)
- Changes in vaginal discharge: amount, color, odor, consistency, presence of blood
- Dyspareunia
- Previous episodes of vulvovaginal disease and setting of diagnosis
- Treatment and response to treatment in previous episodes
- Recent sexual history and medication use

III.   Additional history from a new patient
- Sexual history: new sexual partner(s), number of partners, sexual practices, sexual orientation, contraceptive methods, symptoms in partner(s)
- Estrogenic status of the patient: premenarchal, of childbearing age, pregnant, perimenopausal, menopausal
- Use of oral contraceptives, hormone replacement therapy, selective estrogen receptor modulators (tamoxifen, raloxifene), antibiotics
- Frequency of douching, use of feminine sprays and deodorants, new toiletry products

oral contraceptives, hormone replacement therapy, antiestrogens such as tamoxifen (Nolvadex) and raloxifene (Evista), or antibiotics. The use and frequency of douching, use of "feminine" sprays and deodorants, and new soaps or laundry detergents should also be noted. In an established patient in whom this information has already been documented, current or recent medications and use of "feminine products" should be noted and the sexual history briefly updated.

Table 11-2[20] lists historical factors associated with the most common vaginal conditions, the strength of these associations, and the level of evidence in support of these hypothesized associations. The factors included in Table 11-1 are of a mixed nature, some representing signs and symptoms such as odor or genital itching, others representing behaviors such as oral contraceptive use or receptive oral sex. Many of these factors may be elicited during history taking, but it should be emphasized that none of the factors are uniquely diagnostic of one condition over another.

PHYSICAL EXAMINATION

The physical examination should begin with a visual inspection of the external genitalia, including the perineum. Lesions, erythema, edema, distortions, changes from previous examinations, or trauma (due to scratching, sexual activity, sports activity, or injury) should be noted. Palpation can identify areas of tenderness. Visual inspection of the vagina should include looking for any abnormal coloration, lesions, thinning, or edema. A standard bimanual examination should also be done because vulvovaginal conditions may coexist with upper tract disease. For an established patient, who has been evaluated for vulvovaginal complaints within the last 2 years, the speculum and bimanual examination may be precluded. Instead, a sterile swab may be placed in the vagina to obtain a sample of vaginal secretions.

Different organisms produce characteristic discharges. About 50 percent of women with BV have a homogenous white discharge with a strong, fishy

Figure 11-1

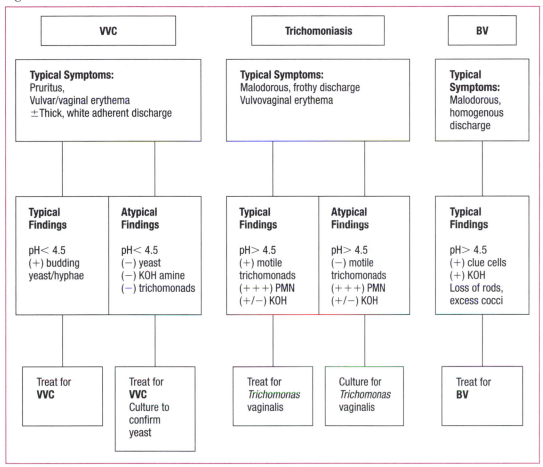

Abnormal vaginal discharge.

odor.[5] The odor may be accentuated during menses and after intercourse due to the elevated pH of blood and semen. VVC is sometimes accompanied (20 percent) by a thick, cottage cheese–like discharge, with little to no odor; more often erythema and swelling are the most salient physical findings. Trichomoniasis typically presents as a frothy yellow-green discharge that is malodorous, and like VVC, evidence of irritation is seen around the labia. In less than 25 percent of cases, the vagina and cervix have a red stippled "strawberry" appearance.[21] These clinical features are not sufficiently sensitive or specific for a definitive diagnosis, and therefore, supporting evidence from laboratory tests is required (Fig. 11-1). Futhermore, some women may be affected by more than one vaginal condition. In a recent study, 14 percent of women with symptomatic vaginitis had mixed infections of VVC, BV, and trichomonas.[22]

LABORATORY TESTS

Table 11-3 provides a summary of diagnostic laboratory tests used to differentiate or rule out the

Table 11-2

Historical Factors Associated with Common Types of Vaginal Infections

Diagnosis	Risk Factor	Strength of Association	Level of Evidence*	Limitations and/or References
Bacterial vaginosis	Ever sexually active	Strong	A	100% of BV patients vs. 94% in those without. Limited value clinically.[a]
	Complaints of genital symptoms	Low (<50%)	A	Presence of odor or discolored discharge helpful; absence not useful.[a–c]
	Complaints of odor	Moderate	B	Often noticed after intercourse.
	Has IUD	Moderate	B	19% in BV patients vs. 5% in non-BV patients.[a]
	New sexual partner	Moderate	C	Increased risk with new partner in past 30 days.[d]
	H/O *Trichomonas* infection	Moderate	C	24% in BV vs. 8% in those without.[a]
Candida vulvovaginitis (CVV)	Taking oral contraceptives	Low	A	Not predictive of diagnosis.[b,e,f]
	Recent use of antibiotics	Low	A	Not predictive of diagnosis.[b,e,f]
	Gastrointestinal carriage	Moderate	A	Relationship of treatment to outcome unclear. Oral nystatin had little effect.[h–k]
	Sexual transmission	Moderate	A	Same strain carriage is common.[i–n] Conflicting data on significance.[o–r] Therapy not associated with outcome.
	Genital itching	Moderate	A	Seen in 22% of those without CVV.[e,t,u]
	Receptive oral sex	Moderate	B	Significance unclear.[p,s]
	Pregnancy	Low	B	Low power of study.[e]
	Diabetes	Low	B	Diabetics have increased risk, but few women with CVV have diabetes mellitus (DM).[e]
	Previous H/O CVV in past year	Moderate	B	Rate 17% in controls, 50% in cases.[f]
	Dietary sugars, milk, or yeasts	Low	C	May be a factor in selected women.[g]
	Tight clothes	Low	C	Reported in one study.[v]

Table 11-2

Historical Factors Associated with Common Types of Vaginal Infections *(Continued.)*

DIAGNOSIS	RISK FACTOR	STRENGTH OF ASSOCIATION	LEVEL OF EVIDENCE*	LIMITATIONS AND/OR REFERENCES
Trichomonas vaginitis	Presence of other STDs	Moderate	A	30% of women with this had other STDs.[w]
	Multiple sexual partners	Moderate	A	

*Level of evidence: A, strong or moderate research-based evidence, consistent across studies; B, limited research-based evidence (less consistent or extensive evidence, but preponderance of evidence supports use of treatment); C, common practice with little or no research-based evidence.

REFERENCES

a. Amsel R, Totten PA, Spiegel CA, Chen KC, Eschenbach D, Holmes KK: Nonspecific vaginitis: Diagnostic criteria and microbial and epidemiologic associations. *Am J Med* 74:14, 1983.

b. Reed BD, Huck W, Zazove P: Differentiation of *Gardnerella vaginalis, Candida albicans,* and *Trichomonas vaginalis* infections of the vagina. *J Fam Pract* 28.673, 1989.

c. Eschenbach DA, Hillier S, Critchlow C, Stevens C, DeRouen T, Holmes KK: Diagnosis and clinical manifestations of bacterial vaginosis. *Am J Obstet Gynecol* 158:819, 1988.

d. Hawes SE, Hillier SL, Benedetti J, et al: Hydrogen peroxide–producing lactobacilli and acquisition of vaginal infections. *J Infect Dis* 174:1058, 1996.

e. Abbott J: Clinical and microscopic diagnosis of vaginal yeast infection: a prospective analysis. *Ann Emerg Med* 25:587, 1995.

f. Geiger AM, Foxman B: Risk factors for vulvovaginal candidiasis: A case-control study among university students. *Epidemiology* 7:182, 1996.

g. Horowitz BJ, Edelstein SW, Lippman L: Sugar chromatography studies in recurrent *Candida* vulvovaginitis. *J Reprod Med* 29:441, 1984.

h. Group NMS: Therapy of candidal vaginitis: The effect of eliminating intestinal *Candida. Am J Obstet Gynecol* 155:651, 1986.

i. Hilton AL, Warnock DW: Vaginal candidiasis and the role of the digestive tract as a source of infection. *Br J Obstet Gynaecol* 82:922, 1975.

j. Miles MR, Olsen L, Rogers A: Recurrent vaginal candidiasis: Importance of an intestinal reservoir. *JAMA* 238:1836, 1977.

k. Davidson F, Mould RF: Recurrent genital candidosis in women and the effect of intermittent prophylactic treatment. *Br J Vener Dis* 54:176, 1978.

l. Schmid J, Rotman M, Reed B, Pierson CL, Soll DR: Genetic similarity of *Candida albicans* strains from vaginitis patients and their partners. *J Clin Microbiol* 3:39, 1933.

m. Lockhart SR, Reed BD, Pierson CL, Soll DR: Most frequent scenario for recurrent *Candida* vaginitis is strain maintenance with "substrain shuffling": demonstration by sequential DNA fingerprinting with probes Ca3, C1, and CARE2. *J Clin Microbiol* 34:767, 1996.

n. Warnock DW, Speller CD, Milne JD, Hilton AL, Kershaw PI: Epidemiological investigation of patients with vulvovaginal candidosis: Application of a resistogram method for strain differentiation of *Candida albicans. Br J Vener Dis* 55:357, 1979.

o. Horowitz BJ, Edelstein SW, Lippman L: Sexual transmission of *Candida. Obstet Gynecol* 69:883, 1987.

p. Buch A, Christensen ES: Treatment of vaginal candidosis with natamycin and effect of treating the partner at the same time. *Acta Obstet Gynecol Scand* 61:393, 1982.

q. Bisschop MP, Merkus JM, Scheygrond H, van Cutsem J: Cotreatment of the male partner in vaginal candidosis: a double-blind randomized control study. *Br J Obstet Gynaecol* 93:79, 1986.

r. Davidson F: Yeasts and circumcision in the male. *Br J Vener Dis* 53:121, 1977.

s. Markos AR, Wade AA, Walzman M: Oral sex and recurrent vulvovaginal candidiasis (letter). *Genitourin Med* 68:61, 1992.

t. Bertholf ME: Symptom diagnosis of *Candida* vaginitis (letter). *J Fam Pract* 17:775, 777, 1983.

u. McCormack WM, Starko KM, Zinner SH: Symptoms associated with vaginal colonization with yeast. *Am J Obstet Gynecol* 158:31, 1988.

v. Elegbe IA, Elegbe I: Quantitative relationships of *Candida albicans* infections and dressing patterns in Nigerian women. *Am J Public Health* 73:450, 1983.

w. Reynolds M, Wilson J: Is *Trichomonas vaginalis* still a marker for other sexually transmitted infections in women? *Int J STD AIDS* 7:131, 1996.

ABBREVIATIONS: BV, bacterial vaginosis; H/O, history of; IUD, intrauterine device; STD, sexually transmitted disease.

SOURCE: Reed BD: Vaginitis. In: Sloane PD, Slatt LM, Curtis P, Ebell MH (eds): *Essentials of Family Medicine,* 3rd ed. Baltimore: Williams & Wilkins; 1998;662, with permission.

three common vaginal conditions, BV, VVC, and trichomonas. First-line tests, such as pH assessment, wet mount, and potassium hydroxide (KOH), are inexpensive and should be readily available in most clinicians' offices. In some clinics, the Gram stain is also used routinely. Newer tests, such as the swab test, are gaining acceptance. Other tests, such as cultures, are reserved for atypical presentations or persistent symptoms despite appropriate treatment.

It is important to note that the sensitivity and specificity of tests for BV are often evaluated in relation to another diagnostic approach such as the Amsel criteria, which is not a true gold standard (see Table 11-3). There is disagreement about the most appropriate gold standard for a polymicrobial condition such as BV. Many investigators favor quantification of *Gardnerella vaginalis* colony-forming units in culture as the reference standard; others prefer the Gram stain.

VAGINAL PH   Vaginal pH is assessed using narrow-range pH paper. One of the products often used in studies of BV is colorpHast® pH 4.0 to 7.0 (EM Science, 480 Democrat Road, Gibbstown, NJ 08027). A pH above 4.5 is consistent with either BV or trichomoniasis. VVC has the normal vaginal pH of 3.5 to 4.5. A vaginal pH of 5.0 to 6.5 in the absence of an abnormal microbial milieu is suggestive of menopause.[23]

MICROSCOPY

Wet Mount.   Examples of the microscopic appearance are shown in Fig. 11-2. A sample of vaginal discharge is diluted with 1 to 2 drops of 0.9% normal saline on one slide and with 10% KOH solution on another slide. The addition of KOH frequently produces a fishy, amine odor when BV is present (whiff test). After placing cover slips on both slides, each is examined under a microscope, using low and high powers. On the saline slide, clue cells, which are vaginal epithelial cells with a uniform grainy appearance resulting from adherent bacteria, are indicative of BV. Clue

cells are a component of the Amsel criteria[24] (Table 11-4).

Trichomonas appears, in the saline preparation, as a fusiform protozoa just slightly larger than a white blood cell. Movement of the three to five flagella extending from the narrow end facilitates identification. About 50 to 70 percent of trichmoniasis is detected by examination of wet mounts.[25] Trichomoniasis is typically accompanied by a large number of polymorphonuclear (PMN) leukocytes visible on the wet mount.

Candida species appear as budding yeast or as hyphal forms and are detected on microscopy in about 50 to 70 percent of women with VVC.[26] Evidence of candidal infection may be seen more readily on the KOH slide because bacterial and eukaryote cells will be lysed. Because many women harbor *Candida* organisms under normal vaginal conditions, the diagnosis of VVC should be reserved for women with accompanying symptoms.

Gram Stain.   A sterile Dacron swab is rubbed against the wall of the vagina, then a smear is made on a slide and air-dried. Reliability studies have shown that the exact location of sampling within the vagina is not important, and it is *not necessary* to use a vaginal speculum, as long as sampling is done well beyond the labia.[27] Gram stain is applied to a slide, which is then examined under a microscope for evidence of lactobacilli, gram-negative and gram-variable bacteria, yeast, and trichomonas. Scoring for the presence/absence of BV is described by Nugent et al.[28] (Table 11-4).

If the Gram stain method is used as a reference standard for diagnosing BV, the Amsel criteria, on average, would have a sensitivity of 70.4 percent and a specificity of 94.4 percent.[7] The Gram stain method requires more experience in slide reading and scoring and is typically a less rapid assessment. Thus, it is more often used in research and not in clinical settings. Recent studies have shown that reliable BV diagnoses can be made when women insert a tampon and either smear it on a slide that is later stained or bring the tampon to the clinician who prepares the smear for Gram staining.[29]

Table 11-3

Diagnostic Tests Used to Diagnose Vaginitis

Clinical Entity	Diagnostic Test	1st Line	2nd Line	Sensitivity	Specificity	LR+ [a]	LR− [a]	Relative Cost	References
Bacterial vaginosis	Whiff test	X		Low (29%)	High (95%)	5.8	.75	+	a
	pH > 4.5	X		Moderate to high (72–89%)	Low-moderate (49–73%)	1.4–3.3	.15–57	+	a (using pH 5), b
	Clue cells present	X		Variable (37–97%)	High (79–92%)	1.8–48.0	0.3–.79	+	a–c
	3 or 4 Amsel criteria	X		Moderate 70%	High (94%)	11.7	.32	+	Compared to Gram stain, b
	Abnormal background flora on gram stain	X	X	High (89–100%)	High (83–97%)	5.2–33	0.1–13	+	Compared to Amsel criteria; b, c
	Culture—*Gardnerella*	—	—	Moderate (88%)	Moderate (86%)	6.3	.14	++	d
	PCR—*Gardnerella*	—	—	High (91–95%)	Low (60–63%)	2.3	.15	+++	e, f
	Proline amino-peptidase assay	—	X	High (93%)	High (91–93%)	10.3–13.3	.08	++	g
Candida vulvovaginitis	Cytology—clue cells	—	X	High (88%)	High (99%)	88	.12	++	c
	pH of secretions ≤ 4.5	X		High (82%)	Low (9%)	.90	2	+	h
	KOH prep	X	X	Low-moderate (22–61%)	Moderate-high (77–94%)	.96–10.2	.41–1.1	+	a, b, i–k
	Candida culture		X	High (93–100%)	High in symptomatic (83%)	5.4	0.1	++	Is the current gold standard; l, m
	Slide latex agglutination	—	—	Moderate (65–81%)	Moderate-high (59–98%)	1.6–40.4	0.2–0.6	++	j, m–o
	Molecular testing—immunologic or PCR	—	X	High (75%)	High in symptomatic (96%)	18.8	0.3	++	e
	Cytology	—	—	Moderate (80%)	High (99+%)	80.0	0.2	Moderate	p

Table 11-3

Diagnostic Tests Used to Diagnose Vaginitis *(Continued.)*

CLINICAL ENTITY	DIAGNOSTIC TEST	1ST LINE	2ND LINE	SENSITIVITY	SPECIFICITY	LR+[a]	LR−[a]	RELATIVE COST	REFERENCES
Trichomonas vaginitis	Normal saline prep	X	—	Low-moderate (37–80%)	High (96–98%)	9.3–40	0.7	+	e, q–t
	Trichomonas culture	—	X	High (80%)	High (100%)	80.0	0.2	++	u
	Enzyme-linked immunosorbent	—	X	Moderate (77–93%)	High (98–100%)	38.5–46.5	0.1–0.2	++	s, t
	Molecular testing (immunologic, PCR)	—	X	High (90%)	High (94–99%)	15.0–90	0.1	++	e, q, u
	Cytology	—	—	Moderate (64%)	Low (55%)	1.4	0.7	++	v

NOTE: LR+ is the relative odds of having the infection versus odds of not having the infection if the characteristic/test is positive; LR− is the relative odds of having the infection versus odds of not having the infection if the characteristic/test is negative.

REFERENCES

a. Reed BD, Huck W, Zazove P: Differentiation of *Gardnerella vaginalis, Candida albicans*, and *Trichomonas vaginalis* infections of the vagina. *J Fam Pract* 28:673, 1989.

b. Schwebke JR, Hillier SL, Sobel JD, McGregor JA, Sweet RL: Validity of the vaginal Gram stain for the diagnosis of bacterial vaginosis. *Obstet Gynecol* 88(4 pt 1):573, 1996.

c. Platz-Christensen JJ, Larsson PG, Sundstrom E, Wiqvist N: Detection of bacterial vaginosis in wet mount, Papanicolaou-stained vaginal smears and in Gram-stained smears. *Acta Obstet Gynecol Scand* 74:67, 1995.

d. Cristiano L, Coffetti N, Dalvai G, Lorusso L, Lorenzi M: Bacterial vaginosis: prevalence in outpatients, association with some micro-organisms and laboratory indices. *Genitourin Med* 65:382, 1989.

e. Ferris DG, Hendrich J, Payne PM, et al: Office laboratory diagnosis of vaginitis. Clinician-performed tests compared with a rapid nucleic acid hybridization test. *J Fam Pract* 41:575, 1995.

f. van Belkum A, Koeken A, Vandamme P, et al: Development of a species-specific polymerase chain reaction assay for *Gardnerella vaginalis*. *Mol Cell Probes* 9:167, 1995.

g. Schoonmaker JN, Lunt BD, Lawellin DW, French JI, Hillier SL, McGregor JA: A new proline aminopeptidase assay for diagnosis of bacterial vaginosis. *Am J Obstet Gynecol* 165:737, 1991.

h. Geiger AM, Foxman B, Sobel JD: Chronic vulvovaginal candidiasis: characteristics of women with *Candida albicans, C. glabrata* and no *Candida. Genitourin Med* 71:304, 1995.

i. McCormack WM, Starko KM, Zinner SH: Symptoms associated with vaginal colonization with yeast. *Am J Obstet Gynecol* 158:31, 1988.

j. Rajakumar R, Lacey CJ, Evans EG, Carney JA: Use of slide latex agglutination test for rapid diagnosis of vaginal candidosis. *Genitourin Med* 63:192, 1987.

k. Oriel JD, Partridge BM, Denny MJ, Coleman JC: Genital yeast infections. *Br Med J* 4:761, 1972.

l. Mendel EB, Haberman S, Hall DK: Isolation of *Candida* from clinical specimens: Comparative study of Pagano-Levin and Nickerson's culture media. *Obstet Gynecol* 16:180, 1960.

m. Hopwood V, Warnock DW, Milne JD, Crowley T, Horrocks CT, Taylor PK: Evaluation of a new slide latex agglutination test for diagnosis of vaginal candidosis. *Eur J Clin Microbiol* 6:392, 1987.

n. Abbott J: Clinical and microscopic diagnosis of vaginal yeast infection: a prospective analysis. *Ann Emerg Med* 25:587, 1995.

o. Reed BD, Pierson CL: Evaluation of a latex agglutination test for the identification of *Candida* species in vaginal discharge. *J Am Board Fam Pract* 5:375, 1992.

p. Siapco BJ, Kaplan BJ, Bernstein GS, Moyer DL: Cytodiagnosis of *Candida* organisms in cervical smears. *Acta Cytol* 30:477, 1986.

q. DeMeo LR, Draper DL, McGregor JA, et al: Evaluation of a deoxyribonucleic acid probe for the detection of *Trichomonas vaginalis* in vaginal secretions. *Am J Obstet Gynecol* 174:1339, 1996.

r. Rubino S, Muresu R, Rappelli P, et al: Molecular probe for identification of *Trichomonas vaginalis* DNA. *J Clin Microbiol* 29:702, 1991.

s. Yule A, Gellan MC, Oriel JD, Ackers JP: Detection of *Trichomonas vaginalis* antigen in women by enzyme immunoassay. *J Clin Pathol* 40:566, 1987.

t. Watt RM, Philip A, Wos SM, Sam GJ: Rapid assay for immunological detection of *Trichomonas vaginalis*. *J Clin Microbiol* 24:551, 1986.

u. Briselden AM, Hillier SL: Evaluation of Affirm VP Microbial Identification Test for *Gardnerella vaginalis* and *Trichomonas vaginalis*. *J Clin Microbiol* 32:148, 1994.

v. Perl G: Errors in the diagnosis of *Trichomonas vaginalis* infections as observed among 1199 patients. *Obstet Gynecol* 39:7, 1972.

ABBREVIATIONS: KOH, potassium hydroxide; PCR, polymerase chain reaction.

SOURCE: Reed BD: Vaginitis. In: Sloane PD, Slatt LM, Curtis P, Ebell MH (eds): *Essentials of Family Medicine*, 3rd ed. Baltimore: Williams & Wilkins; 1998:665–666, with permission.

Figure 11-2

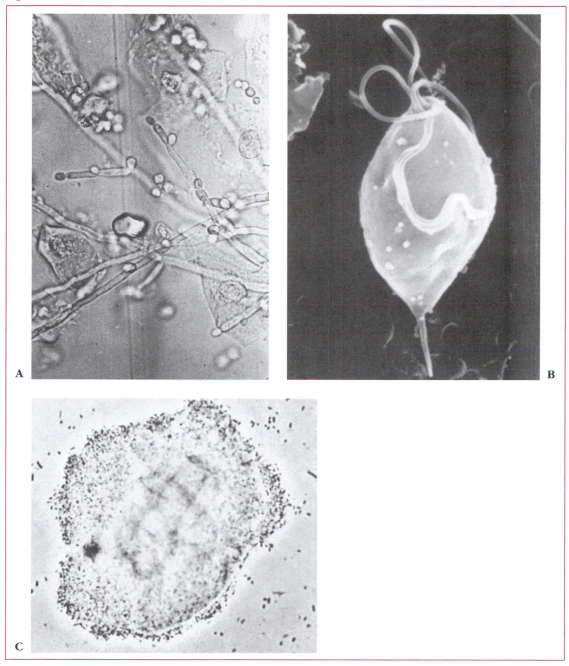

A. Hyphal elements of *C. albicans* seen on high-power magnification during saline microscopy. Patient had florid candidal vaginitis. *(Reproduced with permission from MD Pearlman and JE Tintinalli: Emergency Care of the Woman. New York, McGraw-Hill, 1998.)* **B.** Scanning electron micrograph of *T. vaginalis*. Three of the four anterior flagella (and the origin of the fourth), the undulating membrane with its flagellum, and the axostyle protruding at the end of the body are clearly seen ($\times$ 6000 magnification). *(Reproduced with permission from KK Holmes, PF Sparling, and P Mardh, et al: Sexually Transmitted Diseases, 3rd ed. New York, McGraw-Hill, 1999.)* **C.** Wet mount of vaginal fluid showing a typical clue cell from a woman with bacterial vaginosis. Note that the cell margins are obscured ($\times$ 1000 magnification). *(Reproduced with permission from MD Pearlman and JE Tintinalli: Emergency Care of the Woman. New York, McGraw-Hill, 1998.)*

Table 11-4

Diagnosis of Bacterial Vaginosis

NUGENT GRAM STAIN SCORING SYSTEM				AMSEL CRITERIA
SCORE*	*LACTOBACILLUS* MORPHOTYPES[†]	*GARDNERELLA* AND *BACTEROIDES* SPP. MORPHOTYPES[†]	CURVED GRAM-VARIABLE RODS	Amsel criteria define bacterial vaginosis as being present if three of the four following criteria are found:
0	4+	0	0	1. Homogenous vaginal discharge
1	3+	1+	1+ or 2+	2. Vaginal pH > 4.5
2	2+	2+	3+ or 4+	3. Positive "whiff" test
3	1+	3+		4. The presence of clue cells on wet
4	0	4+		microscopy of the vaginal fluid

*Score: 0–3 normal; 4–6 intermediate; > 7 BV.
[†]Number of morphotypes per oil immersion field: 0 (none); 1+ (<1); 2+ (1–4); 3+ (5–30); 4+ (>30).

VAGINAL CULTURES   When wet mounts are inconclusive, culture offers a more sensitive test for determining the presence/absence of VVC and *Trichomonas vaginalis*. Using Diamond's media culture as the gold standard for identifying *T. vaginalis,* Ohlemeyer et al. reported that the new InPOUCH TV® culture out-performed (sensitivity = 81 percent, specificity = 98.7 percent) wet mount examination alone (sensitivity = 36 percent, specificity = 99.1 percent).[30] Others have shown that the InPOUCH TV® culture approach is equally effective in detecting *T. vaginalis* when the vaginal swab is performed by the clinician or by the woman at home and brought to the clinic.[31]

Culturing for *G. vaginalis,* the most prevalent of the multiple microorganisms that overgrow in the condition of BV, is not recommended. *G. vaginalis* is present in small numbers in a majority of women; thus nonquantitative cultures are "overly sensitive."[32]

NEWER TESTS   There are rapid diagnostic kits that use DNA probes to detect *Candida, T. vaginalis,* and *G. vaginalis.*[22,33] The performance of these tests varies, with sensitivities for candida of 75 percent, for trichomonas 87 to 90 percent, and for BV 95 percent. Specificities range from 61 to 99 percent.[33,34] These tests are gaining acceptance as a rapid and less operator-dependent means of diagnosis. A major disadvantage is their relatively high cost. The

Affirm® VP III (Becton Dickinson, Sparks, MD) requires an initial equipment investment of about $7,500 and then an added per test cost of $12 to $15.

Another recent development is the swab test, which detects the elevated pH and the diamines associated with BV. This approach removes the subjectivity of the whiff test that results from interindividual variability in olfactory sensitivity. The test is performed using a cotton-tipped swab inserted into the vagina to obtain a sample of the discharge. The specimen is then placed within a circle on the card, and a positive test is recorded if the single line changes to an X. The swab test is reported to have a sensitivity of 97 percent and a specificity of 83 percent when compared with presence/absence of clue cells as a standard reference for the diagnosis of BV.[35] One swab test currently available to practitioners, the FemExam® (Cooper Surgical, Shelton, CT) costs about $5 per test.

Diagnosis in the Setting of a Telephone Call to a Pharmacist, Nurse, or Health Care Provider

Screening of vaginal complaints may be handled without an office visit for women who are established patients with medical record documentation of a recent (within the last 2 years) pelvic examination. The medical record should be available at the time of the telephone call or shortly thereafter. The telephone history should be conducted similarly to a face-to-face history and should include information on symptoms and relevant history (see Table 11-1). Of great importance is querying about previous episodes of similar symptoms and treatment regimens. If the woman has had an office evaluation, and was given the diagnosis of VVC with similar symptoms as to those she has currently, it is appropriate for a pharmacist, nurse, or health care provider to recommend nonprescription treatment with an antifungal cream if the woman is not pregnant. However, if the woman has had four or more episodes of VVC in 1 year, or a return of symptoms within 2 months, the woman must be reevaluated in the office to determine whether she has a comorbid condition or a species other than *C. albicans* that could be resistant to most of the nonprescription antifungals. Likewise, an office visit is recommended if the history is not consistent with VVC.

Bacterial Vaginosis

Background

Bacterial vaginosis is a condition of elevated vaginal pH and overgrowth of common vaginal microorganisms, primarily *G. vaginalis*, anaerobic bacilli and cocci (e.g., *Bacteroides, Prevotella, Peptostreptococcus, Mobiluncus*), *Mycoplasma hominis,* and *Ureaplasma urealyticum*.[36,37] The altered vaginal ecology may or may not be accompanied by a homogenous milky vaginal discharge. When BV is present there is a reduction in the vaginal lactobacilli that predominate under normal conditions, particularly H_2O_2-producing lactobacilli.[38] These changes in vaginal ecology produce aromatic amines, often resulting in a fishy odor, most notable after the vagina comes in contact with alkaline semen during intercourse.

Bacterial vaginosis was previously known as nonspecific vaginitis, but this terminology has been replaced in recognition that the vaginal flora imbalance is rarely accompanied by a typical cellular inflammatory response. However, recent investigations of BV in pregnancy suggest that there may be a BV-associated increase in vaginal inflammatory cytokines such as interleukin-1β[39] or interleukin-α.[40] In addition, vaginal discharges from nonpregnant women with BV were noted to have higher than normal levels of lactoferrin, an iron-binding protein contained in granules of PMNs.[41] Authors of this study speculate that the absence of an observed cellular inflammatory response with BV may be due to a rapid destruction of inflammatory cells.

In the vaginal milieu of BV, H_2O_2-producing lactobacilli are reduced, thereby diminishing intrinsic host defense factors in the vagina. Bacteria that predominate produce substances that can interfere with other normal host defenses such as mucous barriers and PMN function.[42] The combined effect may be to allow BV-related organisms, as well as other sexually transmitted organisms (e.g., chlamydia, HIV), to more readily gain access to the upper genital tract. Attempts have been made to identify factors that inhibit H_2O_2-producing lactobacilli because these factors may be the origins of BV. Two recent studies report that H_2O_2-producing lactobacilli are not inhibited by the spermicidal contraceptive, nonoxynol-9,[43] or by antimicrobial agents frequently used to treat vaginal conditions.[44]

Behavioral risk factors associated with BV have been difficult to determine, in part due to the numerous potentially confounding factors. Table 11-2 lists new sexual partner as a factor often linked with BV. A recent study, which controls for multiple confounders, suggests that oral contraceptive use and condom use may be protective for BV when compared with use of an intrauterine device or no contraceptive use.[45] Diagnostic criteria for bacterial vaginosis are listed in Tables 11-3 and 11-4.

Treatment

Guidelines from the Centers for Disease Control and Prevention (CDC) recommend treating both nonpregnant and pregnant women who are troubled by symptoms of BV. It also suggests treating asymptomatic BV after invasive procedures such as endometrial biopsy, hysterectomy, insertion of intrauterine devices, cesarean sections, surgical abortion, and uterine curettage.[46] Tables 11-5 and 11-6 summarize treatment options.

NONPREGNANT WOMEN

Three treatment regiments (see Table 11-5) are commonly used and have been shown to be equally effective (75 to 85 percent cure rate 4 weeks posttreatment). They are metronidazole (Flagyl®) 500 mg orally bid, 7 days; clindamycin cream 2 percent intravaginally once a day, 7 days; and metronidazole gel 0.75 percent, intravaginally bid, 5 days. Abstinence from alcohol use when taking metronidazole in either form is recommended to avoid a possible disulfuram-like reaction. Clindamycin cream may weaken the integrity of latex in condoms or diaphragms, thereby reducing their efficacy.[46] It is recommended that women using these methods for birth control abstain from intercourse during treatment and for 2 to 3 days afterward.

PREGNANT AND LACTATING WOMEN

Drug doses used during pregnancy are lower. Systemic treatment is preferred, particularly in the second and third trimester because of concern for BV-related upper genital tract infections. Empirical evidence suggests that both systemic treatment and intravaginal treatment for BV relieve symptoms, but intravaginal treatment may not reduce the incidence of BV-associated preterm birth among high-risk women.[47] Table 11-6 provides treatment options recommended by the American College of Obstetricians and Gynecologists (ACOG) in 1996[48] and the CDC guidelines of 1998.[46] Alternative modalities include metronidazole 2 g orally in a single dose or oral clindamycin 300 mg bid for 7 days. A 1-month follow-up assessment is indicated to verify treatment success.

Recommendations for treatment of symptomatic BV in the first trimester vary, reflecting concerns about potential teratogenicity of metronidazole. Two recent meta-analyses of observational studies report no association between first trimester metronidazole and birth defects,[49,50] but summary 95 percent confidence intervals include the possibility of a 20 percent increase in risk.

ALTERNATIVE TREATMENTS

Flagyl ER™ 750 mg once a day for 7 days is proposed as an alternative regimen for BV treatment in nonpregnant women, but there are no comparative efficacy trials. Use of lactobacilli suppositories to reestablish a normal vaginal ecology in an effort to treat BV is being explored. In one randomized clinical trial, *Lactobacillus acidophilus* vaginal suppositories lowered BV prevalence at 7 to 10 days posttreatment but had no effect on BV prevalence assessed after a subsequent menses.[51] Hillier et al. identified *L. crispatus* as one species that, when introduced as an intravaginal capsule, can bind to vaginal epithelial cells. Women who had lower baseline levels of endogenous H_2O_2-producing lactobacilli and who refrained from sexual intercourse during treatment were most likely to establish successful colonization of *L. crispatus*.[52]

PERSISTENT OR RECURRING CASES

It is estimated that symptoms will reoccur within 3 months of treatment in 20 to 30 percent of nonpregnant women treated for BV.[53] Among a smaller subset of women, repeated BV treatment is unable to prevent frequently recurring symptoms. These women are more likely to harbor residual abnormalities (e.g., elevated pH, clue cells, imbalance of vaginal flora on Gram stain) even after symptoms subside in response to treatment.[54] One descriptive study noted that women with frequent BV episodes often experience recurrence after menstruation or episodes of VVC.[55] Treatment of recurrent BV has been unrewarding. In a small

Table 11-5

Treatment for Bacterial Vaginosis, Candida Vulvovaginitis, and Trichomonas Vaginitis

CLINICAL ENTITY	MEDICATION	STRENGTH	DOSAGE	EFFICACY	OTC	COST*
Bacterial vaginosis	Metronidazole	500-mg tablet	1 PO bid x 7 days, 4 tablets PO once	87–97%	No	$ 5.70 $ 2.00
	Clindamycin	2% vaginal cream	1 applicatorful in vagina q hs x 7 d	72–94%	No	$23.50
Resistant or recurrent cases of bacterial vaginosis	Metronidazole Clindamycin	0.75% vaginal gel 300-mg tablets	5 g in vagina bid x 5 d 1 PO bid x 7–14 d	79% at 2 wk 94%	No No	$29.71 $13.59–27.17
	Acute regimens above	See above	Extend the course to 14 d	Little data available	No	—
	Povidone-iodine gel or suppositories	5 g	In vagina x 14–28 d	No data found	No	—
Candida vulvovaginitis	Miconazole	200-mg vaginal suppository	1 in vagina q hs x 3 d	—	Yes	$20.89
		2% vaginal cream	1 applicatorful in vagina q hs x 7 d	66%	Yes	$ 7.65
		100-mg vaginal suppository	1 in vagina q hs x 7 d	—	Yes	$11.95
	Clotrimazole	1% vaginal cream	1 applicatorful in vagina q hs x 7 d	—	Yes	$ 9.21
	Butoconazole	2% vaginal cream	1 applicatorful in vagina q hs x 3 d	81–92%; may be useful in non-*C. albicans* species	Yes	$10.39
	Terconazole	80-mg vaginal suppository	1 in vagina q hs x 3 d	See below	No	$17.75
		0.8% vaginal cream	1 applicatorful in vagina q hs x 3 d	In vitro, less effective in non-*C. albicans*	No	$17.75
		0.4% vaginal cream	1 applicatorful in vagina q hs x 7 d	See above	No	$19.75
	Tioconazole	6.5% vaginal ointment	1 applicatorful in vagina once	Note: ointment base will melt or dissolve condoms! Avoid intercourse with condoms for 3 d after use.	Yes	$14.39
	Fluconazole Itraconazole	150-mg tablet 100-mg tablet	1 tablet orally once 2 tablets PO qd x 3 d	56– 98% 74–85% short-term and 51–85% long-term	No No	$ 9.00 $34.06

Table 11-5

Treatment for Bacterial Vaginosis, Candida Vulvovaginitis, and Trichomonas Vaginitis (*Continued.*)

CLINICAL ENTITY	MEDICATION	STRENGTH	DOSAGE	EFFICACY	OTC	COST*
Persistent or recurrent cases of *Candida* vulvovaginitis	Topical treatments above	See above	Prolong the course to 14–21 d	—	Varies	See above
	Oral regimens above	See above	Extended dosing regimens are being studied	No data available	No	See above
	Boric acid†	600 mg in vaginal suppository	1 intravaginally bid for 14 d	Limited data, but anecdotal reports common	No	—
	Terconazole	0.8% vaginal cream	Weekly applicatorful intravaginally	Decreased to 4 episodes per 10 women over 6 mo	No	$26.63/month
Maintenance regimens for recurrent *Candida* vulvovaginitis	Fluconazole or itraconazole	No data available	—	No data available	No	—
	Oral yogurt	Culture positive (10^8/mL) for H_2O_2-producing lactobacilli	240 g (8 oz) daily	0.38 episodes/6 mo compared to 2.54 for placebo	Yes	—
Trichomonas vaginitis	Metronidazole	500 mg	4 tablets PO once for patient and partner(s)	80–90%	No	$2.00/person
Resistant or recurrent cases of *Trichomonas* vaginitis	Metronidazole	500 mg	1 tablet PO bid x 7 d	80–90%	No	$5.70
	Metronidazole	500 mg	Prolong the course to bid 14 or 21 d, and/or increase the dosage to as high as 1500 mg bid	May add intravaginal gel as adjunct	No	$6.00–10.00
	Adjuncts to metronidazole above	Acetic acid vaginal wash 3% or 10% solution	2 x/week	Unknown	No	—
		Povidone-iodine douche‡	Twice a day for 4 days repeated in 2 weeks or 28-day course	92% response to a 28-day course of povidone-iodine suppositories	Yes	$4.00 per douche

*Prices are from the First Data Bank as of April, 1999; cost to the pharmacy.

†Not generally available, can be compounded by pharmacist on request.

‡This item priced from *1998 Drug Topics Redbook*, Montvale, NJ: Medical Economics Data.

SOURCE: Modified with permission from Reed BD: Vaginitis. In: Sloane PD, Slatt LM, Curtis P, Ebell MH (eds): *Essentials of Family Medicine*, 3rd ed. Baltimore: Williams & Wilkins, 1998:662–663.

Table 11-6

Treatment of Vaginal Conditions During Pregnancy and Lactation*

	1ST TRIMESTER	2ND–3RD TRIMESTER	LACTATION
Bacterial vaginosis	Oral clindamycin 300 mg bid for 7 d	Metronidazole 250 mg orally tid for 7 d	Clindamycin cream 2% intravaginally once a day for 7 d
Vulvovaginal candidiasis	Miconazole, butoconazole, terconazole, and clotrimazole topical preparations. 1 applicatorful in vagina and apply externally to labia q hs.[†] Avoid oral medications.	Miconazole, butoconazole, terconazole, and clotrimazole, topical preparations. 1 applicatorful in vagina and apply externally to labia q hs.[†] Avoid oral medications.	Same topical preparations listed for use in pregnancy. May also use tioconazole. 1 applicatorful in vagina and apply externally to labia q hs. Avoid oral medications.
Trichomonas[‡]		Metronidazole 2 g orally, single dose	Metronidazole 2 g orally, single dose, No breast feeding 12–24 h[83]

*Pregnancy categories: B, clindamycin PO and vaginal, metronidazole (trimesters two and three), clotrimazole; C, miconazole, butoconazole, and terconazole. All four of the antifungal topical preparations are listed in the above table because they are recommended in the CDC 1998 treatment guidelines.[46]
[†]Seven to 14 days are recommended.[46,82]
[‡]See text about treatment in 1st trimester and alternative vaginal treatments.

clinical trial, 0.75 percent metronidazole vaginal gel was applied on 2 nonconsecutive days each week for 3 consecutive months; five of six women receiving this treatment were free of BV during the 3-month maintenance phase. However, when treatment was discontinued BV recurred.[56]

Areas of Controversy

Overall, there is a lack of consensus regarding public health strategies for BV. Development of coherent strategies is complicated because: (1) BV is often asymptomatic; (2) the health consequences of asymptomatic BV in nonpregnant and pregnant women are still being studied; (3) BV can be intermittent,[57] with women passing through transitional states of vaginal flora imbalance that may or may not progress to full BV; (4) BV can recur following treatment and spontaneously regress without treatment[55]; (5) in some populations, the prevalence of BV exceeds 20 percent, raising questions about the definitions of normal and abnormal; and (6) there is limited understanding of factors that precipitate BV episodes.

SCREENING NONPREGNANT WOMEN

Up to 50 percent of women who are positive for BV are asymptomatic.[32,58] Little is known about differences between asymptomatic and symptomatic BV with respect to associated adverse health outcomes. Observational studies have reported a link between BV and PID,[12] endometritis,[11] and ectopic pregnancy.[13] It is difficult to conduct clinical trials to test the benefit of BV screening and treatment to prevent PID and endometritis because these conditions are not common, can remain subclinical, and often require invasive techniques to ascertain or confirm the diagnosis. Some clinicians advise routine BV screening for all nonpregnant women of childbearing age, but neither the ACOG nor the CDC advocates this approach.[46,48]

SCREENING PREGNANT WOMEN

The majority of observational studies find that BV diagnosed in pregnancy is associated with an increased risk of preterm delivery.[16,59–61] One study, which used repeat BV screening in pregnancy, demonstrated an elevated risk of preterm birth for both women with persistent BV and women with BV that spontaneously resolved.[62] Because BV is reported to be more prevalent among African American women compared to non-African American women (23 vs 9 percent, respectively),[63] there is speculation that differences in the prevalence of BV may explain up to 40 percent of the difference in preterm delivery rates between African Americans and whites.[64]

Results from clinical trials aimed at treating BV during pregnancy to lower the risk of preterm delivery have been inconsistent. Table 11-7 gives results from four placebo-controlled randomized trials, each with varying systemic treatment protocols. In three of four trials, treatment of BV in *high-risk* pregnant women (previous preterm birth or low pre-pregnancy weight) significantly lowered the risk of preterm delivery.[65–67] However, one trial failed to analyze all women as randomized,[65] and another trial based results on a subgroup analysis.[66] Two of the trials included high- and low-risk asymptomatic women with BV. Both reported that BV treatment in low-risk pregnant women had no significant effect on the rates of preterm delivery.[67,68] Although some clinicians advocate unselected screening for BV in pregnancy,[69] the most recent CDC guidelines,[46] which

were formulated before the negative results of the National Institute of Child Health and Human Development clinical trial, do not recommend BV screening of low-risk pregnant women.[68] With respect to high-risk pregnant women, the CDC guidelines are somewhat noncommittal, stating "high-risk pregnant women who do not have symptoms of BV may be evaluated for treatment."

SEXUAL TRANSMISSION

It remains uncertain whether the condition of BV can develop as a result of sexual transmission. Evidence in favor of transmission includes the finding of BV organisms in the male genitourinary tract,[70,71] a study showing BV concordance among lesbian partners,[72] and studies reporting that BV is associated with having a new sexual partner.[38] Evidence against transmission includes documentation of BV among women who are not sexually active[73] and the ineffectiveness of preventing BV recurrence by treating partners.[74,75] The 1998 CDC guidelines do not recommend routine treatment of sexual partners for BV.[46]

VAGINAL DOUCHING

It has been hypothesized that vaginal douching may influence both growth and ascent of vaginal flora leading to an excess of upper genital tract infections.[76] In a study of 182 women first seen at a STD clinic and followed longitudinally for 2 years, "douching for cleanliness" was positively associated with BV after controlling for age, ethnicity, antibiotic use, and methods of birth control.[38] This observational study was based on a select, high-risk population and did not report on types of douches or on factors that may modify the douching-BV link (e.g., timing of douching in relation to intercourse or menstrual cycle, condom use). Associations between douching and BV are not necessarily causal and may be the result of confounding by social and personal factors related to douching, BV, and adverse health outcomes. Alternatively, BV-related symptoms may promote the use of douches, though women report their motivations to douche

Table 11-7

Randomized Placebo-Controlled Trials for Treatment of Bacterial Vaginosis in Pregnancy to Prevent Preterm Delivery

STUDY	POPULATION	TREATMENT	TIMING OF TREATMENT	RESULTS PRETERM DELIVERY (PTD)
Morales et al.[65] N = 80	High-risk BV+ (previous spontaneous preterm birth)	Metronidazole (250 mg tid for 7 d)	Once between 13–20 wk	**Among BV+ high risk:** 18% PTD in treated* 39% PTD in placebo
Hauth et al.[66] N = 624	High-risk women (previous spontaneous preterm birth or low pre-pregnancy weight)	Metronidazole (250 mg tid for 7 d) and erythromycin (333 mg tid for 14 d)	Once at 22–24 wk Again if BV + at 2–4 w after initial treatment	**Among BV+ high risk:** 31% PTD in treated* 49% PTD in placebo
McDonald et al.[67] N = 879	Asymptomatic, heavy *G. vaginalis* or BV+ on Gram stain: Low risk and High risk (previous spontaneous preterm birth)	Metronidazole (400 mg bid for 2 d)	Once at 24 wks Again if BV + at 4 wk after initial treatment	**Overall:** 7.2% PTD in treated 7.5% PTD in placebo **Among BV+ Gram:** 4.5% PTD in treated 6.3% PTD in placebo **Among high risk:** 9.1% PTD in treated* 41.7% PTD in placebo
NICHD Maternal Fetal Medicine Unit Network 1998[68] N = 1953	Asymptomatic BV+: Low risk and High risk (previous preterm birth)	Metronidazole (2 g repeated at 48 h)	Once at 16–23 wk Repeated at 24–29 wk	**Overall:** 12.2% PTD in treated 12.4% PTD in placebo **Among BV+ high risk:** 29.7% PTD in treated 23.9% PTD placebo

*P < .05.

ABBREVIATIONS: BV+, BV positive; NICHD, National Institute of Child Health and Human Development.

as a more general regard for hygiene. In one of the few published studies of its kind, Onderdonk et al. conducted an experiment in which women were instructed to douche alternately with physiologic saline (control group), 0.04 percent acetic acid, and 0.30 percent providone-iodine and were monitored for vaginal flora. Results showed that only the iodine-based douche significantly reduced the levels of vaginal lactobacillus, the normally dominant microorganism.[77]

Vulvovaginal Candidiasis

Background

Approximately 20 percent of asymptomatic healthy women of childbearing age have vaginal colonization with *C. albicans*, and VVC is the second most common of the vulvovaginal conditions (BV is first). Although most cases of VVC are caused by *C. albicans*, the proportion of nonalbicans *Candida* species has increased to 20 to 35 percent in recent years. Nonalbicans *Candida* species are often more resistant to conventional antifungal therapy. In addition to the risk factors listed in Table 11-2, VVC is also associated with local allergy or hypersensitivity reactions[78] and with a decreased proliferative response of T cells to candidal stimulation, suggesting the importance of host immune factors.[79]

Although VVC is usually considered not to be life-threatening, fatal fetal candidal sepsis has been reported.[80] The inflammatory status that often accompanies VVC can also increase the likelihood of infection after exposure to HIV or hepatitis B. Diagnostic criteria for VVC are listed in Table 11-3.

Treatment

Nonpregnant Women

Topical agents remain appropriate first-line treatment to minimize the potential for adverse reactions and drug interactions (see Table 11-5). A number of preparations are formulated as creams, suppositories, and vaginal tablets. Clinical and mycologic cure rates are 85 to 90 percent with the use of imidazole and triazole derivatives; nystatin (a polyene) has a somewhat lower cure rate of 75 to 80 percent. *C. tropicalis* and *C. glabrata* can be 10 times less sensitive to the older imidazoles than *C. albicans*. Terconazole (Terazol®) is more effective against nonalbicans *Candida* species than the imidazoles and is equally efficacious in the treatment of *C. albicans* infections. However, terconazole is significantly more expensive than the other agents (see Table 11-5), and it is not available as a nonprescription agent.

Previous treatment regimens lasted 7 to 14 days. More recently, additional regimens have become available that are considered equally efficacious and last 1 to 3 days.[9] Tioconazole is the only one-dose topical treatment. Persistence of effective drug concentrations in the vagina results in similar cure rates when compared to 7-day regimens. Treatment regimens including an antifungal cream will result in more rapid relief of labial symptoms. Treatment of severe vulvitis may also include low-potency topical corticosteroids or sitz baths with sodium bicarbonate.[9] All of the topical antifungal preparations are oil based and have the potential to weaken latex condoms and diaphragms.

Oral antifungal agents should rarely be used as first-line treatments. These agents should be reserved for severe, persistent VVC in patients who have been compliant with courses of topical antifungal therapy. Side effects are minimal with topical agents (3 to 7 percent of users) and are for the most part limited to local reactions to the vehicle.[20] However, terconazole has also been associated with headache (21 to 30 percent) and dysmenorrhea (6 percent).[81] Adverse effects reported most often with oral therapy are gastrointestinal symptoms in 5 to 10 percent.[82] Isolated reports of angioedema and anaphylaxis are associated with fluconazole, and hepatotoxicity has been reported with ketoconazole therapy. Significant drug interactions can result when oral azoles are combined with other medications as listed in Table 11-8.[82]

PREGNANT AND LACTATING WOMEN

According to Sobel, a noted authority in vaginitis, "VVC is considered to be more common and difficult to eradicate during pregnancy; however, no recent studies have been performed and the original studies suffered methodologic flaws."[9] The hormonal milieu of late pregnancy results in an increased glycogen concentration in vaginal epithelial cells and secretions, enhancing conditions for overgrowth of *Candida* species. An additional possible mechanism for VVC in pregnancy is the presence of estrogen and progesterone receptors in candidal cells, which result in enhanced proliferation when stimulated.[79] Women with pregestational or gestational diabetes during pregnancy are at even higher risk for VVC. Topical agents are safe in pregnancy and lactation, but oral antifungal agents are contraindicated. Those topical agents with the longest safety record are included in Table 11-6.[83]

Several cases of congenital abnormalities have been reported in children of women who received oral fluconazole during pregnancy.[84]

ALTERNATIVE TREATMENTS

The *Encyclopedia of Natural Medicine* offers several alternative approaches to treating VVC.[85] Not all of these treatments have been evaluated for efficacy through clinical trials. Reestablishing an adequate presence of H_2O_2-producing lactobacilli may be an alternative to antifungal use (see BV alternative treatment). Gentian violet is another traditional treatment. A tampon can be soaked in gentian violet solution and inserted into the vagina. In addition, the vulva can be painted with the solution. One treatment is usually sufficient. Gentian violet is now rarely used because it stains clothing.

In a 1-year cross-over clinical trial, daily oral ingestion of 8 oz of yogurt containing active cultures

Table 11-8

Examples of Drug Interactions with Oral Azoles

DRUG	EFFECT WHEN TAKEN WITH AZOLES
Antacids	Decreased azole levels
Anticoagulants	Increased anticoagulant levels
Astemizole (Hismanal)	Arrhythmia, including torsades de pointes
Carbamazepine (Tegretol)	Decreased itraconazole levels
Cimetidine (Tagamet)	Increased itraconazole levels; decreased ketoconazole levels
Cyclosporine (Sandimmune)	Increased cyclosporine levels
Digoxin (Lanoxin)	Increased digoxin levels
Hydrochlorothiazide	Increased terconazole levels
Histamine H_2-receptor antagonists	Decreased absorption of itraconazole and ketoconazole
Hypoglycemics (oral)	Increased level of hypoglycemic agent
Isoniazid (Laniazid)	Increased ketoconazole, itraconazole levels
Methylprednisolone (Medrol)	Increased plasma concentration of methylprednisolone
Omeprazole (Prilosec)	Decreased absorption of itraconazole and ketoconazole
Oral contraceptives	Decreased contraceptive levels
Phenytoin (Dilantin)	Increased phenytoin levels; decreased itraconazole levels; increased or decreased ketoconazole levels
Rifampin (Rifadin, Rimactane)	Decreased rifampin and azole levels
Theophylline	With fluconazole, increased level of theophylline; with ketoconazole, increased or decreased level of theophylline

SOURCE: Modified with permission from Tobin MJ: Vulvovaginal candidiasis: topical vs. oral therapy. *Am Fam Physician* 51:1719, 1995.

of *L. acidophilus* significantly decreased both candidal colonization and symptoms in 13 women with RVVC. Of note is that 8 women were dropped from the study for refusing to change from the yogurt arm to the nonyogurt arm of the study because of the dramatic symptomatic relief they experienced while eating the yogurt.[86]

PERSISTENT OR RECURRING CASES

Failure to resolve symptoms after an initial course of therapy will occur. Possible causes include noncompliance with the regimen, presence of a mixed infection (most commonly BV and VVC), presence of *Candida* species other than *C. albicans,* sexual reinfection (controversial), and presence of host factors such as immunodeficiency or uncontrolled diabetes. A longer course of topical treatment for 14 to 21 days is then indicated in addition to eliminating cofactors such as hyperglycemia.

Recurrent VVC is defined as four or more microscopically or culture-confirmed episodes in 1 year. Associated risks for recurrence include HIV infection, inadequately controlled diabetes mellitus, cancer chemotherapy, or immunosuppressive therapy.[87] However, in most women the cause of recurrence is not found. RVVC should be treated aggressively with a 14-day course of a topical or oral azole, followed by a maintenance regimen for at least 6 months. In addition to the maintenance regimens in Table 11-5, Sobel suggests the following oral options: ketoconazole 100-mg tablet once per day, itraconazole 50- or 100-mg tablet once per day, fluconazole 100-mg tablet once per week, all for a 6-month period.[87] A small percentage of women may require maintenance azole regimens for several years.[9]

A retrospective review of vaginal boric acid treatment (600 mg/d, 14 days) in a series of patients with *C. glabrata* vaginitis for whom repeated courses of antimycotic therapy with topical and systemic azoles had failed revealed clinical improvement or cure in 21 (86 percent) of 26 episodes and mycologic eradication in 20 of 26 episodes.[88]

The *Encyclopedia of Natural Medicine* also lists boric acid as an alternative treatment for chronic or recurrent VVC (600-mg vaginal suppository capsules, twice a day for 4 months, and may be continued thereafter during menstruation).[85] This treatment has the distinction of being considered "old," "alternative," or "emerging as a promising modality of therapy." Side effects from using boric acid are rare but may include burning of the labia due to boric acid leaking out of the vagina. If this occurs reduce the dose or discontinue use. Women should be advised to refrain from genital sexual activity while using boric acid.

There may be uncommon underlying causes of RVVC. A 38-year-old woman carrier of biotinidase deficiency, with a 14-month history of RVVC despite appropriate therapy, had resolution of symptoms within 2 months of starting pharmacologic doses of biotin (20 mg/d). The carrier rate of this enzyme deficiency is about 1/123 individuals. A trial of biotin or checking the level of biotinidase activity may be warranted in some cases of RVVC.[89]

A study of in vitro lymphocyte proliferative responses demonstrated that in response to *Candida,* macrophages from some women with RVVC produce a prostaglandin that blocks the lymphocyte proliferation response to this organism.[90] Therefore, cotreatment with prostaglandin inhibitor may be indicated in a subgroup of women with RVVC, although no substantive studies have been done to date.

Considerations for Special Populations

DIABETES

Inadequately controlled diabetes mellitus type 1 or 2 is a predisposing factor for VVC. Hyperglycemia can enhance production of protein surface receptors on *C. albicans* organisms that subvert phagocytosis by neutrophils, making VVC more difficult to eradicate.[91] A 14-day course of antifungal topical therapy may be indicated in a woman with uncontrolled diabetes mellitus.

ELDERLY WOMEN

A significant proportion of elderly women may be hesitant to discuss issues related to the genital tract; asking very specific questions about symptoms is crucial. Memory impairment may also limit the validity of the history. The past medical history should be reviewed for factors that would increase the likelihood of VVC, such as diabetes mellitus or glucose intolerance, or conditions such as arthritis or paresis that would impair performance of adequate perineal hygiene.[92] Symptoms consistent with VVC may, in elderly women, be due to atrophic vaginitis (see Chap. 4). Medications such as broad-spectrum antibiotics or corticosteroids can increase the risk for VVC.

Areas of Controversy

SELF-TREATMENT

Because several topical antifungals are now available as nonprescription over-the-counter (OTC) preparations, women may choose to self-medicate without consulting a health care provider. In reality, a number of women have always self-medicated VVC, sometimes by choice, but often because of inaccessibility (financial or geographic) of health care. The overall effect of self-diagnosis and treatment on this disease remains unclear. However, the study by Ferris et al. does confirm the impression that women are likely to use OTC antifungals inappropriately at times to treat more serious gynecologic conditions.[93]

Protection against improper treatment of vaginal symptoms is provided by improved patient education by primary care providers and pharmacists. Women should be able to describe their symptoms by telephone and get appropriate advice as to the advisability of self-treatment versus an office visit. When self-treatment is advisable, patients should be reminded that vaginal antifungals can weaken the integrity of the latex in condoms and diaphragms.[94] It is recommended that women using these methods for birth control abstain from intercourse during treatment and for 2 to 3 days afterward. Women with first or atypical VVC episodes and pregnant women should always be evaluated in the office. Women who have had a pelvic examination within the last 2 years and who have had VVC previously diagnosed in the office and now have symptoms consistent with VVC can usually be safely treated via a telephone call.

TOPICAL VERSUS ORAL TREATMENT

There is an increasing trend, fueled by patient demand, for one dose of fluconazole (Diflucan®) orally as the preferred treatment for even episodic, mild cases of VVC. Indiscriminate use of this agent will result in higher numbers of fluconazole-resistant infections as well as adverse drug effects and drug interactions. It is extremely important that health care providers support the use of topical products for the treatment of the vast majority of episodes of VVC.

SEXUAL TRANSMISSION

Evidence both supports and refutes sexual transmission of VVC.[95] Nearly 10 percent of men examined after sexual contact with women harboring yeast infections developed mycotic balanitis. There is a fourfold increase in yeast colonization in male partners of infected women, and there is isolation of same strains from infected couples. In contrast, there is no direct association between yeast infection and other STDs. Routine treatment of the male partner does not affect cure or recurrence rates in the female. In a study of college women, neither beginning a new relationship nor having multiple sexual partners in a 4-week period was associated with candidiasis after controlling for frequency of sexual intercourse.[96]

ASSOCIATION OF RECURRENT VULVOVAGINAL CANDIDIASIS AND HIV INFECTION

There is an association of RVVC with the impaired cell-mediated immunity of advanced

HIV infection. This should not be misconstrued to imply that all women with RVVC have an underlying HIV infection. However, RVVC is a valid indicator for considering HIV screening.

Trichomoniasis

Background

Trichomoniasis, caused by the protozoan *T. vaginalis*, is primarily transmitted through sexual intercourse. It has been reported that 20 to 50 percent of women with vaginal trichomonads may be asymptomatic.[97] Diagnostic criteria for trichomoniasis are listed in Table 11-3.

Treatment

NONPREGNANT WOMEN

The recommended treatment is metronidazole (Flagyl®) 2 g orally as a single dose (see Table 11-5). If this regimen fails, an alternative is metronidazole 500 mg bid for 7 days. Sexual partners, both men and women, should be treated simultaneously. Clinical cure rates after treatment are comparable for the two regimens (82 to 90 percent), but recurrence rates may be slightly higher with the single dose.[87] As with treatment for BV, women should refrain from alcohol use when taking metronidazole. Women should also be advised to refrain from intercourse until they and their sex partners have completed treatment and are asymptomatic. Advantages of single-dose metronidazole include greater compliance and lower risk of VVC superinfection.

PREGNANT AND LACTATING WOMEN

Because of concern about the teratogenicity of metronidazole, it is typically not prescribed for

women with trichomoniasis in their first trimester (see section on treatment of BV during pregnancy). Women in the second and third trimesters may follow the same treatment regimen as that for nonpregnant women (see Table 11-6).

PERSISTENT OR RECURRING CASES

In the case where women and their sexual partners comply with treatment regimens but fail to clear the trichomoniasis, a culture is indicated to assess drug sensitivity of the organism. Treatment with higher doses of metronidazole has been recommended for these patients (see Table 11-5). There are literature reports of successful treatment of recurrent *T. vaginalis* with paromomycin (250 mg daily for 5 days) suspended in Unguentum Merck and applied intravaginally,[98] and with a combination zinc sulfate douche (1 percent) and metronidazole (500-mg suppository bid and 200 to 400 mg tid orally up to 10 days).[99] Both reports noted that women experienced vaginal irritation secondary to intravaginal treatments. In addition, these therapeutic regimens have not been evaluated using rigorous clinical trial methods; thus, their safety and efficacy remain questionable.

Areas of Controversy

ADVERSE PREGNANCY OUTCOMES

Reports on the relationship between *T. vaginalis* and risk of preterm birth remain inconsistent. The preterm prediction study reported no association.[100] A recent analysis of the Vaginal Infections in Pregnancy (VIP) study showed a modest increase in risk, even after controlling for the presence of BV (adjusted odds ratio =1.3, 95 percent CI 1.1 to 1.4).[10] In the VIP study, the greatest risk of preterm birth (17.3 percent) was among women with both *T. vaginalis* and BV.

Other Causes of Vulvar and Vaginal Disease

Although most cases of vulvovaginal disease are caused by BV, VVC, and trichomoniasis, clinicians should be alert to the possibility of other causes. These include vulvar vestibulitis syndrome (VVS), cyclic vulvovaginitis, cytolitic vaginosis, dysesthetic vulvodynia, skin disorders of the vulva and perineum, and atrophic vaginitis.

Vulvar Vestibulitis Syndrome

Vulvar vestibulitis syndrome is the most common manifestation of vulvodynia, that is, chronic vulvar discomfort often characterized by burning, stinging, irritation, or rawness.[101] In addition, women with VVS also report entry dyspareunia and variable degrees of vestibular erythema. The hallmark physical finding is a report of sharp pain when touching the vulvar vestibulum with a moist cotton swab (sometimes called a positive swab test), with maximal tenderness usually at the 5 o'clock and 7 o'clock positions. The etiology remains unknown. Previous studies have shown an association between human papillomavirus (HPV) infection and VVS. In more recent studies, there is no evidence of HPV being causally linked to VVS.[102]

Treatments for VVS have been unsatisfactory. Topical local anesthetics such as 2 to 5 percent lidocaine applied for 4 to 5 min before coitus may be sufficient treatment for women whose symptoms are limited to entry dyspareunia. In a retrospective case series, 23 patients with VVS were asked to massage the tender areas at least six times a day with alternating applications of Topicort 0.25 percent and either mupirocin (Bactroban) 2.5 percent ointment or erythromycin ophthalmic ointment for at least 1 week or until symptoms abated (median of 3 weeks).[103] Seventeen women responded successfully with complete resolution of their symptoms. Seven women had a recurrence more than 3 months later; reapplication of the therapy had a 100 percent cure rate. Albeit a small study, this is encouraging because this conservative therapy has a success rate at least as high as that reported for invasive treatment modalities such as cryotherapy or perineoplasty of the affected areas.

As with RVVC, underlying causes are occasionally identified. A 32-year-old woman with disabling VVS for more than 2 years despite multiple medical and surgical interventions was found to have transient hyperoxaluria; microscopic oxalate crystalluria and elevated vaginal pH values often preceded her most severe symptoms. Oxalate crystals can cause severe burning and itching when in contact with epithelial surfaces. Calcium citrate given to modify oxalate crystalluria resulted in a significant decrease in pain in 3 months and total alleviation of symptoms after 1 year.[104] Assessments of the metabolic and biochemical factors associated with vulvodynia may be of significant benefit to patients with this disorder.

Cyclic Vulvovaginitis

In this condition, pain is cyclic, often worse during the luteal phase of the menstrual cycle; symptoms may flare up after intercourse, with the worst pain on the next day. The etiology is thought to be a hypersensitivity reaction to *C. albicans* antigen. Treatment with topical azoles for the portion of the luteal phase in which the woman is symptomatic and immediately after intercourse may be sufficient.[105] Prolonged maintenance therapy for 4 to 6 months with topical or oral antimycotics is usually effective if briefer therapy fails.[102]

Cytolytic Vaginosis

Cytolytic vaginosis[18,106] is another cause of cyclic symptoms that are more pronounced in the luteal phase. Although the exact pathophysiology is not known, it is thought to be caused by an overgrowth of the lactobacilli in the vagina, resulting in increased vaginal acidity, with subsequent cytolysis, vaginal discharge, and vulvovaginal irritation. Presenting symptoms are pruritus, dyspareunia, and vulvar dysuria. Physical examination is often similar to that found with VVC. Criteria for diagnosis include absence of *T. vaginalis, Candida,* or clue cells on wet mount with an increased number of lactobacilli; evidence of cytolysis of vaginal epithelial cells; and few white blood cells. The vaginal pH is between 3.5 and 4.5. Therapy includes using pads rather than tampons during menses, discontinuing any antifungal medications, and use of baking soda sitz baths (4 tablespoons in 1 to 2 inches of warm water) twice daily and vaginal douches of 30 to 60 g sodium bicarbonate in a liter of warm water two to three times a week while symptomatic, then every 1 to 3 weeks as needed.

Dysesthetic Vulvodynia

Other names for this entity are essential vulvodynia or pudendal neuralgia. This type of vulvodynia is more common in perimenopausal or postmenopausal women. The patient experiences a constant vulvar burning, often with associated urethral or rectal pain. A hyperesthesia is present and occasionally may be present in the absence of pain. The woman with pudendal neuralgia may report temporary or even permanent relief of symptoms after the stretching of the pudendal nerve during childbirth.[101] The diagnosis of dysesthetic vulvodynia is often one of exclusion. The treatment of choice is amytriptyline 10 mg at bedtime, increasing to 50 to 60 mg.

Skin Disorders

Lichen sclerosus can cause incapacitating pruritus or be asymptomatic. It is more common in elderly than in younger women and is characterized by white vulvar plaques, which are keratinized skin patches. The vulvar skin becomes thin; the labia minora may become atrophic and may fuse with the labia majora. Stenosis of the introitus may make intercourse difficult. Treatment consists of topical 2 percent testosterone

propionate in petrolatum applied bid for 1 to 2 weeks, then twice weekly indefinitely until the lesion resolves or testosterone side effects become problematic.[92]

Contact dermatitis to "feminine hygiene products," soaps, sanitary pads/diapers, and numerous other chemical irritants can cause tenderness, burning, and pruritus. Allergic dermatitis (delayed hypersensitivity reactions) may also cause vulvar symptoms. Removal of the irritant or allergen results in resolution of symptoms.

Atrophic Vaginitis

It is important to recognize that clinically significant atrophic vaginitis is uncommon among postmenopausal women. The majority of women with mild to moderate atrophy are asymptomatic. Atrophic vaginitis can also occur in the following situations: postpartum, especially with breastfeeding (progesterone dominant effect); in association with androgen-producing tumors; among infertility patients taking clomiphene citrate; during and after radiation therapy; with hypothyroidism; excessive exercise associated with amenorrhea; and use of selective estrogen receptor modulators (e.g., tamoxifen). For more information, see Chap. 4.

Patient Education

The following general measures to prevent vulvar/vaginal problems are adapted from the excellent lay resource, *Our Bodies, Ourselves for the New Century* by the Boston Women's Health Book Collective (New York, Simon and Schuster, 1998).

• Gently wash your vulva and anus regularly. Mineral oil is a good cleanser and does not dry out the tissues as soap tends to. Avoid feminine hygiene sprays and irritating soaps.

Avoid talcum powder because studies have linked it to ovarian cancer.[1]

- Always wipe your genital and anal area from front to back, so that bacteria from the anus will not get into the vagina or urethra.
- Make sure your sexual partners are clean. It is a good practice for a man to wash his penis daily and especially before making love. If you or your male partner are being treated for a genital infection, make sure he wears a condom during intercourse. Better yet, avoid intercourse until the infection has been cleared. (*Note:* polyurethane condoms should be worn if vaginal antifungals are used concurrently.)
- Use a sterile, water-soluble jelly if lubrication is needed during intercourse (something like K-Y Jelly or Astroglide, not Vaseline). Recent studies show that birth control spermicidal gels and creams, which usually contain nonoxynol-9, slow down the growth of trichomonads and possibly monilia (yeast). Using these products for lubrication or general prevention is a good idea, especially with a new partner. Most lubricants contain propylene glycol, which may cause irritation to a woman.
- Avoid any form of sexual activity that is painful or abrasive to your vagina.
- Avoid douching of any kind unless specifically recommended by your practitioner. Although you may "feel cleaner," this practice may destroy the "good bacteria" in your vagina.
- Take care of yourself. Not eating well or not resting enough makes you more susceptible to infection. Continue most of these beneficial practices—such as proper diet and rest—even after an infection has been treated.

Acknowledgment

Special acknowledgment is given to Barbara Reed MD, MSPH for Tables 11-2, 11-3, and 11-5.

References

1. Harlow BL: Perineal exposure to talc and ovarian cancer risk. *Obstet Gynecol* 80:19, 1992.
2. Grodstein F, Rothman KJ: Epidemiology of pelvic inflammatory disease. *Epidemiology* 5:234, 1945.
3. Schlech WF, Shands KN, Reingold AL, et al: Risk factors for development of toxic shock syndrome. Association with a tampon brand. *JAMA* 248:835, 1982.
4. Thomason JL, Gelbert SM, Scaglione NJ: Bacterial vaginosis: current review and indications for asymptomatic therapy. *Am J Obstet Gynecol* 165:1210, 1991.
5. Eschenbach DA, Hillier S, Critchlow C, et al: Diagnosis and clinical manifestations of bacterial vaginosis. *Am J Obstet Gynecol* 158:819, 1988.
6. Embree J, Caliando JJ, McCormack WM: Nonspecific vaginitis among women attending a sexually transmitted diseases clinic. *Sex Transm Dis* 11:81, 1984.
7. Schwebke JR, Hillier SL, Sobel JD, et al: Validity of the vaginal Gram stain for the diagnosis of bacterial vaginosis. *Obstet Gynecol* 88:573, 1996.
8. Hurley R: Recurrent candida infection. *Clin Obstet Gynaecol* 8:209, 1981.
9. Sobel JD, Faro S, Force RW, et al: Vulvovaginal candidiasis: epidemiologic, diagnostic, and therapeutic considerations. *Am J Obstet Gynecol* 178:203, 1998.
10. Cotch MF, Pastorek JG, Nugent RP, et al: Trichomonas vaginalis associated with low birth weight and preterm delivery. *Sex Transm Dis* 24:353, 1997.
11. Korn AP, Bolan G, Padian N, et al: Plasma cell endometritis in women with symptomatic bacterial vaginosis. *Obstet Gynecol* 85:387, 1995.
12. Sweet RL: Role of bacterial vaginosis in pelvic inflammatory diseases. *Clin Infect Dis* 20(suppl 2): S271, 1995.
13. Padian NE, Washington AE: Pelvic inflammatory disease: a brief overview. *Ann Epidemiol* 4:128, 1994.
14. Laga M, Manoka AT, Kivuvu M, et al: Non-ulcerative sexually transmitted diseases as risk factors for HIV-1 transmission in women: result from a cohort study. *AIDS* 7:95, 1993.
15. Sewankambo N, Gray RH, Wawer MJ, et al: HIV-1 infection associated with abnormal vaginal flora morphology and bacterial vaginosis. *Lancet* 350: 546, 1997.
16. Hillier SL, Nugent RP, Eschenbach DA, et al: Association between bacterial vaginosis and preterm

delivery of a low-birth-weight infant. *N Engl J Med* 333:1737, 1995.

17. Friedrich EG: Vaginitis. Am Fam Physician 28: 238, 1983.

18. Beckman CR, Ling FW, Herbert WN, et al (eds): Obstetrics and Gynecology, 3rd ed. Baltimore: Williams & Wilkins; 1998;324.

19. Huggins GR, Preti G: Vaginal odors and secretions. Clin Obstet Gynecol 24:355, 1981.

20. Reed BD: Vaginitis, In: Sloane PD, Slatt LM, Curtis P, Ebell MH (eds): *Essentials of Family Medicine,* 3rd ed. Baltimore: Williams & Wilkins; 1998;657.

21. Mclellan R, Spence MR, Brockman M, et al: The clinical diagnosis of trichomoniasis. *Obstet Gynecol* 60:30, 1982.

22. Ferris DG, Hendrich J, Payne PM, et al: Office laboratory diagnosis of vaginitis. *J Fam Pract* 41:575, 1995.

23. Cailouette JC, Sharp CF, Zimmerman GJ, et al: Vaginal pH as a marker for bacterial pathogens and menopausal status. *Am J Obstet Gynecol* 176:1270, 1997.

24. Amsel R, Totten PA, Spiegel CA, et al: Nonspecific vaginitis: diagnostic criteria and microbial and epidemiologic associations. *Am J Med* 74:14, 1983.

25. Krieger JN, Tam MR, Stevens CE, et al: Diagnosis of trichomoniasis: comparison of conventional wet-mount examination with cytologic studies, cultures, and monoclonal antibody staining of direct specimens. *JAMA* 259:1223, 1988.

26. Oriel JD, Partridge BM, Denny MJ, et al: Genital yeast infections. *BMJ* 4:761, 1972.

27. Schwebke JR, Morgan SC, Weiss HL: The use of sequential self-obtained vaginal smears for detecting changes in the vaginal flora. *Sex Transm Dis* 24:236, 1997.

28. Nugent RP, Krohn MA, Hillier SL: Reliability of diagnosing bacterial vaginosis is improved by a standardized method of Gram stain interpretation. *Am J Soc Microbiol* 29:297, 1991.

29. Wilkinson D, Ndovela N, Kharsany A, et al: Tampon sampling for diagnosis of bacterial vaginosis: a potentially useful way to detect genital infections. *J Clin Microbiol* 35:2408, 1997.

30. Ohlemeyer CL, Hornberger LL, Lynch DA, et al: Diagnosis of *Trichomonas vaginalis* in adolescent females: InPOUCH TV® culture versus wet-mount microscopy. *J Adolesc Health* 22:205, 1998.

31. Schwebke JR, Morgan SC, Pinson GB: Validity of self-obtained vaginal specimens for diagnosis of *Trichomonas. J Clin Microbiol* 35:1618, 1997.

32. Hillier SL: Diagnostic microbiology of bacterial vaginosis. *Am J Obstet Gynecol* 169:455, 1993.

33. Briselden AM, Hillier SL: Evaluation of Affirm VP microbial identification test for *Gardnerella vaginalis* and *Trichomonas vaginalis. J Clin Microbiol* 32:148, 1994.

34. DeMeo LR, Draper DL, McGregor JA, et al: Evaluation of deoxyribonucleic acid probe for the detection of *Trichomonas vaginalis* in vaginal secretions. *Am J Obstet Gynecol* 174:1339, 1996.

35. O'Dowd TC, West RR, Winterburn PJ, et al: Evaluation of a rapid diagnostic test for bacterial vaginosis. *Br J Obstet Gynaecol* 103:366, 1996.

36. Thorsen P, Jensen IP, Jeune B, et al: Few microorganisms associated with bacterial vaginosis may constitute the pathologic core: a population-based microbiologic study among 3596 pregnant women. *Am J Obstet Gynecol* 178:580, 1998.

37. Sobel JD: Bacterial vaginosis—an ecologic mystery. *Ann Intern Med* 111:551, 1989.

38. Hawes SE, Hillier SL, Benedetti J, et al: Hydrogen peroxide–producing lactobacilli and acquisition of vaginal infections. *J Clin Infect Dis* 174:1058, 1996.

39. Imseis HM, Grieg PC, Livengood GH, et al: Characterization of the inflammatory cytokines in the vagina during pregnancy and labor and with bacterial vaginosis. *J Soc Gynecol Invest* 4:90, 1997.

40. Platz-Christensen J, Mattsby-Baltzer I, Thomsen P, et al: Endotoxin and interleukin-1α in the cervical mucus and vaginal fluid of pregnant women with bacterial vaginosis. *Am J Obstet Gynecol* 169:1161, 1993.

41. Rein MF, Shih M, Miller JR, et al: Use of lactoferrin assay in the differential diagnosis of female genital tract infections and implications for the pathophysiology of bacterial vaginosis. *Sex Transm Dis* 23:517, 1996.

42. Hillier S: The vaginal microbial ecosystem and resistance to HIV. *AIDS Res Hum Retroviruses* 14: S17, 1998.

43. Richardson BA, Martin HL, Stevens CE, et al: Use of nonoxynol-9 and changes in vaginal lactobacilli. *J Infect Dis* 178:441, 1998.

44. Agnew KJ, Hillier SL: The effect of treatment regimens for vaginitis and cervicitis on vaginal colonization by lactobacilli. *Sex Transm Dis* 22:269, 1995.

45. Shoubnikova M, Hellberg D, Nilsson S, et al: Contraceptive use in women with bacterial vaginosis. *Contraception* 55:355, 1997.

46. Centers for Disease Control and Prevention: 1998 guidelines for treatment of sexually transmitted diseases. *MMWR* 47(RR-1):1, 1998.

47. McGregor JA, French KL, Jones W, et al: Bacterial vaginosis is associated with prematurity and vaginal fluid mucinase and sialidase: results from a controlled trial of topical clindamycin cream. *Am J Obstet Gynecol* 170:1048, 1998.

48. American College of Obstetricians and Gynecologists: *Technical Bulletin, Vaginitis.* 1996:226.

49. Burtin P, Taddio A, Ariburnu O, et al: Safety of metronidazole in pregnancy: a meta-analysis. *Am J Obstet Gynecol* 172:525, 1995.

50. Caro-Paton T, Carvajal A, de Diego IM, et al: Is metronidazole teratogenic? A meta-analysis. *Br J Clin Pharmacol* 44:170, 1997.

51. Hallen A, Jarstrand C, Pahlson C: Treatment of bacterial vaginosis with lactobacilli. *Sex Transm Dis* May-June:146, 1992.

52. Hillier SL, Krohn MA, Meyn L, et al: Recolonization and diagnosis with an exogenous strain of *Lactobacillus crispatus.* Second International Meeting on Bacterial Vaginosis, September 1998, Aspen, Colorado.

53. Blackwell AL, Fox AR, Philips I, et al: Anaerobic vaginosis (non-specific vaginitis): clinical, microbiological, and therapeutic findings. *Lancet* 2:1379, 1982.

54. Cook RL, Redondo-Lopez V, Schmitt C, et al: Clinical, microbiological, and biochemical factors in recurrent bacterial vaginosis. *J Clin Microbiol* 30:870, 1992.

55. Hay PE, Ugwumadu A, Chowns J: Sex, thrush, and bacterial vaginosis. *Int J STD AIDS* 8:603, 1997.

56. Sobel JD, Leaman D: Suppressive maintenance therapy of recurrent bacterial vaginosis utilizing 0.75 percent metronidazole vaginal gel. Second International Meeting on Bacterial Vaginosis, September 1998, Aspen, Colorado.

57. Priestly CJF, Dhar BJ, Goodwin L: What is normal vaginal flora? *Genitourin Med* 73:23, 1997.

58. Ferris DG, Hendrich J, Payne PM, et al: Office laboratory diagnosis of vaginitis. *J Fam Pract* 41:575, 1995.

59. Hay PE, Lamont RF, Taylor-Robinson D, et al: Abnormal bacterial colonization of the genital tract and subsequent preterm delivery and late miscarriage. *BMJ* 308:295, 1994.

60. Gravett MG, Nelson HP, Derouen T, et al: Independent associations of bacterial vaginosis and *Chlamydia trachomatis* infection with adverse pregnancy outcome. *JAMA* 256:1899, 1986.

61. McDonald HM, O'Loughlin JA, Jolley P, et al: Prenatal microbiological risk factors associated with preterm birth. *Br J Obstet Gynaecol* 99:190, 1992.

62. Gratacos E, Figueras F, Barranco M, et al: Spontaneous recovery of bacterial vaginosis during pregnancy is not associated with an improved perinatal outcome. *Acta Obstet Gynecol Scand* 77:37, 1998.

63. Goldenberg RL, Klebanoff MA, Nugent R, et al: VIP Prematurity Study Group. Bacterial colonization of the vagina during pregnancy in four ethnic groups. *Am J Obstet Gynecol* 174:1618, 1996.

64. Goldenberg R, Iams JD, Mercer BM, et al: The preterm prediction study: the value of new vs standard risk factors in predicting early and all spontaneous births. *Am J Public Health* 88:233, 1998.

65. Morales WJ, Schorr S, Albritton J: Effect of metronidazole in patients with preterm birth in preceding pregnancy and bacterial vaginosis: a placebo-controlled, double-blind study. *Am J Obstet Gynecol* 171:345, 1994.

66. Hauth JC, Goldenberg RL, Andrews WW, et al: Reduced incidence of preterm delivery with metronidazole and erythromycin in women with bacterial vaginosis. *N Engl J Med* 333:1732, 1995.

67. McDonald HM, O'Loughlin JAO, Vigneswaran R, et al: Impact of metronidazole therapy on preterm birth in women with bacterial vaginosis flora *(Gardnerella vaginalis)*: a randomized, placebo-controlled trial. *Br J Obstet Gynaecol* 104:1391, 1997.

68. Klebanoff M, Carey JC: Metronidazole did not prevent preterm birth in asymptomatic women with bacterial vaginosis. *Am J Obstet Gynecol* 180:S2, 1999.

69. McGregor JA, French JI: Prevention of preterm birth (letter). *N Engl J Med* 339:1858, 1998.

70. Burdge DR, Bowie WR, Chow AW: *Gardnerella vaginalis*–associated balanoposthitis. *Sex Transm Dis* 13:159, 1986.

71. Hillier SL, Rabe LK, Muller CH, et al: Relationship of bacteriologic characteristics to semen indices in men attending infertility clinic. *Obstet Gynecol* 75:800, 1990.

72. Berger B, Kolton S, Zenilmann J, et al: Bacterial vaginosis in lesbians: a sexually transmitted disease. *Clin Infect Dis* 21:1402, 1995.

73. Bump RC, Buesching WJ: Bacterial vaginosis in virginal and sexually active adolescent females: evidence against exclusive sexual transmission. *Am J Obstet Gynecol* 158:935, 1988.

74. Colli E, Landoni M, Parazzini F: Treatment of male partners and recurrence of bacterial vaginosis: a randomized trial. *Genitourin Med* 73:267, 1997.

75. Vejtorp M, Bollerup A, Vejtorp L, et al: Bacterial vaginosis: a double-blind randomized trial of the

effect of treatment of the sexual partner. *Br J Obstet Gynaecol* 98:920, 1988.

76. Scholes D, Stergachis A, Heiderich FE, et al: Vaginal douching and the risk of *C. trachomatis* infection (abstract). *Am J Epidemiol* 141:96, 1995.

77. Onderdonk AB, Delaney ML, Hinkson PL, et al: Quantitative and qualitative effects of douche preparations on vaginal microflora. *Obstet Gynecol* 80:333, 1992.

78. Faro SF, Apuzzio J, Bahannon N, et al: Treatment considerations in vulvovaginal candidiasis. *Female Patient* 22:21, 1997.

79. Reed BD: Risk factors of candida vulvovaginitis. *Obstet Gynecol Sur* 47:551, 1992.

80. Engelhart CM, van de Vijver NM, Nienhuis SJ, et al: Fetal candida sepsis at midgestation: a case report. *Eur J Obstet Gynecol Reprod Biol* 77:107, 1998.

81. *Drug Facts and Comparisons, 1999 Edition*. St. Louis, MO: Facts and Comparisons; 1999.

82. Tobin MJ: Vulvovaginal candidiasis: topical vs oral treatment. *Am Fam Physician* 51:1715, 1995.

83. Briggs GG, Freeman RK, Yaffe SJ: *Drugs in Pregnancy and Lactation,* 4th ed. Baltimore: Williams & Wilkins; 1994.

84. Pursley TJ, Blomquist IK, Abraham J, et al: Fluconazole-induced congenital anomalies in three infants. *Clin Infect Dis* 22:336, 1996.

85. Murray MT, Pizzorno JE: *Encyclopedia of Natural Medicine,* revised 2nd ed. Rocklin, CA: Prima Publishing; 1998.

86. Hilton E, Isenberg HD, Alperstein P, et al: Ingestion of yogurt containing *Lactobacillus acidophilus* as prophylaxis for candidal vaginitis. *Ann Intern Med* 116:353, 1992.

87. Sobel JD: Vaginitis. *N Engl J Med* 337:1897, 1997.

88. Sobel JD, Dhaim W: Treatment of *Torulopsis glabrata* vaginitis: retrospective review of boric acid therapy. *Clin Infect Dis* 24: 649, 1997.

89. Strom CM, Levine EM: Chronic vaginal candidiasis responsive to biotin therapy in a carrier of biotinidase deficiency. *Obstet Gynecol* 92:644, 1998.

90. Witkin SS, Hirsch J, Ledger WJ: A macrophage defect in women with recurrent *Candida* vaginitis and its reversal in vitro by prostaglandin inhibitors. *Am J Obstet Gynecol* 155:790, 1986.

91. Ryan KJ: *Candida, Aspergillus,* and other opportunistic fungi. In: Ryan KJ (ed): *Sherris Medical Microbiology,* 3rd ed. Norwalk, CT: Appleton & Lange, 1994;595.

92. Nathan L: Vulvovaginal disorders in elderly women. *Clin Obstet Gynecol* 39:933, 1996.

93. Ferris DG, Dekle C, Litaker MS: Women's use of over-the-counter antifungal medications for gynecologic symptoms. *J Fam Pract* 42:595, 1996.

94. Stewart F: Vaginal barriers. In: Hatcher RA, Trussell J, Stewart F, et al (eds): *Contraceptive Technology,* 17th ed. New York: Ardent Media; 1998;371.

95. Johnson CA: Vulvovaginal candidiasis. In: Johnson CA, Johnson BE, Murray JL, et al (eds): *Women's Health Care Handbook.* Philadelphia: Hanley and Belfus; 1996;239.

96. Foxman B: The epidemiology of vulvovaginal candidiasis: risk factors. *Am J Public Health* 80: 329, 1998.

97. Fouts AC, Kraus SJ: *Trichomonas vaginalis*: reevaluation of its clinical presentation and laboratory diagnosis. *J Infect Dis* 141:137, 1980.

98. Coelho DD: Metronidazole-resistant trichomoniasis successfully treated with paromomycin. *Genitourin Med* 73:397, 1997.

99. Houang ET, Ahmet Z, Lawrence AG: Successful treatment of four patients with recalcitrant vaginal trichomonas with a combination of zinc sulfate douche and metronidazole therapy. *Sex Transm Dis* 24:116, 1997.

100. Meis PJ, Goldenberg RL, Mercer B: The preterm prediction study: significance of vaginal infections. *Am J Obstet Gynecol* 173:1231, 1995.

101. Jones KD, Lehr ST: Vulvodynia: diagnostic techniques and treatment modalities. *Nurse Pract* 19:34, 1994.

102. Paavonen J: Vulvodynia—a complex syndrome of vulvar pain. *Acta Obstet Gynecol Scand* 74:243, 1995.

103. White CA, Wiseman BL: Vulvar vestibulitis: case series of conservative topical therapy. Unpublished manuscript.

104. Solomons CC, Melmed MH, Heitler SM: Calcium citrate for vulvar vestibulitis: a case report. *J Reprod Med* 36:879, 1991.

105. Fischer G, Spurrett B, Fischer A: The chronically symptomatic vulva: aetiology and management. *Br J Obstet Gynaecol* 102:773, 1995.

106. Cibley LJ, Cibley LJ: Cytoltic vaginosis. *Am J Obstet Gynecol* 165:1245, 1991.

Leslie A. Shimp
James F. Peggs

Chapter

12

Urinary Incontinence

Overview

Loss of bladder control is a problem that afflicts approximately 13 million women in the United States. It is defined by the Agency for Health Care Policy and Research (AHCPR) Clinical Guideline Panel as "involuntary loss of urine which is sufficient to be a problem."[1]

Prevalence

The prevalence of urinary incontinence among women 15 to 64 years of age is 10 to 30 percent, increasing further with advancing age. Urinary incontinence is most common among homebound and institutionalized elderly, with 40 to 53 percent of these elderly affected.[1,2] In fact, urinary incontinence is among the most common reasons for nursing home admission.[1] Among community-dwelling women, prevalence estimates vary widely based on the age of population surveyed and the frequency criteria used to denote incontinence (e.g., ever experienced urinary incontinence versus number of episodes within a certain time period).[3]

A summary of various studies suggests that urinary incontinence is five to six times more prevalent among younger community-dwelling women than among younger men. However, it is only about twice as common among older women compared to men among those who reside in the community. One community survey of people over the age of 60 years revealed a prevalence among women of 38 percent; many of these patients (25 to 30 percent) reported daily or weekly episodes of incontinence.[4] Urinary incontinence is not a condition that affects only elderly women. In one study of 20,000 patients age 5 years or older, at least 15 percent of women in each decade of life reported this condition.[5]

Relationship to Exercise

Nygaard and DeLancey have studied the relationship between exercise and urinary incontinence and found that among women with an average age of 39 years, 47 percent of those who were regular exercisers reported experiencing some degree of urinary incontinence.[6] Among nulliparous varsity university athletes (mean age 20 years), 28 percent experienced urine loss while participating in their sport.[7] Exercise activities that resulted in incontinence were typically high impact, such as jumping and running. The percent of women experiencing incontinence during various sports is shown in Table 12-1.

Barriers to Diagnosis

Despite its high prevalence, urinary incontinence remains an underreported and underdiagnosed problem. Physicians do not routinely ask about urinary incontinence[8]; most primary care physicians ask fewer than 25 percent of their elderly patients about it.[9] It is equally uncommon for patients to volunteer this information to their health care providers. It has been estimated that less than half of community-dwelling persons with urinary incontinence consult a health care provider about this problem.[1] Studies have shown that 33 to 45 percent of patients with urinary incontinence had never mentioned their symptoms to a physician.[10,11] Further, women seem less likely than men to see a physician for urinary symptoms; in one study 29 percent of men sought care for this symptom, whereas only 13 percent of women did.[12]

A major reason for the lack of self-reporting is embarrassment about hygiene and odor.[13] Such embarrassment may powerfully inhibit social relationships and activities. The psychosocial impact of urinary incontinence may include a decrease in excursions outside the home, troubled family and social interactions, and decreased sexual activity.[14,15] One study found that 19.4 percent of women with urinary incontinence abstained from social activities because of the condition; 14 percent of women described urinary incontinence as a social problem and 60 percent described it as a hygienic problem.[5] Restrictions in social activities were greater for women with more severe leakage

Table 12-1

Relationship Between Types of Exercise and Urinary Incontinence

TYPE OF EXERCISE	NUMBER OF WOMEN PARTICIPATING	NUMBER OF WOMEN INCONTINENT DURING EXERCISE
Running	99	38 (38%)
High-impact aerobics	94	34 (36%)
Tennis	37	10 (27%)
Low-impact aerobics	134	29 (22%)
Walking	164	34 (21%)
Golf	38	7 (18%)
Bicycling	81	13 (16%)
Racquetball	31	4 (13%)
Swimming	87	10 (12%)
Weight lifting	54	4 (7%)

SOURCE: Nygaard I, DeLancey JO: Exercise and incontinence. *Obstet Gynecol* 75:848, 1990.

than those with moderate leakage, and younger women (18 to 45 years) reported more activity restrictions than older women.[16]

Urinary incontinence is often perceived as an inevitable and untreatable consequence of aging. This is due in part to stereotypes of the elderly and perhaps to the insidious onset of this condition. A survey of the membership of Help for Incontinent People (HIP) found that 40 percent of respondents believed their incontinence was due to aging.[17] Adaptation to mild symptoms and progression to different forms of coping with "the problem" may lead incontinence to be viewed as part of what happens as a person ages.[9] Women may also perceive urinary incontinence to be "normal" due to experiences with stress incontinence during pregnancy.[9]

In addition, especially for women, absorbent products that may allow satisfactory self-management of urinary leakage are readily available. Women may believe that urinary incontinence can be managed similarly to menses, concealing urine leakage and odor, without seeking to resolve the incontinence itself.[18] A Swedish study found that 20 percent of women less than 60 years and 29 percent of older women used absorbent pads without ever trying other therapies to reduce urine leakage.[16] Engberg et al. interviewed 147 elderly (67 to 83 years of age) women with urinary incontinence

and asked about how they managed this condition.[19] Sixty-five percent of the women had seven or fewer incontinence episodes per week and 89 percent leaked only a small amount of urine. Most of the patients in this study did not feel that their incontinence was difficult to manage and were generally satisfied with their self-management actions. Common self-care behaviors included locating or staying near a bathroom when out, voiding more frequently, wearing a protective garment, and restricting fluid intake. Fifteen percent of women reported purposefully skipping certain medications (e.g., diuretics) if they were going out.

Economic Cost

In 1995, the economic cost of urinary incontinence in the United States was estimated to be $26.3 billion. These costs included costs associated with the diagnosis, treatment, and routine care of this condition (e.g., absorbent products, laundry) as well as an estimate of the costs of consequences of urinary incontinence (e.g., treatment of urinary tract infections and skin irritation, admission to nursing homes, value of lost earnings).[20] An estimate of the direct costs associated with urinary incontinence (e.g., cost of absorbent products and catheters) found that $11.2 billion is spent annually in managing incontinence among community-dwelling patients, with an additional $5.2 billion spent to provide absorbent products and devices for institutionalized patients.[1] These costs exceed those for treating many other medical conditions that receive considerably more public attention.

Treatment costs vary greatly between behavioral, drug, and surgical interventions. Although urinary incontinence is often an "untreated" or self-managed condition, the long-term cost of untreated incontinence can be significantly higher than successful (results in a "cure") drug or surgical therapy, particularly if persistent urinary incontinence results in nursing home placement.[21]

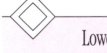

Lower Urinary Tract Anatomy and Physiology

The lower urinary tract consists of the bladder, the urethra, and the internal and external urethral sphincters. The bladder is a hollow muscular organ, which serves as a temporary reservoir for urine that is then eliminated from the body by bladder contraction. The base of the bladder, known as the trigone, is a triangular-shaped fibroelastic muscle located near the attachment of the ureters.

In a woman the urethra is about 1.5 inches long, whereas in a man the length of the urethra is about 8 inches; the greater length of the male urethra provides greater resistance and helps to explain why urinary incontinence is more common in women.

The three major muscular components of the lower urinary tract are the detrusor muscle (the muscular layer of the bladder), the internal urethral sphincter, and the external urethral sphincter. The detrusor muscle is smooth muscle arranged in a helical pattern, which allows the bladder to expand and contract in all directions. The detrusor expands to accommodate the storage of urine; the

normal bladder storage capacity of adults is about 400 to 500 mL of urine.[22] Sensory stretch receptors located throughout the bladder transmit information about bladder fullness to the central nervous system; usually the bladder will accommodate 300 mL of urine before the initial sense of bladder fullness is perceived.[23] The internal sphincter is located at the base of the bladder (also the proximal end of the urethra); the external sphincter is located at the distal end of the urethra.

Innervation

The bladder and internal sphincter are innervated by the autonomic nervous system, whereas the external sphincter is innervated by the somatic nervous system and is under voluntary control (Fig. 12-1). The autonomic nervous system consists of both parasympathetic and sympathetic nerves that innervate the smooth muscle of the bladder and urethra. There are two types of sympathetic receptors present in the bladder and urethra—alpha receptors and beta receptors. Alpha receptors are located primarily in the base of the bladder (trigone) and in the proximal urethra. Stimulation of the alpha receptors, by the transmitter norepinephrine or by medication, causes contraction of the smooth muscles in the trigone and proximal urethra, thus closing the bladder outlet. The innervation of the urethra differs between men and women; the density of urethral alpha receptors is greater in men than in women. Therefore, for women, α-adrenergic agonist agents (e.g., phenylpropanolamine) and α-adrenergic blockers (e.g., doxazosin) may be less effective at increasing or decreasing urethral pressure, respectively.[24]

Beta receptors predominate in the body or fundus of the bladder. Stimulation of beta receptors results in smooth muscle relaxation in the dome of the bladder and allows filling of the bladder. Therefore, activation of the sympathetic system causes urine to be held in the bladder.

Parasympathetic cholinergic receptors are located throughout the bladder. Stimulation of

Figure 12-1

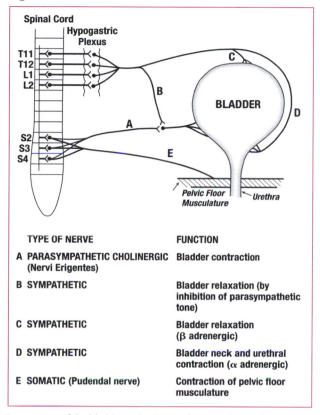

Innervation of the bladder and urinary sphincters. (*Reproduced with permission from JG Ouslander and TM Johnson, Principles of Geriatric Medicine and Gerontology. New York, McGraw-Hill, 1999.*)

these receptors by acetylcholine causes detrusor contraction. Thus, activation of the parasympathetic system causes emptying of the bladder.

The external sphincter is composed of striated muscle innervated by the pudendal nerve of the somatic (voluntary) nervous system. Stimulation of this nerve inhibits urination, thus allowing voluntary control of urination.[25]

In addition to the components of the lower urinary tract, both the spinal cord and brain are involved in control of urination. As the bladder fills, signals are sent to a reflex center located at the sacral level of the spinal cord. The spinal center then returns signals to both the bladder and

external sphincter (indicating either to empty or to continue filling) and also signals the cortical center in the brain. When the signals reach the cortical center an individual becomes aware of the need to urinate.[26]

Micturition

The initiating event for urination is a full bladder. Signals to the cortical center generally occur once bladder volume has reached 250 to 350 mL. When a person is ready to void, the cortical center triggers the inhibition of sympathetic impulses and stimulation of the parasympathetic system, resulting in relaxation of the internal sphincter and contraction of the detrusor. Simultaneously, the trigone closes the ureteral openings and opens the outlet to the urethra, and the external sphincter also relaxes. At this point, intravesicular (internal bladder) pressure is greater than intraurethral pressure, and urination occurs.

Normal urination results in complete emptying of the bladder with little or no residual urine and no back pressure on the kidneys. Bladder emptying should result in a postvoid residual of no more than 50 mL of urine.[22] Normal voiding patterns vary significantly; daytime emptying of the bladder may occur as often as every couple of hours or as infrequently as every 8 to 12 h. Some individuals rarely urinate at night, but nocturia once or twice per night may be regarded as normal.[25,26]

Table 12-2

Age-Related Changes of the Urinary Tract of Women

- Decrease in bladder capacity
- Decrease in the ability to postpone urination
- Decrease in the ability of the kidney to concentrate urine and a resultant increase in urine volume
- Increase in involuntary detrusor contractions
- Decrease in cortical control of the spinal micturition center
- Decrease in muscle tone and bladder contractility, which can lead to both a decrease in urinary flow rates and postvoid residual urine in the bladder
- Decrease in urethral closure pressure and length

Physiologic Effects of Aging

Aging is associated with a number of physical changes that can affect the functioning of the lower urinary tract. (Table 12-2). Urinary incontinence is not a result of aging, nor do aging-related physical changes necessarily cause incontinence. However, these changes do predispose an individual to incontinence and explain why incontinence is more likely to occur in the elderly. Both elderly men and women are most likely to excrete the majority of fluid at night for several reasons including resorption of dependent edema accumulated during the day and a reversal of the day-to-night ratio of urine production (2:1 in young adults) due to an age-related decrease in the nocturnal level of vasopressin.[23,27] Symptoms commonly associated with these changes are frequency, nocturia, urgency, and possibly urinary incontinence.[23,26]

INFLUENCE OF PREGNANCY AND VAGINAL DELIVERY

Urinary incontinence is not uncommon during pregnancy; about 30 to 50 percent of women expe-

rience incontinence during pregnancy.[28] However, for virtually all women, this type of incontinence is transient and resolves quickly after delivery. A smaller percent of women (4 to 8 percent) develop urinary incontinence postpartum, but again, the incontinence is of short duration, with most women regaining continence by 6 months postpartum.[28] Damage of the pudendal nerve and denervation of the pubococcygeus muscle during vaginal delivery have been associated with development of urinary incontinence following pregnancy. Other birthing-related factors potentially related to urinary incontinence are length of second stage labor, episiotomy, pudendal anesthesia, and use of oxytocin.[28]

HYSTERECTOMY

The influence of hysterectomy on urinary incontinence is unclear. Several prospective studies have not found any association up to 2 to 8 years after hysterectomy, whereas a number of epidemiologic studies have found an increased risk of urinary incontinence among women who have had a hysterectomy (RR = 1.3 to 2.1).[28]

MENOPAUSE AND ESTROGEN

Despite the fact that many women report an onset of urinary incontinence about the time of menopause and urethral closure pressure has been found to decrease following menopause, epidemiologic studies have not demonstrated an association between menopause and incontinence.[28] In fact, the prevalence of stress incontinence may decrease after menopause; urge incontinence, however, increases in prevalence after menopause.[28]

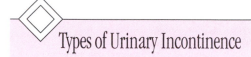

Types of Urinary Incontinence

Urinary incontinence can be classified on the basis of duration or reversibility of symptoms (transient incontinence) or physiologic cause (stress, urge, mixed, and overflow incontinence). There is rarely a single cause of urinary incontinence and no single type is mutually exclusive of any other; that is, a patient with underlying stress incontinence may experience worsening of symptoms from a superimposed bacterial cystitis. Many older individuals suffer from mixed symptoms caused by both urge and stress incontinence. The following paragraphs describe the types in more detail.

Transient Urinary Incontinence

Transient incontinence, as the name implies, appears suddenly and is usually of short duration, lasting only until the precipitating factor is addressed. Transient incontinence occurs in up to half of hospitalized patients and one-third of community-dwelling elderly.[29] Generally this acute incontinence is associated with a medical problem, environmental factors, or drug therapy. Resnick uses the acronym DIAPPERS (purposefully spelled with an extra P) to identify common causes of transient incontinence (Table 12-3).[29] Evaluating the patient for factors associated with transient incontinence and treating those factors identified may allow rapid reestablishment of continence. For example, antibiotic therapy can eliminate incontinence caused by a urinary tract infection, purchase of a bedside commode for nighttime use can eliminate incontinence caused by mobility impairment that precludes ready access to the bathroom, or discontinuation of drug therapy may eliminate incontinence if the drug causes loss of urine control.

MEDICAL CONDITIONS

Medical conditions commonly associated with urinary incontinence are stroke, diabetes mellitus, chronic cough, impaired cognition, constipation or fecal incontinence, obesity, Parkinson's disease, and cardiovascular disease. Over 50 percent of patients with a stroke or a hip fracture develop urinary retention, and subsequent incontinence, during the initial phase of hospitalization.[30] Although these conditions are risk factors for urinary incontinence, a cause-effect relationship has not been established.

MEDICATIONS

Medications frequently contribute to urinary incontinence, such as drugs that alter activity at α-adrenergic, β-adrenergic, or cholinergic receptors; affect the volume of urine; or trigger increases in intra-abdominal pressure (e.g., angiotensin-converting enzyme inhibitor-related cough) (Table 12-4). Two studies found that 62 to 70 percent of elderly patients take medications that have the potential to influence urinary continence.[31,32] Nonprescription and "social" drugs (ethanol, caffeine, tobacco) should be considered along with prescription medications as possible causes of incontinence. The reluctance to report urinary incontinence may obscure the recognition of a medication-related problem. Therefore, all patients prescribed therapy with potential urinary side effects should be questioned regarding the existence of these symptoms and the likelihood of

Table 12-3

Common Causes of Transient Urinary Incontinence

D	Delirium or confusion—can result from either illness (e.g., pneumonia, congestive heart failure, pain) or medication
I	Infection—urinary (symptomatic); asymptomatic bacteriuria does not cause incontinence
A	Atrophic urethritis or vaginitis—responsive to estrogen therapy
P	Pharmaceuticals—includes prescription, nonprescription, and social drugs
P	Psychological disorder—rare; psychological manipulation or severe depression
E	Excessive urine output—may be due to fluid intake, diuretics, mobilization of peripheral edema (nocturia), or metabolic disorders (i.e., hypercalcemia or hyperglycemia)
R	Restricted mobility—due to pain (arthritis) or functional difficulty (stroke, vision impairment)
S	Stool impaction

SOURCE: Reproduced with permission from Resnick NM: Urinary incontinence in the elderly. *Medical Grand Rounds* 3:281, 1984.

drug therapy as a potential causative agent for urinary incontinence should be evaluated when it is suspected.

Drugs with anticholinergic properties may cause urinary retention and associated incontinence of the overflow type. Drugs from many therapeutic classes exhibit such anticholinergic effects. Patients who use more than one agent with anticholinergic properties may experience incontinence due to additive effects. Both nonprescription agents (antihistamines, belladonna alkaloids) and prescription agents (antidepressants, antipsychotics, antihypertensives, anti-Parkinson agents, antiarrhythmics, gastrointestinal antispasmodics) have the potential to create an adverse additive effect. Antihistamines are components of a wide variety of nonprescription agents including allergy products, antitussives, cold preparations, motion sickness agents, and sleep aids.

Diuretics are commonly prescribed agents; about 24 percent of elderly men and 37 percent of elderly women receive diuretic therapy.[33] Loop diuretics, which induce a brisk diuresis, may lead to urgency, frequency, and thus incontinence; thiazide diuretics may also produce incontinence in some patients. A review of medications taken by patients with incontinence found an association between diuretic use and incontinence and nocturia.[34] A study of women with diagnosed urinary incontinence found that those who took diuretics had urinary frequency and significantly more episodes of urine leakage than did women not taking diuretics.[35] Proposed mechanisms by which diuretics adversely affect continence are via an effect on total volume and rate of urine production and a decreased bladder capacity, due to increased frequency of urination to eliminate the greater volume and to protect against incontinence episodes.[35] Pronounced urinary frequency, resulting in a restriction in mobility for several hours after the dose of a loop diuretic, is a common complaint of patients prescribed diuretics. Noncompliance with therapy may result if the restriction in mobility interferes with the performance of common activities or participation in social events. As many as 28 percent of patients on a prescribed diuretic regimen may be noncompliant.[36]

Any agent that impairs cognitive function may result in incontinence. The confusion or lethargy associated with sedative hypnotics and narcotic analgesics can impair the perception of signals from the bladder or cues for appropriate toileting.

The three common social drugs—ethanol, caffeine, and tobacco—may also cause urinary incontinence. Caffeine can adversely affect continence by a diuretic action. Similarly, ethanol may induce incontinence via both diuretic and sedative actions. Bump and McClish report that although

Table 12-4

Drugs Associated with Urinary Incontinence

DRUG CLASS	EXAMPLE MEDICATIONS*	POTENTIAL EFFECT ON URINARY CONTINENCE
α-Adrenergic antagonists[38,39]	Prazosin (Minipress) Terazosin (Hytrin) Doxazosin (Cardura)	Urethral relaxation (decreased proximal urethral pressure)
α-Adrenergic agonists[†,40]	Pseudoephedrine (Sudafed) Phenylpropanolamine (Dexatrim)	Urinary retention (increased proximal urethral pressure)
ACE inhibitors[29]	Captopril (Capoten) Enalapril (Vasotec) Lisinopril (Zestril, Prinivil)	Increased abdominal pressure (secondary to cough)
Anticholinergics[*,40–44] and medications with anticholinergic activity	Dicyclomine (Bentyl) Hyoscyamine (Levsin, Donnagel-PG) Disopyramide (Norpace)	Urinary retention; overflow incontinence (decreased detrusor contractions)
Antidepressants	Amitriptyline (Elavil), doxepin (Sinequan), venlafaxine, (Effexor)	
Antihistamines	Diphenhydramine (Benadryl), hydroxyzine (Atarax)	
Anti-Parkinson agents	Benztropine mesylate (Cogentin), trihexyphenidyl (Artane)	
Anticonvulsants[45–47]	Phenytoin (Dilantin) Gabapentin (Neurontin) Clonazepam (Klonopin)	
Antipsychotics[40–43,48,49]	Haloperidol (Haldol), Thioridazine (Mellaril) Chlorpromazine (Thorazine) Clozapine (Clozaril)	Decreased proximal urethral pressure; dopamine antagonism; urinary retention due to anticholinergic effect
β-Adrenergic agonists[41,42]	Terbutaline (Brethine, Bricanyl)	Urinary retention
β-Adrenergic blocker[*,41]	Propranolol (Inderal)	Urinary retention
Bromocriptine (Parlodel)[40,50,51]		Urinary retention due to dopamine agonist effect
Calcium channel blockers[40–42]	Verapamil (Calan, Isoptin) Nifedipine (Procardia)	Urinary retention (decreased detrusor contractions)

clinicians often view tobacco smoking as a contributing factor for stress urinary incontinence, a relationship between smoking and incontinence is not commonly recognized. Their study of women smokers demonstrated a statistically significant relationship between urinary incontinence and tobacco smoking; current smokers had a 2.5-fold increased risk for stress incontinence.[37] The risk for stress incontinence was related to both current number of cigarettes smoked and the extent

Table 12-4

Drugs Associated with Urinary Incontinence *(Continued.)*

DRUG CLASS	EXAMPLE MEDICATIONS*		POTENTIAL EFFECT ON URINARY CONTINENCE
Diuretics*,[42,43] and medications with diuretic activity	Loop:	Furosemide (Lasix) Bumetanide (Bumex) Torsemide (Demadex)	Urinary frequency and urgency (increased urine volume)
	Thiazide:	Hydrochlorothiazide (HydroDIURIL) Chlorthalidone (Hygroton) Metolazone (Zaroxolyn) Caffeine Theophylline (Theo-Dur)	
Ethanol[40–42]			Frequency (increased urine volume); sedation; delirium
Lithium (Eskalith)[52]			Urgency and incontinence due to cholinergic effects and adrenergic antagonist effects
Misoprostol (Cytotec)[53]			
NSAID[41]		Ibuprofen (Motrin)	Decreased detrusor contractions
Opiates*,[40–43]		Codeine (Tylenol #3) Morphine (MS Contin) Oxycodone (Roxicodone)	Urinary retention (increased) smooth muscle tone); sedation; delirium; constipation
Prokinetic agents[54–56]		Cisapride (Propulsid) Metoclopramide (Reglan)	Urinary frequency; nocturia and incontinence; increased cholinergic activity; decreased urethral pressure
Sedative/hypnotics*,[40–43]		Benzodiazepines[2] Diazepam (Valium), flurazepam (Dalmane)	Sedation: delirium
Skeletal muscle relaxants[42]		Baclofen (Lioresal) Dantrolene (Dantrium)	Urethral relaxation; frequency
Sympatholytics[40–43] (centrally acting antihypertensives)		Methyldopa (Aldomet) Reserpine (Serpasil)	Decreased proximal urethral pressure; α-adrenergic antagonism

*Other drugs in this class may also cause/aggravate urinary incontinence.

†Pseudoephedrine and phenylpropanolamine are present in many nonprescription "cold," allergy, and diet products.

ABBREVIATIONS: ACE, angiotensin-converting enzyme; NSAID, nonsteroidal anti-inflammatory drug.

of lifetime exposure to cigarette smoking (dose). Smoking might increase the risk for stress incontinence by increasing the frequency and intensity of coughing, by causing spontaneous bladder contractions, and by compromising the effectiveness of the sphincters via decreasing collagen synthesis, antiestrogenic effects, and stretching and denervation of the periurethral tissues.[37]

Types of Established Incontinence

The four types of established incontinence are urge, stress, overflow, and functional. A mixed type of incontinence, a combination of urge and stress incontinence, is common in women. The prevalence of the types of incontinence varies by gender and age. In the MESA study of women, aged 60 years and older, the most common form of urinary incontinence was the mixed type (55 percent) followed by stress (27 percent) and then urge (9 percent) incontinence.[57] In women under 75 years of age, stress is the most common form of urinary incontinence.[58] Among women over the age of 75 years, urge incontinence becomes more prevalent than stress and overflow incontinence.

Urge, stress, and overflow incontinence are due to abnormalities in the function of the detrusor, the sphincters, or both. Incontinence occurs when intravesicular (bladder) pressure exceeds intraurethral pressure. However, the symptoms and causes of these types of incontinence are quite different and understanding the features of each type is critical to selecting drug therapy. Urge and stress incontinence are a "failure to store" urine, whereas overflow incontinence is a "failure to empty" urine from the bladder. Poor emptying of the bladder can occur due to detrusor inactivity or outflow obstruction. Urethral obstruction, although common in men, is uncommon in women, and usually occurs only following bladder neck suspension surgery.[29] Functional incontinence is the result of factors outside of the lower urinary tract, such as patient mobility and cognitive impairment.

URGE INCONTINENCE

Urge incontinence is typified by involuntary voiding of moderate to large amounts of urine within a few seconds to minutes of a strong urge to urinate.[1] Patients also commonly experience urgency, frequency, and nocturia. The involuntary voiding occurs secondary to uninhibited bladder contractions. These uninhibited contractions can occur in either the absence (detrusor instability) or presence of neurologic deficits (detrusor

hyperreflexia). Neurologic and genitourinary disorders associated with urge incontinence include diabetes mellitus, stroke, multiple sclerosis, brain tumor, Alzheimer's disease, Parkinson's disease, bladder cancer, cystitis, bladder stones, and diverticuli.[1] However, in some cases, no demonstrable genitourinary or neurologic abnormality can be detected. Behavioral and pharmacologic measures can be used to manage detrusor instability, but detrusor hyperreflexia is managed as a component of a neurologic disorder.[22]

STRESS INCONTINENCE

The term *stress incontinence* applies to the involuntary loss of urine during activities that increase abdominal pressure such as coughing, sneezing, lifting, and laughing.[1] The brief increase in intra-abdominal pressure that occurs during these activities exceeds urethral pressure/resistance and allows leakage of small to moderate amounts of urine immediately concurrent with the increased intra-abdominal pressure. Stress incontinence is more common in women than in men and is associated with estrogen deficiency, weakness of pelvic floor muscles (urethral hypermobility), childbirth, obesity, and urethral sphincter weakness.

MIXED INCONTINENCE

Mixed incontinence has characteristics of both urge and stress incontinence. This type of incontinence is common in women.[1,11]

OVERFLOW INCONTINENCE

Overflow incontinence refers to the almost continual leakage of small amounts of urine associated with overdistention of the bladder. Leakage results when the pressure exerted by the urine accumulated in the bladder overcomes urethral pressure.[1] Overdistention of the bladder can occur secondary to either outlet obstruction or to an underactive and acontractile detrusor (e.g., diabetic neuropathy, vitamin B_{12} deficiency).[27] Outlet obstruction is rare in women but may be associated with severe pelvic prolapse or urethral stricture. Other common symptoms include hesitancy, interrupted or diminished urinary stream, straining to void, and a sense of incomplete emptying.

FUNCTIONAL INCONTINENCE

Finally, involuntary voiding of urine may occur despite normal bladder and urethral function. Functional incontinence can occur due to impairments in cognitive or physical functioning.[1] Some functional incontinence is reversible if environmental barriers to toileting are eliminated. For example, a patient with a handicap such as severe arthritis or blindness may benefit from easy access to a bedside commode chair to regain control over bladder leakage. However, patients unable to recognize bladder cues (e.g., dementia) may need help from caregivers to manage their condition and avoid inappropriate voiding.

Key History

Obtaining a history of urinary incontinence from a patient may be a difficult task. Frequently cited reasons include embarrassment on the part of the patient, assumptions that incontinence is a normal part of aging and disease, and failure of the clinician to inquire about these symptoms. Inquiry about urinary symptoms should become a routine part of the primary care physician's behavior at appropriate times (e.g., complete physical examination, annual pelvic examination). In fact, a recent study found that among women aged 42 to 50 years the cumulative incidence of new-onset urinary incontinence was 8 percent.[59]

Researchers have discovered that the wording of questions to a patient is important in eliciting an accurate response. Asking a "follow-up" question (i.e., probe question) to an initial negative reply identified an additional 10 percent of incon-

Table 12-5

Questions to Identify Urinary Incontinence

1. Can you tell me about any problems you have with your bladder?
2. Do you wear any special padding to protect from urine leakage?
3. Do you avoid certain activities (e.g., church services, exercise) over concern about your bladder?

tinent patients in the study.[3] Table 12-5 provides a sample of suggested questions to use in the office as a way of identifying women with incontinence.

Once a complaint of urinary incontinence has been identified, either at the patient's or health care provider's prompting, evaluation of most patients can be well managed in the office setting. The history elicited from the patient should include a focus on the neurologic and genitourinary systems and on possible reversible causes of incontinence (e.g., infection, excessive or ill-timed fluid intake, or medication effect). Medications, both prescription and nonprescription, that may cause urinary incontinence are listed in Table 12-4.

A detailed history of the symptoms of incontinence should include the timing and amount of urine loss, precipitants of the loss, and use of any efforts to mitigate the problem. A bladder record completed by either the patient or caregiver can prove helpful in understanding the nature of the incontinence problem. Figure 12-2 shows an example of a bladder record.

Physical Examination

A general physical examination should be performed to detect conditions that could contribute to incontinence such as edema, arthritis, dementia, or neurologic disorders. Special attention should be

Figure 12-2

Sample Bladder Record

NAME: _____

DATE: _____

INSTRUCTIONS: Place a check in the appropriate column next to the time you urinated in the toilet or when an incontinence episode occurred. Note the reason for the incontinence and describe your liquid intake (for example, coffee, water) and estimate the amount (for example, one cup).

Time interval	Urinated in toilet	Had a small incontinence episode	Had a large incontinence episode	Reason for incontinence episode	Type/amount of liquid intake
6–8 A.M.					
8–10 A.M.					
10–noon					
Noon–2 P.M.					
2–4 P.M.					
4–6 P.M.					
6–8 P.M.					
8–10 P.M.					
10–midnight					
Overnight					

No. of pads used today: _____ No. of episodes: _____

Comments _____

_____

_____

Bladder record. *(Reproduced from AHCPR Clinical Practice Guideline.)*[1]

paid to the rectal examination for perineal sensation, sphincter tone, and rectal mass. Pelvic examination should assess for vaginal atrophy or pelvic prolapse (cystocele, urethrocele, rectocele). Direct observation to detect stress incontinence via the cough stress test can be performed by having the patient cough vigorously while being observed for urine loss from the urethra. This test should preferably be done with the patient's bladder full, in either the lithotomy position or, if necessary, while standing.

Postvoid residual volume should be measured within 5 to 10 min after the patient voids in a comfortable and private setting. The volume can be determined either by inserting a catheter to drain the residual urine or by using pelvic ultrasound to assess bladder volume. Portable ultrasound devices that estimate postvoid residual volume with dependable accuracy are available and in clinical use. Residual volumes of less than 50 mL are considered normal, those over 200 mL are abnormal, and those between 50 and 200 mL are equivocal but suggestive of inadequate emptying.

Ancillary Tests

Basic laboratory testing should include at least a urinalysis to detect blood, glucose, or infection that could cause or worsen incontinence. Additional blood tests, urine cytology, cystoscopy, and cystometrics may prove helpful only in special circumstances (e.g., suspected cancer, unexplained hematuria).[1] They are not part of the routine evaluation of urinary incontinence.

Treatment

Successful treatment or improvement in the symptoms of urinary incontinence can greatly improve the quality of life for patients with this condition.

One study of elderly women with stress or urge incontinence found that nonpharmacologic therapy alone improved incontinence and consequently the patients' sense of well-being.[60] This is particularly important because self-treatment of urinary symptoms is so prevalent and use of absorbent products can easily conceal urine leakage. However, self-treatment has the potential to aggravate incontinence or to promote problematic health behaviors. Frequent toileting can lead to a reduced bladder capacity and restricting fluid intake can be detrimental, increasing the risk for constipation and dehydration.[19]

Treatment of urinary incontinence can occur via three modes: behavioral, pharmacologic, and surgical. In addition, incontinence aids are helpful in managing incontinence and may be used in conjunction with behavioral techniques and drug therapy. Overflow incontinence must be treated with drainage of the bladder or removal of the obstruction. For other forms of incontinence, behavioral therapy is the preferred initial therapy because it is often effective in reducing symptoms and has the lowest risk of iatrogenic effects. One trial comparing behavioral therapy (contraction of pelvic muscles) in 197 elderly women with urge or mixed incontinence found a greater decrease in incontinence episodes in the behavioral therapy group than in the drug therapy group.[61] Furthermore, 97 percent of patients assigned to behavioral therapy indicated a willingness to continue this therapy indefinitely, whereas only 55 percent of patients assigned drug therapy indicated a willingness to continue with long-term therapy despite improvement in symptoms.

Behavioral Techniques

Behavioral techniques can permit many patients to avoid complications from drug therapy and surgical interventions.[1] Along with the specific behavioral techniques developed for stress and urge incontinence, simple habit modifications can be suggested for patients with incontinence. These habit modifications are to avoid excess fluid intake (limit daily intake to 2 L/d), avoid or limit consumption of caffeine-containing beverages, and void regularly.

A number of behavioral techniques exist for treating urge and stress incontinence. Although overflow incontinence, due to an underactive detrusor (atonic bladder), is not amenable to behavioral treatment, patients with urethral obstruction and symptoms of urgency and frequency may benefit from behavioral techniques used for urge incontinence. These techniques are most likely to be efficacious for patients who are not limited in cognition or mobility, although they have been successfully applied to patients who suffer these limitations.

BLADDER TRAINING TECHNIQUES

Bladder training techniques can be helpful in urge incontinence and include three components: patient education, scheduled voiding, and positive reinforcement. The goal of these programs is to delay voiding between scheduled voiding times and thus to teach patients to postpone urination when the urge to urinate occurs. The AHCPR guidelines suggest that this intervention may be useful for caregivers of home-dwelling elderly. Prompted voiding programs are a type of habit training that have been especially helpful in managing incontinence associated with cognitive impairment. The evidence for effectiveness for both bladder training and prompted voiding is supported by results of controlled trials. Although the evidence of benefit from habit training is weaker, it may be a useful intervention in some circumstances.[1] Bladder training achieved complete continence in 10 to 15 percent of patients and reduced incontinence episodes by 50 percent in 75 percent of patients.[22]

Initially, voiding is scheduled every 1 to 2 h while awake. Once a patient remains "dry" at the initial voiding interval the length of time between voids is increased, usually in 15- to 30-min increments; a 3- to 4-h voiding interval with continence is the goal.[22] Habit training is similar to bladder training in that voiding is done on a scheduled basis. However, the habit training programs do not attempt to postpone voiding; rather an attempt is made to anticipate a patient's natural voiding schedule and encourage toileting to maintain continence. One difficulty in instituting these types of behavioral programs in long-term care facilities is the amount of staff time required and the necessity of changes in patient care routines.[1]

PELVIC MUSCLE EXERCISE

For patients with stress and/or urge incontinence, initial treatment should begin with pelvic muscle exercises (Kegel exercises). Kegel exercises are often described as a "pulling up" or "drawing in" of the perivaginal muscles as if to prevent urination or defecation. Women are instructed to repetitively contract the pubococcygeus and levator ani muscles to strengthen the pelvic and periurethral muscles of the pelvic floor. Strengthening these muscles provides greater urethral closure pressure and greater support for pelvic organs.[1]

Clinical trials have shown that pelvic muscle exercises can provide a 60 percent reduction in the number of incontinence episodes.[1] Wells et al.[62] found that pelvic muscle exercises were comparable in effectiveness to phenylpropanolamine; 77 percent of women using exercises and 84 percent of women taking medication noted an improvement in incontinence symptoms. The benefit from pelvic muscle exercises has been best demonstrated for patients with stress incontinence. However, these exercises may also benefit patients with urge or mixed incontinence and women who have had lower urinary tract surgeries.[1,61,63] The AHCPR guideline panel strongly supported the recommendation that women with stress incontinence be taught pelvic muscle exercises and noted that pelvic muscle exercises may benefit men and women with urge incontinence as well.[1]

The AHCPR guidelines suggest that both sustaining contractions (for 10 s) and repetition (30 to 80 contractions per day for at least 6 to 8 weeks) are important to overall success.[1] Patients may need to continue these exercises indefinitely to sustain improvement. Progressively weighted vaginal cones and biofeedback are sometimes used as tools to enhance pelvic muscle training.[1] Early improvement (reduction of urine leakage within 1 week of beginning pelvic floor muscle exercises) may be achieved by some women who learn "the knack."[64] The knack is a term to describe learning to contract pelvic floor muscles in anticipation of and during increases in intra-abdominal pressure. A small study of this technique found elderly women who could effectively contract their levator ani muscle were able to reduce urine leakage 86 percent during a moderately strong cough.

Biomechanical and Surgical Treatment

Several traditional procedures as well as some innovative biomechanical interventions offer further chance for control of stress incontinence. Traditional surgeries that reestablish a more physiologic angle between the bladder and urethra have long been used to restore bladder control in cases of stress incontinence due to a dropping/prolapse of pelvic organs.[65]

For problems caused by poor urethral sphincter function unrelated to relaxation of pelvic organs (e.g., intrinsic sphincter deficiency), periurethral injections of collagen extract are designed to increase the mass of the distal urethral sphincter, thereby improving the resistance to increased intravesical pressure.[66] Electrical stimulation has also been used to enhance the function of the sphincter mechanism[67,68] as well as suppress detrusor instability in urge incontinence. When used in conjunction with Kegel exercises and well-timed pelvic muscle tightening at the instant of a cough, sneeze, or laugh, these techniques offer hope for sufferers from stress incontinence. Recent trials have shown encouraging results using innovative devices such as adhesive patches over the urethral meatus, endovaginal support rings, and intraurethral inserts to provide improved bladder control to women.[69–72]

Pharmacologic Treatment

A number of nonprescription and prescription medications have been used to improve women's control over urinary incontinence. Figure 12-3 depicts the known receptor sites within the lower urinary tract and provides a scientific basis for the selection of certain pharmaceuticals for treatment.

URGE INCONTINENCE

Pharmacologic therapy for urge incontinence is directed at decreasing uninhibited bladder contractions. The goal of therapy is to increase functional bladder capacity and to decrease the frequency and urgency of urination. A number of anticholinergic and direct-acting smooth muscle relaxants have been evaluated for the treatment of urge incontinence. Unfortunately, the number

Figure 12-3

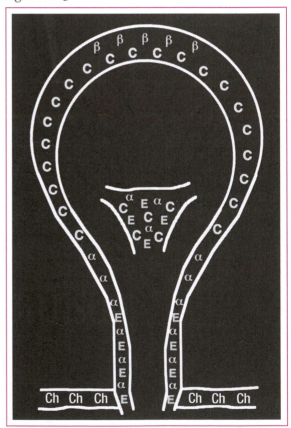

Pharmacologic receptors within the lower urinary tract. α, alpha adrenergic; β, beta adrenergic; E, estrogen; C, acetylcholine (parasympathetic); Ch, acetylcholine (striated skeletal muscle).

of randomized controlled trials is small and there is often little correlation between cystometric and urodynamic tests and symptomatic improvement. A review of the randomized controlled trials, along with expert opinion regarding efficacy, was reported by the AHCPR.[1] The evaluation of agents provided by the Urinary Incontinence Guideline Panel is summarized in Table 12-6.

ANTICHOLINERGIC AGENTS Drugs with a combination of anticholinergic and antispasmodic properties, such as oxybutynin chloride and dicyclomine hydrochloride, are among the most widely used agents. Anticholinergic/antispasmodic agents improve urge incontinence by increasing the volume attained before detrusor contraction, decreasing the strength of bladder contractions, and increasing maximal bladder capacity. However, these agents are not able to suppress detrusor contraction or to increase the time between the perceived need to void and detrusor contraction ("warning time"). Therefore, these medications should be used in combination with behavioral interventions.[1,29]

Tolterodine (Detrol) is a recent addition to the anticholinergic class of agents. Three trials comparing tolterodine 1 to 2 mg bid to oxybutynin 5 mg tid found tolterodine to be equally effective as measured by mean number of voids per day and mean number of incontinence episodes per day. Tolterodine exhibits greater selectivity for bladder tissue than salivary tissue (in contrast to oxybutynin), and clinical trials demonstrated that patients treated with tolterodine experienced less dry mouth than patients treated with oxybutynin.[73] Significant improvement will be seen after 2 weeks of therapy and further improvement may be seen up to 8 weeks after initiation of therapy.

Anticholinergics/antispasmodics have a rapid onset of action and improvement in symptoms should be realized within the first few days of therapy. In general, patients who do not initially respond to therapy are unlikely to benefit from continued therapy.[74] Elderly patients are sensitive to anticholinergic effects and can often be managed on doses that are half of the usual therapeutic dose.[75] The AHCPR panel suggested that selection of an anticholinergic/antispasmodic agent be individualized to patient pattern of use and chosen on the basis of onset of action and duration of effect.[1] Table 12-7 compares the anticholinergic/antispasmodic agents on onset and duration of effect. A drug with fast onset and relatively short duration of effect (e.g., propantheline) might be selected for a woman who desired improved control of symptoms for a relatively short event such as a concert or a church service. A woman who desired a longer period of drug effect, for example, during a work day, may be more appropriately treated with oxybutynin or tolterodine.

Patients frequently experience side effects that limit the usefulness of the anticholinergic/antispasmodic agents. Larger doses of the anticholinergic/antispasmodic agents are generally required to affect bladder function than other organs such as the salivary glands and ciliary muscles of the eye. Potential side effects include dry mouth, constipation, blurred vision, tachycardia, drowsiness, decreased sweating, impotence, and insomnia (see Table 12-6). The frequency of side effects may make long-term therapy intolerable for some patients; one study found that because of side effects, only 18 percent of women were continuing to take oxybutynin 6 months after initiation of therapy.[76] Some patients may be able to benefit from intermittent use of these agents in anticipation of situations known to provoke incontinence or for improved control during important social events.[77] These agents are also relatively contraindicated in the presence of a variety of conditions common in the elderly: cardiac disease, reflux esophagitis, glaucoma, and xerostomia. In addition, these agents must be cautiously added to the regimen of patients with dementia, because they may increase the confusion of patients with cognitive impairment. The anticholinergic/antispasmodic agents have the potential to worsen incontinence by causing urinary retention; subclinical retention can cause an increase in the symptoms of urge incontinence. Incontinence may also worsen if patients increase fluid consumption to manage the side effect of dry mouth.[29]

Table 12-6

Medications Used in the Treatment of Urge and Stress Urinary Incontinence

URGE INCONTINENCE

AGENT	DOSE	COMMON SIDE EFFECTS	AHCPR RATING*	COST†
Oxybutynin (Ditropan)	2.5–5 mg tid–qid	Constipation; dryness of mouth, nose, throat, skin; blurred vision; fatigue; difficulty with urination	Recommended as drug of choice by AHCPR panel. 6/7 trials found oxybutynin superior to placebo. AHCPR rating = A	$ 36 generic
Propantheline (Pro-Banthine)	15–30 mg tid–qid, higher doses required for greatest efficacy	Constipation; dryness of mouth, nose, throat, skin	Probably best for less impaired patients who can tolerate full doses (e.g., 30 mg qid). AHCPR rating = B	$ 53 generic
Dicyclomine (Bentyl)	10–20 mg tid	Constipation; dryness of mouth; nose, throat, skin; blurred vision	Clinical experience suggests it is as effective as other anticholinergics. Recommended as an alternative agent; AHCPR rating = B	$ 21–42 generic
Flavoxate (Urispas)	100 mg tid	Drowsiness, dryness of mouth and throat, constipation, blurred vision, dizziness, fast heart rate	Four trials—none showed benefit; Not recommended by AHCPR.	$ 77–154 brand name
Hyoscyamine (Levsin)	SL tablet (0.125 mg) 0.125–0.25 mg tid SR tablet (0.375 mg) 0.375 mg bid	Dryness of mouth, nose, throat, skin; constipation; blurred vision	No trials meeting the panel's criteria are published. AHCPR makes no recommendation.	SL $ 14 SR $ 33 generic
Imipramine (Tofranil) and doxepin (Sinequan, Adapin)	Initially 10–25 mg qd–tid; total daily dose 25–100 mg	Blurred vision, confusion, constipation, hypotension, irregular heartbeat	Limited studies. AHCPR rating = B	$ 5 generic
Tolterodine (Detrol)	2 mg bid	Dry mouth and eyes, dyspepsia, headache, constipation	Not marketed at time of AHCPR review.	$ 74 brand name

Table 12-6

Medications Used in the Treatment of Urge and Stress Urinary Incontinence (*Continued.*)

STRESS INCONTINENCE

AGENT	DOSE	COMMON SIDE EFFECTS	AHCPR RATING*	COST†
Phenylpropanolamine (PPA) (Prolamine) and Pseudoephedrine (Sudafed)	25–100 mg bid in sustained-release form 15–30 mg tid	Nervousness, restlessness, insomnia, dizziness, dryness of mouth and nose, fast heartbeat	7 trials showed PPA to be somewhat effective. AHCPR rating = A	$ 3–6 generic, non-prescription product
Estrogens (Ogen, Premarin)	Equivalent to 0.3–1.25 mg conjugated estrogen orally or up to 2 g vaginally 1–3 times per week	Breast tenderness, breast enlargement, peripheral edema, abdominal bloating, anorexia, breakthrough bleeding, spotting, dizziness	Meta-analysis of 6 trials found estrogen improved incontinence in postmenopausal women. Estrogen therapy may benefit women with stress and mixed incontinence. AHCPR rating = B	oral $ 14 brand name vaginal 42-g tube $ 39 brand name
Imipramine (Tofranil)	Initially 10–25mg qd-tid; total daily dose 25–100 mg	Blurred vision, confusion, constipation, hypotension, irregular heartbeat	This agent can be considered as an alternative when a patient has not responded to PPA or pseudo-ephedrine. AHCPR rating = C	$ 5 generic

*The Agency for Health Care Policy and Research (AHCPR) published a Clinical Practice Guideline on Urinary Incontinence in Adults: Acute and Chronic Management in 1996 (AHCPR publication number 96-0682). The AHCPR recommendations are primarily based on published scientific literature; when the literature was incomplete or inconsistent the recommendations reflect the professional judgment of panel members and consultants. The panel rated the evidence supported by scientific evidence according to the following criteria: A, recommendation supported by evidence from properly designed and implemented controlled trials; B, recommendation supported by evidence from properly designed and implemented clinical series; C, recommendation supported by expert opinion.

†Prices are average wholesale prices (AWP) to a pharmacy for a 1-month supply of medication; prices were obtained from: *Drug Topics Redbook.*

Table 12-7

Onset and Duration of Action of Anticholinergic Agents

ANTICHOLINERGIC AGENT	ONSET OF ACTION	DURATION OF ACTION
Dicyclomine	1–2 h	≤ 4 h
Hyoscyamine		
Conventional tablet	20–30 min	4–6 h
Extended-release tablet	20–30 min	12 h
Oxybutynin	30–60 min	6–10 h
Propantheline	30–60 min	4–6 h
Tolterodine	≤ 1 h	12 h

TRICYCLIC ANTIDEPRESSANTS The antidepressant medications, imipramine and doxepin, exert an anticholinergic action but also have other actions that may lessen incontinence. They impart both α-adrenergic and β-adrenergic stimulating actions that provide an inhibitory effect on bladder smooth muscle via a local anesthetic-type action. This combination of actions results in decreased bladder contractility and increased sphincter resistance. The benefit from imipramine and doxepin may become apparent only after several weeks of therapy. One study of imipramine found that the average length of time for a responsive patient to attain control of incontinence (dryness) was 2 months, although some patients did respond as early as 1 week after initiation of therapy.[39] Therapy with either imipramine or doxepin is initiated at low doses (e.g., 10 to 25 mg) and titrated upward until clinical benefit or intolerable side effects. The Urinary Incontinence Guideline Panel noted a maximum daily dose of 100 mg.[1] Some clinicians advocate doses up to 150 mg/d for imipramine.[78] Relatively low doses of imipramine may be efficacious in the elderly. Castleden et al. found 50 mg to be the average effective dose for a group of elderly patients.[79] Common potential side effects of the tricyclic antidepressants are dry mouth, fatigue, drowsiness, weakness, postural hypotension (dizziness), and constipation (see Table 12-6). A sudden discontinuation of imipramine may cause adverse effects (e.g., severe nausea and vomiting, lethargy, irritability); therefore, this drug should be withdrawn gradually.

The combination of imipramine and an anticholinergic/antispasmodic agent may provide additive benefit for some patients.[1,29]

CALCIUM CHANNEL BLOCKERS The potential use of calcium channel blockers as smooth muscle relaxants to treat urge incontinence has interested many clinicians. Unfortunately, there are no clinical trials of the calcium channel blockers available in the United States. Terodiline, an agent with both anticholinergic and calcium channel blocking activity, has been studied extensively in Europe; however, ventricular arrhythmia associated with this agent caused trials in the United States to be halted.[1] Chan and Ouslander reported on the use of diltiazem for the treatment of two elderly patients with urge incontinence; neither patient improved and one developed a ventricular arrhythmia.[80] In contrast, a small trial with nifedipine showed an increase in bladder capacity and a decrease in nocturia.[81]

OTHER AGENTS The potential use of the β-adrenergic agonist terbutaline and the nonsteroidal anti-inflammatory drugs (NSAIDs) has also been explored. Two reports suggest terbutaline may decrease urgency and frequency for some patients.[82,83] The majority of patients (14 of 15) in one small trial reported benefit; 9 of 15 also reported side effects from therapy.[83] Prostaglandins produce contractions of the bladder.[81] Several small studies have demonstrated that NSAIDs may decrease the uninhibited contractions that occur with urge incontinence.[81,84,85] However, there is not currently enough evidence to recommend either of these classes of agents for the treatment of urge incontinence.

Another agent suggested as an option for the management of nocturia and nighttime incontinence is desmopressin (DDAVP®). Desmopressin, a synthetic agent that is structurally similar to vasopressin (antidiuretic hormone), acts to decrease urine output via promoting water resorption by the kidney. It is widely used to treat enuresis in children. In two studies, desmopressin was shown to decrease nocturnal urination in adults, but studies are limited and it is unknown if desmopressin will ameliorate nighttime incontinence.[27] Figure 12-4 presents a treatment algorithm.

STRESS INCONTINENCE

Pharmacologic intervention for the treatment of stress incontinence is directed at increasing intraurethral closing pressure. Two classes of agents have the potential to increase intraurethral pressure. The α-adrenergic agonists can increase muscle tone in the trigone, bladder base, and proximal urethra by stimulating alpha receptors at these sites. Estrogens have direct effects on the urethral mucosa and indirect actions in the periurethral area which increase urethral closure pressure.[1] The evaluation of agents provided by the Urinary Incontinence Guideline Panel is summarized in Table 12-6.

α-ADRENERGIC AGENTS   Phenylpropanolamine and pseudoephedrine are the two α-adrenergic agents used for the treatment of stress incontinence. Phenylpropanolamine is the α-adrenergic agent most studied in women with stress incontinence. Many studies have demonstrated a clinical benefit from therapy.[1] However, studies have not been able to correlate either an increase in urethral closure pressure or a specific plasma concentration with clinical efficacy.[86,87] Patients least likely to respond to phenylpropanolamine are women who have had previous surgery to correct urinary incontinence. The lack of response in these women may be partially explained by the replacement of smooth muscle with fibrous scar tissue.[87]

Common side effects of phenylpropanolamine and pseudoephedrine include insomnia, restlessness, anxiety, and headache[1] (see Table 12-6). These agents are also relatively contraindicated in patients with cardiac disease, including hypertension, angina, and arrhythmia; diabetes mellitus; and thyroid disease. Excessive elevation of blood pressure is possible, but unlikely.

ESTROGEN   Estrogen therapy is thought to exert an effect on the functioning of the lower urinary tract due to several factors: the common embryologic origin of the urethra, trigone, and vagina; the prevalence of urinary incontinence in postmenopausal (hypoestrogenic) women and a decrease in maximal urethral closure pressure in postmenopausal women compared to premenopausal women; and the ability of estrogen to reverse atrophic changes, promote maturation of urethral cells, increase vascularization of urethral connective tissue, and stimulate collagen-producing fibroblasts, which have estrogen receptors.[28,88] Postmenopausal estrogen deficiency may lead to atrophic urethritis and decreases in periurethral tissue strength and vascularity. Estrogen therapy reverses these changes and also increases the response of urethral tissue to α-adrenergic stimulation. These changes are thought to explain why estrogen, therapy may provide benefit.[1] However, the effectiveness of estrogen, particularly oral estrogen, is controversial.[28] A meta-analysis of studies examining the effect of oral estrogen on incontinence found that estrogen had a large effect on subjective perception of improvement (64 percent

Figure 12-4

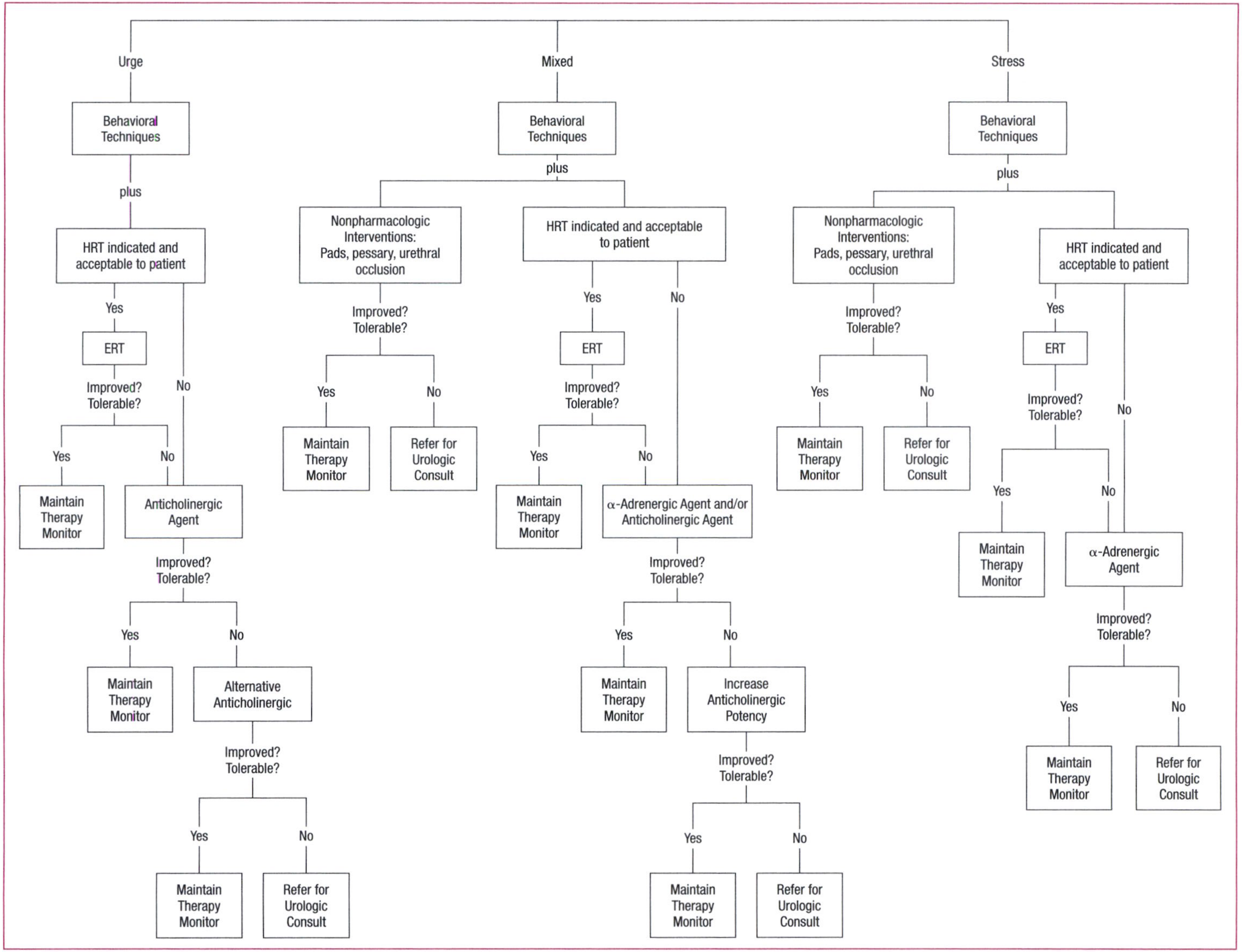

Treatment algorithm for urinary incontinence in women.

improvement compared to placebo); however, no effect of oral estrogen was demonstrated for objective measures (quantity of urine leakage, maximum urethral closure pressure).[88] Topical vaginal estrogen may exert a greater benefit than oral estrogen; several randomized controlled trials of vaginal estrogen have shown a decrease in urgency and incontinence.[28]

Both oral and topical vaginal estrogen can provide effective therapy. The usual dose for oral estrogen therapy is 0.625 mg conjugated estrogen, or the equivalent. Therapy with estrogen vaginal cream is usually initiated with daily application and tapered to several times weekly application. As discussed in Chap. 4, the major risks of chronic estrogen therapy are endometrial cancer and breast cancer. The risk for uterine hyperplasia and cancer can be minimized by the addition of a progestin to therapy. Conversely, estrogens confer protection against osteoporosis and may prevent heart disease and stroke. Patients prescribed estrogen replacement therapy for incontinence should be apprised of both the possible risks and benefits of long-term therapy. Estrogen or hormone replacement therapy is also associated with a number of common side effects including nausea, headache, breast tenderness, and bloating. (see Chap. 4).

The use of phenylpropanolamine in combination with an estrogen can produce a synergistic effect. Estrogen appears to increase the number or the responsiveness of alpha receptors. Combination therapy may be appropriate for women who do not achieve continence with a single agent.[1] Also, imipramine may be useful for patients who have not responded to α-adrenergic agents or estrogen.[1] See Fig. 12-4 for the treatment algorithm.

MIXED INCONTINENCE

Many women suffer from a combination of urge and stress incontinence, thereby requiring a multifaceted approach to therapy.[1,11] For example, a behavioral program may help a woman gain partial control over her urgency and frequency, yet she may continue to leak urine at times of physical strain such as coughing, laughing, or exercising.

Addition of pelvic floor muscle exercises or medication or urethral barriers may afford her even better bladder control. See Fig. 12-4 for the treatment algorithm.

OVERFLOW INCONTINENCE

Overflow incontinence is preferentially managed with nonpharmacologic therapy including intermittent or indwelling catheterization, augmented voiding techniques (e.g., double voiding), use of Credé (suprapubic massage) or Valsalva maneuvers, and surgery.

CATHETERIZATION Catheterization is usually reserved for use as a supportive measure for women with spinal cord injury with urinary retention or persistent overflow incontinence not responsive to behavioral voiding techniques or medications. Intermittent catheterization is preferred over indwelling catheters, particularly among women, due to the high rate of infection and incidence of bladder and renal stones associated with indwelling catheters and the relative ease of performing intermittent catheterization in women. Indwelling catheters may be most appropriate for use in selected patients with incontinence who are terminally ill or for use as a short-term treatment among women with skin irritation or ulcers or during hospitalizations when accurate information on urinary output is important. Additional information about the use of catheterization can be found elsewhere.[1]

DRUG THERAPY Drug therapy may be used acutely, but long-term drug therapy is often lacking in efficacy or limited by adverse drug effects. Pharmacologic therapy for overflow incontinence is directed at facilitating bladder emptying and decreasing residual urine. There are two approaches to pharmacologic therapy. The first is to use a cholinergic agent to increase the strength of detrusor contractions in cases where detrusor atony exists. Bethanechol is the agent most often used. However, the long-term efficacy of this agent is questionable.[23,58] Bethanechol has been used in oral doses ranging from 10 to 50 mg bid to qid. Administration of bethanechol 20 min before a voiding attempt is suggested.[23] This agent is relatively contraindicated in a number of conditions, many of which are common in the elderly, including asthma, coronary artery disease, peptic ulcer disease, Parkinson's disease, and hyperthyroidism. In addition, common side effects of therapy (e.g., stomach pain, diarrhea, dizziness, headache, nervousness) may make therapy intolerable.

A second pharmacologic approach to overflow incontinence may be the use of an α-adrenergic blocking agent (doxazosin, prazosin, terazosin) to decrease relative outflow obstruction. α-Adrenergic receptors are present in the bladder neck, trigone, and urethra and are involved in smooth muscle contractions; a decrease in smooth muscle tone can decrease resistance to bladder emptying. In men α-adrenergic blockers have improved urine flow, bladder emptying, and the symptoms associated with outflow obstruction (e.g., urinary frequency).[29] Interestingly, a recent study of doxazosin in 34 women documented improvement in the symptoms of urgency and frequency.[89] Fifty percent of the women in this study who did not respond to the anticholinergic hyoscyamine responded to doxazosin; in addition, the combination of doxazosin and hyoscyamine led to improvement of a greater number of women than either agent alone. It was postulated that in some cases nonparasympathetic-mediated mechanisms may give rise to the voiding symptoms of urgency and frequency. This suggests an intriguing therapeutic option for the future. In contrast, another trial found terazosin was not effective in treating prostatism-like symptoms in women.[90]

It has also been suggested that estrogen therapy may be helpful in treating women with urethral obstruction due to scarring or fibrosis.[91]

Management Aids

A number of incontinence aids are available. The most common are absorbent pads and garments.

Unfortunately, both patients and practitioners are generally unaware of the variety of commercial products available and health care providers are unlikely to discuss or educate patients regarding their choices.[92,93] This is in contrast to the large number of products marketed and the considerable expense of purchasing these products, $496 million in 1987.[1] A resource guide on incontinence products is available from the National Association for Continence (previously, Help for Incontinent People) of Spartanburg, South Carolina.

Absorbent products are used to "soak up" urine to protect the dignity and comfort of patients and to protect clothing, furniture, and bedding.[92] These products come in the form of underpads, pant liners, and adult diapers and may be either disposable or washable. A number of factors, including the type and severity of incontinence, time of incontinence, ability of the patient/caregiver to use the product, availability, and cost, might be considered when selecting a product.[93] Some absorbent products have special properties (e.g., impregnation with calcium acetate to decrease urine odor, use of a powder that gels when wet to increase leakage protection). However, a recent study with community-dwelling women found that menstrual pads (the least expensive products tested) were as acceptable to women as absorbent products designed to manage urinary incontinence.[94] Desirable properties for the product may vary with the extent of urine leakage. Women with moderate or large volume leakage felt the most essential property of an absorbent product was impermeability in any situation; other desirable characteristics were absence of odor, secure attachment to underwear, nonrustling, and ease of changing.[16]

Women may need to try several types of products before finding one best suited to their needs. In one study of 460 women 40 percent were using the product initially recommended, whereas 52 percent had tried two to four products before finding a satisfactory product and 6 percent found all products tried unsuitable.[16] In addition to the absorbent products, other aids include bedside commodes, urinals, and urine collection devices.

Resources for Clinicians and Patients

Treatment guidelines and patient information and educational materials can be obtained from several organizations (Table 12-8). Information may also be available from the manufacturers of commercial products.

Table 12-8

Educational Resources

National Association for Continence
(Help for Incontinent People)
P.O. Box 8310
Spartanburg, SC 29305-8310
Phone: 800-BLADDER
http://www.nafc.org

Simon Foundation for Continence
P.O. Box 835
Wilmette, IL 60091
Phone: 800-23-SIMON

Bladder Health Council
American Foundation of Urologic Disease
300 W. Pratt Street
Suite 401
Baltimore, MD 21201-2463
Phone: 800-242-2383

AHCPR Clinical Practice Guideline: Urinary
   Incontinence in Adults: Acute and Chronic
   Management, 1996
Superintendent of Documents
U.S. Government Printing Office
P.O. Box 371954
Pittsburgh, PA 15250-7954
Phone: 202-512-1800
http://www.ahcpr.gov/

AHCPR Clinical Practice Guideline: Abbreviated
   report
AHCPR Consumer Guide (Understanding
   Incontinence)
AHCPR Publications Clearing House
P.O. Box 8547
Silver Spring, MD 20907-8547
Phone: 800-358-9295

References

1. Fantl JA, Newman DK, Collings J, et al: *Urinary Incontinence in Adults: Acute and Chronic Management.* Clinical Practice Guideline, No. 2, 1996 Update. AHCPR Publication No. 96-0682. Rockville MD: U.S. Department of Health and Human Services, Public Health Service, Agency for Health Care Policy and Research; 1986.

2. Noelker L: Incontinence in elderly cared for by family. *Gerontologist* 27:194, 1987.

3. Thom D: Variation in estimates of urinary incontinence prevalence in the community: effects of differences in definition, population characteristics, and study type. *J Am Geriatr Soc* 46:473, 1998.

4. Diokno AC, Brock BM, Brown MB, Herzog AR: Prevalence of urinary incontinence and other urologic symptoms in the noninstitutionalized elderly. *J Urol* 136:1022, 1986.

5. Payne CK: Epidemiology, pathophysiology, and evaluation of urinary incontinence and overactive bladder. *Urology* 51(suppl 2A):3, 1998.

6. Nygaard I, DeLancey JO: Exercise and incontinence. *Obstet Gynecol* 75:848, 1990.

7. Wallace K: Female pelvic floor functions, dysfunctions, and behavioral approaches to treatment. *Clin Sports Med* 13:459, 1994.

8. Jeter KF, Wagner DB: Incontinence in the American home—a survey of 36,500 people. *J Am Geriatr Soc* 41:379, 1990.

9. Umlauf MG, Goode PS, Burgio KL: Psychosocial issues in geriatric urology. *Urol Clin North Am* 23:127, 1996.

10. Mitteness LS: The management of urinary incontinence by community-living elderly. *Gerontologist* 27:185, 1987.

11. McGrother C, Resnick M, Yalla SV, et al: Epidemiology and etiology of urinary incontinence in the elderly. *World J Urol* 16(suppl 1):S3, 1998.

12. Roberts RO, Jacobsen SJ, Rhodes T, et al: Urinary incontinence in a community-based cohort: prevalence and healthcare-seeking. *J Am Geriatr Soc* 46:467, 1998.

13. Wyman JF, Choi SC, Harkins SW, Wilson MS, Fantl JA: The urinary diary in the evaluation of incontinent women: a test-retest analysis. *Obstet Gynecol* 71:812, 1988.

14. Harris T: *Aging in the Eighties: Prevalence and Impact of Urinary Problems in Individuals Age 65*

Years and Over. NCHSR Publication No. 21. Rockville, MD: National Center for Health Services Research and Technology Advance Data; 1986; 121 (August 27):1.

15. Wyman JF, Harkins SW, Choi SC, et al: Psychosocial impact of urinary incontinence in women. *Obstet Gynecol* 70:378, 1987.

16. Kinn AC, Zaar A: Quality of life and urinary incontinence pad use in women. *Int Urogynecol J* 9:83, 1998.

17. Lenderking WR, Nackley JF, Anderson RB, Testa MA: A review of the quality of life aspects of urinary urge incontinence. *PharmacoEconomics* 9:11, 1996.

18. Mitteness LS: Social aspects of urinary incontinence in the elderly. *AORN* 56:731, 1992.

19. Engberg SJ, McDowell BJ, Burgio KL, et al: Self-care behaviors of older women with urinary incontinence. *J Gerontol Nurs* 21:7, 1995.

20. Wagner Th, Hu TW: Economic costs of urinary incontinence. *Int Urogynecol J* 9:127, 1998.

21. Ramsey SD, Wagner TH, Bavendam TG: Estimated costs of treating stress urinary incontinence in elderly women according to the AHCPR clinical practice guidelines. *Am J Managed Care* 2:147, 1996.

22. Diokno AC, Atassi O: Urinary incontinence. *Compr Ther* 22:592, 1996.

23. Chutka DS, Fleming KC, Evans MP, et al: Urinary incontinence in the elderly population. *Mayo Clin Proc* 71:93, 1996.

24. Portera SG, Lipscomb GH: Pharmacologic therapy for urinary incontinence and voiding dysfunctions. *Clin Obstet Gynecol* 41:691, 1998.

25. Romanowski GL, Shimp LA, Balson AB, Cahn ML: Urinary incontinence in the elderly: etiology and treatment. *Drug Intell Clin Pharm* 22:525, 1988.

26. Palmer MH: *Urinary Incontinence*. Thorofare, NJ: Slack Publishers; 1985.

27. Nasr SZ, Ouslander JG: Urinary incontinence in the elderly. *Drugs Aging* 12:349, 1998.

28. Thom DH, Brown JS: Reproductive and hormonal risk factors for urinary incontinence in later life: a review of the clinical and epidemiologic literature. *J Am Geriatr Soc* 46:1141, 1998.

29. Resnick NM: Urinary incontinence. *Lancet* 346:94, 1995.

30. Fonda D, Resnick NM, Kirschner-Hermanns R: Prevention of urinary incontinence in older people. *Br J Urol* 82(suppl 1):5, 1998.

31. Gormley EA, Griffiths DJ, McCracken PN, Harrison GM: Polypharmacy and its effect on urinary incontinence in a geriatric population. *Br J Urol* 71:265, 1993.

32. Keister KJ, Creason NS: Medications of elderly institutionalized incontinent females. *J Adv Nurs* 14:980, 1989.

33. Diokno AC, Brown MB, Herzog AR: Relationship between use of diuretics and continence status in the elderly. *Urology* 38:39, 1991.

34. Shimp LA, Wells TJ, Brink CA, et al: Relationship between drug use and urinary incontinence in elderly women. *Drug Intell Clin Pharm* 22:786, 1988.

35. Fantl JA, Wyman JF, Wilson M, et al: Diuretics and urinary incontinence in community-dwelling women. *Neurourol Urodynam* 9:25, 1990.

36. Haynes BR: Determinants of compliance: the disease and the mechanics of treatment. In: Haynes BR, Taylor DW, Sackett DL (eds): *Compliance in Health Care*. Baltimore: Johns Hopkins University Press; 1979.

37. Bump RC, McClish DK: Cigarette smoking and urinary incontinence in women. *Am J Obstet Gynecol* 167:1213, 1992.

38. Marshall HJ, Beevers DG: α-Adrenoceptor blocking drugs and female urinary incontinence: prevalence and reversibility. *Br J Clin Pharmacol* 42:507, 1996.

39. Kiruluta GH, Mercer AR, Winsor GM: Prazosin as cause of urinary incontinence. *Urology* 18:618, 1981.

40. Pannill FC: Urinary incontinence for the primary care physician. *Conn Med* 57:299, 1993.

41. Snella KA, Stach-Klysh AO, Retzky S, et al: *A Profile of Incontinence Diagnosis and Management*. American Council on Pharmaceutical Education written continuing education program #202-999-96-029-H01; 1996.

42. Beizer JL: Urinary incontinence in women: a review for the pharmacist. *J Am Pharm Assoc* NS36(3):196, 1996.

43. Rosenthal AJ, McMurtry CT: Urinary incontinence in the elderly. *Postgrad Med* 95:109, 1995.

44. Cavanaugh GL, Martin RE, Stenson MA, Robinson DD: Venlafaxine and urinary incontinence: possible association. *Ann Pharmacother* 31:372, 1997.

45. Shimp LA: Influence of drug therapy on urinary continence. *Top Geriatr Rehabil* 3:30, 1988.

46. Gil-Nagel A, Gapany S, Blesi K, et al: Incontinence during treatment with gabapentin. *Neurology* 48:1467, 1997.

47. Sandyk R: Urinary incontinence associated with clonazepam therapy. *S Afr Med J* 64:230, 1983.

48. Pollack MH, Reiter S, Hammerness P: Genitourinary and sexual adverse effects of psychotropic medication. *Int J Psychiatry Med* 22:305, 1992.

49. Ambrosini PJ: A pharmacologic paradigm for urinary incontinence and enuresis. *J Clin Psychopharmacol* 4:247, 1984.

50. Sandyk R, Gillman MA: Urinary incontinence in patient on long-term bromocriptine. *Lancet* 2:1260, 1983.

51. Gopinathan G, Calne DB: Incontinence of urine with long-term bromocriptine therapy. *Ann Neurol* 8:204, 1980.

52. Rosenbaum JF, Pollack MH: Treatment-emergent incontinence with lithium. *J Clin Psychiatry* 46:444, 1985.

53. Fossaluzza V, Di Benedetto P, Zampa A, De Vita S: Misoprostol-induced urinary incontinence. *J Intern Med* 230:463, 1991.

54. Pillens PI, Wood SM: Cisapride increases micturition frequency. *J Clin Gastroenterol* 19:336, 1994.

55. Hansen J: Urinary incontinence associated with metoclopramide. *JAMA* 252:3251, 1984.

56. Kumar BB: Urinary incontinence associated with metoclopramide. *JAMA* 251:1553, 1984.

57. Diokno AC: Epidemiology and psychosocial aspects of incontinence. *Urol Clin North Am* 22:481, 1995.

58. Ouslander JG: Geriatric urinary incontinence. *Dis Mon* 38:71, 1992.

59. Holtedahl K, Hunskaar S: Prevalence, 1-year incidence and factors associated with urinary incontinence: a population-based study of women 50–74 years of age in primary care. *Maturitas* 28:205, 1998.

60. Fonda D, Woodward M, D'Astoli M, Chin WF: Sustained improvement of subjective quality of life in older community-dwelling people after treatment of urinary incontinence. *Age Aging* 24:283, 1995.

61. Burgio KL, Locher JL, Goode PS, et al: Behavioral vs drug treatment for urge urinary incontinence in older women. *JAMA* 280:1995, 1998.

62. Wells T, Brink C, Diokno A, et al: Pelvic muscle exercise for stress urinary incontinence in elderly women. *J Am Geriatr Soc* 39:785, 1991.

63. Nygaard IE, Kreder KJ, Lepic MM, et al: Efficacy of pelvic floor muscle exercises in women with stress, urge and mixed urinary incontinence. *Am J Obstet Gynecol* 174:120, 1996.

64. Miller J, Ashton-Miller JA, DeLancey JOL: The knack: use of a precisely-timed pelvic muscle contraction can reduce urine leakage in SUI. *Neurourol Urodyn* 15:392, 1996.

65. Fall M, Pettersson S: The simplified Lapides' operation for stress incontinence. *Scand J Urol Nephrol* 17:27, 1983.

66. Homma Y, Kawabe K, Kageyama S, et al: Injection of glutaraldehyde cross-linked collagen for urinary incontinence: two-year efficacy by self-assessment. *Int J Urol* 3:124, 1996.

67. Brubaker L, Benson JT, Bent A, et al: Transvaginal electrical stimulation for female urinary incontinence. *Am J Obstetr Gynecol* 177:536, 1997.

68. Fall M, Erlandson BE, Nilson AE, Sundin T: Long-term intravaginal electrical stimulation in urge and stress incontinence. *Scand J Urol Nephrol* 44 (Suppl):55, 1977.

69. North BB: A disposable patch for stress urinary incontinence. *Fam Med* 30:258, 1998.

70. Gallo ML, Hancock R, Davila GW: Clinical experience with a balloon-tipped urethral insert for stress urinary incontinence. *Journal of Wound Ostomy and Continence Nursing* 24:51, 1997.

71. Miller JL, Bavendam T: Treatment with the Reliance control insert: one-year experience. *J Endourol* 10:287, 1996.

72. Moore KH, Foote A, Siva S, et al: The use of bladder neck support prosthesis in combined genuine stress incontinence and detrusor instability. *Aust NZ J Obstetr Gynaecol* 37:440, 1997.

73. Hills CJ, Winter SA, Balfour JA: Tolterodine. *Drugs* 55:813, 1998.

74. Bary PR, Moisey CU, Stephenson TP: The urodynamic and subjective results of treatment of detrusor instability with oxybutynin chloride. In: Zinner NR, Sterling AM (eds): *Female Incontinence.* New York: Alan R. Liss; 1981.

75. Diokno AC: Practical approach to the management of urinary incontinence in the elderly. *Compr Ther* 9:67, 1983.

76. Khullar V, Cardozo L: Incontinence in the elderly. *Curr Opin Obstet Gynecol* 10:391, 1998.

77. Walter S, Meyhoff HH, Gerstenberg T: Urinary incontinence in the female. *Acta Obstet Gynecol Scand* 63:159, 1984.

78. American College of Obstetricians and Gynecologists: Urinary incontinence (Technical bulletin, no. 213, October 1995). *Int J Gynecol Obstet* 52:75, 1996.

79. Castleden CM, Duffin HM, Gulati RS: Double-blind study of imipramine: and placebo for incontinence due to bladder instability. *Age Aging* 15:299, 1986.

80. Chan AS, Ouslander JG: Effects of diltiazem on urinary incontinence. *J Am Geriatr Soc* 38:1265, 1980.

81. Brocklehurst JC: Drug effects in urinary incontinence. In: Brocklehurst JC (ed): *Urology in the Elderly*. Edinburgh: Churchill Livingston; 1984.

82. Norlen L, Sundin T, Waagstein F: Beta-adrenoceptor stimulation of the human urinary bladder in vivo. *Acta Pharmacol Toxicol* 43:26, 1978.

83. Lindholm P, Lose G: Terbutaline in the treatment of female urge incontinence. *Urol Int* 41:158, 1986.

84. Cardozo LD, Stanton SL: A comparison between bromocriptine and indomethacin in the treatment of detrusor instability. *J Urol* 123:399, 1980.

85. Palmer J: Report of a double-blind crossover study of flurbiprofen and placebo in detrusor instability. *J Int Med Res* 11(suppl 2):11, 1983.

86. Beisland HO, Fossberg E, Moer A: Urethral sphincter insufficiency in postmenopausal females: treatment with phenylpropanolamine and estriol separately and in combination. *Urol Int* 39:211, 1984.

87. Fossberg E, Beisland HO, Lundgren RA: Stress incontinence in females: treatment with phenylpropanolamine. *Urol Int* 38:293, 1983.

88. Fantl JA, Cardozo L, McClish DK, et al: Estrogen therapy in the management of urinary incontinence in postmenopausal women: a meta-analysis. First report of the Hormones and Urogenital Therapy Committee. *Obstet Gynecol* 83:12, 1994.

89. Serels S, Stein M: Prospective study comparing hyoscyamine, doxazosin, and combination therapy for the treatment of urgency and frequency in women. *Neurourol Urodyn* 17:31, 1998.

90. Lepor H, Theune C: Randomized double-blind study comparing the efficacy of terazosin versus placebo in women with prostatism-like symptoms. *J Urol* 154:116, 1995.

91. Rackley R, Kursh ED: Evaluation and medical management of female urinary incontinence. *Compr Ther* 22:547, 1996.

92. Brink CA: Absorbent pads, garments and management strategies. *J Am Geriatr Soc* 38:368, 1990.

93. Waddell R, Suter F: Incontinence aids in perspective. *Aust Fam Physician* 18:930, 1989.

94. Baker, J, Norton P: Evaluation of absorbent products for women with mild to moderate urinary incontinence. *Appl Nurs Res* 9:29, 1996.

Louise Parent-Stevens
Elizabeth A. Burns

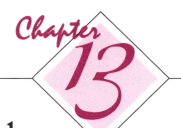

Chapter
13

Menstrual Disorders

Overview

Menstruation is an integral part of a woman's life for the years that span the menarche (onset of menses) to menopause (the final menstrual period). Although a 28-day menstrual cycle is usually considered the norm, there is a wide variation in both the length of the menstrual cycle (ranging from 21 to 45 days) and the duration of blood flow (from 3 to 7 days) in healthy, ovulating women.[1,2] Changes in cycle length can also occur over time within individual women. Adolescents who have recently gone through menarche and women approaching menopause tend to have a greater frequency of very short or very long cycles, which is consistent with a higher incidence of anovulatory cycles in these populations. A number of factors, including weight loss, high levels of physical activity, stress, and smoking may prolong the length of menstrual cycles.[1]

Women's knowledge and understanding of the menstrual cycle appears to be limited and is often colored by myth and misunderstanding. Even among today's young women, who have the benefit of exposure to school-based health education, attitudes toward menstruation are negative and knowledge is poor. A group of 224 sixth-grade girls were surveyed about their knowledge of menstruation.[3] Although most of the participants were able to identify the frequency and length of typical menstruation, the majority were not able to describe adequately why menstruation occurred or quantify the amount of menstrual flow. When the respondents were asked to describe physical or psychological changes that might occur with the onset of menstruation, most identified negative changes, such as cramps, bloating, increased anxiety, tension, and irritability. This lack of knowledge may extend beyond the adolescent years. A survey of 80 college women found that over 30 percent could not provide a basic explanation of menstruation.[4] Understanding normal menstrual function is important in assisting women to identify potential problems and seek medical care when necessary. Knowledge of normal physiology and its relationship to fertility can be a valuable tool for preventing undesired pregnancy and limiting the spread of sexually transmitted disease (STD).[3,5]

Dysmenorrhea

Dysmenorrhea is the presence of pain during or shortly before the onset of a menstrual period. Abdominal pain and cramping and backache are most commonly seen; upper leg pain/ache is also reported. Associated gastrointestinal symptoms include nausea and diarrhea. Headache and fatigue may be present. Pain usually begins on the first day of bleeding, although some women report having symptoms before menses begin or not until the second day of blood flow. In primary dysmenorrhea (no pelvic pathology) pain usually lasts about 2 days and rarely persists beyond 3 days. Primary dysmenorrhea does not occur in the absence of ovulation.[6]

In various surveys, 30 to 60 percent of menstruating women relate having painful menses, with 7 to 15 percent reporting severe pain.[1,7] Among adolescents, the prevalence of dysmenorrhea increases with increasing age, most likely related to its association with ovulatory cycles. It appears to be most common in young adult women between the ages of 17 and 24. After age 24, the prevalence declines, possibly due to the mitigating effect of pregnancy on the condition for many women. Risk for severe dysmenorrhea has been associated with an earlier age at menarche, nulliparity, obesity, smoking, and stress.[1,7]

Etiology

In the past, dysmenorrhea was regarded as an emotional or psychogenic problem.[8] It is now well documented that primary dysmenorrhea is a physiologic entity associated with abnormally increased uterine activity. Higher resting uterine tone and contraction pressures have been documented in women with primary dysmenorrhea as compared to women without significant menstrual pain, suggesting that the pain results from intermittent myometrial ischemia.[6] The main stimulant of this increased uterine activity appears to be the synthesis and release of prostaglandins, specifically prostaglandin E_2 (PGE_2). Elevated endometrial levels of PGE_2 have been documented in women with dysmenorrhea. The production of prostaglandin levels sufficient to trigger pain-inducing uterine contractions occurs only in adequately stimulated endometrial tissue, thus limiting the occurrence of primary dysmenorrhea to ovulatory cycles. In some women with dysmenorrhea, normal levels of prostaglandins with elevated levels of leukotrienes, which also induce uterine contractions, have been demonstrated.[8] An increase in uterine vascularity or a decrease in uterine innervation may be responsible for the decrease in the incidence of dysmenorrhea after pregnancy.[9]

Secondary dysmenorrhea implies an underlying pathology, which may include endometriosis, leiomyomas, endometrial cancer, pelvic inflammatory disease (PID), use of an intrauterine device (IUD), and adhesions.[10,11] Secondary dysmenorrhea often has its onset in the middle to late twenties, may worsen with age, and may persist beyond the first 2 to 3 days of menstrual flow.[10]

Diagnosis

The diagnosis of primary dysmenorrhea is basically one of exclusion. A thorough medical history should be taken to elicit possible causes of secondary dysmenorrhea and to ensure that there are no contraindications to therapy. The menstrual history should include age at menarche, age at symptom onset, and frequency, severity, and relationship of symptoms to the menstrual cycle. Complaints of heavy bleeding, dyspareunia, or pain that occurs at times other than during the menstrual period are suggestive of secondary dysmenorrhea.[12] If a negative history is obtained, a presumptive diagnosis of primary dysmenorrhea may be made. After evaluating prior therapy, including nonprescription and prescription drugs previously used and whether they were effective, a recommendation for therapy can be made. If the pain does not respond to a 3- to 6-month trial of nonsteroidal anti-inflammatory drugs (NSAIDs) or if the history suggests secondary dysmenorrhea, a physical examination, including a pelvic and rectovaginal examination, should be done. Laboratory tests are not usually needed. If further evaluation is needed, a diagnostic laparoscopy may be done to assess for conditions such as endometriosis.[13]

Treatment

Once a diagnosis of primary dysmenorrhea has been made, therapy can be instituted based on the patient's needs. Fortunately, efficacious therapies are available that allow most women to continue their normal activities. The two most commonly used drug therapies are the NSAIDs and combination oral contraceptives (OCs).

NONSTEROIDAL ANTI-INFLAMMATORY DRUGS

For patients not requiring contraception, a trial with NSAIDs as first-line therapy is indicated. NSAIDs exert their therapeutic benefit by decreasing the production of uterine prostaglandins via the inhibition of cyclooxygenase.[6] These agents have been shown in multiple clinical trials to be effective in 80 to 85 percent of women with primary dysmenorrhea. In addition to the relief of cramps, associated symptoms such as headache and muscle aches may respond. Women with IUD-induced dysmenorrhea also appear to have a good response to

NSAID therapy and may also experience a decrease in IUD-related menorrhagia as well.[8]

TYPES Multiple NSAIDs are currently available. Those with an indication for the treatment of dysmenorrhea, approved by the Food and Drug Administration (FDA), are shown in Table 13-1. With the exception of aspirin, which appears to be relatively ineffective, there does not seem to be a significant difference in efficacy between various NSAIDs in the management of dysmenorrhea. It has been postulated that the anthranilic acid derivative NSAIDs (mefenamic acid, meclofenamate) might be more efficacious than other chemical classes due to an additional effect of blocking prostaglandin effects in smooth muscle. However, clinical studies have not shown a consistent benefit over other NSAIDs.[6] Although indomethacin has been shown to be effective, the higher incidence of adverse effects limits its usefulness.[14]

REGIMEN The recommended dosages and treatment regimens for commonly used NSAIDs are shown in Table 13-1. A trial of two to three cycles is reasonable to determine if a particular NSAID is effective. Clinical response and occurrence of adverse effects with NSAIDs are extremely variable. If one agent is not effective or not well tolerated for an individual, it is reasonable to try an alternate NSAID. It is unclear whether giving a higher first dose (loading dose) provides greater benefit than initiation of therapy with a standard dose. For the majority of women, starting treatment with the onset of menstrual flow is equally efficacious to initiating therapy before blood flow and can prevent drug administration to a potentially pregnant woman.[14,15] Because NSAIDs prevent pain rather than just provide analgesia, they are best used on a scheduled basis, not as needed, for the first 2 to 3 days of menstrual flow. An additional advantage to the use of NSAIDs is that several of these agents are available without prescription, albeit at reduced strength compared with prescription-only dosages. Patients should be educated on proper administration to obtain maximal benefit from NSAID therapy.

SIDE EFFECTS NSAIDs in the management of dysmenorrhea are generally well tolerated, most likely due to the intermittent and short-term nature of their use. Among women using these agents for dysmenorrhea, headache, dizziness, and gastric irritation have been most commonly reported.[14] Patients should be advised about these possible adverse effects and instructed to take their NSAID with food to decrease the likelihood of stomach upset. In one study, 25 percent of women treated with NSAIDs noted decreased menstrual bleeding. A delay in the onset of menses has been reported in about 5 percent of women initiating NSAID treatment several days before the expected onset of menses.[14] NSAIDs can cause serious adverse effects including peptic ulcer disease and bronchospasm in patients with asthma or among those with hypersensitivity. These effects are mediated through their inhibition of prostaglandin synthesis. Therefore, NSAIDs are contraindicated in patients with a history of peptic ulcer disease and in patients with a history of wheezing after aspirin or NSAID ingestion.

ORAL CONTRACEPTIVES

The OCs are effective in diminishing symptoms of dysmenorrhea and are reasonable first-line choices for women desiring a contraceptive agent.[16,17] The mechanism of action of OCs in preventing dysmenorrhea is unclear. These agents inhibit ovulation and also reduce menstrual blood prostaglandin content and decrease uterine motility.[16,17] A limited number of studies have documented a 50 to 80 percent efficacy rate for OCs in controlling dysmenorrhea.[18]

Once it has been determined that a woman is a candidate for OC treatment (see Chap. 2 for a complete discussion on the use of OCs), a choice of agents must be made. The clinical data regarding efficacy rates between various OCs in dysmenorrhea are limited. One cross-over study of 22 women found significantly decreased pain while on monophasic OCs compared to triphasic OCs.[17] In an epidemiologic survey of 489 women, no difference was found in the severity of dys-

Table 13-1
NSAIDs for the Treatment of Dysmenorrhea

DRUG NAME	BRAND NAME	GENERIC AVAILABLE	STATUS	DOSAGE FORM/STRENGTH	RECOMMENDED DOSAGE*	MAXIMUM 24-H DOSAGE[†]
DRUGS WITH FDA APPROVED INDICATION FOR TREATMENT OF DYSMENORRHEA						
Diclofenac (immediate release)	Cataflam	N	Rx	Tablet: 50 mg (use immediate release only)	50 mg tid or 100 mg stat then 50 mg tid	150 mg (may give 200 mg on 1st day)
Ibuprofen	Motrin	Y	Rx	Tablets: 300, 400, 600, 800 mg	400–800 mg q4–6h	3.2 g
	Advil, Nuprin, Motrin IB	Y	OTC	Tablets: 200 mg Susp: 100 mg/5 mL	200–400 mg q4–6h	1.2 g (6 tablets)
Ketoprofen	Orudis	Y	Rx	Capsule: 25, 50, 75 mg	25–50 mg q6–8h	300 mg
	Orudis KT, Actron	N	OTC	Tablet: 12.5 mg	12.5 mg q6–8h, may repeat dose in 1 hr if needed	75 mg (6 tablets)
Meclofenamate sodium	Meclomen	Y	Rx	Capsule: 50, 100 mg	100 mg tid, not to exceed 6 d	300 mg
Mefenamic acid	Ponstel	N	Rx	Capsule: 250 mg	500 mg stat, then 250 mg q6h, not to exceed 1 wk	1 g (may give 1.25 g on 1st day)
Naproxen	Naprosyn	Y	Rx	Tablet: 250, 375, 500 mg Susp: 125 mg/5 mL	500 mg stat, then 250 mg q6–8h	1.25 g
Naproxen sodium	Anaprox	Y	Rx	Tablet: 275, 550 mg	550 mg stat, then 275 mg q6–8h	1.375 mg
	Aleve	Y	OTC	Tablet: 220 mg	220 mg q8–12h or 440 mg stat, then 220 mg q8–12h	660 mg (3 tablets)
DRUGS WITH FDA APPROVAL FOR TREATMENT OF MILD-MODERATE PAIN[‡]						
Etodolac	Lodine	N	Rx	Capsule: 200, 300 mg	200–400 mg q6–8h	1.2 g
Fenoprofen	Nalfon	Y	Rx	Tablet: 200, 300 mg Capsule: 600 mg	200–400 mg q6–8h	1.2 g

*Manufacturer recommends prn dosing—for dysmenorrhea, scheduled dosing may be more efficacious.
[†]Maximum 24-h dosage for nonprescription products indicates package labeling instructions.
[‡]Do not use as first-line NSAIDs—may be used as alternates if other NSAIDs not tolerated or effective.
ABBREVIATIONS: OTC, over the counter; Rx, prescription; stat, immediately (first dose).

menorrhea among women using monophasic or triphasic OCs nor was there any difference in dysmenorrhea associated with the progestational potency of the OCs used.[16] Therefore, the choice of OC should be based on other factors. For women on OCs who continue to experience some dysmenorrhea, addition of an NSAID to the regimen may provide additional pain relief.[18]

ALTERNATIVE THERAPIES

Other treatment modalities have been studied in the management of dysmenorrhea and show promise for patients who do not respond to or cannot tolerate the therapies previously discussed. Until further data are available, these agents should be reserved for patients in whom conventional treatment for dysmenorrhea has failed.

Calcium channel blockers block uterine contractions in vitro. In vivo, nifedipine 20 to 90 mg/d, diltiazem 240 mg/d, and nicardipine 60 mg/d (in a single patient) have been effective in decreasing pain associated with dysmenorrhea. Symptoms commonly associated with dysmenorrhea, such as nausea and malaise, were not improved by the calcium channel blockers. In the nifedipine trials, which used immediate-release or sublingual dosing, almost half the patients experienced side effects, including headache, flushing, and palpitations. In addition, there are concerns about the safety of these short-acting agents (see Chap. 17). However, in one study of 36 women, 25 of the women wished to continue therapy after study completion.[19] Diltiazem appears to be better tolerated, with fewer than 10 percent of patients discontinuing the drug because of adverse effects.[20]

β-Adrenergic agonists, which theoretically relax the uterus and thereby decrease uterine tone, have shown some benefit in clinical studies. In a cross-over comparison study, terbutaline inhalation, 6 puffs (1.5 mg) up to six times daily, produced moderate improvement in 12 of 14 women, a significant difference compared to the placebo arm of the study. Adverse drug reactions,

including palpitations, tremor, and flushing, were reported in 4 of the 14 women.[21]

Transcutaneous electrical nerve stimulation (TENS) has been effective in reducing pain associated with primary dysmenorrhea.[22,23] In one study, it produced a more rapid onset of pain relief than naproxen.[22] Some patients may find TENS painful; however, only short periods of stimulation are needed to provide pain relief that persists for several hours. The precise mechanism by which TENS exerts its analgesic effect in dysmenorrhea is unknown but may include a decrease in myometrial ischemia or a direct effect on the nervous system.[22]

Herbal remedies that have been shown to be of possible benefit in the management of dysmenorrhea are listed in Table 13-2.

Patient Education

Dysmenorrhea in many women can be adequately controlled by drug therapy. Unfortunately, due to menstrual myths and a lack of understanding of normal menstruation, many adolescents do not receive adequate treatment despite the availability, without prescription, of effective and relatively inexpensive drugs. In a study of 268 teenage girls who reported menstrual pain, 30 percent did not use any drug therapy for their symptoms even though 36 percent of that group admitted to moderate to severe menstrual pain. Among the 70 percent who self-treated with a nonprescription product, acetaminophen, which is considered less effective than NSAIDs for dysmenorrhea, was the most commonly used agent. Fewer than 20 percent of the study participants reported using the medication to prevent menstrual cramps rather than to treat the pain.[24] Patients, especially to adolescents who are most likely to experience dysmenorrhea, need to be educated about the proper use of nonprescription drugs for this problem and that other therapies can be tried if NSAIDs are ineffective.

Table 13-2

Herbal Medicinals Approved for Menstrual Disorders per the German Commission E

HERBAL (ALTERNATE NAMES)	ACTION	ROUTE	DAILY DOSAGE	APPROVED MENSTRUAL DISORDER USES	CONTRA-INDICATIONS	ADVERSE REACTIONS	DRUG INTERACTIONS
Black cohosh root (*Cimicifugae racemosae* root)	Estrogen-like luteinzing hormone suppressant, binds to estrogen receptors	Oral	40 mg, not to exceed 6 mo	premenstrual discomfort, dysmenorrhea	NK	Gastric irritation CNS side effects at high doses Miscarriage	NK
Bugleweed (lycopi herb, gypsywort)	Antigonadotropic, antithyrotropic, ↓ prolactin levels	Oral	0.02–2 g	Tension and pain in breast	Thyroid disease	Thyroid enlargement with prolonged high doses	Inteferes with diagnostic radioactive isotopes
Chaste Tree fruit (agni casti fructus, vitex fruit)	↓ Prolactin levels	Oral	30–40 mg	Mastodynia, premenstrual complaints, menstrual cycle irregularities	NK	Itching, urticaria	Possible antagonism of dopaminergic antagonists
Potentilla (potentilla anserinae herba, silverweed)	Increased tonus and contraction frequency in uterus (animals)	Oral	4 g	Mild dysmenorrheal disorders	NK	Gastric irritation	NK
Shepherd's Purse (bursae pastoris herba)	Increased uterine contraction	Oral	5–15 g	Mild menorrhagia and metrorrhagia	NK	NK	NK
Yarrow (millefolii herba/flos)	Choleretic, antispasmotic, antibacterial, astringent	Sitz bath	100 g/20 L water	Painful, cramplike conditions of psychosomatic origin (in the lower part of the female pelvis)	Allergy to yarrow	NK	NK

ABBREVIATIONS: CNS, central nervous system; NK, none known.
SOURCE: Adapted from M Blumenthal (ed)[108] and V Schulz et al.[109]

Endometriosis

Endometriosis, the presence of endometrial tissue outside of the uterus resulting in pelvic pain, dysmenorrhea, or infertility, is the most common cause of secondary dysmenorrhea.[25] The incidence of endometriosis has been estimated to range from less than 1 percent to up to 50 percent, depending on the population examined and the method used for diagnosis.[26] Mild endometriosis has frequently been detected in asymptomatic women undergoing laparotomy or laparoscopy; the severity of symptoms may be correlated with the number of ectopic endometrial implants.[27] The endometrial implants of endometriosis are steroid dependent, stimulated by estrogens, and atrophied by androgens or therapies that antagonize estrogenic effects. Therefore, the management of dysmenorrhea and pelvic pain related to endometriosis has focused on surgically removing implants or inducing their atrophy through hormonal manipulation. A decrease in pain symptoms has been achieved through either drug administration or surgical intervention (removal of implants, bilateral oophorectomy),[28–30] and recurrence rates are similar.[26,31]

Treatment Efficacy

Assessment of the benefits of therapy are confounded by the unpredictable nature of the disease; in one study, symptoms of untreated endometriosis worsened in 8 of 17 patients but improved or disappeared in 9 others.[31] Suppressive drug therapy

Table 13-3

Drugs Used in the Medical Management of Endometriosis

DRUG (BRAND NAME)	DRUG CLASS	DOSAGE	COMMENTS
Combination oral contraceptives (various)	Estrogen/ Progestin	One tablet daily PO	Contraceptive benefit, also beneficial for dysmenorrhea
Medroxyprogesterone acetate depot (Depo-Provera)	Progestin	150 mg IM q 3 mo	Contraceptive benefit, spotting early on and amenorrhea after prolonged use very common, delayed return of fertility after discontinuation may occur
Medroxyprogesterone acetate (Provera)	Progestin	10–50 mg/d PO	Irregular bleeding and weight gain common
Danazol (Danocrine)	Synthetic steroid	400–800 mg/d PO	Menstrual irregularities, weight gain, and androgenic effects common
Buserelin	GnRH agonist	900 µg intranasal/d (tid dosing)	Not available in the United States
Goserelin (Zoladex)	GnRH agonist	3.6 mg SC implant every month	FDA approved for monthly dosage form (not for 3-mo dosage)
Leuprolide (Lupron)	GnRH agonist	3.75–7.5 mg IM/mo or 11.25 mg IM q 3 mo	FDA approved in 1- and 3-mo depot forms (7.5 mg/mo dosage is not FDA approved for endometriosis)
Nafarelin (Synarel)	GnRH agonist	200 µg intranasal bid	FDA approved, may cause less bone loss than leuprolide[30]

ABBREVIATIONS: FDA, Food and Drug Administration; GnRH, gonadotropin-releasing hormone.

has a success rate of 70 to 100 percent in managing pain related to endometriosis during active treatment, but the recurrence rate is about 50 percent within 5 years after medication discontinuation.[26,30,31] Table 13-3 lists the agents that have been studied in the management of endometriosis.

Choice of Therapy

Choice of therapy for the management of endometriosis depends on the patient's needs. Women with pain secondary to endometriosis who also desire contraception should be offered a trial of combination OCs or injectable medroxyprogesterone acetate (MPA). If this is unsuccessful, agents that suppress ovarian function, such as danazol or the gonadotropin-releasing hormone (GnRH) agonists, or surgical intervention can be tried. Infertility related to endometriosis does not respond well to medical therapy; surgical intervention may be more successful.[26]

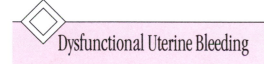

Dysfunctional Uterine Bleeding

Dysfunctional uterine bleeding (DUB) is the category of abnormal uterine bleeding most often seen at the extremes of a woman's reproductive life (adolescence and the perimenopause). Although some authors characterize DUB as bleeding without identifiable structural or systemic cause,[32,33] others also consider anovulation as part of the definition.[11] Indeed, more than 75 percent of the cases of DUB in adolescents are associated with anovulatory cycles.[2]

Abnormal uterine bleeding can be characterized using the following descriptions: hypomenorrhea, menorrhagia, oligomenorrhea, polymenorrhea, metrorrhagia, and menometrorrhagia (Table 13-4).[11,32] Most cases of DUB will fall into the menorrhagia or menometrorrhagia categories. Having the patient keep a menstrual calendar will assist in the classification. Although menorrhagia is defined as blood loss of more than 80 mL/cycle, it is difficult to assess blood loss reliably. About 10 percent of women have menorrhagia, but only half the women who complain of heavy menstrual periods will meet the clinical criteria.

Janssen and her colleagues have developed a visual assessment tool pictorially representing pads or tampons with three saturation options on a grid to be filled in with numbers of each product used and days of bleeding (Fig. 13-1). This can be used to help women discriminate between menorrhagia and normal blood loss.[34]

Etiology

The most common cause of DUB is an anovulatory menstrual cycle. Although anovulatory cycles are frequently associated with amenorrhea,

Table 13-4

Definition of Abnormal Uterine Bleeding Patterns

Amenorrhea (secondary)	No menses for 6 mo in a woman with previously regular cycles
Hypomenorrhea	Decrease in menstrual blood volume
Menorrhagia	Increase in menstrual blood volume and/or length of flow
Oligomenorrhea	Decrease in the number of bleeding episodes or a menstrual interval of > 35 d
Polymenorrhea	Increase in the number of bleeding episodes or a menstrual interval of < 21 d
Metrorrhagia	Irregular bleeding episodes that occur at frequent intervals between menses
Menometrorrhagia	Prolonged heavy bleeding at irregular intervals

Figure 13-1

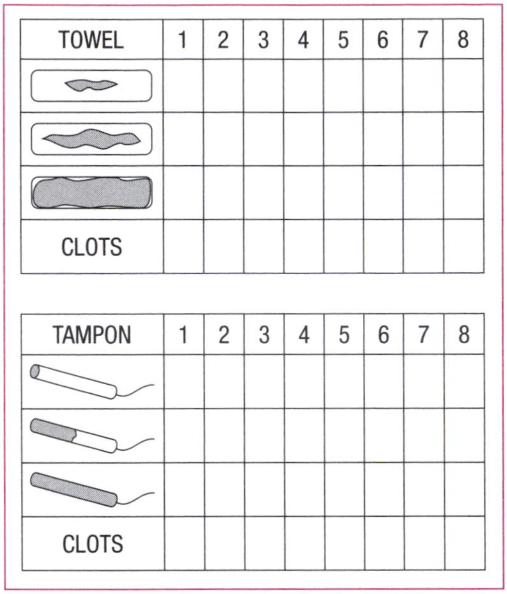

Visual assessment of menstrual blood loss.
(*Reproduced with permission from Janssen et al.[34]*)

anovulation more often results in DUB. At puberty, the hypothalamic-pituitary-ovarian (HPO) axis is immature. Gonadotropins stimulate the production of ovarian estrogen. However, as the estrogen levels rise, they do not trigger an adequate surge of luteinizing hormone (LH). Ovulation does not occur and the resultant menstrual flow may be heavy and prolonged, if estrogen levels fall, or irregular spotting may result from uneven sloughing of the endometrium, if estrogen stimulation persists. Although most young women establish a regular ovulatory menstrual pattern within 2 years, the development of a positive feedback mechanism that triggers the LH surge may take up to 5 years after menarche.[2,32,33]

Stress-related and exercise-induced menstrual abnormalities can result in heavy, irregular bleeding episodes. Sudden weight changes can also interrupt normal menstrual patterns. This may be due to a hypothalamic effect resulting in the disruption of normal GnRH patterns. Obesity-related anovulation and anovulation associated with hyperandrogenic chronic anovulation (commonly called polycystic ovary syndrome) can also cause DUB.[33]

In the perimenopausal period, the ovary is less sensitive to circulating gonadotropins. Although enough estrogen is produced to stimulate endometrial growth, there is not enough to stimulate the LH surge and subsequent ovulation. The anovulatory bleeding pattern that results may either be irregular spotting or heavy intermittent bleeding.[32,33]

Dysfunctional bleeding may also be associated with ovulatory cycles, although this is much less common. A structural (e.g., fibroids, polyps) or systemic (e.g., thyroid, renal, or hepatic disease, coagulopathies) abnormality can result in DUB and should be sought if the patient does not respond to therapy. STDs, vaginal trauma, foreign

Table 13-5

Causes of Abnormal Uterine Bleeding

Reproductive tract disease
  Complications of pregnancy
  Malignancy
  Infections—endometritis, cervicitis, vaginitis
  Benign lesions—leiomyomas, polyps, adenomyosis
  Endometriosis
  Hyperandrogenic chronic anovulation
Systemic disease
  Thyroid disorders
  Adrenal disorders
  Hepatic disease
  Renal disease
  Diabetes mellitus
  Coagulopathy—von Willebrand's, leukemias, thrombocytopenia
  Obesity
Other
  Drug effect—corticosteroids, psychotropic medications, anticoagulants, high-dose aspirin
  Trauma
  Foreign body
  Intrauterine device
  Arteriovenous malformation
  Dysfunctional uterine bleeding

bodies, malignancy, and arteriovenous malformations may also cause vaginal bleeding. A possible etiology for ovulatory cycle DUB is an imbalance between the prostaglandin prostacyclin (PGI_2) (a vasodilator that inhibits platelet aggregation) and thromboxane, which causes vasoconstriction and promotes platelet aggregation.[11,35,36] In these cases, women have sufficient progesterone concentrations that result in a normal secretory endometrium.[11]

Falcone and his colleagues, in a retrospective review of Canadian adolescents admitted for DUB, found that few (3 percent) had undiagnosed hematologic problems. Many (28 percent) had significant past medical and surgical problems. Over half had evidence of anovulatory cycles.[37]

Table 13-5 summarizes the systemic and structural causes of abnormal uterine bleeding.

Diagnosis

Studies should be planned on the basis of age and risk factors. Not every woman with a negative physical and laboratory examination needs invasive testing. Although the diagnosis of DUB is common in adolescents, other causes of abnormal uterine bleeding must be considered. Pregnancy-related bleeding must be considered from the outset. Other etiologies of abnormal uterine bleeding can be worked up in a step-wise fashion (Figs. 13-2 and 13-3).

HISTORY

The initial evaluation (Table 13-6) should include a careful history of the present complaint to quantify and characterize the bleeding episodes, a sexual

Figure 13-2

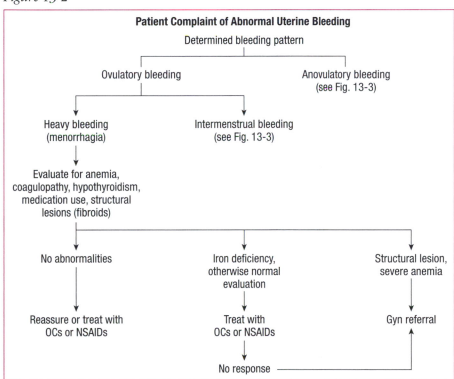

Approach to abnormal uterine bleeding. (*Reproduced with permission from Med Clin N Am 79(2):330, Copyright 1995.*) Abbreviations: OC, oral contraceptive; NSAID, nonsteroidal anti-inflammatory drug.

Figure 13-3

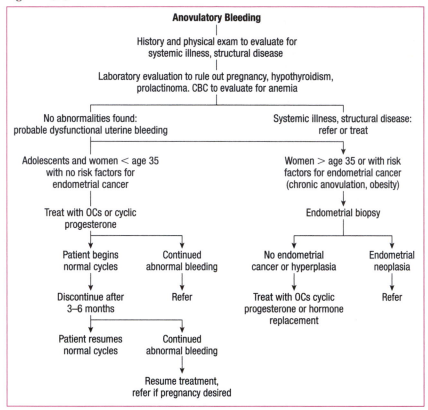

Evaluation of the patient with anovulatory bleeding. (*Reproduced with permission from Med Clin N Am 79(2):330, Copyright 1995.*) Abbreviations: CBC, complete blood count; OCs, oral contraceptives.

Table 13-6

Initial Evaluation of Dysfunctional Uterine Bleeding

EVALUATION	FINDING	TEST
History	Evidence of systemic, chronic	Disease-specific tests
Physical examination	medical illness,	Complete blood count
	pregnancy	Pregnancy test
Pelvic examination	Infection/inflammation	Cultures
	Suspected malignancy	Pap smear, consider biopsy
	Trauma	
	Foreign body	
	Polyp	Biopsy/removal
	Uterine enlargement	Radiologic evaluation/ultrasound
	(or exam not adequate)	
Diagnostic testing	If > 35 y of age, or at high risk	Endometrial biopsy
	for endometrial cancer	and/or hysteroscopy

and reproductive history, a review of current medications (including nonprescription medications) that might contribute to a bleeding problem (e.g., anticoagulants and high-dose aspirin), and a review of systems looking for changes suggestive of thyroid, hepatic, or renal disease or coagulopathies. The history of the bleeding pattern will provide clues as to whether the bleeding is likely ovulatory (bleeding occurs at regular intervals and is preceded by premenstrual symptoms such as breast tenderness or abdominal cramping) or anovulatory (irregular intervals with prolonged bleeding, often following periods of amenorrhea).

PHYSICAL EXAMINATION

To evaluate the severity of bleeding, patients should be screened for evidence of orthostatic hypotension. A physical examination, looking for signs of systemic disease, and a pelvic examination should be done. A Pap smear and cervical cultures should be done as well. Evidence of pelvic infection, vaginal trauma, a foreign body, vaginitis, cervical polyps, or cervicitis will help identify the cause of the bleeding and direct further investigations. A symmetrically enlarged nonpregnant uterus may suggest adenomyosis; if the uterus is enlarged, with an irregular contour, fibroids should be suspected.[33,38]

Although beyond the scope of this chapter, clinicians should keep in mind the sensitive nature of this evaluation and examination. Trauma and foreign bodies may indicate sexual assault (see Chap. 7) or self-mutilation. STDs and pregnancy in the young adolescent may indicate child abuse.

LABORATORY TESTING

Initial laboratory tests should include a pregnancy test, Pap smear, cervical cultures, and a complete blood count (see Table 13-6). Women with significant and long-term DUB will have evidence of iron depletion or iron-deficiency anemia.[33,36] Women with known medical diseases that are associated with abnormal uterine bleeding (renal disease, adrenal insufficiency, or hyperplasia) should have appropriate testing done.

In addition, women suspected of polycystic ovary syndrome/hyperandrogenic chronic anovulation should have serum testosterone, dehydroepiandrosterone sulfate (DHEA-S), and 17-hydroxyprogesterone (17-OHP) levels obtained.[2,11,38] Follicle-stimulating hormone (FSH) and LH levels are not routinely evaluated. Hyperprolactinemia can present as abnormal bleeding, although it is usually associated with amenorrhea, and a serum prolactin level should be considered, especially if there is evidence of galactorrhea. If indicated, coagulation studies, thyroid function tests, and liver function tests can be ordered. There is some disagreement about when to test for coagulation disorders. Some authors would include a coagulopathy profile (platelet count, bleeding time, prothrombin time, partial thromboplastin time, and clotting factors) and thyroid function tests in the initial laboratory investigations; others would advise waiting unless there is a reason to suspect these abnormalities based on the history or physical examination.[2,33,37,38] If the patient does not respond to therapy as anticipated, further testing may be necessary.[38]

ENDOMETRIAL BIOPSY

Women over the age of 35, and those with a history suggestive of chronic, unopposed estrogen exposure (e.g., oligomenorrhea, hyperandrogenic chronic anovulation) that would place them at risk for endometrial cancer, should undergo an endometrial biopsy. Women with obesity, diabetes, early menarche, infertility, and those who bleed after menopause, who are on cyclic postmenopausal hormonal replacement therapy (HRT) and bleed on the days estrogen is taken, or who are on continuous HRT and have continued bleeding after 6 to 9 months should also undergo an endometrial biopsy.[11,38]

Patients who have secretory endometrium identified on biopsy should have further investigations to look for intracavitary uterine lesions (ultrasound or hysteroscopy). If no further abnormalities are discovered during this investigation, the patient can be treated for ovulatory DUB (see Fig. 13-2). If bleeding continues despite treatment, further laboratory investigation, including coagulation studies, should be completed looking for a systemic cause of the bleeding.[38]

ULTRASOUND

A pelvic ultrasound should be ordered when the initial physical examination is not satisfactory to evaluate uterine or ovarian enlargement. Ultrasonography can be used to detect intracavitary endometrial polyps or submucosal fibroids and ovarian pathology and to measure the thickness of the endometrial stripe. Hydroultrasonography can further enhance the identification of intracavitary pathology.[38]

Assessing the thickness of the endometrial stripe is often helpful in planning further investigations, especially in the perimenopausal woman. In a premenopausal woman, the thickness of the stripe varies by phase. The proliferative phase stripe measures 4 to 8 mm; the periovulatory phase stripe measures 6 to 10 mm; and the secretory phase stripe measures 7 to 14 mm. Postmenopausal atrophic endometrium has a stripe measurement of 5 mm or less. HRT can increase this to 10 mm.[39]

In selected patients, combining evaluative modalities may yield better diagnostic results. For women at high risk of endometrial cancer, hysteroscopy with or without biopsy or ultrasonography will be needed to eliminate the possibility of uterine pathology. Hysteroscopy and biopsy has been reported as superior to a dilatation and curettage (D&C) in diagnosing endometrial cancer and its precursors.[40] Women with negative (benign) pathology on biopsy and negative ultrasounds can be diagnosed as having uncomplicated DUB.

In making the diagnosis of DUB, it is important to remember that it is a diagnosis of exclusion and abnormal uterine bleeding has many causes. A careful, step-wise workup will serve patients well.

Treatment

Once the diagnosis of DUB is established, the treatment goals are to control the bleeding and prevent recurrences of the abnormal bleeding episodes (see Fig. 13-2). Treatment for associated disorders, such as iron deficiency, should also be undertaken. Many estrogen/progestin regimens have been used for DUB; treatment choices will also depend on the patient's desire for contraception. In a study of hospitalized adolescents, 92 percent responded to medical (estrogen or estrogen/progesterone) therapy. There was no difference in the control of bleeding between the use of oral versus intravenous hormonal therapy. Fewer than 10 percent of these women had a D&C, the majority for failed medical management.[37] Although hospitalization is not required for most patients, it should be considered if the patient is hemodynamically unstable or if she is anemic and acutely bleeding. Decisions about transfusions should be based on degree of anemia, other medical conditions, and the risk-benefit assessment.

ACUTE HEAVY BLEEDING

In some patients with heavy bleeding, scant uterine endometrial tissue may be present. Despite the fact that the etiology is most likely anovulatory cycles, therapy is started with high-dose estrogen followed by or in conjunction with a progestin (Table 13-7). The first option is to use conjugated equine estrogen either orally (2.5 mg qid) or intravenously (25 mg every 2 to 4 h for 24 h). The majority of women will stop bleeding after the first intravenous dose. After 24 h, those on intravenous therapy can be switched to the oral estrogen dosage for a total of 21 days. Oral MPA, 10 mg, is administered the last 7 days of this treatment cycle. Another option is to start high-dose combination estrogen-progestin therapy by using monophasic OCs. The patient is instructed to take one pill three or four times a day until the bleeding stops, then continue for one more week. After either of these regimens are stopped, the patient will have withdrawal bleeding that may be heavy, but should not be prolonged.[35]

Another regimen for acute bleeding episodes switches the patient to a standard-dose OC pill regimen once the acute bleeding stops. This can be done with a daily pill or by decreasing the numbers

Table 13-7

Treatment Options for Acute Episodes of Dysfunctional Uterine Bleeding

Conjugated equine estrogen (CEE)	25 mg IV q 2–4 h for 24 h, then oral CEE to complete a 21-day course
and	2.5 mg PO qid for 21 d
Medroxyprogesterone acetate (MPA)	10 mg PO daily for the last 7 d of therapy
High-dose estrogen (50 μg) combination OC (monophasic)	3–4 tablets daily until bleeding stops, then continue for another week
Monophasic OC (30–35 μg estrogen)	4 pills daily for 4 d, then 3 pills daily for 3 d, then 2 pills daily for 2 wk
MPA (depot)	150 mg IM
Progesterone in oil	100–200 mg IM
MPA	20–40 mg PO (divide doses) for 5–10 d
D&C for failure of medical therapy	

NOTE: Continue medication regimens for at least 3 months to prevent recurrence.
ABBREVIATIONS: D&C, dilatation and curettage; OC, oral contraceptive.

of pills taken over a 3-week period (4 pills a day for 4 days, 3 pills a day for 3 days, then 2 pills a day for 2 weeks). This is likely to be better tolerated by patients; many women on high-dose estrogens require antiemetics to prevent nausea.[2,11]

For women unable to take estrogen, an intramuscular dose of depot MPA, 150 mg, or 100 to 200 mg of progesterone in oil, intramuscularly, can be used. If oral MPA is used, the dose is 20 to 40 mg/d in divided doses for 5 to 10 days.[11] A D&C may be necessary if hormonal therapy fails to control the acute bleeding episode.

Once the acute episode is over, the patient should continue on standard-dose OC therapy or MPA, 10 mg/d for 10 days each month for the next 2 to 3 months, to prevent a recurrence of another episode of acute heavy bleeding.

RECURRENT BLEEDING EPISODES

HORMONAL THERAPY For the patient with recurrent bleeding episodes, monophasic OCs can be used to control the bleeding and establish regular cycles (Table 13-8). Patients should be warned that the first withdrawal period may be heavy. This therapy should be continued for the next three cycles. If the patient desires contraception, or is not adverse to this therapy, the OCs can be continued on a regular basis. If the patient does not need contraception, MPA, 10 mg/d for 10 days a month or norethindrone, 5 to 10 mg, one to three times a day for 10 days, can be used to stop growth and support and organize the endometrium. A progestin regimen will not delay maturation of the HPO axis.[35] Withdrawal of the progestin will result in regular bleeding episodes. To achieve satisfactory cycling, the progestin therapy may be extended to 14 or even 21 days a month. Associated side effects such as fatigue, mood changes, weight gain, or a change in the lipid profile may limit the usefulness of these therapies. Another option for treatment is the progestin-releasing IUD[2,11,38] (see Chap. 2).

Any of the above medication regimens is suitable for adolescents. The choice often depends on the need for contraception or the willingness to accept hormonal therapy. In addition, compliance with the planned therapy is essential, or irregular spotting and breakthrough bleeding may complicate the original problem of DUB. If the adolescent is not anemic and the bleeding episodes do not lead to social embarrassment, iron supplementation therapy (to maintain iron stores), patient (and parental) education, and close follow-up may be sufficient. Most adolescents will develop ovulatory cycles within 2 years

Table 13-8

Treatment Options for Recurrent Episodes of Dysfunctional Uterine Bleeding

Monophasic OC—28 d	One pill daily for 4–6 mo (continue if contraception desired)
MPA	10 mg PO a day, for 10 d of month to induce withdrawal bleeding*
Norethindrone	5–10 mg PO daily to tid for 10 d a month*
If perimenopausal:	
Low-dose estrogen OC	One pill daily for 4–6 mo (continue if contraception is desired)
CEE and MPA	0.625–1.25 mg CEE PO d 1–25; 10 mg MPA PO daily on d 16–25 of cycle
For NSAID doses, see Table 13-1.	

*Can extend up to 21 days to achieve maximum control of bleeding episodes.

ABBREVIATIONS: CEE, conjugated equine estrogen; MPA, medroxyprogesterone acetate; NSAID, nonsteroidal anti-inflammatory drug; OC, oral contraceptive.

of menarche. Prolonged therapy can be planned with this in mind.[2,41]

Perimenopausal women can be started on low-dose estrogen OCs if there are no contraindications. Alternatively, they can be started on cyclical conjugated equine estrogen, 0.625 mg to 1.25 mg daily, days 1 through 25, with the addition of MPA 10 mg the last 10 days of the cycle. Estrogen dosage can be adjusted to obtain regular bleeding cycles with a minimum of side effects.

PROSTAGLANDIN INHIBITORS   For women with ovulatory DUB, prostaglandin inhibitors may be useful in decreasing menstrual blood loss (see Fig. 13-2). NSAIDs are the drug of choice in treating menorrhagia. Mefenamic acid, naproxen, meclofenamate, indomethacin, and ibuprofen have all been effective in reducing blood loss and menstrual symptoms. Mefenamic acid decreases menstrual blood loss by 30 to 50 percent.[36,42] Most regimens call for the patient to start the medication 3 days before or at the onset of menses and to continue at least the first 3 to 5 days of the period. The course of treatment can be adjusted by the patient to achieve optimal control of the bleeding. Typical recommended dosages are: mefenamic acid, 500 mg tid; ibuprofen 400 mg tid; meclofenamate 100 mg tid; and naproxen sodium 275 mg every 6 h after a 550-mg loading dose[35] (see Table 13-1).

OTHER THERAPEUTIC MEDICAL OPTIONS [2,11,35,36,43]
The above options are those most frequently chosen, have proven over time to be effective, and have side effects that are tolerable to most women. Other medications have been used to decrease menstrual bleeding, but their costs and side-effect profiles make them useful only in rare circumstances. Danazol 200 or 400 mg daily for 12 weeks has been effective in decreasing menstrual blood loss. The drug is expensive and its side effects (weight gain, acne, hot flushes, edema, hirsutism, decreased libido, atrophic vaginitis), reported by 75 percent of women taking the drug, make it poorly tolerated. Danazol is not as effective in controlling DUB long-term if only taken for 1 month, so patients should be instructed to complete a 3-month course.[44]

A medical menopause can be induced using GnRH agonists to reduce estrogen levels. Drugs such as goserelin and leuprolide have been used to control blood loss. They are also expensive ($300 or more for a monthly injection of goserelin) and the adverse side effects (nausea, vomiting, menopausal symptoms, bloating, hair loss) make them a choice of last resort for women who want to preserve fertility. They have also been used preoperatively before uterine surgery to control bleeding. Estrogen/progestin add-back therapy may be needed to control side effects.[45,46] Antifibrinolytic agents have been used (not in the

United States) in the treatment of ovulatory DUB. Their use is limited by side effects (nausea, dizziness, diarrhea, headaches, abdominal pain, allergic manifestations). They have not been shown to be superior to other options.

SURGICAL OPTIONS If medical options fail and the woman has no desire for future fertility, surgical options can be discussed. For women wishing to avoid the risks and morbidity of a hysterectomy, and who cannot tolerate or have failed medical therapy, ablation is a good option, if available. Endometrial ablation or excision can be performed using a laser or electrocautery device.[43] Although very effective for most patients, some will need repeat treatment for continued menorrhagia and some will eventually need a hysterectomy. A D&C is not a long-term treatment option. Hysterectomy is an option for women who no longer desire fertility and have other coexisting conditions such as leiomyomas or pelvic relaxation.

Patient Education

It is important for women to understand how the menstrual cycle works and what is happening to cause these bleeding episodes. For the adolescent, special attention should be paid to the social effects of embarrassing bleeding episodes and the implications of taking hormonal therapy, especially OCs. The clinician may need to intercede with parents who are uncomfortable dealing with the sexual maturation of their daughter and who might be resistant to hormonal therapy, thinking it might dictate future behavior. If life stress, diet regimens, or extreme levels of exercise are contributing to the problem, further counseling specific to those issues will be needed. For older women, the risk of cancer or surgery may weigh heavily. Discussing family history around perimenopausal issues may add a level of understanding for both the patient and clinician. Much has changed in the treatment of DUB over the past generation, and the time spent in reviewing all options will help the woman make an informed choice.

Amenorrhea

Amenorrhea is defined as (1) no menses by age 14 in the absence of growth and development of secondary sexual characteristics, (2) no menses by age 16 even with the development of secondary sexual characteristics (both primary amenorrhea), or (3) no menses for 6 months in a woman who previously experienced regular cycles (secondary amenorrhea). In women with oligomenorrhea, the time period for defining secondary amenorrhea is no menses for three cycle lengths, up to a total of 12 months.[47,48] Secondary amenorrhea is far more common, with a prevalence of 1 to 3 percent. Women who are in college, competitive athletes, or ballet dancers have an even higher prevalence of amenorrhea.[48] Although different studies use varying definitions of amenorrhea, the rates of amenorrhea reported for runners are 5 to 26 percent; for ballet dancers, 37 to 44 percent; and for collegiate swimmers and world-class cyclists, 12 percent.[49]

Etiology

To understand the etiology of amenorrhea, it is important to remember the factors that contribute to a normal menstrual cycle. The woman must have a mature and intact HPO axis, functioning ovaries, a uterus with a functional endometrium, and an unobstructed outflow tract. A disruption at any level can result in amenorrhea or menstrual dysfunction. Pregnancy and lactation are the most common causes for secondary amenorrhea, followed by disorders of the HPO axis.

OUTFLOW TRACT OR UTERINE PATHOLOGY

Several congenital conditions can result in the lack of uterine development. Rokitansky-Küster-Hauser syndrome is characterized by the absence of both the uterus and the vagina due to failure of fusion of the muellerian ducts. The ovaries are normal but there are associated renal abnormalities. Another syndrome that results in the failure of the uterus to develop is androgen insensitivity syndrome (testicular feminization). The affected individuals are phenotypically female, have a 46 XY chromosomal karyotype, and have normally functioning but ectopic testes. A vaginal pouch is present, but no uterus or tubes. The testes, located intra-abdominally or in the inguinal canal, need to be removed due to the risk of malignancy.[50,51]

A septum between the uterus and vagina or an imperforate hymen will also result in primary amenorrhea. This may be associated with cyclic pelvic pain as the endometrium responds to normal hormonal influences.

Obliteration of the uterine cavity due to adhesions (Asherman's syndrome), overzealous curettage, or radiotherapy may also result in amenorrhea. Infection due to tuberculosis, although rare, can also result in endometrial damage and subsequent amenorrhea.[51]

OVARIAN PATHOLOGY

TURNER'S SYNDROME   A patient with primary amenorrhea, delayed puberty, and short stature may have Turner's syndrome (45 XO karyotype). The ovaries are vestigial, but the rest of the anatomy of the genital tract is normal. In other cases, with chromosomal mosaicism, the phenotype may not be typical of Turner's syndrome. Sexual maturation, menarche, and fertility, although rare, can occur spontaneously. The karyotype, 46 XY, can also be found in the case of pure gonadal dysgenesis. In other cases, abnormal X chromosomes have been found.[50]

PREMATURE OVARIAN FAILURE   Premature ovarian failure is frequently associated with autoimmune disorders. Adrenal, pancreatic, and thyroid failure may follow, and the patient should be evaluated for these as well. Radiotherapy and chemotherapy can induce ovarian failure and amenorrhea in the postmenarchal woman. The duration of amenorrhea varies. The younger the patient, the more likely she is to resume regular spontaneous menses.[48,50]

HYPERANDROGENIC CHRONIC ANOVULATION/POLYCYSTIC OVARY SYNDROME   Although there is not ovarian failure per se with hyperandrogenic chronic anovulation (also commonly called polycystic ovary syndrome), characteristic ovarian changes include bilateral multiple cysts, sclerosis, and a hyperplastic theca and stroma. These changes are actually due to many different causes that result in chronic anovulation; the polycystic ovary is a sign, not a disease. Chronic anovulation creates a functional derangement in the ovaries brought about by accumulated and increased androgen. Women with this condition have mild to moderate androgen excess and normal serum estradiol levels, but elevated free estradiol and testosterone levels.

One theory suggests that elevated adrenal androgens, in combination with obesity, result in increased extraglandular estrogen production. The elevated estrogen leads to an acyclic positive feedback on LH secretion and a negative feedback on FSH secretion so that the LH/FSH ratio is increased. These women have higher circulating testosterone, androstenedione, dehydroepiandrosterone (DHA), DHEA-S, 17-OHP, and estrone. For some patients, hyperinsulinemia (secondary to insulin resistance) may precede hyperandrogenism. Hyperinsulinemia can augment thecal cell androgen production in the ovary.

The source of the androgens may be exogenous (e.g., anabolic steroids) or endogenous (from the ovaries or the adrenal glands) and should be identified. The differential diagnosis of hyperandrogenic chronic anovulation includes uncomplicated obesity, stromal hyperthecosis, Cushing's syndrome, thyroid disease, hyperprolactinemia, adrenal hyperplasia (cortisol biosynthetic pathway enzyme deficiencies), and androgen-producing tumors (adrenal or ovarian).[48,51] With a hyperandrogenic state, gonadotropin levels are usually normal, although the LH/FSH ratio may be increased.[51]

PITUITARY PATHOLOGY

Pituitary causes of amenorrhea include congenital syndromes, pituitary adenomas, and secondary causes such as surgery or medication use. Pituitary pathology may result in low or normal levels of gonadotropins.

Kallmann's syndrome is a congenital syndrome associated with an irreversible defect in gonadotropin synthesis. This is sometimes associated with an olfactory sensory defect.[50] Production of FSH can also be decreased in cases of pituitary destruction or, indirectly, by hyperprolactinemia.

Prolactin-secreting adenomas are a common cause of hypogonadotropic amenorrhea. The prolactin acts directly on the hypothalamus to decrease the amplitude and frequency of GnRH pulses. Other causes of hyperprolactinemia are drugs (antipsychotics, antihypertensives, and antidepressants most commonly), pituitary and hypothalamic masses, and hypothyroidism.[48,51]

The empty sella syndrome has been reported in up to 16 percent of patients with amenorrhea and galactorrhea. It is a benign, often congenital, condition that does not always progress to pituitary failure. In this condition, the pituitary is flattened against the floor of the sella by the subarachnoid membrane herniating through a defective sella diaphragm. This also can occur secondary to surgery, radiotherapy, trauma, inflammation, infiltration (sarcoidosis), or infarction (Sheehan's syndrome). Nonfunctioning adenomas are important if they interfere with pituitary function due to their size or because of associated neurologic symptoms.[48,51]

HYPOTHALAMIC PATHOLOGY

Constitutionally delayed puberty due to hypothalamic "failure" is the most common cause of primary amenorrhea. A family history reveals a similar developmental pattern in female relatives. In this condition, breast tissue is normal, but development is delayed. Findings on pelvic examination are normal. Rarely, this delay may be due to child abuse or neglect. In addition, hypothalamic failure may be seen in girls with the premenstrual onset of eating disorders or excessive exercise habits or among those with low body fat stores. Medical illness such as diabetes mellitus, inflammatory bowel disease, juvenile rheumatoid arthritis, chronic infection, and malignancy of the hypothalamus (e.g., craniopharyngiomas) may also result in delayed puberty.[51]

In secondary amenorrhea, women with a normal prolactin level, no withdrawal bleeding from a progesterone challenge test, low or normal gonadotropin levels, and normal sella turcica imaging are considered to have a hypothalamic source of amenorrhea. This usually represents an alteration of the HPO axis in response to psychological stress, eating disorders, strenuous exercise, sudden and severe weight loss, or mental illness. Hypothalamic secondary amenorrhea is a diagnosis of exclusion, however, and other possible etiologies need to be considered prior to making this diagnosis.[48]

Diagnosis

HISTORY

A thorough history and physical examination are essential in identifying the causes of amenorrhea. The history should include questions about the family (maternal/sibling history of menarche, menstrual dysfunction and menopause, autoimmune disease, infertility, congenital anomalies, or endocrinopathies), chronic medical conditions, surgical procedures, current nutritional and dietary status, physical activity patterns, and a detailed menstrual, sexual, and reproductive history. A careful drug history should be taken because many drugs will act to increase prolactin (antipsychotics: phenothiazines, haloperidol; antidepressants: tricyclics, monoamine oxidase inhibitors; antihypertensives: calcium channel blockers, methyldopa), have estrogenic activity, or are toxic to the ovary (chemotherapeutic agents).[48]

PHYSICAL EXAMINATION

A physical examination will screen for abnormal anatomic findings, developmental stage, and evidence of androgen or estrogen imbalance or endocrine abnormalities (e.g., striae, galactorrhea, thyroid enlargement). Inspection of the external genitalia and a pelvic examination are performed to assess hormonal influence, integrity of the outflow tract, and presence of the uterus and ovaries (if palpated). Tanner staging should be done.[41] Body mass index should be calculated to assess the degree of thinness or obesity. The normal range for body mass index is between 20 and 25 kg/m^2 (see Chap. 6).

Patients with primary amenorrhea who are over the age of 14 and without any development of secondary sexual characteristics should be evaluated for a congenital cause of the amenorrhea. With certain chromosomal abnormalities and those conditions associated with muellerian dysgenesis, further evaluation of the renal system for congenital anomalies should also be completed.

INITIAL LABORATORY TESTING

The laboratory evaluation of the patient with amenorrhea starts with a pregnancy test (Table 13-9). Once pregnancy is excluded, the patient should be evaluated for hypothyroidism and hyperprolactinemia (serum thyroid-stimulating hormone [TSH] and prolactin). If the prolactin is elevated, the patient should have radiologic assessment of the sella turcica. If the prolactin level is less than 100 ng/mL a screening view of the sella to rule out tumor is sufficient. If the level is greater than 100 ng/mL or if there are symptoms of an intracranial mass lesion, magnetic resonance imaging (MRI) of the pituitary should be obtained. Many clinicians prefer to order the MRI in all cases of prolactin elevation because it is a more sensitive test.[47,48] If there is evidence of thyroid disease, this

Table 13-9

Laboratory Evaluation of Amenorrhea

TEST	POSITIVE/ELEVATED	NEGATIVE/LOW
1. Pregnancy test	Pregnant, refer/begin appropriate management	Continue to step 2
2. TSH	Hypothyroid	Continue to step 3
Prolactin level	Rule out drug effect	
	Radiologic view of sella/pituitary	
3. Progesterone challenge test	Anovulatory cycles	Continue to step 4
4. Estrogen plus progesterone challenge	Hypoestrogenic amenorrhea	Uterine or outflow tract abnormality, further evaluation for surgery/hysteroscopy
	Continue to step 5	
5. FSH	Ovarian failure	Hypothalamic amenorrhea
LH	Workup for autoimmune disease	Kallmann's syndrome
	If under 30, chromosomal analysis	Imaging studies for pituitary pathology/nonfunctioning adenoma
	Continue to step 6	
6. Testosterone	Hyperandrogenic chronic anovulation	
Dehydroepiandrosterone sulfate	Androgen secreting tumor	
17-hydroxyprogesterone (may do earlier in the workup if there is clinical evidence of androgen excess)	Adrenal tumor/hyperplasia 21-hydroxylase deficiency	

ABBREVIATIONS: FSH, follicle-stimulating hormone; LH, luteinizing hormone; TSH, thyroid-stimulating hormone.

should be further evaluated (with a TSH and free thyroxine) and treated as appropriate.

PROGESTERONE CHALLENGE TEST

If both the prolactin level and thyroid function tests are normal, the next step is to assess the estrogen status using a progesterone challenge test. The standard protocol is to use 10 mg MPA orally, once a day for 10 days. A positive test results if there is any uterine bleeding within 2 to 7 days after the MPA is stopped. A negative test indicates that there may be an outflow tract abnormality, an endometrium that does not respond to progesterone, or inadequate estrogen stimulation of the endometrium. The first two possibilities are eliminated by giving cyclical conjugated equine estrogen (1.25 mg daily days 1 through 21) and MPA (10 mg daily the last 5 days of the 21-day cycle) and obtaining a history of withdrawal bleeding. This challenge can be omitted for women with known normal anatomy and no history of pelvic infection, trauma, or surgery.[48]

Failure to have withdrawal bleeding after both the MPA and the estrogen/MPA challenge results in the diagnosis of an outflow tract or uterine abnormality. In an anatomically normal patient, the woman will need further evaluation (hysteroscopy) to look for adhesions, the most likely cause of secondary amenorrhea in these cases.

EVALUATION OF ANDROGEN EXCESS

Some clinicians would also evaluate patients with evidence of androgen excess by obtaining testosterone, DHEA-S, and 17-OHP levels early in the workup. This will differentiate among the following causes of amenorrhea: hyperandrogenic chronic anovulation syndrome (mild increases in all three tests that are suppressed after dexamethasone administration), an androgen-secreting tumor (high testosterone levels in the clinical setting of rapidly progressive virilization), an adrenal tumor (marked increases in testosterone and DHEA-S that are not suppressed by dexamethasone), adrenal hyperplasia (moderate increases in testosterone and 17-OHP that are suppressed by dexamethasone), or enzyme deficiency. Further evaluations, such as a free testosterone or a corticotropin stimulation test may be necessary to finalize the diagnosis. Because both 17-OHP and DHEA-S are elevated in association with elevated prolactin, a serum prolactin level should be obtained, if not already done. Additionally, an endometrial biopsy may be prudent before inducing a withdrawal bleed in these patients to evaluate for endometrial abnormalities secondary to unopposed estrogen effect.[48,51]

EVALUATION OF ESTROGEN DEFICIENCY

The next step for women with hypoestrogenic amenorrhea (negative progesterone challenge, positive withdrawal bleeding with estrogen-progesterone cycling) is to obtain FSH and LH levels. High gonadotropin levels and low estrogen levels indicate an ovarian problem, most commonly ovarian failure. Ovarian failure is considered premature in women under 40. Women over the age of 30 with ovarian failure do not need a chromosomal evaluation; under age 30, however, this evaluation should be done to rule out testicular feminization syndrome. Because up to 40 percent of women with premature ovarian failure have associated autoimmune disorders, a workup for autoimmune diseases should be done as well. Tests should be guided by the woman's history and physical examination, but might include thyroid function tests, thyroid antibodies, morning cortisol levels, fasting glucose, electrolytes, calcium, phosphorus, complete blood count, sedimentation rate, rheumatoid factor, and antinuclear antibodies.[48]

Normal or low gonadotropin levels and a low estrogen effect indicate pituitary or hypothalamic pathology. If the woman has a history of eating disorders, weight loss, stress, or exercise that corresponds to the amenorrhea, it may not be necessary to perform a pituitary imaging study. Hypothalamic causes are a diagnosis of exclusion and other likely causes should be sought. If the clinical picture does not fit, then an MRI should be done to assess the pituitary.

Treatment

Once the cause of the amenorrhea is identified, appropriate therapy can be initiated. Support, counseling, and subspecialty referral for adolescents and their parents may be needed. The same may be needed for older women, especially those desiring fertility. A working partnership between the subspecialist and the primary care clinician is essential.

For primary amenorrhea, the treatment goal is to initiate pubertal changes if necessary, maintain estrogen status, and start menstruation. Surgical intervention may be needed in patients with outflow tract pathology. If there is gonadal dysgenesis/ovarian failure, the patient will need counseling about infertility. Care should be taken to evaluate the patient, her eating patterns, her exercise regimen, and her living situation before initiating hormonal therapy. No intervention may be needed if the diagnosis is constitutionally delayed puberty. In the case of eating disorders and obesity, dietary and psychological counseling might be tried before hormonal therapy. For girls with short stature, consideration should be given to the effect of hormonal therapy on limiting final height. Subspecialty consultation should be obtained before this is started in patients with Turner's syndrome, for example.[51]

In secondary amenorrhea, the goal is to restore estrogen status, if needed, and treat any underlying causes. Women with sufficient estrogen should have withdrawal bleeding induced at least four to six times a year to avoid endometrial hyperplasia and dysfunctional bleeding patterns and to decrease the risk of endometrial cancer. This can be accomplished by using MPA, 10 mg daily for the first 10 days of the month on a regular basis. OCs can be used for regular cycling if there are no contraindications and contraception is desired.

Women with low estrogen levels need to have estrogen replacement. If there is an intact uterus, progesterone should be added to the medication regimen. If fertility is not desired, OCs are effective. There is a higher dosage of estrogen and progesterone in OCs compared to cyclical conjugated equine estrogen and MPA regimens (given above). Perimenopausal women may prefer the convenience and contraceptive aspect of the combination pills; others may prefer the lower doses of HRT because of fewer medication side effects.

Cyclical HRT is used to prevent bone loss in young women. Depending on their diets, these patients may also need calcium and vitamin D supplementation. Clinicians should consider bone density evaluation and counseling with the goal of minimizing the risk of developing osteoporosis (see Chap. 20). Women with hyperandrogenic conditions may also see additional benefit with use of OCs because the symptoms of androgen excess may decrease with therapy.[48,51]

Women with prolactinomas should be evaluated for medical therapy first. There is a significant risk of hypopituitarism following surgery and a high recurrence rate (up to 20 percent for microprolactinomas and 80 percent for macroprolactinomas). Bromocriptine or cabergoline (as a second-line option if bromocriptine is not tolerated or ineffective) can be used to shrink the tumor or treat idiopathic elevations of prolactin. Medical treatment restores ovulation in 85 percent of patients.[50]

Patient Education

Depending on the cause of the amenorrhea, the problem may be handled easily or require extensive evaluation and treatment. Supportive counseling may be sufficient in some cases; others will require extended intensive psychotherapy. Patients should receive honest assessments of possible future fertility. Clinicians should also be knowledgeable enough to initiate discussions regarding appropriate levels of exercise and assess the need for further nutritional counseling.[41,52]

Premenstrual Syndrome

Premenstrual syndrome (PMS) is commonly used by laypersons as a catch-all term for a variety of symptoms that are experienced, to varying degrees, by the majority of women before the onset of menses. Surveys show that 90 percent of menstruating women have suffered some limited symptoms of PMS, including mood changes, breast tenderness, bloating, and appetite changes. In 30 percent of women, symptoms are described as moderate, and 3 to 8 percent indicate that their symptoms are severe.[53] Until recently, assessing the epidemiology and effectiveness of treatment for PMS was difficult due to the lack of a consistent definition. The most recent *Diagnostic and Statistical Manual of Mental Disorders* (DSM-IV) delineates the research criteria for the diagnosis of Premenstrual Dysphoric Disorder (PMDD)[54] (Table 13-10). Based on these strict criteria, PMDD, the most severe form of premenstrual disorders, occurs in less than 5 percent of menstruating women.[53]

Women with fewer or less severe symptoms are classified as having PMS. (For the purposes of this chapter, the term PMS will be inclusive of PMDD as well as its milder form, PMS, unless otherwise specified.)

Premenstrual syndrome and PMDD must be differentiated from underlying mental disorders, such as somatoform, anxiety, or personality disorders, or general medical conditions, such as seizure disorders and systemic lupus erythematosus. In women with these conditions, symptoms are present throughout the menstrual cycle but are exacerbated by the hormonal changes of impending menses.[54] PMS can occur anytime after the menarche but seems to become more common as women

Table 13-10

Research Criteria for Premenstrual Dysphoric Disorder

A. In most menstrual cycles during the past year, five (or more) of the following symptoms were present for most of the time during the last week of the luteal phase, began to remit within a few days after the onset of the follicular phase, and were absent in the week postmenses, with at least one of the symptoms being either (1), (2), (3), or (4):

1. Markedly depressed mood, feelings of hopelessness, or self-deprecating thoughts
2. Marked anxiety, tension, feelings of being "keyed up," or "on edge"
3. Marked affective lability (e.g., feeling suddenly sad or tearful or increased sensitivity to rejection)
4. Persistent and marked anger or irritability or increased interpersonal conflicts
5. Decreased interest in usual activities (e.g., work, school, friends, hobbies)
6. Subjective sense of difficulty in concentrating
7. Lethargy, easy fatigability, or marked lack of energy
8. Marked change in appetite, overeating, or specific food cravings
9. Hypersomnia or insomnia
10. A subjective sense of being overwhelmed or out of control
11. Other physical symptoms, such as breast tenderness or swelling, headaches, joint or muscle pain, a sensation of "bloating," weight gain

B. The disturbance markedly interferes with work or school or with usual social activities and relationships with others (e.g., avoidance of social activities, decreased productivity and efficiency at work or school).

C. The disturbance is not merely an exacerbation of the symptoms of another disorder, such as Major Depressive Disorder, Panic Disorder, Dysthmic Disorder (although it may be superimposed on any of these disorders).

D. Criteria A, B, and C must be confirmed by prospective daily ratings during at least two consecutive symptomatic cycles. (The diagnosis may be made provisionally before this confirmation.)

NOTE: In menstruating females, the luteal phase corresponds to the period between ovulation and the onset of menses, and the follicular phase begins with menses. In nonmenstruating females (e.g., those who have had a hysterectomy), the timing of luteal and follicular phases may require measurement of circulating reproductive hormones.

SOURCE: Based on information from the *Diagnostic and Statistical Manual of Mental Disorders*, 4th ed. Copyright 1994, American Psychiatric Association, with permission.

reach their thirties and forties. Symptoms progress as a woman ages but disappear at menopause. A hereditary component to PMS has been postulated but not confirmed.[55] Studies suggest that women with PMS have a greater risk for developing a major depressive illness.[56]

Etiology

Numerous etiologies for PMS have been postulated, including deficiencies in hormone secretion, prostaglandins, or nutrient intake.[57] Current research suggests that, in susceptible women, an abnormality in neurotransmitters, specifically serotonin, may be triggered by the normal hormonal changes that occur in the luteal phase of the menstrual cycle.[55,58] The efficacy of both serotonergic drugs and drugs that suppress normal hormonal changes, such as GnRH agonists, support this hypothesis.

Diagnosis

A diagnosis of PMS is not made on the basis of one interview or office visit. Rather, it requires the exclusion of any underlying medical or physiologic condition via a thorough history and complete physical examination. Once other causes have been ruled out, the patient should perform a prospective daily rating of symptoms for at least three menstrual cycles. To warrant a diagnosis of PMDD, there should be at least a 30 percent increase in the severity of symptoms for the week preceding the onset of menses (luteal phase) compared to the week following menses (follicular phase) for two of three cycles.[59]

Treatment

Once a diagnosis of PMS has been made, the clinician should review the patient's daily ratings and identify which symptoms need to be addressed. This is important in the selection of treatment because some therapies (e.g., diuretics) may improve only one or two selected symptoms, whereas others (e.g., GnRH agonists) may provide a wider range of benefits. Women with mild symptoms may wish to attempt a trial of life-style modifications, whereas the more severe symptoms seen in women with PMDD may warrant an immediate trial of drug therapy.

LIFE-STYLE MODIFICATIONS

A woman can try several life-style modifications that may help attenuate her PMS symptoms. High caffeine intake has been associated with increased severity of PMS symptoms; therefore, restriction of caffeine intake during the premenstrual period is recommended. Regular exercise has been shown to improve some PMS symptoms, with aerobic exercise being more effective than strength training at improving mood symptoms.[60] Although it has not been proven in clinical trials, recommending a limitation of salt intake for women who complain of bloating and weight gain is reasonable. A diet high in tryptophan (a serotonin precursor) or complex carbohydrates may also be useful[61] (Table 13-11).

DIETARY SUPPLEMENTS

Calcium supplementation with 1200 mg/d elemental calcium has been shown in a double-blind, placebo-controlled trial to result in a 50 percent decrease in overall symptoms, including mood and physical symptoms.[62] Other dietary supplements that may be of benefit include magnesium, 360 mg/d, and α-tocopherol (vitamin E), 400 IU/d.[53] Vitamin B_6 (pyridoxine) has long been touted as therapy for PMS due to its role as a cofactor in the metabolism of tryptophan to serotonin. Although a review of 12 controlled trials did not support any significant clinical effect and doses of 200 mg/d used chronically may be associated with development of peripheral neuropathy,[63] a recent meta-analysis found vitamin B_6 beneficial for overall PMS symptoms such as nostalgia, irritability, fatigue, and bloating.[63a]

TREATMENT OF MOOD ALTERATION

SEROTONERGIC ANTIDEPRESSANTS   In the early 1990s, it was postulated that antidepressant medications that alter serotonin metabolism might be useful in

Table 13-11

Foods Rich in Tryptophan

Legumes, e.g., kidney/lima/garbanzo/soy beans, lentils, dried peas
Peanuts, cashews, peanut butter
Milk
Whole wheat bread
Oatmeal
Enriched noodles
Hard cheeses, e.g., cheddar, swiss
Eggs
Fish and shellfish
Beef
Pork
Chicken
Lamb

SOURCE: Reproduced with permission from Pennington JAT.[111]

the management of PMDD. Multiple placebo-controlled trials have shown selective serotonin reuptake inhibitors (SSRIs) and other serotonergic antidepressants to be significantly better than placebo, with response rates ranging from 50 to 80 percent. However, it is important to note that in many of the trials there was a substantial placebo response. Table 13-12 lists the agents that have been studied. Affective symptoms, such as mood swings, anger/irritability, anxiety, and guilt, were most improved, but physical symptoms, such as bloating and breast tenderness, also significantly improved with serotonergic therapy.[64–66] One study found a significant decrease in functional impairment in women receiving active drug.[65] In general, relatively low doses are sufficient for the treatment of PMDD—a study of 20 mg daily versus 60 mg daily of fluoxetine found no significant difference in efficacy but a higher adverse effect rate in patients receiving the 60-mg dose.[67] Although the initial studies used daily dosing, subsequent studies have confirmed that intermittent dosing during the luteal phase (the last 2 weeks of the menstrual cycle) is equally efficacious and better tolerated.[68,69] Even with intermittent dosing, the beneficial effects of serotonergic drugs are seen within the first cycle of treatment.[65,67,70]

Side effects from the serotonergic drugs are common; headache, insomnia, nervousness, and gastrointestinal distress occurred in more than 10 percent of patients taking SSRIs.[65,68,71,72] These effects generally subside with continued therapy. Decreased libido has also been commonly reported and may not abate over time.[65,72–75] One study found significant alterations, either lengthening or shortening, of the menstrual cycle in a group of women taking fluoxetine for PMDD.[76]

OTHER ANTIDEPRESSANTS Antidepressants that affect noradrenaline, with little to no effect on serotonin, including desipramine, maprotiline, and bupropion, have been studied in comparison with the serotonergic drugs (see Table 13-12). Although some improvement in mood symptoms was seen with the nonserotonergic antidepressants, the SSRIs were significantly more effective.[66,72,77]

Clomipramine, a tricyclic antidepressant (TCA) that inhibits reuptake of serotonin, and nortriptyline, has been shown to improve PMDD symptoms.[70,78,79] Other TCAs with predominantly serotonergic effects (e.g., amitriptyline and doxepin) may also be beneficial, although clinical studies are lacking (see Table 13-12). The anticholinergic effects of the TCAs, including dry mouth, sedation, and constipation, may limit their usefulness. Intermittent dosing of clomipramine has also been shown to be efficacious. Adverse effects occurred in approximately two-thirds of the women.[70] In women using TCAs during the luteal phase, tolerance to adverse effects may not develop due to the intermittent dosing. However, for women with symptom duration of less than 1 week, intermittent use may be more tolerable than chronic medication administration.

The majority of studies using serotonergic agents have been short-term, less than six menstrual cycles; however, PMDD is a chronic, long-term problem for women who suffer from it. Two studies of daily fluoxetine treatment for an average of 18 months demonstrated continued benefit from the drug, whereas women who discontinued the medication had a recurrence of their symptoms.[73,74] Reinstituting medication resulted in relief from PMDD symptoms.[74]

Table 13-12

Psychotropic Drugs for Mood Symptoms Related to Premenstrual Syndrome

Drug (Brand Name)	Dosages Studied	Comments
Selective Serotonin Reuptake Inhibitors		
Fluoxetine (Prozac)	Daily: 20–60 mg Intermittent*: 20 mg/d	Most studied,[64,66–68,72–74] 4 of 5 randomized, placebo-controlled trials showed benefit with daily use, can start at 10 mg/d to decrease side effects
Sertraline (Zoloft)	Daily: 50–150 mg Intermittent: 100 mg/d	1 open-label trial and 1 DBPC trial of daily, 1 DBPC trial of intermittent dosing[65,69,71]
Paroxetine (Paxil)	Daily: 5–30 mg	1 open-label study and one randomized, DBPC trial[75,77]
Fluvoxamine (Luvox)	Daily: 100 mg	Single pilot study[113]
Other Serotonergic Agents		
Venlafaxine (Effexor)	Daily: 25 mg bid	Unpublished data
Nefazodone (Serzone)	Daily: 200–600 mg in divided doses	Open-label study[114]
Tricyclic Antidepressants		
Clomipramine (Anafranil)	Daily: 25–75 mg Intermittent: 25–75 mg/d	2 placebo-controlled trials[70,78]; anticholinergic side effects common
Nortriptyline (Aventyl, Pamelor)	Daily: 50–125 mg/d	Single pilot study[79]
Anxiolytics		
Buspirone (BuSpar)	Intermittent: 30–60 mg/d	2 DBPC trials[83,84] Non-sedating, no dependence
Alprazolam (Xanax)	Intermittent: 1–2 mg/d	2 out of 3 DBPC trials showed benefit[80–82] Concern with abuse potential, especially with daily dosing; with intermittent dosing, taper over a few days after OM to avoid withdrawal symptoms

*Intermittent dosing: during luteal phase (e.g., d 14–28 of cycle).
ABBREVIATIONS: DBPC, double-blind, placebo-controlled; OM, onset of menses.

ANXIOLYTICS Because anxiety can be a major component of PMDD symptoms, anxiolytic agents have been studied (see Table 13-12). Alprazolam, a benzodiazepine, has been shown in some but not all double-blind, placebo-controlled trials to be effective for many of the mood symptoms as well as some physical symptoms (headache, abdominal bloating/cramps) of PMDD.[80–82] The majority of studies have dosed the drug only during the luteal phase, which may decrease the risk of drug dependence. Intermittent dosing regimens should include dosage tapering (e.g., decrease dosage by one tab-let per day after the onset of menses) to minimize withdrawal symptoms.[81] The most common side effect of alprazolam is drowsiness, which may be controlled by giving a small dose on a frequent (tid to qid) basis. Other benzodiazepines may offer similar relief from PMDD symptoms, but clinical data are not available at this time. Buspirone, a non-sedating, nonbenzodiazepine anxiolytic, has been clinically effective at doses of 25 to 60 mg/d (given in divided doses) when taken during the luteal phase.[83,84] Side effects were primarily neurologic, including lightheadedness and weakness. An advantage of buspirone over alprazolam is its lack of potential for dependence.

TREATMENT OF PHYSICAL SYMPTOMS

FLUID RETENTION AND BLOATING   Diuretics have been used with equivocal results in the management of bloating and weight gain secondary to PMS.[57] Spironolactone is a mild, nonthiazide diuretic with antiandrogenic effects. Several double-blind, placebo-controlled trials using spironolactone, 100 mg/d during the luteal phase, demonstrated a significant decrease in the subjective symptom of swelling/bloating as well as improvement in some of the negative mood changes associated with PMS.[85,86] Short-term spironolactone is generally well tolerated. Other diuretics have also been tried. Because there are limited clinical data on their use in PMS, these agents are generally reserved for patients for whom spironolactone fails.

OTHER PHYSICAL SYMPTOMS   Evening primrose oil (EPO), whose active ingredient, γ-linoleic acid is a prostaglandin precursor, has been investigated in the management of PMS. A review of clinical trials suggests that this agent has little or no clinical benefit.[87] Tamoxifen has been effective for the treatment of severe breast pain.[88,89] There is a concern about the risk of endometrial cancer with long-term use of tamoxifen; intermittent dosing, which was shown efficacious in one study, may decrease this risk.[88] For more severe cases of mastalgia, bromocriptine at doses of 1.25 to 7.5 mg/d during the luteal phase can be used.[53] Side effects, including gastrointestinal distress, headache, and fatigue, are more common at the higher doses.[57] Menstrual migraine can be treated with nonprescription or prescription NSAIDs, which may also improve mood symptoms associated with PMS.[13]

MENSTRUAL CYCLE MODULATION

HORMONAL THERAPY   Deficiency in progesterone synthesis during the luteal phase, one of the earliest theories for the etiology of PMS, resulted in the use of natural and synthetic progestins for PMS

management. This hypothesis is unproven; indeed, the majority of well-controlled trials with progesterone have not shown any significant benefit over placebo.[53,57] Women on either estrogen replacement therapy or GnRH therapy reported a return in their PMS symptoms when progesterone supplementation was given.[57,90] Suppression of ovulation by estradiol implants or patches has been shown to be clinically effective.[91] However, to prevent endometrial hyperplasia, a progestational agent is generally added to the regimen, which may result in a recurrence of some PMS-like symptoms.

Oral Contraceptives.   The data regarding the effects of combination OCs on PMS symptomatology are conflicting. A survey of women with PMS symptoms found that women taking OCs were likely to have more severe symptoms.[92] Conversely, in a small placebo-controlled trial, women reporting moderate to severe PMS symptoms experienced a decrease in breast pain and edema but no significant change in mood symptoms while taking a triphasic OC.[93] OCs may be tried for patients with mild symptoms before moving to more aggressive therapy. (see Chap. 2 for a complete discussion of OCs.)

Danazol.   A suppressor of ovarian activity, danazol has been shown to be beneficial in the treatment of PMS; however, it is not FDA approved for this indication. In double-blind, placebo-controlled trials, both physical symptoms (e.g., breast pain, lethargy, and abdominal swelling) as well as psychological symptoms (e.g., irritability, depression, anxiety, and mood swings) were significantly improved in 40 to 75 percent of the women.[94–96] Doses of 100 to 200 mg bid have been studied; the optimal dose has not been determined. Although the clinical effects of danazol are thought to be related to its ability to suppress ovulation, there are conflicting data as to the relationship between anovulatory cycles and symptom relief.[97,98] Adverse effects in clinical studies have been mild, including gastrointestinal distress, oily skin, and weight gain, but the studies have all been short-term, less than 6 months. Altered menses occurred in about 50 percent of women in one study.[94] Long-term use (6 months or longer) of danazol for other disorders has been associated with menstrual abnormalities and weight gain in over half the women followed. Androgenic adverse effects, including acne, hirsutism, and deepening of the voice as well as antiestrogenic effects, such as hot flashes, have been reported in up to 12 percent of patients.[99] Liver toxicity has been rarely reported.[32] Intermittent dosing, from the onset of symptoms to the onset of menses, has been shown in one small trial to be effective and may minimize the risk of long-term use.[97] Danazol may be useful in women with a combination of physical and psychological symptoms.

Gonadotropin-Releasing Hormone Agonists.　Due to their ability to suppress endogenous hormone production, GnRH agonists have been widely studied in the treatment of PMS. Table 13-13 lists the agents currently available. None of these agents are currently approved by the FDA for the treatment of PMS. Studies have shown that both psychological symptoms (e.g., irritability, anxiety, and depression) and physical symptoms (e.g., breast swelling and fluid retention) respond to treatment with GnRH agonists.[100–102] Results with monthly injections have been more consistently positive than those seen with agents that must be given intranasally on a daily basis.[57] This may be a compliance issue. There may be a lag time of several menstrual cycles before benefits are seen.[100] Women with premenstrual exacerbation of underlying mood disorders did not respond as well to treatment with GnRH agonists as women who had symptoms only during the premenstrual period.[100,101]

Side effects with long-term use of GnRH agonists are of considerable concern, especially the reported decrease in bone mineral density.[57] Other symptoms of estrogen deficiency such as hot flashes have also been reported. The hypoestrogenic state induced by GnRH agonists may put patients at increased risk for cardiovascular disease. To minimize these risks, therapy with GnRH agonists alone should be limited to less than 6 months. Alternately, replacement doses of estrogen and progesterone (add-back therapy) or a bisphosphonate can be given along with the GnRH agonist; this has been shown to minimize bone loss while maintaining drug benefits.[33,35,37,103–106] However, some women may experience recurrence of their PMS symptoms when add-back therapy is used.[90]

SURGICAL MANAGEMENT　Bilateral oophorectomy eliminates the symptoms of PMS. However, it is associated with serious long-term risks of osteoporosis and premature heart disease as well as adverse effects such as vasomotor flashes and decreased libido. Before oophorectomy is considered, the patient should have demonstrated a response to "medical ovariectomy" with GnRH

Table 13-13

Gonadotropin-Releasing Hormone Agonists Used in the Management of Premenstrual Syndrome

DRUG (BRAND NAME)	DOSAGE	COMMENTS
Buserelin	400 µg intranasal/d (bid dosing)	DBPC trial[102]: buserelin better than placebo Not currently available in the United States
Goserelin (Zoladex)	3.6 mg SC implant every month	DBPC trial[115]: improvement in physical symptoms, little change in psychologic symptoms
Leuprolide (Lupron)	3.75–7.5 mg IM/mo or 11.25 mg IM q 3 mo	2 DBPC trials[100,101]: improvement in physical and psychologic symptoms, placebo-controlled cross-over study[116] no difference vs placebo (2 cycles only)

ABBREVIATIONS: DBPC, double-blind, placebo-controlled; GnRH, gonadotropin-releasing hormone.

agonists and should understand the irreversibility and potential consequences of the procedure.[57] If a hysterectomy is done concomitantly, estrogen replacement therapy (without addition of a progestin) may be given to minimize the risks of the hypoestrogenic state. In one small study, this regimen was not associated with recurrence of PMS symptoms.[107]

Patient Education

Premenstrual syndrome carries a certain connotation that often evokes jokes or implies excuses. Understandably, therefore, a woman may be concerned about receiving such a diagnosis. However, she should be educated that it is a true illness that, in the majority of cases, can be controlled by therapy. Both the patient and her family should be educated about PMS/PMDD so that they can better understand and deal with the condition. A woman should be taught about the importance of dietary and life-style modification; these changes may give the patient a beneficial sense of control over the condition. Patients who are candidates for drug therapy must understand that no single drug is effective for all symptoms in all women. Identifying the best therapy for an individual may require a trial of several different agents over a period of months. If necessary, self-help material, individual or family counseling, and professional support groups can be recommended.[53]

Herbal Therapies for Menstrual Disorders

Herbal preparations have long been touted for the management of menstrual disorders. Unfortunately, controlled trials are lacking for many of these agents, including angelica (*Dong quai*), blue cohosh, pasque flower, and black haw. In 1978, the Commission E, as directed by Germany's Federal Institute for Drugs and Medical Devices, undertook an extensive, 12-year review of 360 herbal products.[108] Their monographs can serve as a source of information regarding herbal products. Table 13-2 summarizes the agents the Commission determined are probably effective in the management of menstrual disorders.

Herbal medicines may be valuable in the treatment of menstrual disorders; however, patients must understand that these agents are not without toxicity and may cause drug-drug or drug-disease interactions. For example, women with PMS may attempt self-treatment with St. John's Wort, which is widely used for its antidepressant effects. This herb is reported to have mild monoamine oxidase inhibitor properties and probably affects norepinephrine and serotonin metabolism; therefore, it may be of benefit in PMS. However, patients should be aware that the concurrent administration of St. John's Wort and serotonergic agents, such as fluoxetine, may induce serious side effects due to a drug interaction between these agents. Until further data are available, herbs should be used cautiously and only products from well-established companies should be purchased. To minimize the risk of drug interactions, health care providers should routinely question their patients about use of herbal and alternative therapies.

References

1. Harlow SD, Ephross SA: Epidemiology of menstruation and its relevance to women's health. *Epidemiol Rev* 17:265, 1995.
2. Lavin C: Dysfunctional uterine bleeding in adolescents. *Curr Opin Pediatr* 8:328, 1996.
3. Koff E, Rierdan J, Stubbs ML: Conceptions and misconceptions of the menstrual cycle. *Womens Health* 16:119, 1990.
4. Koff E, Rierdan J: Early adolescent girls' understanding of menstruation. *Womens Health* 22:1, 1995.
5. Cumming DC, Cumming CE, Kieren DK: Menstrual mythology and sources of information about menstruation. *Am J Obstet Gynecol* 164:472, 1991.

6. Shapiro SS: Treatment of dysmenorrhea and premenstrual syndrome with non-steroidal anti-inflammatory drugs. *Drugs* 36:475, 1988.

7. Harlow SD, Park M: Longitudinal study of risk factors for the occurrence, duration and severity of menstrual cramps in a cohort of college women. *Br J Obstet Gynaecol* 103:134, 1996.

8. Dawood MY: Nonsteroidal anti-inflammatory drugs and changing attitudes towards dysmenorrhea. *Am J Med* 84(Suppl 5A):23, 1988.

9. Sjoberg NO: Dysmenorrhea and uterine transmitters. *Acta Obstet Gynecol Scand Suppl* 87:57, 1979.

10. Toth PP, Jothivijayarani A: Gynecology. In: Graber MA, Toth PP, Herting RL Jr (eds): *University of Iowa: The Family Practice Handbook,* 3rd ed. St. Louis: Mosby; 1997.

11. Apgar BS: Dysmenorrhea and dysfunctional uterine bleeding. *Prim Care* 24:161, 1997.

12. Smith RP: Cyclic pelvic pain and dysmenorrhea. *Obstet Gynecol Clin North Am* 20:753, 1993.

13. Parsons LH, Stovall TG: Surgical management of chronic pelvic pain. *Obstet Gynecol Clin North Am* 20:765, 1993.

14. Jacobson J, Cavalli-Bjorkman K, Lundstrom V, et al: Prostaglandin synthetase inhibitors and dysmenorrhea: a survey and personal clinical experience. *Acta Obstet Gynecol Scand Suppl* 87:73, 1979.

15. Chan WY, Dawood MY, Fuchs F: Prostaglandins in primary dysmenorrhea: comparison of prophylactic and nonprophylactic treatment with ibuprofen and use of oral contraceptives. *Am J Med* 70:535, 1981.

16. Milsom I, Sundell G, Andersch B: The influence of different combined oral contraceptives on the prevalence and severity of dysmenorrhea. *Contraception* 42:497, 1990.

17. Nabrink M, Birgersson L, Colling-Saltin AS, Solum T: Modern oral contraceptives and dysmenorrhoea. *Contraception* 42:275, 1990.

18. Jacobson J, Lundstrom V, Nilsson B: Naproxen in the treatment of OC-resistant primary dysmenorrhea: a double-blind cross-over study. *Acta Obstet Gynecol Scand Suppl* 113:87, 1983.

19. Sandahl B, Ulmsten U, Anersson KE: Trial of the calcium antagonist nifedipine in the treatment of primary dysmenorrhea. *Arch Gynecol* 227:147, 1979.

20. Andersson KE: Calcium antagonists and dysmenorrhea. *Ann NY Acad Sci* 522:747, 1988.

21. Kullander S, Svanberg L: Terbutaline inhalation for alleviation of severe pain in essential dysmenorrhea. *Acta Obstet Gynecol Scand* 60:425, 1981.

22. Milsom I, Hedner N, Mannheimer C: A comparative study of the effect of high intensity transcutaneous nerve stimulation and oral naproxen on intrauterine pressure and menstrual pain in patients with primary dysmenorrhea. *Am J Obstet Gynecol* 170:123, 1994.

23. Dawood MY, Ramos J: Transcutaneous electrical nerve stimulation (TENS) for the treatment of primary dysmenorrhea: a randomized crossover comparison with placebo TENS and ibuprofen. *Obstet Gynecol* 74:656, 1990.

24. Campbell MA, McGrath PJ: Use of medication by adolescents for the management of menstrual discomfort. *Arch Pediatr Adolesc Med* 151:905, 1997.

25. Bromham DR: Endometriosis in primary medical care. *Br J Clin Pract Suppl* 72:54, 1991.

26. Falcone T, Goldberg JM, Miller KF: Endometriosis: medical and surgical intervention. *Curr Opin Obstet Gynecol* 8:178, 1996.

27. Perper MM, Nezhat F, Goldstein H, et al: Dysmenorrhea is related to the number of implants in endometriosis patients. *Fertil Steril* 63:500, 1995.

28. Barbieri RL: Endometriosis and the estrogen threshold theory: relation to surgical and medical treatment. *J Reprod Med* 43(3 Suppl):287, 1998.

29. Vercellini P, De Giorgi O, Oldani S, et al: Depot medroxyprogesterone acetate versus an oral contraceptive combined with very-low dose danazol for long-term treatment of pelvic pain associated with endometriosis. *Am J Obstet Gynecol* 175:396, 1996.

30. Afarwal SK: Comparative effects of GnRH agonist therapy: review of clinical studies and their implications. *J Reprod Med* 43(3 Suppl):293, 1998.

31. Evers JL, Dunselman GA, Land JA, Bouckaert PX: Is there a solution for recurrent endometriosis? *Br J Clin Pract Suppl* 72:45, 1991.

32. Brenner PF: Differential diagnosis of abnormal uterine bleeding. *Am J Obstet Gynecol* 175:766, 1996.

33. Wathen PI, Henderson MC, Witz CA: Abnormal uterine bleeding. *Med Clin North Am* 79:329, 1995.

34. Janssen CA, Scholten PC, Heintz APM: A simple visual assessment technique to discriminate between menorrhagia and normal menstrual blood loss. *Obstet Gynecol* 85:977, 1995.

35. Chuong CJ, Brenner PF: Management of abnormal uterine bleeding. *Am J Obstet Gynecol* 175:787, 1996.

36. Rosenfeld JA: Treatment of menorrhagia due to dysfunctional uterine bleeding. *Am Fam Physician* 53:165, 1996.

37. Falcone T, Desjardins C, Bourque J, et al: Dysfunctional uterine bleeding in adolescents. *J Reprod Med* 39:761, 1994.

38. Long CA: Evaluation of patients with abnormal uterine bleeding. *Am J Obstet Gynecol* 175:784, 1996.

39. Weissman AM, Barloon TJ: Transvaginal ultrasonography in nonpregnant and postmenopausal women. *Am Fam Physician* 53:2065, 1996.

40. Gimpelson RJ, Rappold HO: A comparative study between panoramic hysteroscopy with directed biopsies and dilatation and curettage. A review of 276 cases. *Am J Obstet Gynecol* 158(3 Pt 1):489, 1988.

41. Johnston E, Saenz RB: Care of adolescent girls. *Prim Care* 24:53, 1997.

42. Fraser IS, McCarron G, Markham R, et al: Long-term treatment of menorrhagia with mefenamic acid. *Obstet Gynecol* 61:109, 1983.

43. Taylor PJ, Gomel V: Endometrial ablation: indications and preliminary diagnostic hysteroscopy. *Bailliere's Clin Obstet Gynecol* 9:251, 1995.

44. Higham JM, Shaw RW: A comparative study of danazol, a regimen of decreasing doses of danazol, and norethindrone in the treatment of objectively proven unexplained menorrhagia. *Am J Obstet Gynecol* 169:1134, 1993.

45. Candiani GB, Vercellini P, Fedele L, et al: Use of goserelin depot, a gonandotropin-releasing hormone agonist, for the treatment of menorrhagia and severe anemia in women with leiomyomata uteri. *Acta Obstet Gynecol Scand* 69:413, 1990.

46. Thomas EJ, Okuda KJ, Thomas NM: The combination of a depot gonadotrophin releasing hormone agonist and cyclical hormone replacement therapy for dysfunctional uterine bleeding. *Br J Obstet Gynaecol* 98:1155, 1991.

47. Johnson CA: Amenorrhea. In: Johnson CA, Johnson BE, Murray JL, et al (eds): *Women's Health Care Handbook.* Philadelphia: Hanley & Belfus; 1996;117.

48. Kiningham RB, Apgar BS, Schwenk TL: Evaluation of amenorrhea. *Am Fam Physician* 53:1185, 1996.

49. DeSouza MJ, Metzger DA: Reproductive dysfunction in amenorrheic athletes and anorexic patients: a review. *Med Sci Sports Exerc* 23:995, 1991.

50. Crosignani PG, Vegetti W: A practical guide to the diagnosis and management of amenorrhoea. *Drugs* 52:671, 1996.

51. McIver B, Romanski SA, Nippoldt TB: Evaluation and management of amenorrhea. *Mayo Clin Proc* 72:1161, 1997.

52. Monteleoner GP Jr, Browning DG: Nutrition in women. *Prim Care* 24:37, 1997.

53. Korzekwa MI, Steiner M: Premenstrual syndromes. *Clin Obstet Gynecol* 40:564, 1997.

54. American Psychiatric Association: Premenstrual dysphoric disorder. In: *Diagnostic and Statistical Manual of Mental Disorders,* 4th ed. Washington, DC: American Psychiatric Association 1994:715.

55. Rubinow DR: The premenstrual syndrome: new views. *JAMA* 268:1908, 1992.

56. Yonkers KA: Antidepressants in the treatment of premenstrual dysphoric disorder. *J Clin Psychiatry* 58(Suppl 14):4, 1997.

57. Severino SK, Moline ML: Premenstrual syndrome: identification and management. *Drugs* 49:71, 1995.

58. Steiner M: Premenstrual syndromes. *Annu Rev Med* 48:447, 1997.

59. National Institute of Mental Health. *NIHM Premenstrual Syndrome Workshop Guidelines.* Rockville, MD, April 14–15, 1983.

60. Steege, JF, Blumenthal JA: The effects of aerobic exercise on premenstrual symptoms in middle-aged women: a preliminary study. *J Psychosom Rev* 37:127, 1993.

61. Sayegh R, Schiff I, Wurtman J, et al: The effect of a carbohydrate-rich beverage on mood, appetite, and cognitive function in women with premenstrual syndrome. *Obstet Gynecol* 86:520, 1995.

62. Thys-Jacobs S, Starkey P, Bernstein D, et al: Calcium carbonate and the premenstrual syndrome: effects on premenstrual and menstrual symptoms. *Am J Obstet Gynecol* 179:444, 1998.

63. Kleijnen J, Riet GR, Knipschild P: Vitamin B_6 in the treatment of the premenstrual syndrome: a review. *Br J Obstet Gynecol* 97:847,1990.

63a. Wyatt KM, Dimmock PW, Jones PW, Shaughn O'Brien PM: Efficacy of vitamin B_6 in the treatment of premenstrual syndrome: systematic review. *BMJ* 318:1375, 1999.

64. Wood SH, Mortola JF, Chan YF, et al: Treatment of premenstrual syndrome with fluoxetine: a double-blind, placebo-controlled, cross-over study. *Obstet Gynecol* 80:339, 1992.

65. Yonkers KA, Halbreich U, Freeman E, et al: Symptomatic improvement of premenstrual dysphoric disorder with sertraline treatment: a randomized controlled trial. *JAMA* 278:983, 1997.

66. Pearlstein TB, Stone AB, Lund SA, et al: Comparison of fluoxetine, bupropion, and placebo in the treatment of premenstrual dysphoric disorder. *J Clin Psychopharmacol* 17:261, 1997.

     steiner M, Steinberg S, Stewart D, et al: Fluoxetine in the treatment of premenstrual dysphoria. *N Engl J Med* 332:1529, 1995.

68. Steiner M, Korzekwa M, Lamont J, et al: Intermittent fluoxetine dosing in the treatment of women with premenstrual dysphoria. *Psychopharmacol Bull* 33:771, 1997.

69. Halbreich U, Smoller JW: Intermittent luteal phase sertraline treatment of dysphoric premenstrual syndrome. *J Clin Psychiatry* 58:399, 1997.

70. Sundblad C, Hedberg MA, Eriksson E: Clomipramine administered during the luteal phase reduces the symptoms of premenstrual syndrome: a placebo controlled trial. *Neuropsychopharmacology* 9:133, 1993.

71. Freeman EW, Rickels K, Sondheimer SJ, et al: Sertraline versus desipramine in the treatment of premenstrual syndrome: an open-label trial. *J Clin Psychiatry* 57:7, 1996.

72. Ozeren S, Corakci A, Yucesoy I, et al: Fluoxetine in the treatment of premenstrual syndrome. *Eur J Obstet Gynecol Reprod Biol* 73:167, 1997.

73. de la Gandara MJJ: Premenstrual dysphoric disorder: long-term treatment with fluoxetine and discontinuation. *Actas Luso Esp Neurol Psiquiatr* 25:235, 1997.

74. Pearlstein TB, Stone AB: Long-term fluoxetine treatment of late luteal phase dysphoric disorder. *J Clin Psychiatry* 55:332, 1994.

75. Sundblad C, Wikander I, Andersch B, et al: A naturalistic study of paroxetine in premenstrual syndrome: efficacy and side-effects during ten cycles of treatment. *Eur Neuropsychopharmacol* 7:201, 1997.

76. Steiner M, Lamont J, Steinberg S, et al: Effect of fluoxetine on menstrual cycle length in women with premenstrual dysphoria. *Obstet Gynecol* 90:590, 1997.

77. Eriksson E, Hedberg MA, Andersch B, et al: The serotonin reuptake inhibitor paroxetine is superior to the noradrenaline reuptake inhibitor maprotiline in the treatment of premenstrual syndrome. *Neuropsychopharmacology* 12:167, 1995.

78. Sundblad C, Modigh K, Andersch B, et al: Clomipramine effectively reduces premenstrual irritability and dysphoria: a placebo-controlled trial. *Acta Psychiatr Scand* 85:39, 1992.

79. Harrison WM, Endicott J, Nee J: Treatment of premenstrual depression with nortriptyline: a pilot study. *J Clin Psychiatry* 50:136, 1989.

80. Freeman EW, Rickels K, Sondheimer SJ, et al: A double-blind trial of oral progesterone, alprazolam, and placebo in treatment of severe premenstrual syndrome. *JAMA* 274:51, 1995.

81. Schmidt PJ, Grover GN, Rubinow DR: Alprazolam in the treatment of premenstrual syndrome. A double-blind, placebo-controlled trial. *Arch Gen Psychiatry* 50:467, 1993.

82. Harrison WM, Endicott J, Nee J: Treatment of premenstrual dysphoria with alprazolam: a controlled study. *Arch Gen Psychiatry* 47:270, 1990.

83. Brown CS, Ling FW, Farmer RG, et al: Buspirone in the treatment of premenstrual syndrome. *Drug Ther Suppl* 90:112, 1990.

84. Rickels K, Freeman EW, Sondheimer SJ: Buspirone in treatment of premenstrual syndrome (letter). *Lancet* 1(8641):777, 1989.

85. Wang M, Hammarback, S, Lindhe B-A, et al: Treatment of premenstrual syndrome by spironolactone: a double-blind, placebo-controlled study. *Acta Obstet Gyncol Scand* 74:803, 1995.

86. O'Brien PM, Craven D, Selby C, et al: Treatment of premenstrual syndrome by spironolactone. *Br J Obstet Gynaecol* 86:142, 1979.

87. Budeiri D, Po AL, Dornan JC: Is evening primrose oil of value in the treatment of premenstrual syndrome? *Control Clin Trials* 17:60, 1996.

88. Grio R, Cellura A, Geranio R, et al: Clinical efficacy of tamoxifen in the treatment of premenstrual mastodynia. *Minerva Ginecol* 50:101, 1998.

89. Kontostolis E, Stefanidis K, Navrozoglou I, et al: Comparison of tamoxifen with danazol for treatment of cyclical mastalgia. *Gynecol Endocrinol* 11:393, 1997.

90. Schmidt PJ, Nieman LK, Vdanaceau MA, et al: Differential behavioral effects of gonadal steroids in women with and in those without premenstrual syndrome. *N Engl J Med* 338:209, 1998.

91. Smith RNJ, Studd JWW, Samblera D, et al: A randomized comparison over 8 months of 100 mcg and 200 mcg twice weekly doses of transdermal oestradiol in the treatment of severe premenstrual syndrome. *Br J Obstet Gynecol* 102:475, 1995.

92. Bancroft J, Rennie D: The impact of oral contraceptives on the experience of perimenstrual mood, clumsiness, food craving and other symptoms. *J Psychosom Res* 37:195, 1993.

93. Graham CA, Sherwin BB: A prospective treatment study of premenstrual symptoms using a triphasic oral contraceptive. *J Psychosom Res* 36:257, 1992.

94. Hahn PM, Van Vugt DA, Reid RL: A randomized, placebo-controlled, crossover trial of danazol for the treatment of premenstrual syndrome. *Psychoneuroendocrinology* 20:193, 1995.

95. Deeny M, Hawthorn R, McKay-Hart D: Low dose danazol in the treatment of premenstrual syndrome. *Postgrad Med J* 67:450, 1991.

96. Watts JF, Butt WR, Logan-Edwards R: A clinical trial using danazol for the treatment of premenstrual syndrome. *Br J Obstet Gynaecol* 94:30, 1987.

97. Sarno AP Jr, Miller EJ Jr, Lundblad EG: Premenstrual syndrome: beneficial effects of periodic, low-dose danazol. *Obstet Gynecol* 70:33, 1987.

98. Halbreich U, Rojanski N, Palter S: Elimination of ovulation and menstrual cyclicity (with danazol) improves dysphoric premenstrual syndromes. *Fertil Steril* 56:1066, 1991.

99. Zurlo JJ, Frank MM: The long-term safety of danazol in women with hereditary angioedema. *Fertil Steril* 54:64, 1990.

100. Freeman EW, Sondheimer SJ, Rickels K: Gonadotropin-releasing hormone agonist in the treatment of premenstrual symptoms with and without ongoing dysphoria: a controlled trial. *Psychopharmacol Bull* 33:303, 1997.

101. Brown CS, Ling FW, Andersen RN, et al: Efficacy of depot leuprolide in premenstrual syndrome: effect of symptom severity and type in a controlled trial. *Obstet Gynecol* 84:779, 1994.

102. Hammarback S, Backstrom T: Induced anovulation as treatment of premenstrual tension syndrome. A double-blind cross-over study with GnRH-agonist versus placebo. *Acta Obstet Gynecol Scand* 67:159, 1988.

103. Mortola JF, Girton L, Fischer U: Successful treatment of severe premenstrual syndrome by combined use of gonadotropin-releasing hormone agonist and estrogen/progestin. *J Clin Endocrinol Metab* 72:252A, 1991.

104. Mezrow G, Shoupe D, Spicer D, et al: Depot leuprolide acetate with estrogen and progestin add-back for long-term treatment of premenstrual syndrome. *Fertil Steril* 62:932, 1994.

105. Studd J, Leather AT: The need for add-back with gonadotropin-releasing hormone agonist therapy. *Br J Obstet Gynaecol* 103(Suppl 14):1, 1996.

106. Mukherjee T, Barad D, Turk R, et al: A randomized, placebo-controlled study on the effect of cyclic intermittent etidronate therapy on the bone mineral density changes associated with six months of gonadotropin-releasing hormone agonist treatment. *Am J Obstet Gynecol* 175:105, 1996.

107. Casper RF, Hearn MT: The effect of hysterectomy and bilateral oophorectomy in women with severe premenstrual syndrome. *Am J Obstet Gynecol* 62:105, 1990.

108. Blumenthal M (ed): *The Complete German Commission E Monographs: Therapeutic Guide to Herbal Medicinals.* Austin, TX: American Botanical Council; 1998:27,90,98,108,188,208,214,233,347,391.

109. Schulz V, Hansel R, Tyler VE: *Rational Phytotherapy: A Physicians' Guide to Herbal Medicine* (3rd ed). New York: Springer; 1998;241.

110. Black Cohosh. In: *Lawrence Review of Natural Products.* St. Louis: Facts & Comparisons; 1998.

111. Pennington JAT: *Brown and Church's Food Values of Portions Commonly Used* (17th ed). Philadelphia: Lippincott-Raven; 1998.

112. Yonkers KS, Gullion C, Williams A, et al: Paroxetine as a treatment for premenstrual dysphoric disorder. *J Clin Psychopharmacol* 16:3, 1996.

113. Freeman EW, Rickels K, Sondheimer SJ: Fluvoxamine for premenstrual dysphoric disorder: a pilot study. *J Clin Psychiatry* 57(Suppl 8):56, 1996.

114. Freeman EW, Rickels K, Sondheimer SJ, et al: Nefazodone in the treatment of premenstrual syndrome: a preliminary study. *J Clin Psychopharmacol* 14:180, 1994.

115. West CP, Hillier H: Ovarian suppression with the gonadotrophin-releasing hormone agonist goserelin (Zoladex) in management of the premenstrual tension syndrome. *Hum Reprod* 9:1058, 1994.

116. Helvacioglu A, Yeoman RR, Hazelton JM, et al: Premenstrual syndrome and related hormonal changes: long-acting gonadotropin releasing hormone agonist treatment. *J Reprod Med* 38:864, 1993.

Charles D. Ponte
Karen M. Gross

Chapter

14

Sexually Transmitted Diseases and Pelvic Inflammatory Disease

Overview

Sexually transmitted diseases (STDs) pose a continuing challenge for society and health care providers alike. There are over 13 million new cases of STDs, excluding HIV infection, reported each year in the United States[1] Most persons diagnosed with STDs are under the age of 25. The overall economic, social, and personal impact of STDs is impossible to calculate. However, the cost in the United States of treating pelvic inflammatory disease (PID) and its complications alone has been estimated at more than $4 billion annually.[2] Despite the substantial number of diagnosed cases, underreporting of new cases continues to be a significant problem. Syphilis, gonorrhea, chancroid, lymphogranuloma venereum, granuloma inguinale, and HIV/AIDS are the only diseases that are reportable in every state.[3] Nonreportable STDs include infectious vaginitis, molluscum contagiosum, nongonococcal urethritis, mucopurulent cervicitis, hepatitis A and B, human papillomavirus (HPV) infection, epididymitis, and the ectoparasitic infections (pubic lice and scabies). In the interest of public health, STDs must be accurately diagnosed, treated, and reported in a timely fashion.

Although more men than women are affected by STDs, women are more likely to suffer from complications.[4] These include increased fetal/perinatal morbidity and mortality, PID, infertility, ectopic pregnancy, chronic abdominal/pelvic pain, and even neoplasia. This higher complication rate is attributed to the difficulties in diagnosing STDs in women; many women are asymptomatic, resulting in diagnostic and treatment delays. In addition, due to the vaginal milieu during intercourse, a woman is more likely to acquire an STD during any one single sexual encounter.[5]

To reduce the consequences of STDs and PID, preventive strategies must be promoted by the public and health care providers. Men and women are encouraged to be proactive regarding preventive measures, which can dramatically reduce the like-

Table 14-1

STD Prevention Strategies

Abstinence
Avoid intercourse with a known infected partner
Use a new condom with each episode
 of intercourse
Strive for a mutually monogamous relationship
 with an uninfected partner
Examine your partner for the presence of lesions
Talk about your partner's past sexual history
Refrain from partners who have had multiple
 sexual partners
Practice genital self-examination
Avoid illicit drug use that may be associated
 with unsafe sexual practices

lihood for infection. Suggested approaches to reduce the chances of acquiring an STD are listed in Table 14-1.[3,5]

This chapter describes the most common STDs affecting women in the U.S. today. Emphasis is placed on a contemporary evidence-based approach to the epidemiology, diagnosis, and management of these disorders. Diagnostic and treatment guidelines are provided to assist the clinician in the therapeutic decision-making process. The information contained in this chapter will allow clinicians to better inform their patients about cost-effective treatment options and their inherent benefits and risks. Women must be empowered to exercise preventive health practices and take an active role in treatment decisions.

Genital Human Papillomavirus Infection

Condylomata acuminata, or genital warts, is a common STD. Despite its increasing prevalence, the exact number of persons in the United States afflicted with this disorder is difficult to determine. Many individuals with HPV infection are asymptomatic or have subclinical disease. Furthermore, estimates are limited by the inability to accurately and reliably diagnose HPV infection. The best estimate suggests that about 10 to 20 percent of men and women between the ages of 15 and 49 have evidence of the disease based on colposcopic/cytologic, serologic, or DNA/RNA probe findings.[6]

Only 1 percent of sexually active individuals have clinical manifestations of HPV infection. The disease poses a particular threat to women because HPV infection is associated with the development of cervical cancer.[7] Risk factors associated with genital HPV infections in women include a higher number of sexual partners, greater frequency of intercourse, and the presence of condylomata on the partner.[6] Use of condoms can reduce but not eliminate the likelihood of infection with HPV. Importantly, despite treatment of symptomatic warts, contemporary regimens do not cure or eliminate the disease.

Pathophysiology

There are many types of HPV that are responsible for the development of clinical disease. The HPV types associated with visible genital warts are 6, 11, 42, 43, and 44.[8] In addition, over 20 HPV types have been associated with cervical cancers, although most do not cause visible warts. Types 16 and 18 are associated with most cases of high-grade cervical intraepithelial neoplasia and invasive cervical cancer.[6] Malignant transformation cofactors include cigarette smoking, use of oral contraceptives, immunosuppression, other STD pathogens, and certain vitamin deficiencies.[8]

The lesions associated with genital warts can appear anywhere in the genital tract of women. They can be localized or they can spread through the entire genital tract. Skin or mucous membrane trauma, often clinically undetectable, appears necessary for viral penetration and intraepithelial

replication.[8] Exophytic lesions may be seen by the naked eye (Fig. 14-1), but subclinical infections typically go unnoticed by the patient. Common sites include the external genitalia and the perineum. The vagina and cervix may also be affected. The patient is often asymptomatic, although mild discomfort (including pruritus) is reported with lesions of the labia, introitus, or perianal areas.[9] Interestingly, spontaneous remissions have occurred with untreated genital warts.[8]

Diagnosis

Direct visual inspection (see Fig. 14-1), colposcopy (with and without biopsies), and the

Figure 14-1

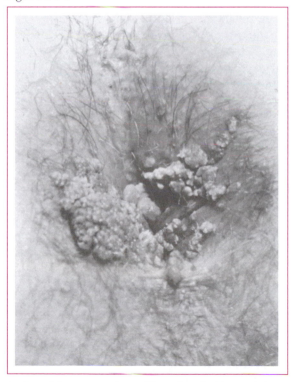

Anal condylomata acuminata. *(Reproduced with permission from KK Holmes et al [eds]: Sexually Transmitted Diseases, 3rd ed. New York: McGraw-Hill, Copyright 1999.)*

results of Pap smears are the most clinicallly useful methods to detect the presence of HPV infection in women. Viral DNA probes are valuable in the research setting but are not practical in the clinical arena.[8] No confirmatory serology tests are available to definitively establish HPV infection in humans.

Treatment

The treatment of genital warts can be discouraging for both the clinician and the patient. There is no universally effective curative treatment method, recurrence rates are high, and subclinical infection can persist despite therapy (Table 14-2). However, the presence of genital warts may be unsightly and can cause physical and emotional discomfort. Thus, all women with known HPV infection should be offered an appropriate treatment regimen.

The treatment of genital warts is usually divided into cytotoxic, physical ablation, and immunologic modes.[10] Because no clearly superior drug is currently available for all patients, choice of therapy is based on a number of factors. These include patient and provider preferences; size, number, and location of warts; wart morphology; cost; adverse effects; and convenience.[3]

CYTOTOXIC DRUGS

Cytotoxic drugs include trichloroacetic acid, bichloroacetic acid, podophyllin, podofilox, and 5-fluorouracil. These agents destroy the infected tissue and are applied topically. Dose and duration of therapy vary with the agent used. Only podofilox 0.5 percent solution or gel and imiquimod 5 percent cream are recommended for patient self-administration to visible genital warts.[3] Patients can usually apply these products at home after minimal training by their health care provider. Importantly, local anesthesia is seldom needed with these therapies. Trichloroacetic acid is the only cytotoxic agent safe to use during pregnancy. Local skin reactions and recurrences are common with these preparations.

PHYSICAL ABLATION

Physical ablation methods include cryotherapy, laser therapy, electrodesiccation, loop electrosurgical excisional procedure, and surgical excision. These methods are often painful and require local or general anesthesia. As with cytotoxic drugs, these methods are associated with high recurrence rates. These methods are reserved for patients in whom topical therapies have failed or who have a large number or surface area of warts.

IMMUNOLOGIC THERAPY

Intralesional interferon and topical imiquimod are newer methods used to treat genital warts. These agents possess immunomodulator and antiviral effects that aid in the resolution of genital lesions. Intralesional therapy is a time-consuming procedure and its utility is limited by pain, flulike symptoms, and rare leukopenia. Topical imiquimod is a relatively safe and effective alternative to the traditional topical preparations available on the market. Local reactions tend to be mild. It is also easy to apply and may be more effective for lesions in women.[10]

COUNSELING

Counseling women about HPV infection should be considered as important as the treatment itself. A diagnosis of genital warts can be especially frightening for the patient because of its association with cervical cancer. Thus, it is important for the health care provider to develop effective counseling strategies to help women with HPV infection cope with their disease and its consequences. Table 14-3 includes information that should be conveyed to all women with genital warts.[11]

Table 14-2

Success and Recurrence Rates for Selected HPV Treatments

TREATMENT TYPE	SUCCESS RATES	RECURRENCE RATES	SUGGESTED REGIMEN
CYTOTOXIC AGENTS			
Trichloroacetic acid	64–81%	36%	80–90% solution: Apply to warts, allow to dry. Repeat weekly, if needed.
Podophyllin	38–79%	21–65%	10–25% solution in compound tincture of Benzoin: Apply to wart, allow to dry. Wash off in 1–4 h. May apply weekly for up to 6 wk.
Podofilox	68–88%	16–34%	0.5% solution or gel: Apply twice daily for 3 d followed by 4 d of no therapy. May repeat for up to 4 cycles.
5-Fluorouracil	68–97%	0–8%	5% cream: Apply cream 1–3 times per wk. Wash off in 3–10 h. May apply for several weeks.
PHYSICAL ABLATION			**AVERAGE NUMBER OF TREATMENTS**
Cryotherapy	70–96%	25–39%	1.9
CO$_2$ laser	72–97%	6–49%	1.3
Electrodesiccation	94%	25%	1.4
LEEP	72%	51%	1.0
Surgical excision	89–93%	19–22%	1.1
ANTIVIRAL AGENTS			
Interferon: Intralesional	36–53%	21–25%	1 million units per wart (up to 5 warts) 3 times a week on alternate days for 3 wk (Alpha-2b); 250,000 units twice a week for up to 8 wk (Alpha-n3).
Topical	33%	NR	
Systemic	7–82%	23%	
Imiquimod: Topical	37–52%	13–19%	5% cream: Apply cream 3 times per wk at bedtime. Wash off in 6–10 h. May repeat for up to 16 wk.

ABBREVIATIONS: LEEP, loop electrical excisional procedure; NR, not reported.
SOURCE: Adapted from references 3,10,107–109.

Table 14-3

Counseling Strategies for Women with HPV Infections

1. Advise condom use and limiting the number of sexual partners
2. Stress that visible warts can be treated and removed (but not cured)
3. Make the patient an active participant in treatment decisions
4. Describe the natural history and course of HPV infection
5. Stress the need for regular Pap smears and follow-up
6. Help the patient inform her partner(s)
7. Refer to support group if necessary

Genital Herpes Simplex

Genital herpes simplex virus infection is an STD caused by herpes simplex virus type 2 (HSV-2) or herpes simplex virus type 1 (HSV-1). Although both types can cause genital or oral infection, most cases of genital herpes are caused by HSV-2 (estimated 70 percent).[12] There are 200,000 to 500,000 new symptomatic cases of genital herpes per year in the United States. At least 45 million people in the United States have been infected with HSV-2.[3] HSV-2 is more common in women (one in four) than in men (about one in five), possibly due to more efficient male-to-female transmission.[13] The number of persons infected with HSV-2 is increasing in the United States and worldwide, despite increased promotion of safer sex practices.[12,14,15]

Genital HSV infection can result from oral-genital or genital-genital contact with an infected person. Most persons with HSV-2 are unaware that they are infected. Simple education with pictures of lesions and pamphlets allows over 50 percent of undiagnosed HSV-2 seropositive persons to recognize the signs and symptoms of genital her-

pes.[16] Most persons seropositive for HSV-2 shed virus from urogenital and perianal skin. Asymptomatic shedding is more frequent in the first year after symptomatic primary infection and with HSV-2 infection (3.3 to 4.3 percent of days) compared to HSV-1 (0.6 to 1.2 percent of days).[17] Estimates of overall rates of subclinical shedding range from 2 to 3 percent of days (as determined by cultures)[17,18] to 10 to 12 percent of days (as determined by polymerase chain reaction [PCR] methods), with some persons shedding on over 50 percent of days.[19] Over two-thirds of HSV-2 infections are transmitted to partners during periods of asymptomatic shedding.[20]

The transmission rate with regular intercourse has been estimated to be 10 percent per year in studies of serodiscordant couples (one partner is HSV-2 positive and the other is not).[20,21] Annual transmission rates were significantly higher in couples with a female susceptible partner (18.9 to 22 percent) compared to a male susceptible partner (0 to 4.5 percent) and in women without past HSV-1 infection (32 percent). Use of barrier contraception, such as a diaphragm, condom, or both, reduced the overall rate to 5.7 percent compared to a rate of 13.6 percent associated with nonuse (though only 15 percent of couples used barrier methods).[20] Studies have shown that HSV-2 infection is a risk factor for the acquisition of HIV infection in heterosexuals.[22,23]

Pathophysiology

Primary genital herpes occurs when virus comes in contact with susceptible mucosal surfaces or skin. HSV ascends peripheral sensory nerves and enters the sacral nerve ganglion, becoming latent with intermittent episodes of symptomatic or asymptomatic reactivation.

In primary herpes simplex infection, there is often a prodrome of malaise, myalgias, headache, and low-grade fever. Symptoms usually occur within 3 to 7 days of exposure.[24] Systemic symptoms peak in the first 3 to 4 days and then wane. Painful lesions, itching, and burning in the genital area begin in the first few days after onset of the pro-

Figure 14-2

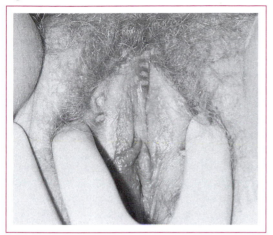

Primary genital herpes of the vulva. *(Reproduced with permission from KK Holmes et al [eds]: Sexually Transmitted Diseases, 3rd ed. New York: McGraw-Hill, copyright 1999.)* (See Color Plate 1.)

Figure 14-3

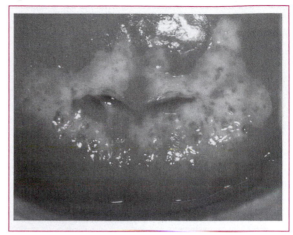

Severe primary HSV-2 cervicitis. *(Reproduced with permission from KK Holmes et al [eds]: Sexually Transmitted Diseases, 3rd ed. New York: McGraw-Hill, copyright 1999.)* (See Color Plate 2.)

drome. Typical lesions are groups of small painful vesicles on the vulva, perineum or perianal skin, or cervix (Figs. 14-2 and 14-3). Vesicles quickly become ulcers, especially on mucosal surfaces, which become crusted in later stages of healing. Lesions are usually painful to touch (unlike syphilis chancres, which are typically painless). Atypical presentations with nonulcerative genital lesions, such as vulvar erythema, fissures, or furuncle-like lesions, are common.[25] Tender inguinal nodes, dysuria, vaginal discharge, and cervical ulcerations are often present in the primary infection stage, but are infrequent with recurrences. Viral shedding lasts for a mean of 12 days, with a mean of 20 days required for lesion healing.[26]

Pharyngeal infection with HSV is common in primary HSV-1 or HSV-2 infection, with or without concurrent genital symptoms, but is rare with recurrent disease.[27] Anorectal HSV may cause perianal or rectal lesions, rectal pain, or discharge in about 20 percent of women with primary HSV.[26] Rare serious complications may occur with primary HSV infection. Aseptic meningitis occurs in up to 5 percent of patients with primary HSV-2. Sacral autonomic radiculopathy, with constipation, urinary retention, and sacral anesthesia, occurs in 1 percent of cases.[26] Herpes keratocon-

junctivitis, acute salpingitis,[28] transverse myelitis,[29] encephalitis,[30] and disseminated, bloodborne infection (with cutaneous or visceral involvement) occur rarely.

In recurrent genital herpes, 85 percent of women note itching or burning in the genital or perianal area 30 min to 2 days before lesions develop. Lesions tend to be fewer and less painful than in the primary outbreak. Lesions become culture-negative in 2 to 7 days and heal in 7 to 10 days on average.[31] Recurrences of genital herpes occur less frequently with HSV-1 infection compared to HSV-2 (median recurrence rates per month: 0.06 for HSV-1 and 0.31 for HSV-2).[18] Identification of the type of HSV (by culture or by serotyping) can provide important prognostic information.

Diagnosis

Because many patients with genital herpes have mild symptoms, it is important to maintain a high level of suspicion for HSV whenever a woman has any painful genital lesion. Differential diagnosis of genital ulcers must include syphilis and chancroid (Fig.14-4).[3, 32] Viral culture is the gold standard for diagnosis, but false-negative results are common.[25] A positive culture is more likely when obtained in the earlier vesicular stage of disease rather than later and in primary rather than recurrent disease. Sensitivity of cultures during a primary episode in women was increased

Figure 14-4

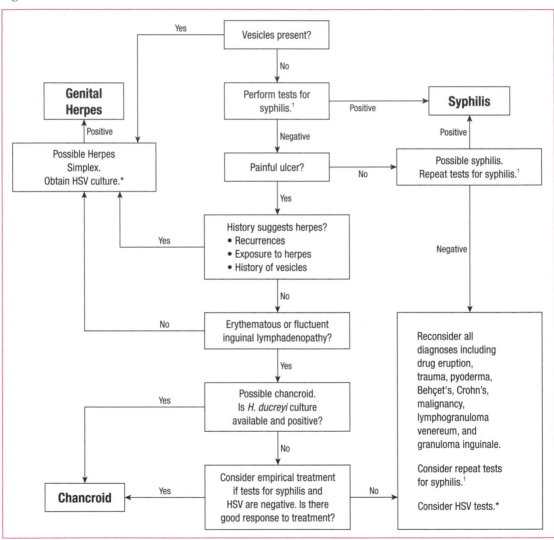

Evaluation of the patient with genital ulcer(s). A negative HSV culture does not exclude the diagnosis of herpes. *If high index of suspicion, consider repeat cultures with next occurrence, or acute and convalescent HSV antibody titers. Consideration of alternate diagnosis is also advisable. †Darkfield microscopic examination or direct fluorescent antibody tests of chancre exudate are best initial tests for primary syphilis. (*Adapted with permission from Centers for Disease Control and Prevention, 1998, and L Corey and KK Holmes, Ann Intern Med 98:973, copyright 1983.*)

from 59 to 77 percent by sampling multiple urogenital sites rather than a single site.[25] Sensitivity of cultures during recurrent disease is only about 50 percent.[33] If the culture is negative with clinical suspicion of HSV, repeat culture at the next occurrence of symptoms or antibody titers (acute and convalescent) should be considered. Several antigen kits are available with sensitivity and specificity comparable to culture; however, they do not allow differentiation of viral types.[12]

Treatment

Three antiviral drugs are available for the treatment of genital herpes: acyclovir (Zovirax), valacyclovir hydrochloride (Valtrex), and famciclovir (Famvir) (Table 14-4). Systemic therapy (oral or intravenous) is more efficacious and better tolerated than topical therapy (topical application of acyclovir can cause a genital burning sensation). Acyclovir is a synthetic purine nucleoside analogue with inhibitory activity against HSV-1 and HSV-2. Valacyclovir hydrochloride is an inactive prodrug of acyclovir with higher bioavailability. It is rapidly converted to acyclovir by first-pass intestinal and hepatic metabolism. Famciclovir is rapidly converted to penciclovir, an antiviral compound with the same mechanism of action as acyclovir. Acyclovir, famciclovir, and valacyclovir are Pregnancy Category B drugs, but there are no adequate well-controlled studies to establish safety in pregnant women.

INITIAL EPISODE

Acyclovir and valacyclovir have been studied in the treatment of initial episodes of genital herpes. Acyclovir significantly reduced duration of infection and time to lesion healing compared to placebo.[34] Valacyclovir has similar efficacy compared to acyclovir.[35] Median times to lesion healing, cessation of pain, and viral shedding were 9 days, 5 days, and 3 days, respectively. Famciclovir does not currently have an indication for the initial treatment of HSV.

Table 14-4

Antiviral Drugs for Genital Herpes Simplex

RECOMMENDED DOSAGES AND COST* (G/B)*	INITIAL EPISODE	RECURRENT EPISODES[†]	CONTINUOUS SUPPRESSION
Acyclovir (Zovirax®) (Generic available)	200 mg five times daily for 10 d ($50-G) OR IV 5 mg/kg tid for hospitalized patients with severe disease	200 mg five times daily for 5 d ($25-G)	400 mg bid ($3.78/d-G) Alternate dosing: 200 mg tid ($2.94/d-G) or 200 mg five times daily ($4.90/day-G)
Valacyclovir (Valtrex®)	1 g bid for 10 d ($72.83-B)	500 mg bid for 5 d ($28.91-B)	1 g qd[‡] ($3.64/d-B)
Famciclovir (Famvir®)	Not indicated	125 mg twice daily for 5 d ($25.46-B)	250 mg bid ($6.36/d-B)

*Costs reflect 1998 (Drug Topics) Red Book average wholesale prices (AWPs) per therapy course unless otherwise noted. Actual patient cost may vary considerably. G, generic; B, brand name.
[†]Therapy should be initiated at first sign or symptom of infection.
[‡]For patients with nine or fewer recurrences per year, valacyclovir 500 mg daily was equally effective.

RECURRENT EPISODES

Acyclovir and valacyclovir were compared to placebo for the treatment of recurrent genital herpes.[36] Both drugs hastened lesion healing and reduced duration of pain by 1 day and stopped viral shedding twice as rapidly as placebo. In addition, famciclovir reduced time to healing of lesions by 1 day and reduced time to cessation of viral shedding by over 45 percent.[37] All three drugs are generally well tolerated, with nausea, headache, or dizziness occurring in a small percentage of patients. Patients should be taught to recognize early prodromal symptoms and begin medication immediately to ensure greatest efficacy.

SUPPRESSION

Individuals who experience more than six recurrences per year benefit from suppressive therapy.[38] Acyclovir, valacyclovir, or famciclovir taken continuously have each been shown to significantly reduce recurrences. Daily suppressive therapy with acyclovir reduced the amount of asymptomatic shedding of HSV-2 in women by 94 percent (from 28 percent of days without therapy to 8 percent with therapy).[19] Because most HSV-2 transmission occurs during asymptomatic shedding of virus, suppressive therapy may play an important role in reducing transmission to partners.[12] Actual transmission rates during suppressive therapy have not been determined by clinical trials. Continuous use of acyclovir for 5 years is well tolerated,[39] but the effects of long-term use of valacyclovir and famciclovir are not yet known. After the first year of suppressive therapy, the need for suppressive medication should be reevaluated because recurrences tend to become less frequent over time. The decision to discontinue suppressive therapy should be individualized, taking into account the patient's preferences, frequency of breakthrough recurrences while on suppressive therapy, and risk of transmitting HSV to a susceptible partner. Women who discontinue suppressive therapy should be offered 5-day antiviral therapy to be used as needed for recurrences.

Herpes in Pregnancy

Genital herpes in pregnancy causes significant fetal and newborn morbidity and mortality.[40] Primary HSV-2 infection occuring in early to midgestation is likely to result in spontaneous abortion (45 percent) or congenital anomalies. Neonatal herpes occurs in 33 to 50 percent of infants born to women with primary HSV in pregnancy (whether symptomatic or not), in 3 to 5 percent of those with recurrent lesions at delivery, and in less than 3 percent with recurrent asymptomatic shedding. It is important to note that most newborns with neonatal HSV are born to asymptomatic mothers with no history of genital herpes. Overall, neonatal mortality is 17 percent with neurologic sequelae in 33 percent of survivors. Weekly surveillance cultures in late pregnancy are no longer recommended; a single culture at the time of delivery from an asymptomatic HSV-infected mother is useful to guide neonatal treatment. Cesarean delivery is recommended only if active lesions are present at the time of delivery.[41] Acyclovir suppression for HSV-infected women in late pregnancy did not reduce the cesarean section rate in one clinical trial and is not recommended.[42]

Empirical therapy with intravenous acyclovir should be considered in HSV-exposed newborns who develop signs of infection, such as vesicular skin lesions, hepatitis, pneumonitis, or encephalitis. Infants suspected of sepsis who show clinical deterioration despite antibiotic treatment, especially with negative bacterial cultures, should be cultured for HSV and considered for empirical treatment with acyclovir.[43]

Education and Prevention

The psychological impact of being diagnosed with an incurable STD should not be underestimated. Providing information and emotional support in a sensitive, nonjudgmental manner can help the patient adjust more easily to the diagnosis (Table 14-5). Several promising vaccines are being studied for primary prevention of HSV-2.[44] The vaccines have also demonstrated some therapeutic benefit in reducing frequency of recurrences in animal models and in HSV-2-infected humans.[45,46]

Gonococcal Infection

Gonorrhea is among the most frequently reported communicable diseases in the United States, causing an estimated 600,000 new infections per year.[3] In women, *Neisseria gonorrhoeae* causes urogenital, rectal, and pharyngeal infection as well as upper genital tract disease. It is estimated that up to 80 percent of women infected with gonorrhea are asymptomatic.[47] The infection rate for women with gonococcus in 1996 was 118/100,000 population, declining since 1975.[48] Adolescent women have rates five times higher than other age groups. About 85 percent of all gonococcal infections occur in African American and Hispanic populations. Other risk factors include exposure to multiple partners and use of nonbarrier methods of contraception.

Antibiotic-resistant strains of gonococci have been steadily increasing, with an estimated 30

Table 14-5
Counseling Women with Genital Herpes

General information:
  It is a common infection, affecting 1 in 4 women and 1 in 5 men.
  Many persons who transmit the virus are not aware of their infection.
  Transmission is mainly by sexual contact (genital-genital contact or oral-genital contact).
  Most people with genital herpes have recurrences (often every few months).
  Medication is available to treat or suppress the recurrences.
  Avoid handling the lesions, and wash your hands after contact (to avoid spreading the infection to
    other skin or eyes.)
To decrease the chances of giving your partner herpes:
  Use condoms consistently.
  Using a diaphragm or a vaginal spermicide may also decrease risk.
  Avoid having sex when any symptoms are present.
  Objects may rarely spread the virus, so avoid sharing towels, razors, etc. when symptoms are present.
It is important to talk to your current and future sexual partners about your infection:
  About 5% of male partners of women with genital herpes will become infected in 1 y when the
    above precautions are used (but not all 5% will develop symptoms).
Herpes in pregnancy:
  Greatest risk occurs with primary herpes during pregnancy.
  Pregnant women with herpes should inform their doctor of their diagnosis.
  Women with herpes lesions at delivery should be delivered by cesarean section to decrease the risk
    of transmission of herpes infection to the infant.
More information is available:
  CDC's National STD hotline: 919-361-8488 (Mon–Fri, 9 A.M.–7 P.M. EST)
  Internet: www.herpesweb.net
  Many areas have support groups for people with herpes.

percent of strains now resistant to penicillin and tetracycline. Quinolone-resistant strains are becoming widespread in Asia, but to date occur only rarely in the United States (< 0.05 percent in 1996).[3] Patients infected with *N. gonorrhoeae* are often co-infected with *Chlamydia trachomatis* (20 to 40 percent in some populations), leading to the recommendation that patients with gonococcus be routinely treated with a regimen effective against *C. trachomatis.*[3]

Pathophysiology

The endocervical canal is the primary site of gonococcal infection in women. Urethral colonization is present in the majority of women, but is rarely the sole site of infection.[49] Common symptoms include increased vaginal discharge, dysuria, menorrhagia, and intermenstrual bleeding.[50] Physical examination may be normal or may reveal cervical abnormalities, such as mucopurulent discharge, increased erythema, edema, or friability of the cervix.[51] Gonococcal organisms may be recovered by culture from the rectum of 35 to 50 percent of women with gonococcal cervicitis, but are only rarely associated with proctitis symptoms in women.[52] Pharyngeal infection (usually asymptomatic) is present in 10 to 20 percent of heterosexual women with gonorrhea, usually in association with urogenital disease.[53] Gonococcal conjunctivitis is rare in adults, occurring by autoinoculation from concomitant urogenital disease. Ophthalmia neonatorum can occur in newborns of infected mothers.

The most common serious complication of *N. gonorrhoeae* is PID. More than half of the approximately 1 million cases of PID per year are associated with this organism.[2] Long-term sequelae from a single episode of PID, including infertility, chronic pelvic pain, dyspareunia, and ectopic pregnancy, occur in about 18 to 20 percent of women.[54] Gonococcal bacteremia can result in disseminated gonococcal infection (DGI), a rare syndrome of acute arthritis, tenosynovitis, and dermatitis. Over 80 percent of patients with DGI will have gonococci cultured from the primary site of infection (anogenital or pharynx) or from a sexual partner. Only 50 percent of patients with DGI will have positive cultures from blood, synovial fluid, or skin lesions. Most have arthralgias or tenosynovitis, with frank arthritis only in 30 to 40 percent.[55] Skin lesions occur in two-thirds of cases, but can be easily overlooked (Fig. 14-5). They are classically described as tender necrotic pustules on an erythematous base, usually on the distal extremities. Gonococcal endocarditis and meningitis are extremely rare.

Diagnosis

The gold standard test for gonococcal infection in asymptomatic persons is culture from the sites of exposure (urethra, endocervix, rectum, throat). A single endocervical culture in women has an estimated sensitivity of 80 to 95 percent in carefully controlled conditions.[56] Sensitivity may be lower if inadequate specimen collection, transport, or laboratory processing occurs. A number of non-

Figure 14-5

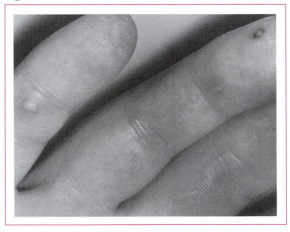

Skin lesions in disseminated gonococcal infection. *(Reproduced with permission from KK Holmes et al [eds]: Sexually Transmitted Diseases, 3rd ed. New York: McGraw-Hill, copyright 1999.)* (See Color Plate 3.)

culture tests have also been evaluated. The DNA probe has become increasingly favored in settings where handling and storage of culture media are difficult. When studied in patients in STD clinics (prevalence of gonorrhea 9 to 10 percent), the DNA probe had a very high sensitivity and specificity (97 to 99 percent), high positive predictive value (> 90 percent), and was more sensitive than a single culture.[57,58] Enzyme immunoassay (EIA, Gonozyme) yields too many false-positive results to be useful for screening, particularly in populations with low prevalence of gonococcus (positive predictive value 55 percent if prevalence is 3.6 percent).[59] Tests based on the ligase chain reaction (LCR) and polymerase chain reaction (PCR) of first-void urine and endocervical swabs are being studied.[60–62] They appear to have sensitivity equal to or greater than culture when used in populations with 8 to 9 percent prevalence or higher, but their usefulness in screening populations with low prevalence remains to be determined.

Treatment

Both broad-spectrum cephalosporins and quinolones remain highly effective against *N. gonorrhoeae* when given as a single dose. Table 14-6 lists the regimens currently recommended by the Centers for Disease Control and Prevention (CDC) for therapy of uncomplicated gonococcal infections (see the CDC guidelines[3] for therapy for complicated infections). Choice of therapy is guided by consideration of adherence issues, allergy history, contraindications, and cost. Oral formulations are generally more acceptable to patients and are

Table 14-6

Therapy for Uncomplicated Gonococcal Infections of the Cervix, Urethra, Rectum, and Pharynx[†3]

CDC Recommended Regimens and Cost*	Alternative Regimens
Cefixime 400 mg orally in a single dose ($7.21-B)	Spectinomycin 2 g IM in a single dose (expensive, for patients who cannot tolerate quinolones or cephalosporins). ($21.18-B)
or	or
Ceftriaxone 125 mg IM in a single dose*** ($6.66-B)	Single-dose cephalosporin (ceftizoxime 500 mg IM) [$6.48-B],
or	cefotaxime 500 mg IM [$5.77-B],
Ciprofloxacin 500 mg orally in a single dose*** ($3.74-G)	cefotetan 1 g IM [$11.72], or
plus	cefoxitin 2 g IM [$19.66-B] with probenecid 1 g PO [$3.54-G])
Azithromycin 1 g orally in a single dose ($19.83-G)	or
or	Single-dose quinolone regimens (enoxacin 400 mg orally [$3.11-B], lomefloxacin 400 mg PO [$6.60-B], norfloxacin 800 mg PO [$5.08-G])[‡]
Doxycycline 100 mg orally twice daily for 7 d ($1.78-G)	

*Cost reflects 1998 (Drug Topics) Red Book average wholesale prices (AWPs) per regimen. Actual patient cost may vary considerably. G, generic; B, Brand.

†Gonococcal infections of the pharynx are more difficult to eradicate than from urogenital sites. CDC recommended regimens include drugs with *** above *or* ofloxacin 400 mg orally in a single dose *plus* azithromycin or doxycycline as above.

‡Pregnant women should **not** be treated with quinolones (ciprofloxacin, enofloxacin, lomefloxacin, norfloxacin) or tetracyclines. Cephalosporins *or* spectinomycin intramuscularly *plus* erythromycin base or amoxicillin (see Table 14–7 for doses) are acceptable alternatives in these patients.

more cost-effective. Quinolones (e.g., ciprofloxacin, enofloxacin, lomefloxacin, norfloxacin) are contra-indicated in pregnancy, during lactation, and in persons under age 18 due to risk of arthropathy. Sucralfate, ranitidine, antacids, and some mineral supplements may interfere with absorption of quinolones. A single 2-g dose of azithromycin has been shown in clinical trials to be effective against *N. gonorrhoeae*, but it is not recommended due to high cost and a high incidence of gastrointestinal distress (35 percent).[3]

Patients should be advised to avoid sexual intercourse until therapy is completed (or for 7 days after a single-dose regimen) and both the patient and their sex partner(s) are free of symptoms. Patients should refer all sex partners with whom they have had sexual contact in the last 60 days for evaluation and treatment. Gonorrhea must be reported to public health officials (state health departments can provide information about each state's reporting process). If the patient's last sexual contact was more than 60 days before the diagnosis or onset of symptoms, the most recent partner should be evaluated and treated. Patients with uncomplicated gonorrhea who are treated with recommended regimens need not return for a test of cure. Any patients with persistent symptoms after treatment should be evaluated by culture for gonococcus and tested for *C. trachomatis*. Infections after treatment usually result from reinfection rather than treatment failure.

Screening and Prevention

The CDC recommends annual screening of asymptomatic women in the following groups: (1) women with mucopurulent cervicitis, (2) sexually active adolescents, (3) women aged 20 to 24 who have new or multiple partners or who do not consistently use barrier contraception (Fig. 14-6).[3] In areas of high prevalence of disease, broader screening of sexually active young women may be advisable. Screening endocervical culture is recommended at the first prenatal visit for pregnant women at risk or living in a geographic area with high preva-

lence of gonorrhea, with repeat testing in the third trimester for those at continued risk of acquiring infection.

Chlamydia Trachomatis

Chlamydia trachomatis infection is the most common bacterial STD in the United States, with an estimated 4 million cases annually.[63] As many as 1 in 10 sexually active adolescent girls tested for chlamydia are infected. Prevalence is 5 percent or greater for most populations tested, but tends to be higher among those who are younger, live in inner cities, have lower socioeconomic status, or are African American.[63] Other risk factors include recent new sexual partner, use of nonbarrier method of contraception, prior infection with gonorrhea or chlamydia, and cervical ectopy.[64]

Pathophysiology

Chlamydiae are gram-negative bacteria with an obligate intracellular life cycle. *C. trachomatis* is transmitted to partners by sexual intercourse and to neonates through childbirth. The organism infects columnar epithelial cells of the cervix, urethra, or rectum. The cervix is the usual inital site of infection. Most infections are asymptomatic, but vaginal discharge and dysuria may occur. Signs of infection include cervical erythema, ectopy, or mucopurulent discharge. Lower abdominal pain and menstrual abnormalities may occur as infection ascends to the upper genital tract. It is not known what proportion of women with chlamydial infection will develop PID.[63] *C. trachomatis* is associated with 7 to 51 percent of cases of PID,[65] with a more insidious onset than nonchlamydial PID. Risk of PID increases with the number of chlamydial infections (with three or more infections, the risk is up to 10 times greater than for women with a first infection).[66]

Figure 14-6

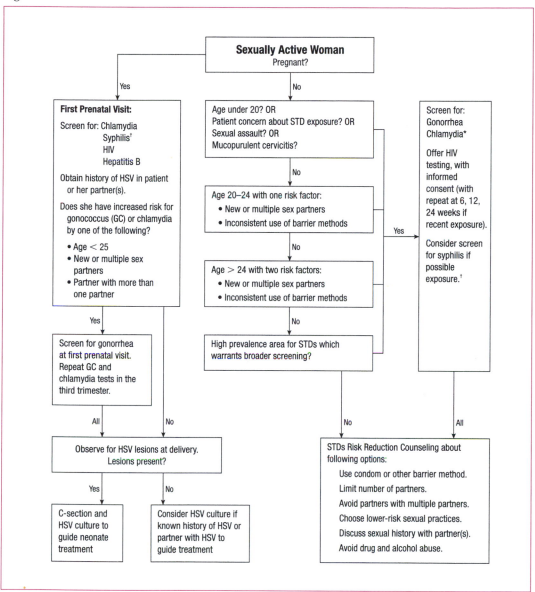

STD screening algorithm. *Chlamydia culture is the preferred test in cases of sexual assault. If not available, nonculture tests (ligase chain reaction or polymerase chain reaction) are acceptable alternatives. A positive nonculture test must be verified by a second nonculture test based on a different diagnostic principle. Enzyme immunoassay (EIA) and direct fluorescent antibody (DFA) are not acceptable first tests due to higher false-negatives and false-positives. †Serologic nontreponemal tests (e.g., VDRL or RPR) are used for screening. Sequential tests using the same method, preferably by the same lab, should be done at 6, 12, 24 weeks when evaluating recent exposure (as in sexual assault). *(Adapted with permission from Centers for Disease Control and Prevention, 1998.)*

Diagnosis

Cell culture of *C. trachomatis* is nearly 100 percent specific but has a relatively low sensitivity of 70 to 85 percent.[67] Due to its high specificity, cell culture is the preferred method for use in investigations of sexual assault. Culture may be obtained from the endocervix using a Dacron, rayon, or cotton swab or cytobrush, after initially wiping away cervical secretions. Swabs with wooden shafts are toxic to *C. trachomatis* and must be avoided. Specimens for chlamydia tests should be obtained after *N. gonorrhoeae* culture or Pap smear. Because *C. trachomatis* organisms live in columnar epithelial cells, it is important that the sample be obtained from within the endocervix. Specimens should be refrigerated after collection and processed in the laboratory within 48 h. Urethral, nasopharyngeal, and rectal specimens should be tested by cell culture because reliability of other methods has not yet been established.[3] Pooling of a urethral swab specimen with an endocervical specimen increases culture sensitivity by 23 percent.[68]

A variety of nonculture tests are available for *C. trachomatis*, with the advantage of easier handling and laboratory processing and with sensitivities higher than culture.[67] EIA (Chlamydiazyme or Microtrak) is an antigen detection method with sensitivity for endocervical specimens approaching that of culture. Direct fluorescent antibody test (DFA) is a method for detecting antigen with sensitivity of 80 to 90 percent and specificity of 98 percent. It is a rapid but labor-intensive test that may best be used as a confirmatory test for other nonculture techniques. Rapid tests (such as Clearview, TestPack, SureCell) use EIA methods, but are much less sensitive and specific than EIAs performed in a laboratory. DNA probes (PACE 2 Gen-probe) have a sensitivity of 72 to 96 percent and specificity of 97 to 99 percent, with the advantage that a single swab specimen can be tested for *C. trachomatis* and *N. gonorrhoeae*.[69] The most promising development in *C. trachomatis* testing has been the nucleic acid amplification tests, PCR (Amplicor by Roche) and LCR (LCx by Abbott). Both tests are more sensitive

than culture (> 92 percent) with high specificity (99 to 100 percent) using endocervical or urethral specimens.[60] PCR and LCR tests on first-voided urine specimens in both men and women are highly sensitive, offering a method for noninvasive screening.[61,70] They cost two to three times as much as the other nonculture tests.[71] They may detect chlamydial DNA long after viable organisms have been eradicated, so they should be used with caution when performing tests of cure. The PCR-positive state after treatment with doxycycline appears to last up to 3 weeks.[72]

A recommended approach for populations with low to moderate prevalence of infection (< 6 percent) would be to use EIA or DNA probe testing, with a confirmatory test such as DFA or nucleic acid amplification (commercial PCR or LCR) on those with reactive or equivocal test results.[71] Many labs will perform confirmatory tests on the same specimen. For screening populations with high (≥6 percent) prevalence (such as adolescents, STD clinic patients, patients with a history of exposure or with clinical findings suggesting infection), commercial PCR or LCR is the most cost-effective test.[73] If PCR or LCR is not available, EIA or DNA probe with confirmatory testing with DFA is recommended. In medicolegal settings, such as child abuse or sexual assault, culture is required to prove infection, but may be combined with PCR or LCR.

Treatment

Table 14-7 summarizes the CDC recommendations for treatment of chlamydial infections in adolescents and adults.[3] Azithromycin is four times as costly as doxycycline; however, because it may be given as a single, directly observed dose, it may be more cost-effective due to improved compliance, thereby preventing more cases of PID.[74] Patients do not require retesting for chlamydia after completing treatment with doxycycline or azithromycin unless symptoms persist. After treatment with erythromycin, retesting more than 3 weeks after treatment is recommended due to lower cure rates. Nonculture tests

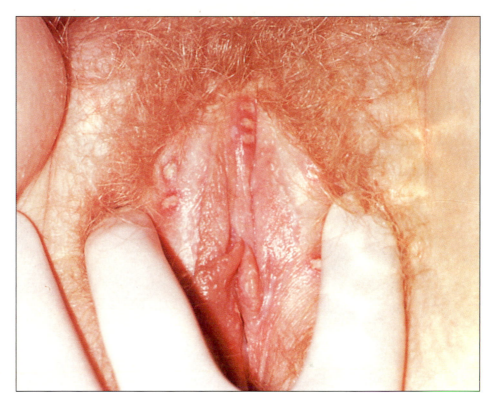

Plate 1 (Figure 14-2)

Primary genital herpes of the vulva.

(Reproduced with permission from KK Holmes et al, [eds]: Sexually Transmitted Diseases, 3rd ed. New York, McGraw-Hill, 1999.)

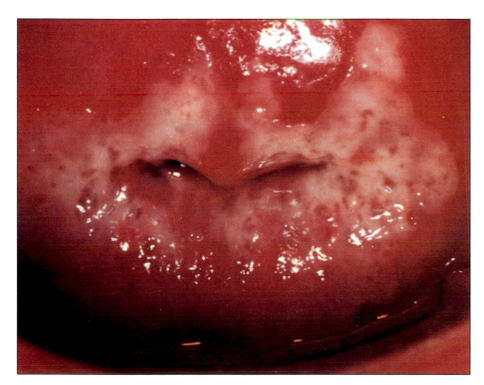

Plate 2 (Figure 14-3)

Severe primary HSV-2 cervicitis.

(Reproduced with permission from KK Holmes et al, [eds]: Sexually Transmitted Diseases, 3rd ed. New York, McGraw-Hill, 1999.)

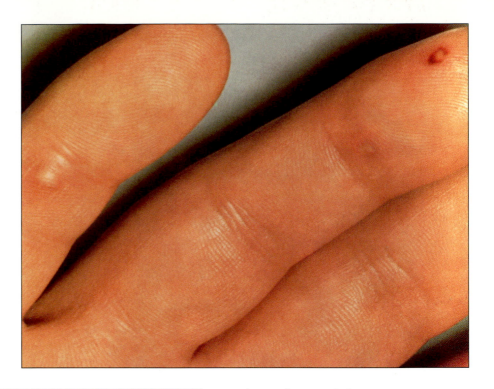

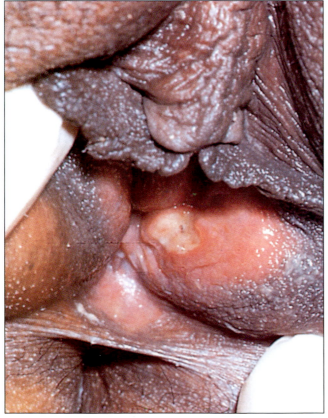

Plate 3 (Figure 14-5)
Skin lesions in disseminated gonococcal infection.

(Reproduced with permission from KK Holmes et al, [eds]: Sexually Transmitted Diseases, 3rd ed. New York, McGraw-Hill, 1999.)

Plate 4 (Figure 14-7)
Chancroid ulcer of the fourchette in a female.

(Reproduced with permission from KK Holmes et al, [eds]: Sexually Transmitted Diseases, 3rd ed. New York, McGraw-Hill, 1999.)

Table 14-7

CDC Recommended Treatment for Chlamydial Infections[3]

RECOMMENDED REGIMENS	RECOMMENDED REGIMENS FOR PREGNANT WOMEN
Azithromycin 1 g PO in a single dose ($19.83-G) *or* Doxycycline 100 mg PO twice daily for 7 d ($1.78-G)	Erythromycin base 500 mg PO qid for 7 d ($12.88-G) *or* Amoxicillin 500 mg PO tid daily for 7 d ($4.72-G)
ALTERNATIVE REGIMENS	**ALTERNATIVE REGIMENS FOR PREGNANT WOMEN***
Erythromycin base 500 mg PO qid for 7 d ($12.88-G) *or* Erythromycin ethylsuccinate 800 mg PO qid for 7 d ($15.09-G) *or* Ofloxacin 300 mg bid for 7 d ($67.49-G)	Erythromycin base 250 mg PO qid for 14 d ($5.68-G) *or* Erythromycin ethylsuccinate 800 mg PO qid for 7 d ($15.09-G) *or* Erythromycin ethylsuccinate 400 mg PO qid for 14 d ($7.55-G) *or* Azithromycin 1 g PO in a single dose ($19.83-G)

*Erythromycin estolate is contraindicated in pregnancy because of hepatotoxicity. Preliminary data indicate azithromycin may be safe and effective in pregnancy, but data are insufficient to recommend its routine use in pregnant women.

performed prior to 3 weeks after therapy may give false-positive results. Rescreening in several months is advisable if likelihood of reinfection is high (e.g., in adolescents).

Patients should be instructed to refer their sex partners for evaluation and treatment. Any sex partner within 60 days before the onset of symptoms or diagnosis (or the most recent sex partner if the last sexual contact was over 60 days before onset or diagnosis) should be evaluated, tested, and treated. Patients should avoid sexual intercouse until they and their partners have completed treatment (or for 7 days after a single-dose regimen) and are symptom-free.

Prevention

Screening asymptomatic women is an important strategy to reduce the prevalence of chlamydia infections (see Fig. 14-6). Pregnant women at increased risk for chlamydia (i.e., age under 25, or women with new or more than one sex partner or whose partners have other partners) should have a screening test in the third trimester to prevent postpartum endometritis and chlamydia infection in the infant. There is little evidence that chlamydia causes adverse effects in early pregnancy, so screening in the first trimester may not be beneficial.[3]

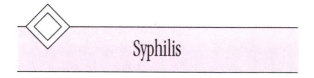

Syphilis

The prevalence of syphilis for men and women of all racial and ethnic groups has been on the steady decline since 1990.[4] Reported cases of primary and secondary syphilis have dropped 84 percent from 1990 to 1997. This may be attributed to enhanced federal and state syphilis control programs, the emergence of HIV prevention programs, the decline in crack cocaine use, and the presence of acquired immunity in at-risk populations.[75] In 1992, females between the ages of 10 and 29 years had a higher rate of syphilis versus comparably aged males.[4] African American women have the highest rates for all women.[11,75] Heterosexual contact, linked to crack cocaine use, is the most frequent source of transmission.[76] The southern United States continues to have the highest rate of syphilis compared to other regions of the country.[75]

Pathophysiology

Syphilis is caused by the spirochete *Treponema pallidum*. The organism can invade intact mucous membranes or damaged skin. It gains entry into the bloodstream via the lymphatics and then disseminates throughout the body. The disease exists in primary, secondary, latent, and tertiary forms (Table 14-8). Congenital syphilis may result if the disease goes untreated during pregnancy. In areas with a high prevalence of HIV infection, all persons with primary syphilis should be tested for HIV with a follow-up HIV test in 3 months for those who initially test negative.[3]

Fifty percent of persons with untreated primary syphilis will progress to the secondary stage; the remainder will enter the latent stage.[9] Tertiary syphilis is associated with serious and potentially life-threatening sequelae including cardiac, neurologic, ophthalmic, auditory, bone, liver, and skin lesions.[3]

Table 14-8
Clinical Characteristics of Syphilis Stages

Primary:	Mean incubation period of 21 d (10–90 d)
	Solitary, painless, indurated lesion (chancre) at infection site
	Women may be unaware of vaginal/cervical lesion
	Phimosis may occur in males due to edema
	Inguinal lymphadenopathy may be present
	Chancre may persist for 3–6 wk
Secondary:	Occurs 9 wk following initial exposure (persists 2–12 wk)
	Stage may develop earlier in AIDS patients
	Generalized lymphadenopathy
	Flulike symptoms
	Cutaneous eruptions (early lesions—macular; late lesions—maculopapular)
	Minimal symptoms with cutaneous lesions
	Neurosyphilis may present with vague neurologic complaints
	Resolution of stage occurs spontaneously
Latent:	Essentially no symptoms
	Early phase— < 1 y following inoculation (secondary symptoms may recur)
	Late phase— > 1 y following inoculation (no symptoms)
	30% of persons enter tertiary phase
Tertiary:	Can occur at any time following latency
	Superficial and/or deep tissue gummas
	Cardiovascular, neurologic, and other organ infiltration

SOURCE: Adapted from references 9,110,111.

Diagnosis

The clinical diagnosis of primary syphilis is made on the basis of darkfield microscopic examination or direct fluorescent antibody tests of chancre exudate or tissue and/or serologic tests. Serology is not valuable during the primary stage of syphilis. A presumptive diagnosis of syphilis can be made using both nontreponemal and treponemal serologic tests.[3] Nontreponemal tests include the VDRL and rapid plasma reagin (RPR) and the treponemal tests include the fluorescent treponemal antibody absorbtion (FTA-ABS) and microhemagglutination assay-T. pallidum (MHA-TP). The nontreponemal tests correlate with disease activity and are reported quantitatively. Following adequate therapy, nontreponemal tests revert back to normal. However, a small number of persons maintain a low antibody titer, probably for life. This is called the serofast reaction.[3] Reactive treponemal tests remain so for life, regardless of treatment status or disease activity. Thus, they should not be used to determine treatment efficacy. It is important to note that nontreponemal tests may be used to diagnose syphilis in most persons infected with HIV. However, serologic testing in persons with concomitant HIV infection and syphilis may result in higher than usual titers, false-negative results, or delayed seroreactivity.[3]

Patients with syphilis who also have signs or symptoms of neurologic disease (e.g., meningitis) or uveitis should be evaluated for neurosyphilis with lumbar puncture for cerebrospinal fluid (CSF) evaluation and ocular slit-lamp examination. The VDRL-CSF is the standard test used to aid in the diagnosis of neurosyphilis. However, some experts consider the CSF FTA-ABS test to be more specific.[3] Lumbar puncture is not routinely recommended for patients with primary or secondary syphilis in the absence of neurologic or ocular signs and symptoms.[3]

Treatment

The treatment of syphilis requires the parenteral administration of an appropriate bactericidal antibiotic. Regardless of the stage or clinical manifestation of the disease, the drug of choice has remained parenteral penicillin G.[3] Partners of persons with documented syphilis should be evaluated, both clinically and serologically, and treated accordingly. Recommendations for testing of partners have been recently published.[3]

The current guidelines for the treatment of syphilis are summarized in Table 14-9.[3] Because no well-established alternative therapies exist for the management of syphilis, patients allergic to penicillin must be carefully evaluated and desensitized, if necessary. Any patient receiving parenteral penicillin may experience the Jarisch-Herxheimer reaction. This allergic flulike reaction results from the release of antigen from the lysis of the T. pallidum spirochetes during therapy. Patients should be informed about this reaction before treatment. Antipyretics or corticosteroids may be helpful in ameliorating this reaction. The reaction typically abates within 24 h following the initiation of therapy. The Jarisch-Herxheimer reaction can also induce labor and cause fetal distress.[3] Pregnant women should be counseled to promptly report symptoms of labor or any abnormal fetal activity to her primary care provider.

Pelvic Inflammatory Disease

Pelvic inflammatory disease is the clinical syndrome resulting from infection of the uterus, fallopian tubes, ovaries, peritoneum, and contiguous structures. PID is the most common serious complication of STDs in women.[77] Approximately 1 million women per year in the United States develop symptomatic PID.[3] Asymptomatic PID is known to occur because many women with PID sequelae and serologic evidence of previous STDs have no history of previous PID symptoms.[77] One-third of women hospitalized with acute PID and over 90 percent hospitalized for chronic PID will undergo surgery.[77] In 1990, the total cost of

Table 14-9

Current Guidelines for the Treatment of Syphilis[3]

PRIMARY AND SECONDARY STAGES

Benzathine penicillin G 2.4 million units IM (single dose) or
Doxycycline 100 mg orally bid for 2 wk* (penicillin allergy history) or
Tetracycline 500 mg orally qid for 2 wk* (penicillin allergy history)
    Treat for 4 wk if duration of infection exceeds 1 year
    Doxycycline and tetracycline are contraindicated during pregnancy

LATENT STAGE

Early Latent:
    Benzathine penicillin G 2.4 million units IM (single dose)
Late Latent or Latent of Unknown Duration:
    Benzathine penicillin G 7.2 million units total (3 doses—2.4 million units IM weekly)

TERTIARY STAGE
Benzathine penicillin G 7.2 million units total (3 doses—2.4 million units IM weekly)
NEUROSYPHILIS
Aqueous crystalline penicillin G 18–24 million units a day (3–4 million units IV q4h for 10–14 d) Procaine penicillin 2.4 million units IM daily, plus probenecid 500 mg PO qid, both for 10–14 d   (alternative)

PID in the United States was estimated to be over $4.2 billion, with $2.73 billion for direct medical care.[2] During the 1980s, an average of 276,000 women/year were hospitalized for PID (two-thirds for acute PID, one-third for chronic PID). Sexually active younger women, minority women, and unmarried or separated women have higher rates of hospitalization and outpatient visits for acute PID than other women.[77] Most women with PID are under age 25, are nulliparous, and have never been pregnant.[78]

Risk factors for PID include young age at first intercourse, multiple sex partners, high frequency of sexual intercourse, and increased rate of acquiring new partners within the previous 30 days.[3] IUD usage increases a woman's risk of PID (relative risk 1.6, 95 percent CI 1.2 to 2.0), with the highest risk in the first month after insertion.[79] Vaginal douching,[80] smoking,[81] and substance abuse are also associated with increased risk of

PID. Use of a barrier contraceptive or oral contraceptive reduces the risk of PID.[65]

Pathophysiology

Most cases of PID are polymicrobial. *N. gonorrhoeae* and *C. trachomatis* as well as endogenous anaerobic and aerobic bacteria (including Bacteroides spp., *Peptostreptococcus* and *Peptococcus* spp., streptococci, enterococci, *Escherichia coli, Haemophilus influenzae,* and *Gardnerella vaginalis*) have been implicated in the etiology of PID.[82] *Mycoplasma hominus* and *Ureaplasma, urealyticum* might be etiologic agents in some women with PID. *N. gonorrhoeae* is isolated from 27 to 80 percent of women with acute PID, and *C. trachomatis* is isolated in up to 51 percent.[65] The current favored hypothesis for the mechanism of PID is that *N. gonorrhoeae* and *C. trachomatis* initiate tubal infection with secondary invasion of other bacteria from the cervix and vagina. Gonococcal or chlamydial cervical infection may alter the cervicovaginal environment, resulting in an overgrowth of endogenous flora and coexistent bacterial vaginosis. Altered host defenses then allow cervical pathogens to ascend into the uterus and establish infection. Reduced cervical defenses during menses are implicated because symptoms of gonococcal and chlamydial salpingitis occur within 7 days of onset of menses in over 50 percent of cases.[83]

Diagnosis

The clinical diagnosis of PID is often inaccurate. There can be wide variation in the presenting signs and symptoms of PID. A clinical diagnosis of PID is confirmed by laparoscopy about 75 percent of the time.[84,85] The differential diagnosis of PID includes ectopic pregnancy, appendicitis, hemorrhagic or ruptured ovarian cyst, ovarian torsion, and gastroenteritis.[86] Delay in diagnosis and treatment contributes to the development of long-term sequelae;

therefore, the clinician should maintain a "low threshold" for the treatment of suspected PID.[3] Table 14-10 lists the CDC criteria for the clinical diagnosis of PID.[3] Using CDC's highly sensitive criteria will mean that some women who do not have PID will be misdiagnosed and treated for PID. It is important to explain to the patient the uncertainty of the diagnosis and the reason for empirical treatment. All women with suspected PID should have cervical cultures for *N. gonorrhoeae* and cervical culture or a nonculture test for *C. trachomatis*. Perihepatitis (Fitz-Hugh–Curtis syndrome), either asymptomatic or manifested by pleuritic right upper abdominal pain, occurs in up to 27 percent of patients with PID.[66] Perihepatitis can occur in the absence of other PID symptoms in some patients.[78]

Treatment

All PID treatment regimens must provide broad-spectrum coverage of likely pathogens, including *N. gonorrhoeae*, *C. trachomatis*, anaerobes, gram-negative bacteria, and streptococci. No available

Table 14-10

CDC Criteria for the Diagnosis of PID[3]

Empirical treatment of PID should be initiated in sexually active young women and others at risk for STDs if all of the following **MINIMUM CRITERIA** are present, and no other cause(s) for the illness are identified:
- Lower abdominal tenderness
- Adnexal tenderness, and
- Cervical motion tenderness

ADDITIONAL CRITERIA that support a diagnosis of PID include the following:
- Oral temperature > 101°F (38.3°C)
- Abnormal cervical or vaginal discharge
- Elevated erythrocyte sedimentation rate
- Elevated C-reactive protein, and
- Laboratory documentation of cervical infection with *N. gonorrhoeae* or *C. trachomatis*

The **DEFINITIVE CRITERIA** for diagnosing PID which are warranted in selected cases include the following:
- Histopathologic evidence of endometritis on endometrial biopsy
- Transvaginal sonography or other imaging studies showing thickened fluid-filled tubes with or without free pelvic fluid or tubo-ovarian complex, and
- Laparoscopic abnormalities consistent with PID

Table 14-11

CDC Criteria for Hospitalization for PID

- Surgical emergencies such as appendicitis cannot be excluded
- Pregnant patients
- Patients not responding clinically to oral antimicrobial therapy
- Patients with severe illness, nausea and vomiting, or high fever
- Patients with tubo-ovarian abscess or
- Immunodeficient patients (e.g., HIV with low CD4 counts, taking immunosuppressive therapy, or with another disease)

NOTE: Clinical experience should guide decisions about transition to oral therapy, which may be accomplished within 24–48 h of clinical improvement.

studies compare parenteral versus oral therapy or inpatient versus outpatient therapy. Table 14-11 lists CDC criteria for hospitalization. Recommendations for treatment of PID are listed in Table 14-12. Treated patients should demonstrate substantial improvement within 3 days (such as defervescence and reduction in abdominal and uterine/adnexal/cervical motion tenderness). Patients who do not respond require reevaluation with additional diagnostic tests or surgical intervention.

Sex partners of patients with PID should be examined and treated if they had sexual contact with the patient in the 60 days prior to the onset of symptoms. Partners should be treated empirically for *N. gonorrhoeae* and *C. trachomatis*, regardless of the apparent etiology of the PID or pathogens isolated from the infected woman. Without treatment of infected partners, risk of reinfection is high.

Complications

An estimated 15 to 20 percent of women with PID will suffer from long-term sequelae such as infertility, ectopic pregnancy, chronic pelvic pain, dys-

pareunia, pyosalpinx, tubo-ovarian abscess, and pelvic adhesions.[87] Risk of infertility after one episode of PID is between 8 and 12 percent,[88] but may be as high as 21 percent if the episode was severe. With two episodes, infertility risk increases to about 20 percent and to 40 percent with three episodes or more.[88] Delay in seeking medical care (> 3 days after onset of symptoms) and age over 25 are associated with higher rates of impaired fertility.[89] Risk of ectopic pregnancy increases 10-fold after PID.[87] Women with PID should be counseled about STD risk reduction and periodically rescreened for STDs.

Prevention

Screening women at risk for *N. gonorrhoeae* and *C. trachomatis* is an important prevention strategy for PID (see Fig. 14-6). Screening of high-risk women has decreased the risk of PID by over 60 percent.[90] An estimated 10 to 40 percent of women not treated for gonococcal or chlamydial cervicitis will develop acute PID.[91] The risk of PID increases with the number of chlamydia infections (5-fold increase with two infections, 10-fold increase with three or more infections).[92] Any woman diagnosed with chlamydia or PID should be counseled about her increasing risk of complications (such as infertility) with repeated infection and about measures to protect herself.

HIV Infection

The face of HIV infection has been changing since the first reported cases in the early 1980s. Whereas in the past the predominant groups affected were men having sex with men and injecting-drug users, the virus has now become increasingly prevalent in the heterosexual population. Consequently, women are at an increased

Table 14-12

CDC Recommended Treatment for PID[3]

ORAL REGIMEN A	ORAL/PARENTERAL REGIMEN B
Ofloxacin 400 mg PO bid for 14 d ($142.25-G)	Ceftriaxone 250 mg IM once ($6.66-B),
plus	or
Metronidazole 500 mg PO bid for 14 d ($9.28-G).	Cefoxitin 2 g IM ($19.66-B) plus probenecid 1 g orally ($3.54-G), in a single dose, given concurrently once
ALTERNATIVE ORAL REGIMENS	or
Amoxicillin/clavulanic acid plus doxycycline was evaluated in a single clinical trial. Azithromycin has been evaluated in treatment of PID but data are insufficient to recommend this agent.	Other parenteral third-generation cephalosporin (e.g., ceftizoxime or cefotaxime)
	plus
	Doxycycline 100 mg PO bid for 14 d ($3.56-G) (with one of the above regimens).
PARENTERAL REGIMEN A*	**ALTERNATIVE PARENTERAL REGIMENS**
Cefotetan 2 g IV q12h ($46.04/day-B)	Ofloxacin 400 mg IV q12h ($52.80/d-B),
or	plus
Cefoxitin 2 g IV q6h ($80.38/day-B),	Metronidazole 500 mg IV q8h ($46.02/d-G).
plus	or
Doxycycline 100 mg IV or orally† q12h ($37.78/d-IV-G; $0.25/d-oral-G).	Ampicillin/sulbactam 3 g IV q6h ($54.60/d-B),
	plus
PARENTERAL REGIMEN B‡	Doxycycline 100 mg IV or PO‡ q12h ($37.78/d-IV-G; $0.25/d-oral-G).
Clindamycin 900 mg IV q8h ($60.22/d-G),	or
plus	Ciprofloxacin 200 mg IV q12h ($28.80/d-B),
Gentamicin loading dose IV or IM, 2 mg/kg body weight, followed by maintenance dose of 1.5 mg/kg q8h	plus
	Doxycycline 100 mg IV or PO‡ q12h
	plus
	Metronidazole 500 mg IV q8h

*Parenteral therapy may be discontinued 24 h after patient improves clinically. Continuing oral therapy should consist of doxycycline 100 mg PO bid to complete a total of 14 d of therapy.

†Because of pain with IV infusion, doxycycline should be administered orally when possible, even when the patient is hospitalized. Both oral and IV doxycycline have similar bioavailability.

‡Parenteral therapy may be discontinued 24 h after patient improves clinically. Continuing oral therapy should consist of doxycycline 100 mg PO bid or clindamycin 450 mg PO qid to complete a total of 14 d of therapy. When tubo-ovarian abscess is present, clindamycin is preferred to doxycycline due to better anaerobic coverage.

risk of acquiring the virus, underscoring the importance of implementing prevention programs for individuals at high risk. High-risk behaviors for women include having unprotected sex with infected partners, injecting illicit drugs, and using crack cocaine.[93] The presence of concomitant STDs such as gonorrhea, syphilis, and genital ulcer disease may also predispose an individual to acquiring HIV.[94]

In 1996, the incidence of deaths from AIDS-opportunistic infection (AIDS-OI) declined for the first time in the United States.[96] This decline was ascribed to the use of antiretroviral therapies, which improved the survival of individuals with HIV infection, ongoing prevention strategies, and AIDS-OI prophylaxis. In 1996, AIDS-OIs were diagnosed in approximately 56,730 persons, a 6 percent decline from 1995. The overall prevalence of AIDS acquired from heterosexual contact among women over 13 years of age rose 23 percent from 1995 to 1996.[95] There was a 12 percent disproportionate rise in the AIDS-OI incidence in heterosexual non-Hispanic black women. Further, among women over 50 years of age with AIDS-OI, cases increased 106 percent (340 to 700 cases) from 1991 to 1996.[96] Disturbingly, a recent study reported that older women with heterosexually acquired AIDS were less likely to use condoms and to have been tested for HIV infection prior to hospitalization for opportunistic infections.[96]

It is now recognized that women, including pregnant women, experience the same natural course of HIV-1 infection as men.[97] Furthermore, pregnancy does not affect the morbidity or mortality outcomes of HIV-infected women.[3,98] A number of distinctive clinical conditions may occur in women as the disease progresses. These include severe mucocutaneous candidiasis, genital warts, herpes simplex infections, PID, cervical dysplasia, carcinoma in situ, and invasive cervical carcinoma.[9, 97] Many of these diseases are serious, resistant to conventional therapy, may frequently recur, or require aggressive treatment approaches. Treatment-resistant or recurrent vaginal candidiasis may be the initial presentation of clinical HIV-1 infection in women.[97]

Diagnosis

The diagnosis of HIV-1 infection in women poses several challenges to health care providers. Many adolescent or young adult women who practice high-risk sexual behaviors or inject illicit drugs and are at risk for acquiring an HIV-1 infection have limited access to health care. The diagnosis of HIV-1 infection is often delayed until overt

clinical manifestations ensue or when the woman is found to be pregnant.[97] Providers must identify high-risk women and offer education, counseling, and testing, if appropriate. HIV-1 infected women should be encouraged to openly discuss reproductive options and pregnancy, if necessary.[3] The CDC has recommended that all pregnant women receive counseling and HIV testing.[99] If an HIV-infected woman becomes pregnant, there is a 15 to 25 percent risk of the infant being born with the infection. The use of antiretroviral therapy during pregnancy and labor, with subsequent administration to the infant, can reduce the risk of neonatal infection to 8 percent.[3] Women with HIV-1 infection should be discouraged from breast-feeding because transmission of the virus via breast milk has occurred.[3]

Antibody tests are used to diagnose HIV-1 infection. A common screening test is the EIA. Screening should be offered to identified high-risk individuals or to whomever requests the test. Any woman diagnosed with an STD should be offered HIV testing. Informed consent must be obtained, and in some jurisdictions written consent is required.[3] A positive screening test must be confirmed with an additional test, such as the Western blot or an immunofluorescence assay. A positive confirmatory test indicates that the person is infected and capable of transmitting the virus.

Treatment

The management of HIV-1 infection and its complications, including opportunistic infections, is both complicated and costly. A full discussion of treatment options for the person with HIV-1 infection or AIDS is beyond the scope of this review. However, the current use of antiretroviral agents and the management of HIV-infected pregnant women and children have been addressed in two recent publications.[97,100] The reader is encouraged to review this and other information concerning the primary management of HIV infection.[101,102] Updated guidelines for the treatment of HIV infection may be found at the CDC-sponsored HIV/ AIDS Treatment Information Service Web site, www.hivatis.org (or 1-800-HIV-0440).

Other Uncommon Sexually Transmitted Diseases

Chancroid, lymphogranuloma venereum, and granuloma inguinale are STDs that cause genital ulcers. They are rare in the United States but are endemic in tropical and semitropical regions of the world. Genital ulcer disease, particularly chancroid, is an important cofactor for the transmission of HIV.[103]

Chancroid

Chancroid is caused by *H. ducreyi*, a gram-negative streptobacillus.[104] After a 1- to 5-day incubation period, one to several small, tender, indurated papules or pustules appear on the vulva, vagina, cervix, or anogenital skin of an infected woman. Papules quickly erode into tender ulcers, which are soft with deep ragged edges (Fig. 14-7). Thirty to 60 percent of patients will have enlarged, firm, tender regional lymph nodes, usually unilateral. Nodes are usually firm but can become fluctuent. Definitive diagnosis requires culture isolation of *H. ducreyi*, but culture is not widely available and is insensitive. A probable diagnosis may be made if the following criteria are met: (1) the presence of one or more painful ulcers, (2) no evidence of *T. pallidum* infection by darkfield examination of ulcer exudate or serologic testing at least 7 days after the onset of ulcers, and (3) the clinical presentation, appearance of the ulcers, and regional lymphadenopathy are typical of chancroid and a test for HSV is negative.[3] Painful ulcer and suppurative inguinal lymphadenopathy are almost pathognomonic for chancroid.[3] Recommended treatment

regimens are (1) azithromycin 1 g orally in a single dose, or (2) ceftriaxone 250 mg intramuscularly in a single dose, or (3) ciprofloxacin 500 mg bid for 3 days, or (4) erythromycin base 500 mg orally qid for 7 days.[3] Fluctuent nodes should be drained. Patients should be seen within 7 days of beginning treatment to ascertain objective improvement. Failure to improve should prompt reevaluation of the diagnosis, testing for HIV, and evaluation for other STD. An estimated 10 percent of chancroid patients are coinfected with syphilis or HSV.[3] Also, high rates of HIV among patients with chancroid have been noted in the United States.[3] Sexual partners should be examined and treated for chancroid, regardless of whether symptoms of the disease are present, if they had sexual contact with the patient 10 days preceding the onset of symptoms.

Figure 14-7

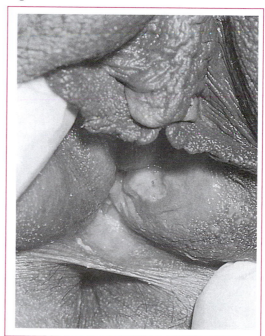

Chancroid ulcer of the fourchette in a female. *(Reproduced with permission from KK Holmes et al [eds]: Sexually Transmitted Diseases, 3rd ed. New York: McGraw-Hill, copyright 1999.)* (See Color Plate 4.)

Lymphogranuloma Venereum

Lymphogranuloma venereum is caused by the L1, L2, or L3 serotypes of *C. trachomatis*.[104] After a 5- to 7-day incubation period, one to several labial or cervical lesions (or rarely a nongenital lesion) form. Usually the lesions are papules or pustules that rapidly ulcerate. Over 50 percent of the genital lesions are asymptomatic and resolve without scarring. Subsequently, unilateral or bilateral tender lymph nodes enlarge and coalesce into bubos. Bubos above and below the inguinal ligament can produce a near-pathognomonic "groove" sign. The bubos may resolve without treatment or may become fluctuent with rupture and sinus formation. Proctitis and involvement of perianal lymphatic tissues occurs rarely in women and can result in perianal fistulas and strictures. The diagnosis can be made clinically, but may be confirmed by *C. trachomatis* culture of aspirate of involved nodes or by complement fixation serologic testing for *C. trachomatis*.[100] Treatment is doxycycline 100 mg bid or erythromycin base 500 mg orally qid, each given for 21 days.[3] Sexual partners should be examined, tested for urethral or cervical infection, and treated if they have had contact with the patient in the 30 days prior to onset of symptoms.

Granuloma Inguinale

Granuloma inguinale (or donovanosis) is a chronic, painless, ulcerative granulomatous disease caused by *Calymmatobacterium granulomatis*, a gram-negative rod.[105] There is a debate over whether this is primarily an STD, but the genitalia are the usual site of infection. A painless irregular, beefy-red, hard ulcer forms initially and gradually enlarges (Fig. 14-8). Labial, vaginal, and cervical lesions occur in women and can be mutilating. Cervical lesions can mimic invasive cervical cancer. Regional lymphadenopathy is usually absent, unless the lesion is secondarily infected. Adjacent skin in contact with an ulcer may develop a similar "kissing" lesion.[105] Diagnosis requires visualization of dark-staining Donovan

Figure 14-8

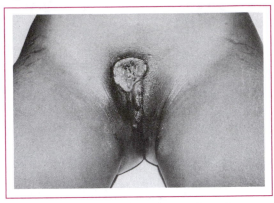

Deep necrotic ulcer caused by *Calymmatobacterium granulomatous* resulting in tissue destruction. (*Reproduced with permission from KK Holmes et al [eds]: Sexually Transmitted Diseases, 3rd ed. New York: McGraw-Hill, copyright 1999.*)

bodies within mononuclear cells on tissue crush preparation or biopsy specimens.[3] Treatment is with trimethoprim-sulfamethoxazole, one double-strength tablet orally bid or doxycycline 100 mg bid, for a mimimum of 3 weeks. Alternatives include ciprofloxacin 750 mg bid or erythromycin base 500 mg qid for a minimum of 3 weeks.[3] Sexual partners who have had contact with the patient in the last 60 days or who have symptoms should be treated.

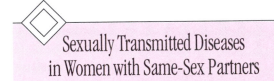

Sexually Transmitted Diseases in Women with Same-Sex Partners

Little research has been done to investigate transmission of STDs among women with same-sex partners. Although most STDs occur less frequently in lesbians, it should not be assumed that these women are not at risk for STDs. As many as 90 percent of lesbian women have a history of sex with men at some time in their lives. Genital herpes, genital warts, gonorrhea, and chlamydia occur less frequently among lesbians, but have been found in lesbians despite not having had heterosexual intercourse for many years.[106] In one retrospective case-control study, bacterial vaginosis occurred significantly more frequently among lesbian women compared to heterosexual women (33 versus 13 percent).[106] There are a few case reports of female-to-female transmission of HIV. Dental dams (latex squares, available at medical supply stores) may be used to decrease the risk of STDs acquired during oral sex. Nonlubricated condoms can be cut to form latex squares as an alternative. A careful sexual history, physical examination, and assessment of other risk behaviors (such as intravenous drug use) should guide decisions about testing for STDs. Lesbian patients should receive periodic Pap smears, especially if there is a history of intercourse with men. Recognizing that risk of HIV transmission among same-sex female partners is probably very low, HIV testing should be offered to women with multiple partners of either gender, a history of unprotected heterosexual intercourse, or other high-risk behaviors such as intravenous drug use.

Chapter 14

Summary

The STDs, including PID, continue to affect the medical community, patients, and society at large. The public health consequences of undetected and untreated cases mandate the development and implementation of effective strategies for targeted populations, which will lessen the personal and socioeconomic costs associated with these disorders. Furthermore, because women are disproportionately affected, health care providers must advocate and encourage empowerment of women to practice prevention measures to reduce the likelihood of infection. Likewise, clinicians are encouraged to enhance their knowledge and skills in the detection and management of STDs and PID and to adopt an evidence-based approach to their practice.

Despite advances in the diagnosis and treatment of these diseases, many unanswered questions remain regarding the most appropriate and cost-effective approach to the patient. It is anticipated that the outcomes of ongoing research efforts will answer these remaining questions.

References

1. Quinn TC, Cates W Jr: Epidemiology of sexually transmitted diseases in the 1990's. In: Quinn TC, Gallin JI, Fauci AS (eds): *Advances in Host Defense Mechanisms: Sexually Transmitted Diseases,* vol. 8. New York: Raven; 1992:1.
2. Washington AE, Katz P: Cost of and payment source for pelvic inflammatory disease. Trends and projections, 1985 through 2000. *JAMA* 266:2565, 1991.
3. Centers for Disease Control and Prevention: 1998 Guidelines for treatment of sexually transmitted diseases. *MMWR* 47(RR-1):1, 1998.
4. Horton JA: Chapter 2. Infectious diseases. In: Horton JA (ed): *The Women's Health Data Book,* 2nd ed. Washington, DC: The Jacobs Institute of Women's Health; 1995; Chap. 2.
5. Sexually transmitted diseases. In: Hatcher RA, Trussell J, Stewart F et al. (eds). *Contraceptive Technology,* 16th ed. New York: Irvington; 1994; Chap. 4.
6. Koutsky L: Epidemiology of genital human papillomavirus infection. *Am J Med* 102(5A):3, 1997.
7. Bosch FX, Manos MM, Munoz N, et al: Prevalence of human papillomavirus in cervical cancer: a worldwide perspective. *J Natl Cancer Inst* 87:796, 1995.
8. Verdon ME: Issues in the management of human papillomavirus genital disease. *Am Fam Physician* 55:1813, 1997.
9. Miller KE: Sexually transmitted diseases. *Prim Care* 24:179, 1997.
10. Beutner KR: Therapeutic approaches to genital warts. *Am J Med* 102(5A):28, 1997.
11. Centers for Disease Control and Prevention: *Sexually Transmitted Disease Surveillance, 1992.* Atlanta, GA: Division of STD/HIV Prevention; 1993.
12. Schomogyi M, Wald A, Corey L: Herpes simplex virus-2 infection. An emerging disease? *Infect Dis Clin North Am* 12:47, 1998.

13. Centers for Disease Control and Prevention: *Genital Herpes*. Atlanta, GA: National Center for HIV, STD and TB Prevention, Division of STD Prevention; 1997.

14. Johnson RE, Nahmias AJ, Magder LS, et al: A seroepidemiology survey of the prevalence of herpes simplex virus type 2 infection in the United States. *N Engl J Med* 321:8, 1989.

15. Johnson RE, Lee F, Hagdy A, et al: US genital herpes trends during the first decade of AIDS—prevalence increased in young whites and elevated in blacks. *Sex Transm Dis* 21(Suppl):109, 1994.

16. Langenberg A, Beneditti J, Jenkins J, et al: Development of clinically recognizable genital lesions among women previously identified as having "asymptomatic" herpes simplex virus type 2. *Ann Intern Med* 110:882, 1989.

17. Koelle DM, Benedetti J, Langenberg A, Corey L: Asymptomatic reactivation of herpes simplex virus in women after the first episode of genital herpes. *Ann Intern Med* 116:433, 1992.

18. Brock BV, Selke S, Benedetti J, et al: Frequency of asymptomatic shedding of herpes simplex in women with genital herpes. *JAMA* 263:418, 1990.

19. Wald A, Corey L, Cone R, et al: Frequent genital herpes simplex virus 2 shedding in immunocompetent women: effect of acyclovir treatment. *J Clin Invest* 99:1092, 1997.

20. Mertz GJ, Benedetti J, Ashley R, et al: Risk factors for the sexual transmission of genital herpes. *Ann Intern Med* 116:197, 1992.

21. Bryson Y, Dillon M, Berstein DI, et al: Risk of acquisition of genital herpes simplex virus type 2 in sex partners of persons with genital herpes. A prospective couple study. *J Infect Dis* 167:942, 1993.

22. Hook EW, Cannon RO, Nahmias AJ, et al: Herpes simplex virus infection as a risk factor for human immunodeficiency virus infection in heterosexuals. *J Infect Dis* 165:251, 1992.

23. Holmberg SD, Stewart JA, Gerber AR, et al: Prior herpes simplex virus type 2 infection as a risk factor for HIV infection. *JAMA* 259:1048, 1988.

24. Kaufman RH: Clinical feature of herpes genitalis. *J Reprod Med* 31(5 Suppl):379, 1986.

25. Koutsky LA, Stevens CE, Holmes KK, et al: Underdiagnosis of genital herpes by current clinical and viral-isolation procedures. *N Engl J Med* 326:1533, 1992.

26. Corey L: Genital herpes. In: Holmes KK, Mardh PA, Sparling PF, Wiesner PJ (eds): *Sexually Transmitted Diseases*, 3rd ed. New York: McGraw-Hill; 1999.

27. Glenzen WP, Fernal GW, Lohr JA: Acute respiratory disease of university students with special reference to the etiologic role of *Herpesvirus hominum*. *Am J Epidemiol* 101:111, 1975.

28. Lehtinen M, Rantala I, Teisala K, et al: Detection of herpes simplex virus in women with acute pelvic inflammatory disease. *J Infect Dis* 152:78, 1985.

29. Shturman-Ellstein R, Borkowsky W, Fish I, Gershon AA: Myelitis associated with genital herpes in a child. *J Pediatr* 88:523, 1976.

30. Lipton JD, Schafermeyer RW: Central nervous system infections. The usual and the unusual. *Emerg Med Clin North Am* 13:417, 1995.

31. Guinan ME, MacCalman J, Kern ER, et al: Course of an untreated episode of recurrent genital herpes simplex infection in 27 women. *N Engl J Med* 304:759, 1981.

32. Corey L, Holmes KK: Genital herpes simplex virus infections: current concepts in diagnosis, therapy, and prevention. *Ann Intern Med* 98:973, 1983.

33. Lafferty WE, Coombs RW, Benedetti J, et al: Recurrences after oral and genital herpes simplex virus infection: influence of site of infection and viral type. *N Engl J Med* 316:1444, 1987.

34. Mertz GJ, Critchlow CW, Benedetti J, et al: Double-blind placebo-controlled trial of oral acyclovir in first-episode genital herpes simplex virus infection. *JAMA* 252;1147, 1984.

35. Fife KH, Barbarash RA, Rudolph T, et al: Valacyclovir versus acyclovir in the treatment of first-episode genital herpes infection. Results of an international, multicenter, double-blind, randomized clinical trial. The Valacyclovir International Herpes Simplex Virus Study Group. *Sex Transm Dis* 24:481, 1997.

36. Tyring SK, Esmann J, Spruance SL, Corey L: A randomized, placebo-controlled comparison of oral valacyclovir and acyclovir in immunocompetent patients with recurrent genital herpes infections. The Valacyclovir International Study Group. *Arch Dermatol* 134:185, 1998.

37. Sacks Sl, Aoki FY, Diaz-Mitoma F, et al: Patient-initiated twice daily oral famciclovir for early recurrent genital herpes. A randomized, double-blind, multicenter trial. Canadian Famciclovir Study Group. *JAMA* 276:44, 1996.

38. Mattison HR, Reichman RC, Benedetti J, et al: Double-blind, placebo-controlled trial comparing long-term suppressive with short-term oral acyclovir therapy for management of recurrent genital herpes. *Am J Med* 85(2A):20, 1998.

39. Goldberg LH, Kaufman RH, Kurtz TO, et al: Continuous five-year treatment of patients with frequently recurring genital herpes simplex infection with acyclovir. *J Med Virol* 45(Suppl 1), 1993.

40. Overall JC Jr: Herpes simplex virus infection of fetus and newborn. *Pediatr Ann* 23:131, 1994.

41. American Academy of Pediatrics, American College of Obstetricians and Gynecologists (ACOG): *Guidelines to Perinatal Care*, 3rd ed. Elk Grove Village, IL: American Academy of Pediatrics, American College of Obstetricians and Gynecologists; 1992.

42. Brocklehurst P, Mindel A, Cowan F, et al: A randomized placebo-controlled trial of suppressive acyclovir in late pregnancy in women with recurrent genital herpes infection. *Br J Obstet Gynaecol* 105:275, 1998.

43. Jacobs RF: Neonatal herpes simplex virus infections. *Semin Perinatol* 22:64, 1998.

44. Langenberg AG, Burke RL, Adair SF, et al: A recombinant glycoprotein vaccine for herpes simplex type 2: safety and immunogenicity. *Ann Intern Med* 122:889, 1995.

45. Strauss SE, Wald A, Kost RG, et al: Immunotherapy of recurrent genital herpes with recombinant herpes simplex virus type 2 glycoproteins D and B: results of a placebo-controlled vaccine trial. *J Infect Dis* 176:1129, 1997.

46. Fricker J: Herpes vaccines: spinning a new DISC. *Lancet* 348(9041):1576, 1996.

47. Hook EW, Handsfield HH: Gonococcal infections in the adult. In: Holmes KK, Mardh PA, Sparling PF, Wiesner PJ (eds): *Sexually Transmitted Diseases*, 2nd ed. New York: McGraw-Hill; 1990:149.

48. Division of STD Prevention. *Sexually Transmitted Disease Surveillance*, 1996. Atlanta, GA: Centers for Disease Control and Prevention; 1997.

49. Schmali JD, Martin JE Jr, Domescik G: Observation on the culture diagnosis of gonorrhea in women. *JAMA* 210:312, 1969.

50. Curran JW, Rendtorff RC, Chandler RW, et al: Female gonorrhea: its relation to abnormal uterine bleeding, urinary tract symptoms, and cervicitis. *Obstet Gynecol* 45:195, 1975.

51. Brunham RC, Paavonen JA, Stevens CE, et al: Mucopurulent cervicitis—the ignored counterpart in women of urethritis in men. *N Engl J Med* 311:1, 1984.

52. Klein EJ, Fisher LS, Chow AW, Guze LB: Anorectal gonococcal infection. *Ann Intern Med* 86:340, 1997.

53. Tice AW, Rodriguez VL: Pharyngeal gonorrhea. *JAMA* 246:2717, 1981.

54. Weström L: Effect of acute pelvic inflammatory disease on fertility. *Am J Obstet Gynecol* 121:707, 1975.

55. Kerle KK, Mascola JR, Miller TA: Disseminated gonococcal infection. *Am Fam Physician* 45:209, 1992.

56. U.S. Preventive Services Task Force: *Guide to Clinical Preventive Services*, 2nd ed. Alexandria, VA: International Medical Publishing; 1996.

57. Stary A, Kopp W, Zahel B, et al: Comparison of DNA-probe test and culture for the detection of *Neisseria gonorrhoeae* in genital samples. *Sex Transm Dis* 20:243, 1993.

58. Vlaspolder F, Mutsaers JA, Blog F, et al: Value of DNA probe assay (Gen-Probe) compared with that of culture for diagnosis of gonococcal infection. *J Clin Microbiol* 31:107, 1993.

59. Lieberman RW, Whelock JB: The diagnosis of gonorrhea in low-prevalence female population: enzyme immunoassay versus culture. *Obstet Gynecol* 69:743, 1987.

60. Buirner M, van Doornum GJ, Ching S, et al: Detection of *Chlamydia trachomatis* and *Neisseria gonorrhoeae* by ligase chain reaction-based assays with clinical specimens. *J Clin Microbiol* 34:2395, 1996.

61. Oh MK, Smith KR, O'Cain M, et al: Urine-based screening of adolescents in detention to guide treatment for gonococcal and chlamydial infections. Translating research into intervention. *Arch Pediatr Adolesc Med* 151:52, 1998.

62. Mahoney JB, Luinstra KE, Tyndall M, et al: Multiplex PCR for detection of *Chlamydia trachomatis* and *Neisseria gonorrhoeae* in genitourinary specimens. *J Clin Microbiol* 33:3049, 1995.

63. Centers for Disease Control and Prevention: Recommendations for the prevention and management of *Chlamydia trachomatis* infections. *MMWR* 42(RR 12):1, 1993.

64. Handsfield HH, Jasman LL, Roberts LP, et al: Criteria for selective screening for *Chlamydia trachomatis* infection in women attending family planning clinics. *JAMA* 255:1730, 1986.

65. Cates W, Rolfs RT, Aral SO: Sexually transmitted diseases, pelvic inflammatory disease and infertility: an epidemiologic update. *Epidemiol Rev* 12:199, 1990.

66. Gjønnaess H, Dalaker K, Ånestad G, Mårdh P, et al: Pelvic inflammatory disease. Etiological studies with an emphasis on chlamydial infection. *Obstet Gynecol* 59:550, 1982.

67. Black CM: Current methods of laboratory diagnosis of *Chlamydia trachomatis* infections. *Clin Microbiol Rev* 10:160, 1997.

68. Jones RB, Katz BP, van der Pol B, et al: Effect of blind passage and multiple sampling on recovery of *Chlamydia trachomatis* from urogenital specimens. *J Clin Microbiol* 24:1029, 1986.

69. LeBar WD: Keeping up with new technology: new approaches to diagnosis of *Chlamydia* infection. *Clin Chem* 42:809, 1996.

70. Pasternak R, Vuorinen P, Pitkajarvi T, et al: Comparison of manual Amplicor PCR, Cobas Amplicor PCR and LCx assays for the detection of *Chlamydia trachomatis* infection in women using urine specimens. *J Clin Microbiol* 35:402, 1997.

71. Dean D, Ferrero D, McCarthy M: Comparison of performance and cost-effectiveness of direct fluorescent-antibody, ligase chain reaction and PCR assays for verification of chlamydial enzyme immunoassay results for populations with a low to moderate prevalence of *Chlamydia trachomatis* infection. *J Clin Microbiol* 36:94, 1998.

72. Bauwens JE, Clark AM, Stamm WE: Diagnosis of *Chlamydia trachomatis* endocervical infections by a commercial polymerase chain reaction assay. *J Clin Microbiol* 31:3023, 1993.

73. Genç M, Mårdh PA: A cost-effectiveness analysis of screening and treatment for *Chlamydia trachomatis* infection in asymptomatic women. *Ann Intern Med* 124:1, 1996.

74. Magid D, Douglas JM Jr, Schwartz JS: Doxycycline compared with azithromycin for treating women with genital *Chlamydia trachomatis* infections: an incremental cost-effectiveness analysis. *Ann Intern Med* 124:389, 1996.

75. Centers for Disease Control and Prevention: Primary and secondary syphilis—United States, 1997. *MMWR* 47:493, 1998.

76. Centers for Disease Control and Prevention: Relationship of syphilis to drug use and prostitution — Connecticut and Philadelphia, PA. *MMWR* 37:755, 1998.

77. Centers for Disease Control and Prevention: Policy guidelines for prevention and management of pelvic inflammatory disease (PID). *MMWR* 40(RR-5):1, 1991.

78. Weström L, Mirth P: Acute pelvic inflammatory disease (PID). In: Holmes K, Mirth P, Sparling PF (eds): *Sexually Transmitted Diseases*, 2nd ed. New York: McGraw-Hill; 1990.

79. Burkman RT: Intrauterine devices and pelvic inflammatory disease: evolving perspectives on the data. *Obstet Gynecol* 51(Suppl 12):S35, 1996.

80. Wølner-Hanssen P: Association between vaginal douching and PID. *JAMA* 263:1936, 1990.

81. Scholes D, Daling JR, Stergachis AS: Cigarette smoking and risk of pelvic inflammatory disease. *Am J Epidemiol* 132:759, 1990.

82. Sweet RL: Use of laparoscopy to determine microbial etiology of acute salpingitis. *Am J Obstet Gynecol* 134:68, 1979.

83. Sweet RL, Blankfort-Doyle M, Robbie MO, Schacter J: The occurrence of chlamydial and gonococcal salpingitis during the menstrual cycle. *JAMA* 255:2062, 1986.

84. Morcos R, Frost N, Hnat M, et al: Laparoscopic versus clinical diagnosis of acute pelvic inflammatory disease. *J Reprod Med* 38:53, 1993.

85. Arrendondo JL, Diaz V, Gaitan H, et al: Oral clindamycin and ciprofloxacin versus intramuscular ceftriaxone and oral doxycycline in the treatment of mild-to-moderate pelvic inflammatory disease in outpatients. *Clin Infect Dis* 24:170, 1997.

86. Newkirk GR: Pelvic inflammatory disease: a contemporary approach. *Am Fam Physician* 53:1127, 1996.

87. Weström L: Incidence, prevalence and trends of acute PID and its consequences in industrialized countries. *Am J Obstet Gynecol* 138:880, 1980.

88. Weström L, Joesoef R, Reynolds G, et al: Pelvic inflammatory disease and fertility. A cohort study of 1,844 women with laparoscopically verified disease and 657 control women with normal laparoscopic results. *Sex Transm Dis* 19:185, 1992.

89. Hillis SD: Delayed care of pelvic inflammatory disease as a risk factor for impaired fertility. *Am J Obstet Gynecol* 168:1503, 1993.

90. Scholis D, Stergachis A, Heinrich FE, et al: Prevention of pelvic inflammatory disease by screening for cervical chlamydial infection. *N Engl J Med* 334:1362, 1996.

91. Platt R, Rice PA, McCormack WM: Risk of acquiring gonorrhea and prevalence of abnormal adnexal findings among women recently exposed to gonorrhea. *JAMA* 250:3205, 1983.

92. Hillis SD, Owens LM, Marchbanks PA, et al: Recurrent chlamydial infections increase the risks of hospitalization for ectopic pregnancy and pelvic inflammatory disease. *Am J Obstet Gynecol* 176(1 Pt 1):103, 1997.

93. Kahn JO, Walker BD: Acute human immunodeficiency virus type 1 infection. *N Engl J Med* 339:33, 1998.

94. Cohen MS: Sexually transmitted diseases enhance HIV transmission: no longer a hypothesis. *Lancet* 351(Suppl 3):5, 1998.

95. Centers for Disease Control and Prevention. Update: trends in AIDS incidence—United States, 1996. *MMWR* 46:861, 1997.

96. Centers for Disease Control and Prevention: AIDS among persons aged ≥ 50 years—United States, 1991–1996. *JAMA* 279:575, 1998.

97. Andiman WA: Medical management of the pregnant woman infected with human immunodeficiency virus type 1 and her child. *Semin Perinatol* 22:72, 1998.

98. MacDonald MG, Ginzburg HM, Bolan JC: HIV infection in pregnancy: epidemiology and clinical management. *J Acquir Immune Defic Syndr Hum Retrovirol* 4:100, 1991.

99. Centers for Disease Control and Prevention: U.S. Public Health Service recommendations for HIV counseling and volunteer testing of pregnant women. *MMWR* 44(RR-7):1, 1995.

100. Chaudry MN, Shepp DH: Antiretroviral agents — current usage. *Dermatol Clin* 15:319, 1997.

101. Kakuda TN, Struble KA, Piscitelli SC: Protease inhibitors for the treatment of human immunodeficiency virus infection. *Am J Health Syst Pharm* 55:233, 1998.

102. Carpenter CC, Fischl MS, Hammer SM, et al: Antiretroviral therapy for HIV infection in 1998: updated recommendations of the International AIDS Society—USA Panel. *JAMA* 280:78, 1998.

103. Dickerson MC, Johnston J, Delea TE, et al: The causal role for genital ulcer disease as a risk factor for the transmission of human immunodeficiency virus. An application of the Bradford Hill criteria. *Sex Transm Dis* 23:429, 1996.

104. Goens JL, Schwartz RA, DeWolf K: Mucocutaneous manifestations of chancroid, lymphogranuloma venereum and granuloma inguinale. *Am Fam Physician* 49:415, 1994.

105. Hart G: Donovanosis. *Clin Infect Dis* 25:24, 1997.

106. Skinner CJ, Stokes J, Kirlew Y, et al: A case-controlled study of the sexual health needs of lesbians. *Genitourin Med* 72:277, 1996.

107. Beutner KR, Tyring SK, Trofatter KF Jr, et al: Imiquimod, a patient-applied immune-response modifier for treatment of external genital warts. *Antimicrob Agents Chemother* 42:789, 1998.

108. Beutner KR, Spruance SL, Hougham AJ, et al: Treatment of genital warts with an immune-response modifier (imiquimod). *J Am Acad Dermatol* 38(2 Pt 1):230, 1998.

109. Mayeaux EJ, Harper MB, Barksdale W, et al: Noncervical human papillomavirus genital infections. *Am Fam Physician* 52:1137, 1995.

110. Hansen M: Disorders of the male reproductive system. In: Hansen M (ed): *Pathophysiology-Foundations of Disease and Clinical Intervention*. Philadelphia: Saunders; 1998:866–889.

111. Sexually transmitted diseases. In: Andreoli TE, Bennett JC, Carpenter CCJ, Plum F (eds): *Cecil's Essentials of Medicine*, 4th ed. Philadelphia: Saunders; 1997; 741–748.

Louise Acheson

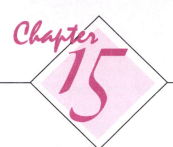
Chapter
15

Miscarriage

"Your absence is inconspicuous
Nobody can tell what I lack."

—*Sylvia Plath*[1]

Overview:
Miscarriage as a Life Event

When a miscarriage occurs, the events have a different significance for different women in different situations. Spontaneous abortion (SAB) may be a hoped-for event or a source of intense grief. It is wise to start from a neutral position to learn from each woman herself the value of this pregnancy at this time in her life. Most women who miscarry for the first time "never thought that they might have a miscarriage." About one-fourth of women after a miscarriage express a need to have another baby quickly.[2] Grieving is usual after a miscarriage. Many women and couples feel that others did not validate the grief they felt after an early miscarriage, assuming that it would not be as intense or long-lasting as, for example, grieving after a relative's death. In general, that may be true, but the loss of a much-desired, irreplaceable pregnancy can be a major life event.[3]

Recurrent pregnancy loss and miscarriage after the first trimester of pregnancy are likely to be particularly difficult experiences. Recurrent spontaneous abortion squelches the woman's hopes for a "normal" reproductive history and raises questions about whether there is "something wrong" with her—questions that are not easily dispelled. The assumption that people will be able to have children when and if they want to is part of our culture's image of adulthood. Not being able to reproduce has a potentially serious effect on self-esteem.[4] The later in pregnancy that a loss occurs, the more intense may be the grief for the expected pregnancy, experience of birth, and imagined child for whom the woman has already made room in her life. A pregnant woman is said to be "expecting," and miscarriage is a story of unrealized expectations. Many couples who have lost a pregnancy express bitterness and a sense of irony at the unexpected conflation of birth and death, and at medicine's inability to influence the course of events despite the use of sophisticated techniques for diagnosis. "Gone is the thought that pregnancy means you will have a baby."[5]

Studies involving interviews with women who have experienced miscarriages, and with their significant others, suggest that emotional reactions such as grief, anxiety, and depression occur with nearly equal frequency and last equally long whether the pregnancy was or was not desired.[2,6] Some people experience distress related to seemingly insensitive language used by clinicians, including the term "spontaneous abortion" instead of miscarriage, use of mechanistic terms such as "evacuation" of the uterus and "products of conception" "when to us it was a baby," and sexist terms implying failure on the woman's part but not the man's, such as "blighted ovum" rather than "blighted spermatozoan."[2,5,7] A few male partners blame the woman and dissociate themselves from the process of miscarriage.[7] Many women blame themselves. Almost universally, people desire from clinicians answers to the questions: What caused the pregnancy loss? How should the woman care for herself immediately after the miscarriage? How long to wait before attempting to conceive again (if desired)? Many women and men feel that clinicians treat their miscarriage and the associated procedures as routine and address these questions, if at all, in a perfunctory manner.[5,7,8] Although clinicians may be uncomfortable at having no specific or scientific answer to give and at having no measures to offer for prevention of pregnancy loss in most cases, they need to anticipate and prepare to respond to these questions at a planned follow-up visit (Table 15-1).

Miscarriage

Prevalence

Approximately 10 to 15 percent of clinically recognized pregnancies end in miscarriage, but a greater

Table 15-1

Questions Women Ask After a Miscarriage

QUESTION	RESPONSES
How long will I bleed afterward?	Up to 1 week of bleeding is usual. Repeatedly soaking a pad more than once every 2 h is not normal. A clinician should be contacted.
Can tampons be used?	It is customary to recommend pads, not tampons, but this has not been studied scientifically.
How soon can I return to usual activities, such as work?	Usually within 1 or 2 d. However, difficulty concentrating and trouble sleeping are common and the feelings associated with losing the pregnancy may take more time to resolve.
When can we resume sexual intercourse?	It is wise to wait a few days to be sure that the cervix is closed, or until the bleeding has stopped. Contraception will be needed right away because, on the average, women ovulate about 2 wk after a miscarriage.
How long should we wait before attempting pregnancy again?	There is no one right answer to this question. Many people need time to resolve the grief of losing a pregnancy and decide to wait 3–6 mo. Some people want to attempt pregnancy as soon as possible; they should wait until the first menses after the miscarriage. Women trying to conceive should take folic acid, at least 0.4 mg daily.
What caused the miscarriage?	Most miscarriages result from a defect in the chromosomes of the embryo, so that it could not develop normally past the very early stages. A miscarriage after 12 weeks' gestation or after a fetal heartbeat was observed may be due to other causes and may prompt further medical investigation.

number of pregnancies are lost earlier, before the missed menses and diagnosis of pregnancy. Early data from hysterectomy specimens found to contain fertilized zygotes before the missed menses suggested that 29 percent were morphologically abnormal and nonviable.[9] The development of sensitive tests for β-human chorionic gonadotropin (β-HCG), allowing for the biochemical detection of pregnancy within several days from conception, led to the discovery that 21 to 56 percent of prospectively followed pregnancies end before the missed menses. An additional 6 to 14 percent of pregnancies miscarried after the conventional time of pregnancy detection (6 to 12 weeks' gestation), for a total early pregnancy loss rate of 31 to 62 percent.[10–12] Thus, miscarriage is a spectrum of clinical events, from the shedding of an undetected conceptus in what appears to be menstruation, to the expulsion of a well-established pregnancy accompanied by painful uterine cramps and hemorrhage, perhaps requiring surgical intervention.

Not only are many pregnancies lost before detection, but conversely many women (30 percent) with a viable pregnancy experience bleeding in the first trimester and are diagnosed with "threatened SAB." A little more than half of these women go on to miscarry or have a tubal pregnancy, whereas the others carry the pregnancy, often without a specific diagnosis of the cause of the bleeding.[13]

Etiology

The majority of first trimester pregnancy losses result from chromosome abnormalities.[14] The most often detected chromosomal problem is aneuploidy (the presence of an abnormal number of chromosomes). Most trisomies, for example, are incompatible with fetal viability (except for trisomy 21, 13, 18 or an abnormal number of sex chromosomes) and result in early miscarriages. Because of the difficulty and expense of studying spontaneously aborted fetal tissues, especially from miscarriages completed at home, there is no definitive estimate of the proportion with an abnormal number of chromosomes, but it is probably on the order of 60 to 70 percent.[15,16] Miscarriages occurring later in gestation (in the second trimester or after fetal development to 8 weeks' size) are less likely to have abnormal embryonic karyotypes and are more likely to be due to other maternal causes.

The risk of miscarriage, in parallel with the risk of most chromosome abnormalities, increases with maternal age. Monosomy X (Turner's syndrome), unlike other aneuploidies, is associated with younger maternal age. Smoking is a risk factor for SAB when age and obstetric history are controlled.[17] Sporadic miscarriages may rarely be caused by infection in early pregnancy with viruses such as herpes simplex, rubella, varicella, parvovirus B19, or HIV, and by syphilis or malaria. Where professional abortions are illegal, many miscarriages actually are incomplete abortions nonprofessionally induced, and many of those coming for emergency care are infected. This situation skewed and obscured lay and medical perceptions about SAB for generations. Most studies of the etiology of miscarriages have been conducted in women with recurrent pregnancy losses; therefore the section on recurrent miscarriages includes discussion of less common etiologies.

Prognosis

Decades ago, on the basis of statistical calculations rather than empirical data, it was believed that women who had had one or two miscarriages were at markedly increased risk of subsequent pregnancy loss.[18] Empirical data, however, show that after one, two, or even more miscarriages (depending on the etiology and maternal age), the risk of miscarriage with the next pregnancy is only moderately elevated over that of other women of childbearing age (an estimated 24 to 30 percent compared with 10 to 15 percent). After one miscarriage, 80 to 95 percent of couples attempting pregnancy conceive and give birth to a living child within 2 years.[14,19] This is similar to the reproductive "success" rate of the general population.

Diagnosis

TYPICAL PRESENTATION

A large number of early pregnancy losses occur within a few days of conception and pass unnoticed. This section discusses the diagnosis of miscarriage in a clinically recognized pregnancy prior to 20 weeks' gestation. Initially, the pregnancy appears to be normal. Typically at 7 to 10 weeks since the last menstrual period (LMP), vaginal bleeding begins, either painlessly or with mild cramps. If the fetus is nonviable, in most cases the arrest of fetal development has occurred before any sign of a problem. Although bleeding from a closed cervical os is called a "threatened SAB," by the time bleeding begins nothing can be done to prevent a miscarriage. In pregnancies that go on to miscarry, painful uterine contractions usually begin within 4 days of the onset of bleeding.[20] Contractions cause dilation of the cervix (the SAB is termed "inevitable" if the cervix is dilated > 1 cm or tissue is passed from the os). This is followed by an increase in bleeding and expulsion of the gestational sac and placental tissue either completely or incompletely. If the entire sac and placenta have been expelled, the uterus usually contracts firmly and heavy bleeding subsides within minutes. Early in gestation, the gestational sac and placental tissue are usually expelled together because the chorionic villi surround the sac, but after 8 to 10 weeks separate and incomplete expulsion of the placenta may occur. Incomplete SAB usually presents with persistent, profuse bleeding. A "missed abortion" is diagnosed when fetal components without a fetal heartbeat are present after 7 weeks' gestation. The clinical features include persistent amenorrhea, lack of growth or shrinkage of the uterus, and the woman's perception that she no longer "feels pregnant." The nonviable pregnancy may remain in the uterus for several weeks, but uterine bleeding and cramping eventually begin. Only 12 percent of all pregnancy losses occur after 16 weeks' gestation; 90 percent of miscarriages seen in general practice occur in the first 13 weeks.[13,21,22]

DIFFERENTIAL DIAGNOSIS

When vaginal bleeding occurs in the first trimester of pregnancy, the clinician's first task is to diagnose its cause. The differential diagnosis is presented in Table 15-2. Because an ectopic pregnancy is potentially life-threatening if it ruptures, the diagnostic workup of early pregnancy bleeding is directed initially toward detecting or excluding ectopic pregnancy and also to distinguishing a normal, early pregnancy from an abnormal one. If the diagnosis of normal intrauterine pregnancy is established (e.g., by observing fetal cardiac motion on sonography), the chances of a subsequent miscarriage are less than 5 percent.[23,24]

HISTORY

The history, obtained when a woman presents with vaginal bleeding in early pregnancy, should include the duration of amenorrhea, whether the LMP was normal, the dates of the prior menses, her history of recent pregnancies, and whether hormonal contraception was used just before conception—all information needed for determining the expected gestational age and whether to suspect trophoblastic disease. Gestational trophoblastic disease would be more likely if the woman had miscarried within the past year and had irregular bleeding without normal menses since. Risk factors for ectopic pregnancy, including a history of pelvic infection, ruptured appendix, previous ectopic pregnancy, or tubal surgery, may increase the suspicion for this diagnosis.

Table 15-2
Etiology of First Trimester Vaginal Bleeding

Miscarriage (50 to 60%)
Ectopic pregnancy (5%)
Normal light bleeding at the time of implantation
Molar pregnancy or other gestational trophoblastic disease
Subchorionic hemorrhage in the presence of a viable fetus
Arrested development of one fetus in multiple gestation
Cervicitis or other reason for friability of the cervix (common)
Endocervical polyp
Vaginal trauma or ulceration

Inquiry about nausea, vomiting, and other symptoms of pregnancy may be helpful, particularly if the woman states that she no longer feels pregnant. There is a lower incidence of miscarriage in first trimester pregnancies with moderate to severe nausea and vomiting (2 percent SAB), compared to those with no or mild nausea (22 percent SAB).[25] The woman should be asked about the amount and duration of vaginal bleeding (number of pads or tampons used per hour or per day, size of clots, comparison with her usual menstrual flow) and symptoms of volume depletion such as orthostatic faintness, syncope, or palpitations to determine how urgently she needs medical evaluation. In addition, it is worth asking whether the bleeding was postcoital and about the presence of a purulent or malodorous vaginal discharge or a penile discharge in the partner, any of which may suggest a diagnosis of cervicitis rather than miscarriage.

The presence of abdominal pain may help to distinguish a bleeding ectopic pregnancy or an impending or recently completed miscarriage from more benign causes of bleeding, which are most often painless. Finally, the woman should be asked to describe any tissue that she has passed other than blood, for example, pink tissue (decidua) or whitish tissue (chorionic villi or gestational sac). If a period of observation is planned, she can be alerted to retrieve, place in a clean container, and bring for inspection any tissue other than blood or blood clots that passes from her vagina.

PHYSICAL EXAMINATION

Physical examination first involves assessment of hemodynamic stability: orthostatic pulse and blood pressure, skin color, and level of consciousness. The presence or absence of fever should be documented. If the patient is hemodynamically unstable, fluid resuscitation; cross-matching of red blood cells; a quick pelvic examination, possibly with bedside ultrasound or culdocentesis[26]; and preparation for evacuation of the uterus and possible laparotomy for ectopic pregnancy should commence without delay.

In hemodynamically stable patients, the abdominal and pelvic examinations may provide clues to the diagnosis of vaginal bleeding. Bimanual examination should be done to assess the size and contours of the uterus and adnexae. If the duration of amenorrhea or size of the uterus is consistent with an estimated gestational age of 10 weeks or more, an attempt should be made to detect the fetal heartbeat using a portable Doppler device, if one is available. Hearing a normal fetal heartbeat makes the diagnosis of a viable intrauterine pregnancy with near certainty. However, bleeding usually presents before 10 weeks, when, if a fetal heartbeat were present, it would not be detectable using this device.

Marked abdominal or uterine and adnexal tenderness may be a sign of peritoneal irritation from intraabdominal bleeding. Cervical motion tenderness may also be present in such cases. These should lead to a high suspicion of ectopic pregnancy. During a miscarriage, the uterus is typically mildly or moderately tender and may be boggy or firm. In early pregnancy, an adnexal mass may be normal, representing a corpus luteum cyst, or abnormal, representing a tubal pregnancy, pedunculated uterine leiomyoma, or ovarian tumor. Marked localized tenderness suggests torsion of an ovarian mass (more common in the early second trimester), necrosis of a fibroid, or possibly an early ectopic pregnancy.

On speculum examination, bleeding from a vaginal source or from a friable cervix or endocervical polyp may be directly visible. When bleeding appears to come from inside the os, it is important to see whether the cervical os is closed or open. If this is not apparent, a sterile large cotton swab or ring forceps can be used to gently and shallowly probe the os. In this situation an internal os that is dilated 1 cm indicates an inevitable or very recently completed miscarriage. If gestational tissue is visibly being extruded from the os but is not attached to the cervix (as in the rare cervically implanted pregnancy, which should *not* be manipulated in the office because of the risk of inducing hemorrhage), ring forceps can be used to grasp and gently remove the tissue.

LABORATORY AND OTHER DIAGNOSTIC TESTS

URINARY CHORIONIC GONADOTROPIN   A urine pregnancy test should be performed initially to confirm pregnancy. Tests now in common use, both in medical settings and for home testing, detect HCG at a threshold of 10 to 50 mIU/mL, corresponding to the level present at 1 to 7 days after implantation. Implantation occurs 5 days after fertilization; therefore, the urine pregnancy test is likely to be positive by the time of the missed menses. After termination of a pregnancy in the first trimester, it may take up to 3 weeks for the HCG level to become undetectable. Thus, a positive urine pregnancy test is not helpful for determining whether a miscarriage will occur or has recently occurred, but during the first trimester a negative test after an initial diagnosis of pregnancy usually means that the pregnancy has ended.

TRANSVAGINAL ULTRASOUND   The most helpful diagnostic test for bleeding in early pregnancy is the transvaginal ultrasound (TVUS) examination. TVUS has higher resolution than transabdominal ultrasound and can reliably detect a gestational sac and fetal pole at 4 to 6 weeks, about 1 week earlier than transabdominal ultrasound.[27] In a normal pregnancy at 5 weeks from the LMP, a 5- to 8-mm gestational sac is visible in the uterus, surrounded by a bright echogenic ring that represents the chorionic villi. At 6 weeks, a yolk sac and embryo (fetal pole) can be seen in a 1.6-cm chorionic sac. At 7 weeks, the chorionic sac is 2.5 cm in diameter and fetal heart motion should be detectable.[27,28] If an intrauterine gestational sac with fetal cardiac motion is seen after 7 weeks of amenorrhea, the chance of a miscarriage is less than 5 percent. Occasionally, an abnormally slow (< 85 beat/min) fetal heart rate is noted (normal 100 to 170); anecdotally, this may indicate impending fetal death that will later result in a miscarriage.[27]

In the presence of a viable intrauterine pregnancy, the source of bleeding may sometimes be visible sonographically. One of the most common findings is a subchorionic lucency representing subchorionic hemorrhage. The hemorrhage may be self-limited and often resorbs, causing miscarriage in only 30 percent of cases,[27] but a follow-up ultrasound examination after 3 to 4 weeks is warranted to assess the stability and resolution of the hematoma, as is careful observation for normal fetal growth later in pregnancy. Sometimes more than one gestational sac is observed. Arrested development can lead to SAB of one fetus, or one of the so-called gestational sacs may be an artifact of subchorionic bleeding. The majority of multiple gestations sonographically diagnosed in the first trimester end up as singletons at delivery, unless the diagnosis is deferred until two hearts are seen.[27]

If an empty or irregularly shaped gestational sac larger than 1.6 to 2.5 cm in diameter is seen, this indicates an anembryonic pregnancy (sometimes said to result from a "blighted ovum"), which will either be resorbed or will end in a symptomatic miscarriage. If a gestational sac of more than 16 mm diameter and fetal pole with crown-rump length at least 5 mm are seen without cardiac motion, an impending miscarriage or missed abortion is likely. If the chorionic sac is larger than 2.5 cm, cardiac motion ought to be visible; if it is absent, a miscarriage is virtually certain to occur. If a fetal pole without cardiac motion is visible in a gestational sac smaller than 1.6 cm, this may represent either a nonviable pregnancy or a normal pregnancy prior to 46 days' gestation, and further observation is indicated.[19,27,28] If there is no

sign of an intrauterine pregnancy (but the urinary chorionic gonadotropin [UCG] is positive), either the woman has recently undergone a complete miscarriage or there is a pregnancy of less than 5 weeks' gestation or there is an ectopic pregnancy. Ectopic pregnancy, if suspected on clinical grounds, should remain part of the differential diagnosis even if a tubal pregnancy is not visualized on ultrasound examination. It is rare but not impossible to have both intrauterine and ectopic pregnancies (estimated incidence of this, termed *heterotopic pregnancy*, is too variable to be useful: from 1/1000 to 1/30,000 pregnancies).

QUANTITATIVE HUMAN CHORIONIC GONADOTROPIN   If sonography does not determine the diagnosis unequivocally, measurement of the level of HCG in the woman's serum as it changes over a period of days may be of great value in determining whether a viable early pregnancy exists. The expected serum level of HCG has been determined for normal pregnancies at each stage of gestation. A level markedly lower than that expected for the duration of amenorrhea is cause for concern, but the range of normal levels and the possibility of error in dating the pregnancy combine to decrease the predictive value of a single HCG level (unless it is undetectable). However, a single serum HCG level may be of great diagnostic value when correlated with the expected normal findings on TVUS.

Allowing for some variability in HCG measurement and the sonographer's expertise, a gestational sac should be visible at levels above 1800 mIU/mL (by International Reference Preparation), a fetal pole at 7200 mIU/mL, and cardiac motion at 21,000 mIU/mL.[27] Serial quantitative HCG determinations have further diagnostic value because during the first 6 weeks of a normal pregnancy, regardless of the absolute level initially, the level should rise exponentially, nearly doubling every 48 h.[29]

When maternal serum is sent for an initial quantitative HCG level as part of the initial workup of first trimester bleeding, another sample should be obtained if the diagnosis is still in doubt 2 days later to check for the expected rise. A rise of at least 66 percent in 48 h is within 1 standard deviation for a normal pregnancy; a plateau or a decrease suggests

Figure 15-1

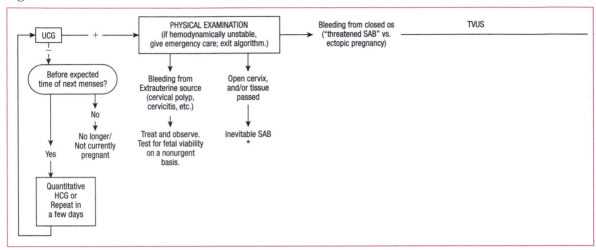

Algorithm for the diagnosis of early pregnancy bleeding.

*Expectant management or consider D&C, follow-up in 1 week.

ABBREVIATIONS: CRL, crown-rump length; FHR, fetal heart rate; SAB, spontaneous abortion; D&C, dilatation and curettage; IUP, intrauterine pregnancy; HCG, human chorionic gonadotrophin; UCG, urinary chorionic gonadotropin; IRP, International Reference Preparation; TVUS, transvaginal ultrasound.

Figure 15-1 (Continued.)

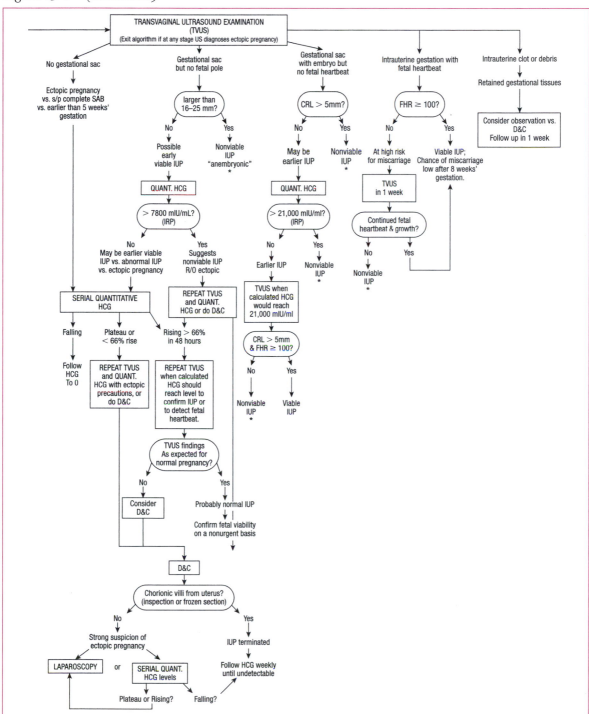

a nonviable pregnancy but cannot reliably distinguish an ectopic from an intrauterine pregnancy nor an impending from an incomplete miscarriage. A spontaneously resorbed or completely expelled gestational sac and placenta should result in a rapidly falling level of HCG, which will become undetectable after varying lengths of time depending on the initial level ($t_{1/2}$ approximately 48 h).[28]

Figure 15-1 shows an algorithm for the diagnosis of early pregnancy bleeding that relies heavily on early TVUS in conjunction with quantitative HCG levels. Because sonographic visualization of the uterine contents during early pregnancy depends on the sonographer's skill and the equipment, one should be cautious in diagnosing a nonviable pregnancy on the basis of a single ultrasound examination at less than 7 weeks' gestation.

SERUM PROGESTERONE LEVEL   Maternal serum progesterone has also been tested as a means of distinguishing normal from abnormal early pregnancy. Initially, progesterone is produced by the corpus luteum, but by the time of the missed menses, it is being produced by the trophoblast, as is HCG. After the missed menses, 70 percent of viable pregnancies will have a serum progesterone level greater than 25 ng/mL, but only 1.5 percent of ectopic or nonviable pregnancies will have levels this high.[28] A serum progesterone level less than 5 ng/mL occurs in only 1/1500 normal pregnancies. An abnormally low progesterone level does not indicate whether a pregnancy is ectopic or whether a miscarriage is complete. A single progesterone level higher than 25 ng/mL or lower than 5 ng/mL has strong predictive value in early pregnancy, but many values will be in the "gray zone" between. Serial quantitative HCG levels are widely available and more likely to provide information about whether a pregnancy is developing normally.

EXAMINATION OF TISSUE FROM THE UTERUS   If tissue is spontaneously expelled from the uterus and recovered or if the uterine contents are evacuated surgically, the tissue should be examined by the clinician. The best way is to float the specimen in a small container of normal saline. Blood is washed from the surface of the specimen by gentle agitation. The shed endometrial lining or decidual tissue appears meaty and pink or rose-colored, often in shreds or sheets. Decidua will form regardless of the location of the pregnancy, so its presence does not exclude ectopic pregnancy. To be sure that the specimen is from an early intrauterine pregnancy, it is necessary to see the delicate, white, frondlike chorionic villi. These will often appear in a clump, surrounding the gestational sac. Later in the first trimester one may see a gestational sac containing fetal tissue and sometimes amniotic fluid, with chorionic villi attached to one side of the sac. When an apparently intact gestational sac is retrieved, one can be fairly sure that a miscarriage is complete. Thus, the reasons for asking women to save tissue that has been passed and for clinicians to examine it are to ascertain that bleeding is not likely to be caused by an ectopic pregnancy (if chorionic villi are passed from the uterus) and to diagnose completed miscarriages that are not likely to require surgical intervention (dilatation and curettage [D&C]). Formal pathologic examination of tissue from an early SAB or from suction curettage may resolve uncertainty if chorionic villi or a gestational sac are not apparent on the clinician's gross examination.

Should the gestational products be sent for chromosome analysis? In sporadic miscarriages, although chromosomal abnormalities that explain the pregnancy loss are frequently found, this will not add much prognostic information for the next pregnancy. Fetal chromosome analysis is an expensive test that is not necessary in most cases. However, in cases of recurrent miscarriage or second trimester pregnancy loss, the finding of a normal fetal karyotype may direct the diagnostic workup toward a search for maternal causes. Karyotyping of gestational tissues should be considered in a second trimester miscarriage or a pregnancy lost after documentation of a fetal heartbeat and possibly in a second consecutive miscarriage.[15,30]

Management Strategies

ACUTE CARE: EXPECTANT MANAGEMENT VERSUS INTERVENTION

When early pregnancy bleeding is determined to be due to a nonviable intrauterine pregnancy, the woman and clinician must decide whether and when to proceed with an intervention to remove the gestational tissues from the uterus. Some clinically recognized, nonviable, intrauterine pregnancies may spontaneously resorb, as do some early ectopic pregnancies, but no published data were found for estimating how often this may occur. Usually it is predictable that a nonviable pregnancy will lead at some point to cramping, heavier bleeding, and the passage of tissue. Typically, this occurs within days of the initial onset of vaginal bleeding, but it may be weeks.[20] It is rare for a missed abortion to result in a coagulopathy or infection in the absence of uterine instrumentation, so waiting for spontaneous onset of the symptoms of a miscarriage is not likely to be dangerous. However, waiting several days for the occurrence of painful cramps and unpredictably heavy uterine bleeding may be anxiety provoking and inconvenient, leading some women to request uterine evacuation as soon as they know that a miscarriage is inevitable. Such a course of action may be preferable for women who live far from a source of emergency care or have less reliable transportation, who have less prospect of help at home, or who have a lower tolerance for blood loss (e.g., are already anemic or would refuse transfusions). Women may choose this option because it gives them some control over the timing of pregnancy completion, because they anticipate better pain relief and comfort measures with a scheduled D&C compared to undergoing the miscarriage at home or at work, and because they wish for an emotionally painful process of pregnancy loss to be over as soon as possible.

Clinical features do not enable prediction of the severity of pain and bleeding that will be associated with first trimester miscarriages. In general, spontaneous abortions after 10 weeks' gestation are more likely to be incomplete and to require D&C. For clinicians, a scheduled procedure is undoubtedly more convenient than attendance in an emergency, but perhaps less so than follow-up care in the office after a spontaneous miscarriage at home. Whether by deliberate choice or because they did not come to medical attention earlier, an estimated 25 to 50 percent of women miscarry outside the hospital and about 50 percent do not undergo D&C.[13,22,31]

Women with miscarriages often present for emergency care while experiencing heavy vaginal bleeding or painful uterine contractions. These symptoms can indicate that expulsion of the gestational sac and placental tissue is about to occur spontaneously or that the process has in fact been incomplete. Logically, it is the latter situation that is more likely to require intervention to evacuate the uterus to stop the bleeding, but in practical terms, no distinction is usually made. Women presenting to emergency departments with severe symptoms due to a miscarriage usually receive the diagnosis incomplete abortion and undergo suction curettage.[13,31] It appears that this usual practice (rather than, for example, several hours of observation with analgesics) developed before the legalization of elective abortion when many women presenting in this fashion were experiencing complications of an incomplete or septic criminal abortion and delay in seeking professional care. In that context, a policy of immediate D&C is likely to have saved lives. In modern context, D&C for all women presenting with severe cramping and bleeding may be seen as expedient, saving time in the emergency department, providing rapid relief of symptoms, and ensuring that removal of the gestational tissues is complete.

Scientific data for deciding which women, presenting during the acute phase of a miscarriage, should have vacuum aspiration are scarce. The Ambulatory Sentinel Practice Network (ASPN) study was the first in the United States to document that many women seen by family physicians for miscarriages do well without a D&C.[22] In this case series from multiple practices, 40 percent of those with SABs were managed at home or in the doctor's office, 20 percent visited the emergency department but were not hospitalized, and 40 percent were hospitalized. About 48 percent of the miscarriages reported to the ASPN study were managed without a D&C. Clinicians reported that a D&C was usually performed because of persistent or excessive bleeding; pain, the patient's request, or "customary practice" were factors in some cases.

Based on a survey of a nationally representative sample of Finnish women in 1994, Hemminki estimated that in the 1990s 30 percent of miscarriages were treated in outpatient settings, but only 1.5 percent without a visit to a physician.[31] Eighty-eight percent of those seen at clinics, emergency departments, and hospitals had a D&C. Similarly, in a small, population-based prospective study of early pregnancy bleeding in Britain, 29 percent of women who miscarried did so at home without a D&C, whereas 89 percent of those hospitalized had a D&C.[13]

Two randomized, controlled trials of immediate D&C versus expectant management were found. Neilsen and Hahlin[32] randomized 155 patients with first trimester inevitable or incomplete SAB diagnosed by ultrasound, excluding those with a diameter of tissue inside the uterus of less than 15 or more than 50 mm, to expectant management with oral analgesics and D&C 3 days later if ultrasound still showed intrauterine tissue, versus immediate D&C. Twenty-one percent of those managed expectantly had a D&C, only 2 percent as an emergency; 69 percent did not have retained products at the 3-day follow-up examination. Those with expectant management had an average of 1.3 days longer of bleeding (8.8 versus 7.5 days) but no difference in blood count 2 weeks later and no difference in duration of pain or of convalescence. Chipchase and James[33] randomized 35 women with retained products of conception less than 50 mm diameter by TVUS during first trimester miscarriages to D&C versus expectant management with analgesics. The small

number of subjects reduced the power to detect differences, but there were no significant differences between groups in days of bleeding (4 with expectant management versus 2 with D&C), duration of sick leave (4 days versus 6.5 days), satisfaction, complications (infection), or subsequent conceptions (75 percent within 1 year). None of the 19 women managed expectantly needed a D&C. Based on the observational data and these small randomized trials, it seems desirable to offer women with first trimester miscarriages who are hemodynamically stable a choice of observation at home with analgesics or D&C. Follow-up visits should be scheduled within about 1 week, with provision for as-needed emergency evaluation should hemorrhage or increased pain occur.

SURGICAL PROCEDURES　The current procedure for evacuating gestational tissues from the uterus is vacuum aspiration (also called suction curettage) using a plastic cannula of approximately the same diameter in millimeters as the number of weeks gestation (up to 12 mm), attached to a suction device that supplies 600 mmHg negative pressure. Although it is usually referred to as a D&C, dilation of the cervical os may not be required if it is already open, and sharp curettage of the uterine lining is often unnecessary. The procedure is usually accomplished with paracervical anesthesia (if dilation is required), parenteral analgesia and sedation, or general anesthesia. Antibiotics (e.g., doxycycline 100 mg orally or cefoxitin 2 g intravenously), are often given prophylactically during or immediately after the procedure.

The main complications of suction curettage are those related to anesthesia, retained products of conception (sometimes leading to hemorrhage), and infection. Rare complications include cervical stenosis following instrumental dilation of the os, perforation by dilators or by sharp curettes, and partial endometrial ablation or synechiae (Asherman's syndrome). The procedure is a safe one. The best data on complication rates come from large case series of elective first trimester suction curettage for pregnancy termination; it is plausible that these do not differ substantially from the complications of suction curettage for first trimester miscarriages. They include: death, 0.5 to 2/100,000; retained placental tissue, 3/1000; perforation, less than 2/1000; cervical stenosis, 2/1000; infection, 2/100.[34] The ASPN study found that endometritis was diagnosed at follow-up in 5 percent of first trimester miscarriages without D&C and 7 percent with D&C, but because 7 percent of the women were considered to have endometritis prior to undergoing D&C, the rate of endometritis resulting from the procedure cannot be determined.[22]

MEDICAL PROCEDURES   Effective medical means are being developed for elective termination of early pregnancies. Methotrexate has been used successfully to terminate ectopic pregnancies without surgery[28] and as an initial agent in elective abortion of intrauterine pregnancies. Prostaglandins combined with progesterone antagonists (e.g., mifepristone) are effective abortifacients in the first 49 days of gestation, inducing a miscarriage-like series of events. At the time of this writing, these same agents have not been fully studied as alternatives to expectant management or suction curettage in cases of SAB, but preliminary reports suggest that future options may include pharmacologic management.[35–38]

RH SENSITIZATION   It is a standard of care for Rh-negative women, not previously sensitized, to receive Rh immune globulin (Rhogam) within 72 h of a spontaneous abortion to prevent Rh sensitization. This is based on the finding of a 2 percent incidence at 8 weeks and a 9 percent incidence of Rh sensitization with abortion at 12 or more weeks' gestation prior to the use of Rhogam and a much lower incidence since its institution.[39] Use of the "micro" dose of 50 μg before 12 weeks' estimated gestational age is less expensive and as effective as the larger dose used later in pregnancy. There is little scientific evidence on which to base a decision about whether to give Rh immune globulin in cases of early pregnancy bleeding whose cause is initially undetermined; examination of bleeding women and controls in early pregnancy showed nonsignificant differences in the incidence of detectable

fetomaternal hemorrhage.[40,41] If the woman is seen during the first days of bleeding, it seems appropriate to ascertain her blood type and screen for antibodies and to consider administering Rh immune globulin, but this practice is based only on indirect evidence that Rh sensitization can occur prior to the expulsion of gestational products or even in a viable early pregnancy with retroplacental hemorrhage.[14] However, sensitization may occur as early as 4 weeks' gestation, when production of fetal blood cells begins.

CARE AFTER THE MISCARRIAGE

British women surveyed after being treated by their general practitioner for a miscarriage expressed a need for more specific information on caring for themselves afterward.[8] Table 15-1 lists common questions and suggested answers. Clinicians should recognize that there is little scientific evidence with which to answer these questions.

EVALUATION OF BLEEDING   Usually, women bleed for about 1 week after complete spontaneous abortion or D&C. Bleeding is usually less than a normal menstrual period and should not be heavier than six to eight pads per day. Prolonged bleeding or repeatedly saturating more than one pad in 2 h should lead to concern about retained products of conception (or an undiagnosed tubal pregnancy or trophoblastic neoplasm) and should prompt further evaluation of the patient. This evaluation should include measurement of serum or urine HCG, blood count, and hemodynamic status. Physical examination in case of retained products may reveal a boggy (rather than firm) uterus with the os still open (rather than closed). Sonographic examination may show retained echogenic material in the uterus (clot or placenta) and is also useful for excluding retained products (if the endometrial thickness is 10 mm or less).[16] If available, a report of the pathologic examination of the uterine contents should be reviewed for the presence of chorionic villi or evidence of a molar pregnancy. Suction curettage may need to be performed or repeated if retained gestational tissue appears to be causing significant bleeding. Many clinicians also perform a urine pregnancy test to ensure that it is negative at follow-up; HCG levels will remain elevated with an undiagnosed ectopic pregnancy or gestational trophoblastic disease.

EMOTIONAL CONSIDERATIONS At the time of a threatened miscarriage, or when pregnancy is diagnosed for women who have had a previous abnormal pregnancy, anxiety is a common experience. Uncertainty about whether the pregnancy is normal and whether it will continue can go on for days or weeks. The woman may worry that pain and hemorrhage could begin when she does not have help or transportation easily available. Usual activities may to some extent be postponed. A tubal pregnancy is potentially life-threatening, giving extra cause for anxiety until the location of the pregnancy can be ascertained. The anxiety is compounded for many women by their beliefs that miscarriages can be caused by their actions and circumstances. This belief conflicts with the realistic perception that the outcome is usually beyond their control and that of clinicians.[5,6] In the face of uncertainty about whether the pregnancy will develop normally, it may be difficult or impossible to fully accept and invest emotional energy in the pregnancy.

After the completion of a miscarriage, women can resume normal activities within 1 day, unless severely anemic from blood loss or otherwise unusually ill. However, the grief and anxiety commonly associated with loss of the pregnancy are apt to impair concentration and decrease performance to a variable degree.[5] Women, and others who have gone through the experience with them, should be assured that vivid recollections of events and the associated emotions are common, as are sleep disturbance and feelings of disbelief, sadness, bitterness, anger, or guilt and uncertainty about where to go from here. Sexual intercourse should be deferred for a few days or until the bleeding has stopped.

Women should meet or talk with a clinician sometime within the month after an uncompli-

cated miscarriage, both for medical follow-up and to discuss family planning and the etiology of the miscarriage. It appears to be helpful to state explicitly that miscarriages are not generally caused by a person's actions during the pregnancy but, as far as is known, by errors or defects very early in development of the embryo.[8] The woman, or those close to her, may have in mind specific events or exposures that they see as potential causes for what happened; it is desirable to ask about these and to address their concerns as specifically as possible. If smoking or substance abuse or (rarely) a hazardous occupational exposure is identified, the miscarriage may provide a powerful motivation for the woman to avoid these harmful exposures in the next pregnancy. The clinician should be ready to provide specific advice and referrals for the woman who is now ready for action to stop smoking or drinking.

If loss of a pregnancy precipitates a major depression or anxiety disorder, the symptoms almost always begin in the first month after the loss.[42] Thus it may be practical to screen for depression and anxiety at the initial follow-up visit, scheduling further visits for supportive care if symptoms are significant and referring the woman for treatment if they persist. Depression is more common in the months following a miscarriage than among women who have not recently been pregnant.[6,42] Neugebauer et al. found that 11 percent of 229 women seen for SAB at a medical center and followed prospectively met criteria for a major depressive disorder during the 6 months after SAB.[6] This was compared to 4 percent of a population-based matched sample of women in the same community. A prior history of major depression, childlessness, and age over 35 were predictive of depression. Prettyman et al. screened 65 British women who underwent D&C for first trimester miscarriages and found that 12 weeks afterward 32 percent were anxious and 6 percent were depressed.[43] Chalmers found that most women "had not recovered emotionally" by 3 months after a miscarriage.[2]

FUTURE CHILDBEARING AND FAMILY PLANNING At least 75 percent of women attempting pregnancy after one miscarriage will have a viable pregnancy within 1 to 2 years. About 25 percent of women feel a need to attempt pregnancy as soon as possible after having miscarried.[2] There is no substantiated biologic basis for recommending a period of waiting before trying to conceive again after a miscarriage, except in cases of major depression or anxiety or in the weeks following a major hemorrhage while anemia is resolving. Those desiring another pregnancy immediately should abstain from intercourse or use barrier contraception until the follow-up UCG is negative. They should be advised that it is normal for the resumption of menses to be somewhat variable, although, on the average, women resume ovulating about 2 weeks after a completed miscarriage and have their first menstrual period within 1 month.[13,16]

Many women and couples desire another pregnancy but feel that they need time to resolve their feelings and to heal physically and emotionally after the miscarriage. Barrier contraception or oral contraceptive hormones are good choices in this situation. Those choosing fertility awareness methods may need to abstain or use barrier contraception until the first menses because the resumption of ovulation is somewhat unpredictable following a miscarriage. Because injection of a slowly-released progestagen (Depo-Provera) can diminish fertility for several months, this is not a good choice for those desiring to conceive again within the coming year.

Finally, some women will feel that the miscarriage offered them a "reprieve" from an inopportune pregnancy. Conflicting expectations about childbearing between the woman and her partner may be revealed. The clinician's task is to help the woman deal with her ambivalent feelings in such a way as to be able to use an effective contraceptive method of her choice. When the lost pregnancy was unwanted, it may be wise to select a contraceptive method that is simple and does not require repeated actions by the woman or her partner to be effective. Methods such as progesterone injections or implants or an intrauterine device (IUD) may be especially appropriate in such situations. Insertion of an IUD is usually deferred until 3 to 6 weeks after the miscarriage.

Recurrent Pregnancy Loss

Definition and Prevalence

Recurrent SAB has been variably defined: strictly as three or more consecutive pregnancy losses before 20 weeks' gestation, sometimes more loosely as two or more losses, not necessarily consecutive. Whatever the definition, sporadic miscarriage is common, but a small subpopulation of women (0.5 to 3 percent) experience multiple miscarriages and a dearth of normal pregnancies.[14,44] The experience of these women has not been studied from the perspective of primary care. Most published medical information originates from subspecialty referral centers with a selected clientele. Recurrent SAB is often associated with subfertility. This may include very early loss of unrecognized conceptions, or an increased risk of preterm delivery, placenta previa, breech delivery, and fetal malformations in subsequent pregnancies, depending on the etiology of the reproductive problems.[14] Many couples (up to 50 percent) with subfertility and recurrent pregnancy loss do not find an etiology despite extensive workup.

Etiology

The various etiologies and management of recurrent SABs are presented in Table 15-3.

CHANCE PHENOMENA

If the chance of a miscarriage in each pregnancy is independent, and estimated at 15 percent, then the chance of a second miscarriage is 2.3 percent and of a third miscarriage 0.34 percent. This is nearly identical to the proportion found in a study of women doctors.[14]

Table 15-3

Etiologies and Management of Recurrent Spontaneous Abortions

CAUSE	DIAGNOSTIC FINDINGS	MANAGEMENT OPTIONS	RECURRENCE RISK
Unknown	Nonspecific	Expectant	2.3% of women will have two consecutive miscarriages, 0.3% will have three by chance alone.
Genetic			
Fetal chromosomal aneuploidy due to error in gametogenesis	Older mother; father >55 y Abnormal karyotype of abortus Early pregnancy losses	Consider chromosome analysis in subsequent pregnancies	Sporadic occurrence; depends on maternal age
Heritable genetic factors:	Highly likely if couple has a genetically abnormal child	Based on genetic consultation	Depends on inheritance pattern
Parent carries a balanced translocation	Parental karyotype shows translocation; abortus has unbalanced translocation. Early pregnancy losses.	Reproduction with donor gametes Chromosome analysis in subsequent pregnancies	High
Single-gene defect	Analysis of pedigree. Genetic diagnosis of previously affected family members. Carrier testing of parents.	Prenatal diagnosis Reproduction with donor gametes	Depends on inheritance pattern: 25% for autosomal recessive; 50% for autosomal dominant; most males if X-linked lethal trait
Abnormal uterine anatomy			
Incompetent cervix	Painless dilation or PROM. Second trimester loss of normal fetus.	Cervical cerclage in subsequent pregnancies Surveillance of cervix by TVUS	High if no cerclage. 30% or less with cerclage
Congenital anomaly (septate, bicornuate, unicornuate, etc.)	Association with conization, DES. Second trimester loss of normal fetus. Premature labors, malpositions more common. Ultrasound shows abnormal shape. Hysteroscopy ± laparoscopy	Surgical or hysteroscopic resection	High if not corrected Low if corrected
Leiomyomata (fibroids) Intrauterine synechiae	Loss of normal fetus at any stage Sonography, hysteroscopy	Myomectomy Hysteroscopic resection	Moderate: depends on placental implantation site Low if abnormality corrected

Table 15-3

Etiologies and Management of Recurrent Spontaneous Abortions (*Continued.*)

CAUSE	DIAGNOSTIC FINDINGS	MANAGEMENT OPTIONS	RECURRENCE RISK
Endocrine: Insufficient luteal phase	Early pregnancy losses. History of anovulation, LH hypersecretion disorders, hyperandrogenism. Endometrial biopsy shows asynchronous endometrium.	Progesterone in first trimester Clomiphene for ovulation induction and to stimulate folliculogenesis	30% without treatment 10–30% with treatment
Infections: Not a proven cause of recurrent SAB	Ureaplasma, mycoplasmas, group B streptococcus	Treat if infection is diagnosed.	Unknown
Immunologic factors			
Humoral: Antiphospholipid antibodies	Anticardiolipin antibodies and lupus anticoagulant; false + syphilis serology. Premature births, preeclampsia, SABs Thrombotic and autoimmune phenomena	Low-dose aspirin 80 mg/d plus heparin wk 7–34.	50–90% if untreated 10–40% with treatment
Cell-mediated immunity	High serum levels of interleukin 2 and tumor necrosis factor Increased type 1 helper T-cell response to trophoblast antigens	Experimental: Immunosuppression	Unknown
Toxic agents: Drugs, ionizing radiation	Exposure history	Avoid exposure: smoking cessation, etc	Depends on continued exposure
Maternal medical conditions: e.g., thrombocytosis, inherited thrombophilia	Impaired uterine perfusion; Vasculopathy; very high platelet count or recurrent thrombosis and clotting diathesis (e.g., factor V Leiden, Protein C deficiency)	Treat maternal condition if possible; consider anticoagulation	Unknown

ABBREVIATIONS: DES, diethylstilbestrol; LH, luteinizing hormone; PROM, premature rupture of membranes; SAB, spontaneous abortion; TVUS, transvaginal ultrasound.

GENETIC ABNORMALITIES

CHROMOSOMAL ANEUPLOIDY   Stern et al. reported from two referral centers in the United States and Mexico that 60 percent of recurrent miscarriages and 60 percent of sporadic miscarriages had abnormal embryonic karyotypes.[15] The proportion of spontaneously aborted fetuses that are chromosomally abnormal increases with increasing maternal age and is also higher with paternal age over 55 years. Most embryonic chromosomal abnormalities are of maternal origin and cause SAB in the first trimester of pregnancy. Chromosomal abnormalities are less common among second trimester SABs compared to early pregnancy losses. With a history of recurrent SAB, the finding of a normal embryonic karyotype somewhat increases the probability of SAB in the next pregnancy (23 percent compared to 15 to 17 percent when the embryo was karyotypically abnormal). This suggests that nonrandom (probably maternal) causes are more likely to account for repetitive losses of genetically normal fetuses.[15,45]

HERITABLE GENETIC ABNORMALITIES   Heritable genetic abnormalities account for 1 to 5 percent of recurrent miscarriages.[14,44] The likelihood is much higher if the parents have also borne a genetically abnormal child.[46] A small proportion (approximately 1 to 5 percent) of couples with recurrent SAB carry a balanced translocation of part of their chromosomal material. Balanced translocations are present in 0.1 to 0.2 percent of individuals in the general population. During gametogenesis, some offspring may inherit normal chromosomes, some may inherit the balanced translocation, but in many the translocation can become unbalanced, resulting in a lethal duplication or omission of part of a chromosome. Both members of a couple who have experienced two or more SABs should consider having karyotyping to detect such a balanced translocation.[30,47]

Some recurrent pregnancy losses are due to single-gene defects discernable from the family history such as α-thalassemia (homozygotes die of fetal hydrops) or Gaucher's disease. Analysis of the pedigree may rarely reveal that all live births are females, suggesting an X-linked disorder lethal to affected male fetuses. Examples of such X-linked disorders are focal dermal hypoplasia, incontinentia pigmenti, and Rett syndrome.[30]

STRUCTURAL ABNORMALITIES OF THE UTERUS

Ten to 16 percent of recurrent pregnancy losses are attributed to structural abnormalities in the uterus, including cervical incompetence, congenital mullerian defects such as bicornuate or septate uterus, or acquired abnormalities such as uterine synechiae and leiomyomata.[44,47] Painless dilation (incompetence) of the cervix can result in repeated second trimester losses of otherwise viable pregnancies. Cervical incompetence is more common in women exposed to diethylstilbestrol during fetal development, and after cervical conization; however, in most cases the etiology is unknown.[14] Cases are difficult to distinguish from other causes of second trimester pregnancy loss. The woman may initially present with spontaneous rupture of the membranes or may be found to have a dilated (and usually effaced) cervix on examination while asymptomatic. The situation tends to recur in subsequent pregnancies. It is unclear to what degree shortening or internal dilation (funneling) of the cervix, visualized in early pregnancy on ultrasound examination, is predictive of subsequent cervical dilation and pregnancy loss, or whether sonography can be useful in following women with a history of cervical incompetence to detect recurrence and the need for intervention.[14,48]

Spontaneous abortion related to uterine anomalies is thought to result from implantation over an abnormal part of the uterine wall or septum. The obstetric history may also include premature birth or malposition, such as breech presentation, owing to intrauterine constraint by a septum or fibroids.[14]

ENDOCRINE PROBLEMS

Maintenance of early pregnancy requires the presence of sufficient progesterone, which is produced by the corpus luteum until 7 to 9 weeks' gestation and thereafter by the trophoblast. Insufficient progesterone or inability of the endometrium to respond will result in early miscarriage (exemplified by the abortive effect of the progesterone antagonist mifepristone in early gestation). Although a large proportion of women with recurrent SAB (15 to 30 percent) can be shown by endometrial biopsies to have dyssynchronous endometrial development, treatment with progesterone has never been proven to prevent recurrent miscarriages.[18,47] Measurement of progesterone levels during the luteal phase does not distinguish these women from those with normal endometrium and no pregnancy losses.[18]

Other endocrine disorders, such as hypothyroidism, autoimmune thyroiditis, and diabetes mellitus have not been conclusively proven to cause miscarriages. If discovered, these disorders should be treated before conception.

MATERNAL INFECTIONS

There is no proven association of recurrent SAB with any type of maternal infection.[47] Culture or serologic evidence of mycoplasma, ureaplasma, and group B streptococci have been associated in some studies but not in others.[14] Evidence does not support a causal role for chlamydia, listeria, or toxoplasmosis in recurrent SAB.

IMMUNOLOGIC FACTORS

HUMORAL IMMUNITY Antiphospholipid antibodies are associated with adverse pregnancy outcomes including recurrent SAB, premature labor, intrauterine growth retardation, stillbirth, and preeclampsia. They are present in 3 to 5 percent of women with recurrent SAB and are rare in women with normal reproductive histories.[47] These may be IgG or IgM antibodies against cardiolipin or phosphatidylserine. They are theorized to lead to decreased synthesis of prostacycline and increased production of thromboxane in blood vessels, including placental vessels, resulting in thrombosis.[47] When antiphospholipid antibodies are the cause of recurrent SAB, the prognosis is poor without treatment.

Other hypotheses involving causation of recurrent SAB by abnormal maternal antibodies have been disproved. Theories that recurrent SAB results from antibodies against sperm or trophoblast tissue have also been disproved.[47]

CELL-MEDIATED IMMUNITY A more recent hypothesis for explaining immunologically mediated reproductive failure involves activation of specific types of cell-mediated immune responses that result in immune rejection of the conceptus. Support for this hypothesis includes the finding of high levels of tumor necrosis factor and interleukin 2 in the serum of women having miscarriages and observations that 60 to 80 percent of nonpregnant women with a history of unexplained recurrent SAB (versus only 3 percent of women with normal reproductive histories) have abnormal TH1 immune responses to trophoblast antigens.[47,49] The practical significance of these observations remains to be elucidated. It is not certain that the increased cytokine production is the cause, rather than the result, of miscarriage.

MISCELLANEOUS FACTORS

Toxic agents associated with miscarriages include alcohol (more than one drink a day), tobacco (1 to 40 cigarettes a day),[17] heavy metal poisoning, prolonged exposure to organic solvents, arsenic, drugs including antineoplastic agents, antiprogesterone agents, ergots, inhalation anesthetics, and ionizing radiation but not microwaves, shortwaves, or ultrasound.[14] Spermicides, oral contraceptives, caffeine less than that in 4 cups of coffee (400 mg caffeine) per day, and video display terminals have been shown not to be associated with miscarriages.[14] Maternal medical conditions that cause diminished uterine perfusion, including thrombocytosis with platelet counts over 1 million/mL, may cause recurrent pregnancy losses.[47]

AGING GAMETES

This hypothesis asserts that early pregnancy loss and perhaps teratogenesis can result from fertilization that occurs late in the period of viability of ova or sperm after ovulation or ejaculation, as might occur with infrequent intercourse or use of periodic abstinence for contraception. There are limited data addressing this hypothesis.[14]

Future Reproductive Potential

Most couples with recurrent SAB, regardless of treatment, are able to have live births subsequently. Overall, the chance after three consecutive miscarriages is about 70 percent in 2 years for couples with a previous live birth and 40 to 50 percent with no previous children.[18] Many treatments have been claimed to be effective because they resulted in about 75 percent of couples successfully carrying a pregnancy. However, when studies are appropriately controlled, the same rate applies to untreated groups. A few conditions carry a worse prognosis. The chances of successful childbearing after recurrent SAB decline with advancing maternal age to about 45 percent at age 40 or more.[45] Miscarriage due to trisomy as a result of a parental balanced translocation has a high likelihood of recurrence. Cervical incompetence also tends to recur time after time, but early pregnancy loss can be prevented by cerclage, with a greater than 70 percent live birth rate. Once antiphospholipid antibodies and recurrent SAB are present, the chance of a live birth without treatment is 10 to 50 percent; 71 percent of 45 such women treated with heparin plus low-dose aspirin in a randomized trial, however, bore infants who survived.[50–52]

Diagnosis

HISTORY

The history is similar to that for any patient with a threatened miscarriage. Special attention should be paid to the woman's menstrual and prior infertility or pregnancy history, with as many details as possible about any previous pregnancy losses. Her medical history should include information about exposure to diethylstilbestrol in utero or to toxins, symptoms of endocrine disorders or gynecologic infection, history of thrombosis (e.g., stroke), autoimmune phenomena, or a false-positive syphilis test

(suggestive of antiphospholipid syndrome). The chronic sorrow of recurrent pregnancy losses and the effects of uncertainty on the couple deserve empathic attention. The family history should include multiple pregnancy losses in the extended family, heritable disorders, and consanguinity. Records of any previous diagnostic testing, fetal autopsies and karyotyping, and pedigrees from genetic counseling should be requested.

PHYSICAL EXAMINATION

The general physical examination may detect signs of systemic illness or increased androgen effect. On pelvic examination, an abnormal size and shape of the uterus may be palpable. One should also seek signs of genital infection.

LABORATORY EVALUATION AND IMAGING

Laboratory evaluation of women with recurrent miscarriage between pregnancies should aim to detect causes of recurrent SAB that can be treated or circumvented. The workup might reasonably include the tests shown in Table 15-4.[47,51] Tests that are not useful in the workup of recurrent miscarriage include human leukocyte antigen typing, mixed lymphocyte culture reactions, antipaternal antibody titers, and antinuclear antibodies.[47]

When a woman who has had recurrent miscarriages becomes pregnant, it may be important to her to establish fetal viability as early as possible. This can be done by measuring serial HCG levels until the level reaches 1500 or 2000 mIU/mL, then performing a transvaginal ultrasound examination, which should show a gestational sac. Ultrasound can be repeated every 1 or 2 weeks until fetal viability or nonviability is established. If another miscarriage occurs, fetal karyotyping and pathologic examination of fetus and placenta should be ordered.[44] If a clinical diagnosis of incompetent cervix is suspected, serial cervical examinations may detect the onset of dilation. In viable pregnancies after SABs with previously abnormal or unknown fetal karyotypes, most experts recommend fetal karyotyping by amniocentesis at 15 to

Table 15-4

Suggested Laboratory Investigations for Patients with Recurrent Miscarriages

Blood tests
  Complete blood count (to rule out thrombocytosis)
  Hemoglobin electrophoresis (if hemoglobinopathy is suspected)
  Lead level (if a source of exposure is identified)
  Fasting blood glucose or glycohemoglobin
  Thyroid-stimulating hormone and antithyroid antibodies
  Syphilis serology
  Anticardiolipin antibodies and a lupus anticoagulant test
Genital cultures
  Mycoplasma and ureaplasma
Genetic testing
  Karyotyping (both parents or mother first, followed by the father if mother's karyotype is normal)
Invasive procedures
  Endometrial biopsy (performed on d 24–25 of a 28-d cycle (or about 10 d after ovulation), followed by measurement of serum testosterone, dihydroepiandrosterone sulfate, and prolactin if the endometrial histology lags ≥ 2 d behind the dates. Some experts advocate a second, confimatory endometrial biopsy if the first is abnormal[20,47]
  Hysteroscopy or hysterosalpingogram to assess the anatomy of the endometrial cavity

19 weeks' gestation (this way of sampling fetal genetic material carries a slightly lower risk of procedure-related pregnancy loss than chorionic villus sampling or early amniocentesis).[51]

Management Strategies

GENETIC DISORDERS

A number of management strategies can be used, based on the presumed etiology of the recurrent miscarriages and the level of expertise of the clinician. If a genetic abnormality, such as a balanced translocation, is detected in one parent, the couple has the option of substituting donor gametes for those of the affected person or of having in vitro fertilization with embryo biopsy and karyotyping before implantation. In cases of spontaneous abortions of karyotypically abnormal fetuses without a detectable parental chromosome abnormality, synchronizing intercourse with ovulation may be beneficial (according to the "aging gamete"

hypothesis).[14] In cases of X-linked or other single-gene disorders, genetic counseling and prenatal diagnosis by fetal DNA testing may be an option if pregnancy reaches the stage of viability.

CERVICAL CERCLAGE

Cervical incompetence is a clinical diagnosis based on the history of the circumstances and symptoms preceding previous second trimester pregnancy losses. Cervical cerclage procedures, ideally performed between 14 and 18 weeks' gestation, can enable the woman to carry a pregnancy to term (when the cerclage is removed or a cesarean delivery is scheduled). Placement of the cerclage, however, can lead to ruptured membranes, premature labor, or amniotic infection. The operation should be preceded by cervical cultures and treatment of pathogens and by sonographic confirmation of fetal viability.[14] Emergency cerclage, late in the second trimester, is more likely to lead to complications and premature delivery.

SURGICAL CORRECTION OF ANATOMIC ABNORMALITIES

If anatomic abnormalities of the uterus are suspected, sonography may show fibroids or abnormal cornua but often a septum will be missed. Abnormalities of the endometrial cavity can be evaluated by hysterosalpingogram or by hysteroscopy; simultaneous laparoscopy may be indicated depending on the diagnosis. Ultrasound-guided, transcervical metroplasty or hysteroscopic resection of a septum, lysis of synechiae, or resection of submucous fibroids can be offered to correct the abnormal uterine shape, resulting in term gestation rates of 70 to 80 percent.[47,51] Estrogen therapy (e.g., 1.25 mg conjugated equine estrogen per day) is recommended during healing to prevent synechiae. Conventional myomectomy, with a full-thickness scar of the uterine fundus, would necessitate cesarean delivery without labor.

ENDOCRINE DISORDERS AND LUTEAL PHASE INSUFFICIENCY

Hypothyroidism should be treated and diabetes or hyperprolactinemia controlled before conception. When endometrial biopsies suggest an inadequate luteal phase, progesterone is commonly given during early gestation, but its benefit has not been substantiated in controlled trials. The dose is 25 to 50 mg bid in vaginal suppositories from the day of ovulation until 10 weeks' gestation.[51] Synthetic progestins (e.g., medroxyprogesterone acetate) are ineffective. In disorders of luteinizing hormone hypersecretion or hyperandrogenism, ovulation induction and stimulation of folliculogenesis with clomiphene citrate may be helpful. The initial dose is 50 mg/d on days 5 through 9 of the cycle; in subsequent cycles the dose is increased by 50 mg/d to a maximum of 200 mg/d.[18]

IMMUNOTHERAPY

Immunization of the woman with paternal leukocytes is an unproven therapy with potential risks of graft-versus-host disease, intrauterine growth retardation, and fetal thrombocytopenia from the induction of antiplatelet antibodies. This type of treatment is not recommended.[47] Other immunoregulatory treatments not well substantiated by controlled studies include cyclosporine, plasmapheresis, and intravenous immunoglobulins.

ANTICOAGULATION

Women with antiphospholipid antibodies causing miscarriages have a poor prognosis without treatment. There is evidence, based on controlled trials, in support of anticoagulation with low-dose aspirin (80 mg daily from the time of the positive pregnancy test) plus heparin (10,000 IU subcutaneously bid from 7 to 34 weeks' gestation, adjusted to maintain the partial thromboplastin time about twice the control).[47,50] The observed rate of live birth was 70 percent when selected patients were treated with both heparin and aspirin, compared to 40 percent with aspirin alone.[50] The complications of anticoagulation include bone demineralization and bleeding, including placental abruption. Data on the use of low-molecular-weight heparin in pregnant women with antiphospholipid antibodies are not available at the time of this writing. Prednisone with aspirin has been studied and found no more effective than placebo.[52]

Supported Decision-Making

At each juncture, the woman/couple and the clinician should revisit the issue of whether to actively pursue pregnancy, "let nature take its course," or opt for contraception. Those deciding to attempt adoption face potentially discouraging hurdles in qualifying and waiting for adoption, especially through agencies, and may decide to pursue private adoption. The cost of adoption or assisted reproductive technology is typically tens of thousands of dollars. Those confronting childlessness, especially in their forties, will naturally go through all the stages of grieving and must find a source of generativity and self-esteem apart from parenting.[4]

All couples with recurrent miscarriage require psychological support throughout the uncertainty and burdensome diagnostic and therapeutic process if they continue to attempt pregnancy, or through the process of adapting to the loss of fertility and reorganization of their life goals. Professional psychological support and also support from self-help groups can make a difference. RESOLVE is a national support organization for couples who have experienced pregnancy losses or infertility.[53] Another large support group in the United States for people who have experienced pregnancy losses is SHARE (Source of Help in Airing and Resolving Experiences).[54] These groups can be contacted by telephone or the Internet [RESOLVE: (617) 623-0744 or resolveinc@aol.com and SHARE: (800) 821-6819 or share@national shareoffice.com]. The chronic, sometimes cyclic, depression experienced by some women with infertility or reproductive losses may benefit from specific therapy (cognitive or pharmacologic).[4]

References

1. Plath S: Parliament Hill Fields. In: Hughes T (ed): *Sylvia Plath: Collected Poems*. London: Faber & Faber; 1981.

2. Chalmers B: The psychosocial import of spontaneous abortion. In: Cecil R (ed): *The Anthropology of Pregnancy Loss: Comparative Studies in Miscarriage, Stillbirth, and Neonatal Death*. Washington, DC: Berg; 1996.

3. Woods JR Jr, Esposito JL (eds): *Pregnancy Loss: Medical Therapeutics and Practical Considerations*. Baltimore: Williams & Wilkins; 1987.

4. Rosenthal M: Infertility. In: Rosenfeld JA, Alley N, Acheson LS, Admire JB (eds): *Women's Health in Primary Care*. Baltimore: Williams & Wilkins; 1997:351.

5. Layne L: Never such innocence again: irony, nature, and technoscience in narratives of pregnancy loss. In: Cecil R (ed): *The Anthropology of Pregnancy Loss: Comparative Studies in Miscarriage, Stillbirth, and Neonatal Death*. Washington, DC: Berg; 1996:131.

6. Neugebauer R, Kline J, Shrout P, et al: Major depressive disorder in the six months after miscarriage. *JAMA* 277:383, 1997.

7. Puddifoot JE, Johnson MP: The legitimacy of grieving: the partner's experience at miscarriage. *Soc Sci Med* 45:837, 1997.

8. Friedman T: Women's experiences of general practitioner management of miscarriage. *J R Coll Gen Pract* 39:456, 1989.

9. Hertig AT, Rock J, Adams EC, Menkin M: Thirty-four fertilized human ova, good, bad, and indifferent, recovered from 210 women of known fertility: a study of biologic wastage in early human pregnancy. *Pediatrics* 23:202, 1959.

10. De Luca MA, Leslie PW: Variation in risk of pregnancy loss. In: Cecil R (ed): *The Anthropology of Pregnancy Loss: Comparative Studies in Miscarriage, Stillbirth, and Neonatal Death*. Washington, DC: Berg; 1996:113.

11. Wilcox AJ, Weinberg CR, O'Connor JF, et al: Incidence of early loss of pregnancy. *N Engl J Med* 319: 189, 1988.

12. Edmonds DK, Lindsay KS, Miller JF, et al: Early embryonic mortality in women. *Fertil Steril* 38:447, 1982.

13. Everett C: Incidence and outcome of bleeding before the 20th week of pregnancy: prospective study from general practice. *BMJ* 315:32, 1997.

14. Abortion. In: Cunningham FG, MacDonald PC, Gant NF, et al. (eds): *Williams Obstetrics*, 20th ed. Stamford, CT: Appleton & Lange; 1997;579.

15. Stern JJ, Dorfmann AD, Gutierrez-Najar AJ, et al: Frequency of abnormal karyotypes among abortuses from women with and without a history of recurrent spontaneous abortion. *Fertil Steril* 65:250, 1996.

16. Apgar BS, Churgay CA: Spontaneous abortion. *Prim Care* 20:621, 1993.

17. Kline J, Stein ZA, Susser M, Warburton D: Smoking: a risk factor for spontaneous abortion. *N Engl J Med* 297:793, 1977.

18. Speroff L, Glass RH, Kase NG: *Clinical Gynecologic Endocrinology and Infertility*, 4th ed. Baltimore: Williams & Wilkins; 1989:535.

19. Stone L: Pregnancy losses. In: Lemcke DP, Pattison J, Marshall LA, Cowley DS (eds): *Primary Care of Women*. Norwalk, CT: Appleton & Lange; 1995:531.

20. Boyd ME: Spontaneous abortion. *Can J Surg* 32: 260, 1989.

21. Andelusi B: Prognosis in pregnancy after threatened abortion. *Int J Gynaecol Obstet* 18:444, 1980.

22. Ambulatory Sentinel Practice Network: Spontaneous abortion in primary care. *J Am Board Fam Pract* 1:15, 1988.

23. Cashner KA, Christopher CR, Dysert GA: Spontaneous fetal loss after demonstration of a live fetus in the first trimester. *Obstet Gynecol* 70:827, 1987.

24. Simpson JL, Mills JL, Holmes LB, et al: The Diabetes in Early Pregnancy Study: low fetal loss rates after ultrasound-proved viability in early pregnancy. *JAMA* 258:2555, 1987.

25. Medalie JH: Relationship between nausea and/or vomiting in early pregnancy and abortion. *Lancet* 273(6986):117, 1957.

26. Eisinger SH: Culdocentesis. *J Fam Pract* 13:95, 1981.

27. Deutchman M: Advances in the diagnosis of first-trimester pregnancy problems. *Am Fam Physician* 44(5)Suppl:15S, 1991.

28. Stovall TG, McCord ML: Early pregnancy loss and ectopic pregnancy. In: Berek JS, Adashi EY, Hillard PA (eds): *Novak's Gynecology*, 12th ed. Baltimore: Williams & Wilkins; 1998:487.

29. Pittaway DE, Reish RL, Wentz AC: Doubling times of human chorionic gonadotropin increase in early viable intrauterine pregnancies. *Am J Obstet Gynecol* 152:299, 1985.

30. Trott EA, Russell JB, Plouffe L Jr: A review of the genetics of recurrent pregnancy loss. *Del Med J* 68:495, 1996.

31. Hemminki E: Treatment of miscarriage: current practice and rationale. *Obstet Gynecol* 91:247, 1998.

32. Nielsen S, Hahlin M: Expectant management of first-trimester spontaneous abortion. *Lancet* 345:84, 1995.

33. Chipchase J, James D: Randomised trial of expectant versus surgical management of spontaneous miscarriage. *Br J Obstet Gynaecol* 104:840, 1997.

34. Hern WM: *Abortion practice*. Philadelphia: Lippincott; 1984.

35. Egarter C, Lederhilger J, Kurz C, et al: Gemeprost for first trimester missed abortion. *Arch Gynecol Obstet* 256:29, 1995.

36. Henshaw RC, Cooper K, El-Refaey H, et al: Medical management of miscarriage: non-surgical uterine evacuation of incomplete and inevitable spontaneous abortion. *BMJ* 306:894, 1993.

37. Lelaidier C, Baton-Saint-Mleux C, Fernandez H, et al: Mifepristone (RU486) induces embryo expulsion in first trimester non-developing pregnancies: a prospective randomized trial. *Hum Reprod* 8:492, 1993.

38. de Jonge ET, Makin JD, Manefeldt E, et al: Randomised clinical trial on medical evacuation and surgical curettage for incomplete miscarriage. *BMJ* 311:662, 1995.

39. Keith LG, Berger GS: The risk of Rh immunization associated with abortion, spontaneous and induced. In: Frigoletto F Jr, Jewett JF, Konugres A (eds): *Rh Hemolytic Disease*. Boston: Hall Medical Publishers; 1982.

40. Kuller JA, Laifer SA, Portney D, Rulin M: The frequency of transplacental hemorrhage in patients with threatened abortion. *Gynecol Obstet Invest* 37:229, 1994.

41. Von Stein GA, Munsick RA, Stiver K, Ryder K: Fetomaternal hemorrhage in threatened abortion. *Obstet Gynecol* 79:383, 1992.

42. Tharpar AK, Tharpar A: Psychological sequelae of miscarriage: a controlled study using the general health questionnaire and the hospital anxiety and depression scale. *Br J Gen Pract* 42:94, 1992.

43. Prettyman RJ, Cordle CJ, Cook GD: A 3-month follow-up of psychological morbidity after early miscarriage. *Br J Med Psychol* 66:363, 1993.

44. Stephenson MD: Frequency of factors associated with habitual abortion in 197 couples. *Fertil Steril* 66:2, 1996.

45. Boue J, Boue A, Lazar P: Retrospective and prospective epidemiological studies of 1500 karyotyped spontaneous human abortions. *Teratology* 12:11, 1975.

46. Byrd JR, Askew DE, McDonough PG: Cytogenetic findings in 55 couples with recurrent fetal wastage. *Fertil Steril* 28:246, 1977.

47. Hill JA: Recurrent spontaneous early pregnancy loss. In: Berek JS, Adashi EY, Hillard PA (eds): *Novak's Gynecology*, 12th ed. Baltimore: Williams & Wilkins; 1998:963.

48. Iams JD, Johnson FF, Sonek J, et al: Cervical competence as a continuum: a study of ultrasonographic cervical length and obstetric performance. *Am J Obstet Gynecol* 172:1097, 1995.

49. Hill JA, Polgar K, Anderson DJ: T Helper 1-type immunity to trophoblast antigens in women with recurrent spontaneous abortion. *JAMA* 273:1933, 1995.

50. Rai R, Cohen H, Dave M, Regan L: Randomised controlled trial of aspirin and aspirin plus heparin in pregnant women with recurrent miscarriage associated with phospholipid antibodies (or antiphospholipid antibodies). *BMJ* 314:253, 1997.

51. Palumbo A, Ginsburg E: Spontaneous and recurrent abortion. In: Carr PL, Freund KM, Somani S (eds): *The Medical Care of Women*. Philadelphia: Saunders; 1995;271.

52. Laskin CA, Bombardier C, Hannah M, et al: Prednisone and aspirin in women with autoantibodies

and unexplained recurrent fetal loss. *N Engl J Med* 337:148, 1997.

53. RESOLVE, Inc., 1310 Broadway, Somerville, MA 02144-1779. National Helpline (617) 623-0744. http://resolve.org/ E-mail: resolveinc@aol.com

54. National SHARE Office, St. Joseph's Health Center, 300 First Capitol Dr., St. Charles, MO 63301-2893. (800) 821-6819. http://www.nationalshareoffice.com/ E-mail: share@nationalshareoffice.com

Mindy A. Smith
Linda Boyd
Janet R. Osuch
Kendra Schwartz

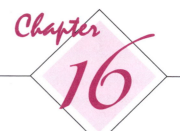

Chapter

16

Breast Disorders

Overview of Women's Concerns

There is a great deal of focus on breasts in our society. This is seen in the media, in fashion design, and in the women often selected to model. American women seek to enhance small breasts or minimize large breasts and, overall, are rarely satisfied with their natural breasts. Juxtapose this anatomic focus with the fact that breast cancer is the most common cancer in women and one will begin to understand the tremendous amount of distress caused by breast disorders.

Over the past 10 years, with the dramatic increase in the attention to the topic of breast cancer in the lay press and media, many women have a heightened awareness and concern about breast cancer. When a breast problem develops, fear of cancer can manifest in speedy consultations for even minor breast complaints or may provoke such anxiety that medical care is avoided. The worry about and response to breast cancer is a complex issue that involves a woman's sexuality, psychological make-up, background, and many other individual factors. Many women feel that they would rather die than lose a breast. Other women place a higher value on life even with disfigurement. Health care providers often assume that patients want to have everything done to evaluate a problem and will be compliant with therapeutic recommendations. However, it is important to remember that not all patients see value in seeking medical care, and indeed there are a variety of responses to dealing with a breast problem.

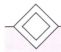

Breast Anatomy and Physiology

Anatomy

The basic components of the breast are the parenchyma, consisting of breast lobes (which secrete milk) and ducts (which transport the milk to the nipple), and the surrounding adipose and connective tissue (Fig. 16-1). The breasts rest on top of the pectoralis major muscle. The connective tissue, or fascia, extends anteriorly to the second rib near the clavicle, inferiorly to the inframammary ridge near the fifth rib, medially to the lateral edge of the sternum, and laterally to the latissimus dorsi muscle. Cooper's ligaments, also composed of connective tissue, are supporting ligaments for the breast and attach to the fascia below the skin and to the fascia of the pectoralis major muscle.

The lobes of the breast consist of lobules that consist of hollow alveoli (milk glands) lined by a single layer of milk-secreting epithelial cells. Each lobule is encased in a crisscrossing mantle of contractile myoepithelial strands and a capillary network.[1] The lumen of the alveolus connects to a

Figure 16-1

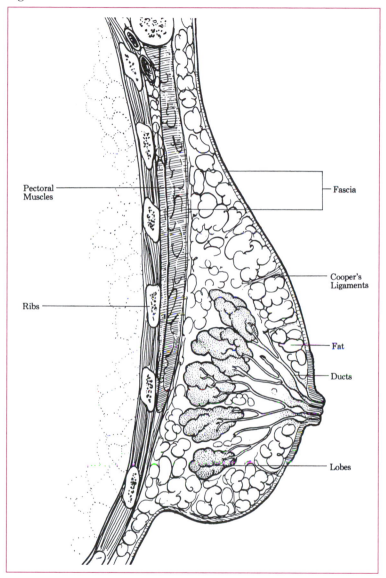

Pectoral
Muscles

Fascia

Cooper's
Ligaments

Ribs

Fat

Ducts

Lobes

Breast anatomy. The internal anatomy of the breast can be viewed as a system of branching treelike structures embedded in adipose and connective tissue. The parenchymal tissue is composed of two types: the lobes, which secrete milk, and the ducts, which transport the milk to the nipple. Each lobular element is drained by a small duct, which enlarges as it courses toward the nipple and ends as a lactiferous sinus, whose function is to store milk. These structures are located posterior to the areola and often can be palpated as a bumpiness at that location. Circular muscle contraction of the nipple stimulated by suckling empties the lactiferous sinuses to initiate lactation. *(Reproduced with permission from the Breast Cancer Digest: A Guide to Medical Care, Emotional Support, Educational Programs, and Resources, 2nd ed. U.S. Department of Health and Human Services, Public Health Service, National Institutes of Health.)*

nonmuscular duct that empties into a series of intra-lobular collecting ducts lined by contractile muscle cells. These reach the exterior by 12 to 20 major collecting ducts arranged radially. The collecting ducts end in lactiferous sinuses, whose function is to store milk. These structures are located posterior to the areola and can often be palpated as a bumpi-ness. Circular muscle contraction of the nipple, stimulated by suckling, empties the sinuses to ini-tiate lactation. Montgomery glands are visible as bumps around the areola; these become more prominent during pregnancy.

The majority of the breast tissue is drained by the axillary lymph nodes that extend along the axillary vein into the infraclavicular and supra-clavicular nodes.

Physiology

The major influence on growth of the breast tissue at puberty is estrogen. The initial response to estro-gen is an increase in size and pigmentation of the areola and the formation of a mass of breast tissue, consisting primarily of elongated ducts and con-nective tissue, beneath it. Removal of this breast nodule in the adolescent will result in a failure of breast development on that side. Lobular forma-tion is dependent on progesterone and is absent until the onset of ovulation. Full differentiation of the breast requires insulin, cortisol, thyroxine, prolactin, and growth hormone.[1] Full maturation of the breast epithelium depends on full-term preg-nancy, in the presence of prolactin, which stimu-lates marked proliferation of duct and lobular cells. The number of breast cells recedes after delivery and weaning, but remains elevated above that of nulliparous women. In the perimenopausal period, lobules begin to recede, leaving mostly ducts and fibroconnective tissue. As these lobular elements recede, women often develop cysts. At meno-pause the lobules atrophy, leaving primarily ducts, adipose, and connective tissue. Use of hormone replacement therapy (HRT), however, will convert breast tissue back to the premenopausal state.

Changes in the breast occur routinely in re-sponse to the estrogen-progesterone fluctuations of the menstrual cycle. Fluid secretion, mitotic activity, and DNA production of glandular epithe-lium and nonglandular tissue peak during the luteal phase[2]; this accounts for the premenstrual changes of nodularity and tenderness reported by many women.

Classification of Breast Disease

A basic scheme classifies breast disease as benign or malignant. Malignant disease is further divided by the location from which the cancer arises, duc-tular or lobular. It is then further subdivided into in situ or invasive cancer.

In contrast, confusion about the classification of benign breast disease is pervasive. In addition, normal physiologic processes in the breast are often described as diseases, leading to further confusion on the part of the clinician and fear in women labeled as having breast disease. A classi-fication system recently introduced by Hughes, Aberrations of Normal Development and Involu-tion (ANDI), can be helpful in understanding benign breast conditions in the context of normal breast development and involution.[3] The ANDI classification organizes breast problems into three reproductive periods (Table 16-1). The classifica-tion system ends at age 55 because it is uncom-mon for postmenopausal women to have benign breast problems.

The normal process and aberrations noted in each stage are shown in Table 16-1, along with the clinical presentation and associated disease states. In this classification, the breast condition commonly referred to as fibrocystic represents a heterogeneous group of benign breast disorders, including exaggerated cyclic effects, proliferative effects, and involutional effects on lobules and ducts. Proliferative effects are seen histologically as epithelial proliferation, ductular branching and intraductal epithelial proliferation (papillomatosis), lobular hyperplasia, and proliferation of intralobular

Table 16-1

The ANDI Classification of Benign Breast Disease

STAGE (PEAK AGE)	NORMAL PROCESS	ABERRATION		
		UNDERLYING CONDITION	CLINICAL PRESENTATION	DISEASE STATE
Early reproductive period (15–25 y)	Lobule formation	Fibroadenoma	Discrete lump	Giant fibroadenoma Multiple fibroadenomas
	Stroma formation	Juvenile hypertrophy	Excessive breast development	
Mature reproductive period (25–40 y)	Cyclic hormonal effects on glandular tissue and stroma	Exaggerated cyclic effects	Cyclic mastalgia and nodularity, generalized or discrete	
Involution (35–55)	Lobular involution (including microcysts, apocrine change, fibrosis and adenosis)	Macrocysts Sclerosing lesions	Mastalgia Lumps Mammogram abnormalities	
	Ductal involution (including periductal round cell infiltrates)	Duct dilation Periductal fibrosis	Nipple discharge Nipple retraction	Periductal mastitis with bacterial infection and abscess formation
	Epithelial turnover	Mild epithelial hyperplasia	Histologic report	Epithelial hyperplasia with atypia

SOURCE: Modified with permission from Hughes LE: A unifying concept for benign disorder of the breast: ANDI. In: Donegan WL, Spratt JS (eds): *Diseases of the Breast.* Philadelphia: Saunders; 1995.

connective tissue. Involutional effects on lobules produce cysts and sclerosing lesions, and involutional effects on ducts produce duct dilation and periductal fibrosis, occasionally producing nipple discharge.

Key History

Questions to ask in the course of a routine evaluation of a woman presenting for care, often in the context of an annual examination, focus on risk factors for breast cancer and breast symptoms.

Risk Factors

A number of factors influence the risk of breast cancer. These include heredity, personal experience of breast disease, reproductive experience, alcohol intake, and use of hormones. The incidence of breast cancer increases with age. The single most important risk factor is female gender; 75 percent of women with breast cancer have no risk factors other than gender and age. Red flags from the patient history for increased risk of breast cancer are noted in Table 16-2 by an asterisk.

HEREDITY

Family history of breast or ovarian cancer increases the risk of breast cancer. In a recent meta-analysis of 74 published studies, Pahroah et al. developed pooled relative risks (RR) of breast cancer based on the number or type of family member affected.[4] For a single first-degree relative (mother, sister, daughter) the pooled RR was 2.1 (range, 1.2 to 8.8), for two first-degree relatives the pooled RR was 3.6 (range, 2.5 to 13.6),

Table 16-2
Focused History for Common Breast Disorders

QUESTION/MANEUVER	PURPOSE
BREAST PAIN HISTORY	
Location	Within breast, chest wall, or neck
Duration	Coincides with event; acute/chronic
Severity (scale of 1–10)	Quality; need for intervention
Unilateral or bilateral	Bilateral is more often physiologic
Relationship to hormones	Cyclic or noncyclic; use of hormones
Previous breast problems or surgery	Trauma, tumor, infection
Lifestyle altering	Need for intervention
Worry	Perceived need for testing/reassurance
PALPABLE BREAST MASS HISTORY	
Location	Unilateral,* bilateral symmetrical
Method of discovery	Self, provider, mammogram
Size	May relate to duration
Duration	Acute/chronic, change in size
Hormonal influences	Cyclic or noncyclic,* postmenopause*
Characteristics (changing, pain)	Soft vs. hard,* mobile vs. fixed*
Nipple discharge	Spontaneous,* color (watery,* bloody*)
Personal history	Previous breast cancer or biopsies*
Family history	Breast or ovarian cancer*
NIPPLE DISCHARGE HISTORY	
Spontaneous	Nonspontaneous is physiologic
Color	Milky, green, yellow, red,* watery*
One duct or more than one	Single duct is more concerning
Unilateral or bilateral	Unilateral more concerning
Duration, persistence	Note pregnancy or breast-feeding
Hormonal status	Pre- or postmenopause
Medications	Use of those that increase prolactin
Recent surgery or trauma	Relationship to onset
Sexual activity	Relationship to discharge

*Red flags more suggestive of breast cancer than other signs or symptoms; however, any persistent symptom needs a workup.

and for a single second-degree relative (grand-mother, aunt, niece) the pooled RR was 1.5 (range, 1.2 to 1.9). The increased risk, however, is also dependent on whether the relative was pre- or postmenopausal at diagnosis (risk increases if the relative was premenopausal) and whether one or both breasts are involved (risk increases if both breasts are involved). For example, a woman whose mother was diagnosed after menopause with breast cancer on one side has a risk of breast cancer that is very similar to that of a women with no such family history (RR = 1.2 versus 1.0).[5]

Two genetic mutations increase the risk of breast cancer. Mutations in BRCA-1 (located on chromosome 17) and BRCA-2 (located on chromosome 13) are inherited in an autosomal dominant pattern. Having one of these genetic mutations increases the lifetime risk of breast cancer to 60 to 90 percent. There is also an increased absolute risk of ovarian cancer (15 to 60 percent) and colon cancer (6 percent) among women with one of these genetic mutations.[6] The prevalence of these genes, however, in the general population is likely to be small. Based on a case-control study including women with a first invasive breast cancer and age-matched controls, the proportion of patients with breast cancer with disease-related genetic variants was only 3.3 percent (0 to 7.2 percent of white women and 0 percent of black women).[7]

PERSONAL HISTORY

A personal history of breast, ovarian, or endo-metrial cancer is also associated with an increased risk of subsequent breast cancer. Among women with prior breast cancer, the 5-year absolute risk of developing a second breast cancer is 2 to 5 percent.[8] In addition, an increased risk of breast cancer is also associated with breast tissue biopsies showing proliferative disease (e.g., moderate or florid hyperplasia or papilloma [RR = 1.5 to 2.0] or atypical hyperplasia [RR = 3 to 5]).[9] A summary, based on current literature, of the risk of breast cancer with benign lesions on biopsy is shown in Table 16-3.

REPRODUCTIVE HISTORY

With respect to reproductive experience, a first pregnancy resulting in a live birth before age 30 and a fewer number of years menstruating (i.e., years of exposure to endogenous ovarian hormone including later menarche, early menopause, and greater amount of time spent while pregnant or lactating and not cycling) are protective against breast cancer.[10] Lactation does not appear to be associated with a decrease in breast cancer risk,[11] but should be encouraged because of the nutritional and other benefits to the infant. There is

Table 16-3

Risk of Breast Cancer with Benign Breast Lesions

PATHOLOGIC CRITERIA	INCIDENCE	RELATIVE RISK OF BREAST CANCER
Nonproliferative	70%	1.0
Proliferative without atypia	26%	1.6 (1.3–1.9)
Atypical hyperplasia	4%	4.4 (3.7–5.3)

SOURCE: Dupont WD, Page DL: Risk factors for breast cancer in women with proliferative breast disease. *N Engl J Med* 312:146, 1985.
Dupont WD, Parl FF, Hartman WH, et al: Breast cancer risk associated with proliferative breast disease and atypical hyperplasia. *Cancer* 71:1258, 1993.
London SJ, Connolly JL, Schnitt SJ, et al: A prospective study of benign breast disease and the risk of cancer. *JAMA* 267:941, 1992.

also no association between breast cancer and induced abortion or miscarriage.[12]

ALCOHOL INTAKE

Alcohol intake appears to increase the relative risk of breast cancer by about 30 to 40 percent (RR = 1.3 to 1.4) for moderate drinkers (1 or more alcoholic beverages per day) compared with non-drinkers of alcohol.[13]

USE OF HORMONES

There is a small increase in the risk of breast cancer among current users of either oral contraceptives (OCs) or HRT (RR = 1.24 and 1.35, respectively) (see Chaps. 2 and 4). The increased risk for both appears to return to baseline 5 years after discontinuing use.[14,15]

THE GAIL MODEL

A useful method of estimating individual probabilities of developing breast cancer among white women who are being examined yearly was developed by Gail et al.[16] The probabilities are based on data derived from over 280,000 women who participated in the Breast Cancer Detection Demonstration Project (BCDDP). The model uses five factors (age at menarche, number of previous breast biopsies, presence or absence of atypical hyperplasia on biopsy, age at first live birth, and number of first-degree relatives [mother or sisters] with breast cancer) to determine an absolute 5-year and lifetime risk of breast cancer for an individual woman. A computer disk or computer program that can be used to calculate this risk estimate based on individual patient data can be obtained through the National Cancer Institute Web site: http://www.nci.nih.gov.

Use of the information derived from this method may be helpful both in planning clinical trials and in assisting selected women in decision-making for future treatment and surveillance. However, there are a number of problems with this model including a tendency to overestimate risk for younger women and an absence of consideration of other risk factors such as inherited genetic mutations, personal history of breast or ovarian cancer, relative's menstrual status at time of diagnosis of breast cancer, and use of hormones. The former was demonstrated in a study attempting to replicate the predictive ability of the model on a second population, women enrolled in the Nurses' Health Study, a group not engaged in annual screening.[17] They found that the model overpredicted absolute breast cancer risk by 33 percent, with an overprediction of more than twofold among premenopausal women, among women with extensive family history of breast cancer, and among women with age at first birth younger than 20 years.

Symptoms

Women should be asked whether they have any breast symptoms including pain, identified lumps, nipple discharge, or skin changes. These specific symptoms will be discussed in detail in the following sections.

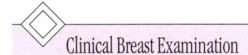

Clinical Breast Examination

The clinical breast examination (CBE) should include inspection and careful palpation of the entire breast region (bordered by the sternum in the middle, the inframammary crease inferiorly, the clavicle superiorly, and the anterior axillary line laterally) and the associated lymph node chains (Table 16-4). Breasts should be inspected initially with the patient in the sitting position, looking for differences between the breasts in size, symmetry, and shape in addition to skin abnormalities, such as color change, dimpling or puckering (peau d'orange), and unilateral and new nipple inversion or scars. Two additional maneuvers, having the woman raise her arms (thus exposing the lateral sides and inferior portion of the breasts) and having her contract her

Table 16-4

Components of the Clinical Breast Examination

Observation (three positions*)
  Size
  Symmetry
  Shape
  Skin color
  Skin texture
  Nipple/areola
  Skin retraction
Palpation of lymph nodes (woman sitting)
  Supraclavicular
  Infraclavicular
  Axillary
Palpation of breast (woman sitting and supine;
  select pattern†)
  Background nodularity
  Dominant mass/thickening
  Nipple compression if spontaneous nipple
    discharge reported

*Positions are sitting with arms at sides, with arms raised, and with hands on hips while pushing inward to contract the pectoralis muscles.

†Three patterns are recommended: wedge, vertical strip, and circular (see Fig. 16-2).

pectoralis muscles (by placing her hands on her hips and pushing in tightly) may reveal underlying contour changes in breast tissues that would not otherwise be seen. The latter maneuver is particularly useful in detecting skin retraction from tumors involving Cooper's ligaments.

The next step, while the woman is seated, is to palpate the supraclavicular and infraclavicular lymph node regions for the presence of enlarged lymph nodes. The latter areas can be palpated simultaneously while the examiner is standing in front of the woman. The axillary lymph nodes are then palpated with the examiner supporting the woman's elbow. Examining the axillary nodes in this manner allows the axillary fat pad to move forward, allowing better access to this lymph node chain.

The breasts may then be palpated while the woman is sitting, using a bimanual approach. This is not necessary in every woman, but may be helpful in examining a woman with pendulous breasts. The breasts are palpated to identify areas of breast tissue thickening or nodularity or the presence of masses. Once the woman is supine, it is important that the breast tissue be palpated against the firm background of her chest wall. To achieve this with a woman who has large breasts, she may have to be rotated slightly with a pillow under her scapula to allow for the breast tissue to spread out across the chest wall. Alternatively, manual displacement of the breast tissue, to centralize the portion to be examined against the chest wall, can be done.

Three patterns of breast palpation may be used to ensure that the entire breast is systematically examined (Fig. 16-2). The pattern of palpation is a matter of choice, although adopting some pattern is recommended over random palpation. One study of breast self-examination (BSE) showed that the vertical strip method may be more effective.[18] Whatever pattern is chosen, the main objective is to systematically palpate the whole area using both light touch and deep palpation to assess the entire volume of breast tissue, including the retroareolar area. This is done using the pads of the first three fingers of the examiner's hand, covering a dime-sized area for each examining finger. When assessing the breasts for nodularity and tissue thickening, it is helpful to examine the symmetry between the two breasts. In this way, subtle thickenings felt on palpation of one breast can be compared to the opposite breast in the mirror image location. Symmetry on examination is usually an indication of the examination being normal. Palpation of the nipple in a woman who does not have a history of persistent spontaneous nipple discharge is not recommended. In women with a history of spontaneous nipple discharge, the last step of the examination is to compress the nipple gently in the horizontal and vertical direction to check for discharge. If this technique fails to elicit the discharge, firm pressure should be applied from the periphery toward the nipple.

Congenital abnormalities that may be seen on CBE include nipple inversion, hypomastia, Poland's syndrome (hypomastia of one breast with absence

Figure 16-2

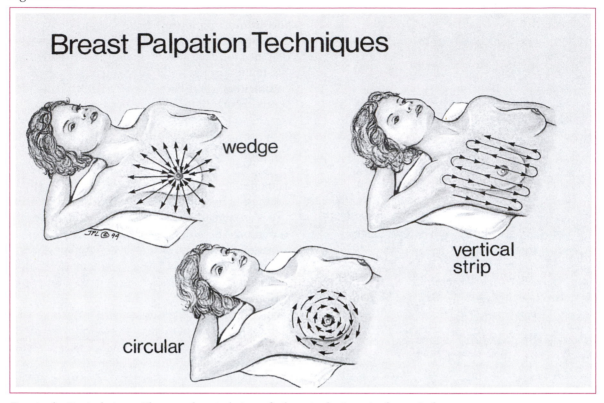

Breast palpation techniques. There are three techniques for breast palpation: circular, vertical strip, and wedge. Any of these methods are appropriate as long as the entire pentagon-shaped area of the breast is examined. *(Reproduced with permission from JR Osuch et al. Alexandria, VA: American Medical Women's Association, copyright 1994.)*

of the pectoralis major muscle), and supernumerary breast/nipples. With respect to nipple inversion, the nipples evert as one of the final steps in breast development. If a woman indicates that her nipple has been inverting over time from an everted state, the clinician should be alerted to the possibility of periductal mastitis or subareolar carcinoma. Hypomastia can be congenital or acquired, the latter caused by ill-placed chest tubes in the neonatal period, chest wall radiation therapy prior to pubescence, or inappropriate surgical resection of the breast bud.

Supernumerary breasts or nipples occur in about 10 percent of the population and are inherited as an autosomal dominant characteristic. Super-

numerary breasts are most frequently found in the axilla. Because the tissue is hormonally responsive, it can become engorged and painful during cycling or pregnancy. Polythelia, or extra nipples, may occur with or without associated breast tissue usually in an inframammary location anywhere from groin to neck. These may be mistaken for skin tags or moles.

The CBE may be challenging in women with breast implants. The natural breast tissue may be palpated using a displacement technique.[19] With the patient sitting, examination of the breast tissue may be accomplished by having the woman lean forward, allowing the breast tissue to be gently examined in the transverse and longitudinal planes.

When supine, the implant can often be systematically displaced away from the examining hand using the wedge pattern of palpation, allowing for examination of the natural breast tissue. This may not be possible in all areas if the implant is firm or fixed. The integrity of the implants should also be assessed, if possible, and changes in size, shape, and compressibility (usually bilaterally symmetric and soft). Pain, however, may be the only sign of rupture, and axillary lymphadenopathy may be present.

It is important to spend an adequate amount of time doing the CBE because the time spent is correlated with accuracy of findings.[20] It may be helpful for the clinician to remember the steps in terms of seven P's. These are positions, palpation (including perimeter, pattern of search, palpation with pads, and pressure), and patient education. This is a part of a step-by-step approach to the CBE that can be found on Medscape.[21] An ideal time to teach BSE to a woman is while performing the CBE.

Breast Pain

Breast pain, also known as mastalgia or mastodynia, is a common condition most often affecting women in their middle thirties. Many women experience some degree of breast discomfort during their lives, especially in relationship to their menstrual cycle. In one primary care study of 443 women, 47 percent reported cyclic breast pain.[22] Breast pain is the most common presenting breast complaint in primary care practice.[23] Breast pain can interfere with daily activities, and a woman's sexuality can be affected if her breasts are too tender to be touched. In addition, many women are concerned about cancer, although breast pain alone is not a frequent presenting symptom in patients with breast cancer. In one study, although 15 percent of women with breast cancer presented with pain, only 7 percent had pain as their only

symptom.[24] This study was conducted before the availability of screening mammography, however, and in most patients, masses were detected on CBE; in the remainder of the cases, masses were palpated on follow-up. Although breast pain is self-limited in up to 85 percent of the cases, the complaint should be addressed and the woman should be carefully evaluated.

Etiology

The etiology of breast pain is often unclear. Most commonly breast pain is cyclic. A hormonal etiology is assumed to be present; studies have shown alterations in prolactin response to thyrotropin-releasing hormone,[25] and increased fatty acid profiles are seen in women with breast pain.[26] However, studies of levels of circulating progesterone, estrogen, and prolactin have yielded conflicting results. Cyclic mastalgia is typically bilateral and starts when a woman is in her thirties, although similar symptoms may be seen among postmenopausal women on HRT. The breasts are tender in the week or two before the onset of menses, with the pain gradually subsiding during the menses. For some women there is mild sensitivity; to others it can be quite painful. In one study, cyclic breast pain was reported by 66 percent of women, with 21 percent of women reporting severe pain.[27]

Breast pain can also be continuous or noncyclic in about one-third of the cases. This type of mastalgia is typically unilateral and usually affects women in their forties. The pain is not temporally related to the menstrual cycle. The pain can interfere with activities because movement will often worsen the breast pain. Most often, a specific cause for breast pain is not found. However, it is important to keep in mind that although pain is not a common presenting symptom of breast cancer, this diagnosis must still be considered. Of women presenting with breast pain who have a normal CBE and radiologic studies, cancer will be found in about 0.5 percent on follow-up.[11] This necessitates 3- to 6-month follow-up examinations in all women with persistent mastalgia.

Other causes of noncyclic breast pain include costochondritis (Tietze's syndrome), reported to occur in approximately 7 percent of cases,[28] and rare causes including prior breast surgery or radiation, trauma, duct ectasia, Mondor's disease (phlebitis of the thoracoepigastric vein), and cervical radiculopathy causing referred pain.

Diagnosis of Breast Pain

HISTORY

Aspects of a focused history for the problem of breast pain are shown in Table 16-2. Because women do not often complain of breast pain to their clinician unless the symptoms are severe, it may be helpful to routinely ask about breast tenderness in the general history. This question may fit comfortably when asking about other premenstrual symptoms or just before the CBE. When breast tenderness is revealed, the clinician should attempt to determine the location, duration, and severity of the discomfort and whether the pain is unilateral or bilateral. Asking whether the pain changes with her menstrual cycle will help to establish whether the pain is cyclic or noncyclic. The clinician should also evaluate the degree to which the pain worries the patient and in what ways the pain affects the woman's life (e.g., interference with exercise, hugs, sexual activity, and sleep).

The history should also include current use of OCs and HRT. Rarely, other agents can cause breast pain (e.g., reserpine). Pregnancy should also be considered with bilateral pain of recent onset. Information about previous breast problems or surgery should be sought.

Women with cyclic mastalgia often describe their pain as dull, aching, heavy, or sore and located in the upper outer quadrants of both breasts. Women with noncyclic pain often describe the pain as sharp, burning, or drawing, more commonly located in the subareolar or medial portions of the breast. Nonbreast causes may result in symptoms such as pain radiating down the arm or axilla or pain with deep inspiration.

PHYSICAL EXAMINATION

A CBE should be performed during the office visit with particular attention to areas of focal pain. Sometimes women will have significant pain during the examination and may be reluctant to let the clinician perform a thorough and adequate examination. For these women, premedication with a nonsteroidal anti-inflammatory drug (NSAID) or narcotic agent could be helpful. Inspection is directed at searching for evidence of trauma or old surgical scars; both are related to noncyclic mastalgia. Although nodularity is common to both cyclic and noncyclic breast pain, the presence of a dominant mass should prompt a workup to rule out malignancy (see next section). Pain reproduced by palpation of the lateral chest wall or costochondral junction suggests a musculoskeletal etiology, as does pain with neck motion.

DIAGNOSTIC PROCEDURES

If the woman is 35 years of age or older and has unilateral/focal pain, diagnostic mammography should be considered. For other women, mammography should be performed based on screening guidelines (see Chap. 1). Mammography requires that each individual breast be pressed between two metal plates to get an adequate image; it may, therefore, cause excruciating discomfort for a woman whose breasts are already painful. Premedication with an NSAID or narcotic agent can be helpful for relieving some of the discomfort if mammography is planned, and the mammogram technician should be alerted about the pain before the test. For women with cyclic pain, planning the test during days 3 to 10 of the menstrual cycle should be considered. If any masses or cysts are found, the appropriate workup should be completed (see next section).

Management

Mastalgia is a frustrating condition for both patient and provider because little is known about it and there is little scientific basis for treatment. Most important is to be supportive of the woman's experience of pain and to acknowledge what she is saying about its effects on her life. Discussing a step-wise approach to different treatment modalities, as described here, is also helpful. It is reassuring to note that mastalgia will often spontaneously resolve; in one study of the long-term course of mastalgia in 212 women, 43 percent of women with cyclic mastalgia and 46 percent of women with noncyclic mastalgia reported resolution of pain.[29] For women with cyclic mastalgia, resolution was commonly associated with menopause, whereas in women with noncyclic mastalgia resolution more often seemed spontaneous. Improvement, however, often occurred over many years, and the average duration of pain was long (median 12 years).[29] For some women, just knowing that the pain is not a likely sign of cancer is helpful. In fact, reassurance after a negative evaluation may be all that is needed. The algorithm presented in Fig. 16-3 presents an approach to the diagnosis and management of mastalgia. Cyclic mastalgia is generally more responsive to treatment than noncyclic breast pain.

BREAST PAIN DIARY

Sometimes additional information will assist in making a diagnosis. As with many types of pain, it is helpful for the patient to rate the pain subjectively in a prospective manner, noting situations that seem to improve or worsen the pain. This information contributes to a better understanding of the level of discomfort and can help to differentiate cyclic from noncyclic mastalgia. An example of a breast pain diary is shown in Fig. 16-4. After 2 to 3 months of baseline recording, a repeat CBE is performed if pain persists. If the examination does not reveal an abnormality, treatment may be initiated as described below. The breast pain diary should be continued after treatment to determine more accurately the effectiveness of therapy by comparing pre- and posttreatment information.

PHYSICAL MODALITIES

Wearing a properly fitting brassiere may be helpful in minimizing breast movement and, therefore, reducing overall pain. In an English study of 100 women with breast pain, 75 experienced relief after being professionally fitted, regardless of their age, cup size, or underlying breast disease.[30] Sometimes, a brassiere can be worn at night to improve sleep.

DIETARY ADJUSTMENTS

Controlled studies have not been able to confirm any benefit to caffeine reduction for mastalgia. Anecdotally, however, many women do report improvement with limiting caffeine intake, and an active intervention may provide women with a sense of control over the disorder and is therefore perceived as helpful.

Restriction of fat intake to 15 percent of total calories was shown to be effective in reducing breast tenderness after 6 months in one study.[31] This level of fat restriction, however, is difficult to achieve. Here again, there are overall health benefits to fat intake restriction, and if the woman is willing, she can try this as a treatment modality for her breast pain. Vitamin B and E supplements have not been proven to be of benefit.

MEDICATION ADJUSTMENT OR ELIMINATION

Consider reducing or eliminating the hormonal content of OCs or HRT regimens (see Chaps. 2 and 4). Encourage the woman to continue her breast pain diary and review any changes in reported pain before and after the medicine is reduced or discontinued.

PHARMACOLOGIC TREATMENT

If pain persists after an initial attempt at nonpharmacologic therapy, six medications have been shown to be beneficial; the first five have been confirmed as helpful in controlled clinical trials. These medications, along with the suggested doses, response rates, and side effects are listed in Table 16-5. Bromocriptine and tamoxifen, although shown to be of benefit, are not generally recommended because of their adverse effects. In addition, the lack of information about the long-term

Figure 16-3

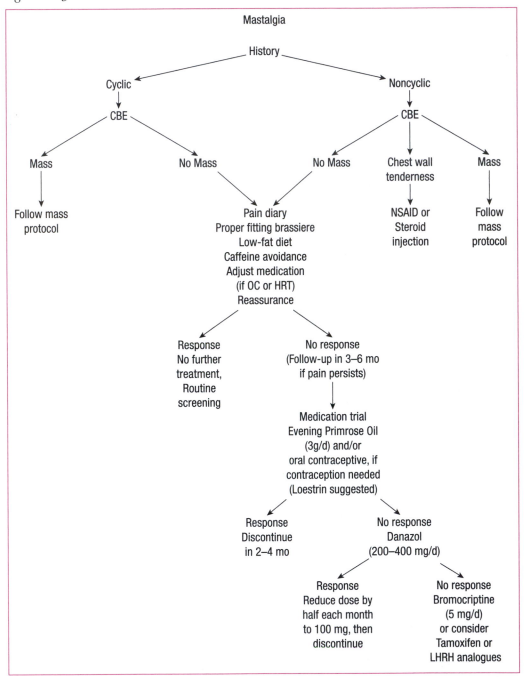

Algorithm for mastalgia. CBE, clinical breast examination; HRT, hormone replacement therapy; LHRH, luteinizing hormone-releasing hormone; NSAID, nonsteroidal anti-inflammatory drug; OC, oral contraceptive. (*Modified with permission from Schwartz K: Breast problems. In: Sloane PD, Slatt LM, Curtis P, Ebell MH [eds]: Essentials of Family Medicine, 3rd ed. Baltimore: Williams & Wilkins; 1998;340.*)

Figure 16-4

	Breast Pain Diary	
Day of month	Pain Scale (0=no pain, 10=worst pain)	Comments (things that make it better/worse)
1	0_____10	
2	0_____10	
3	0_____10	
4	0_____10	
5	0_____10	
6	0_____10	
7	0_____10	
8	0_____10	
9	0_____10	
10	0_____10	
11	0_____10	
12	0_____10	
13	0_____10	
14	0_____10	
15	0_____10	
16	0_____10	
17	0_____10	
18	0_____10	
19	0_____10	
20	0_____10	
21	0_____10	
22	0_____10	
23	0_____10	
24	0_____10	
25	0_____10	
26	0_____10	
27	0_____10	
28	0_____10	
29	0_____10	
30	0_____10	
31	0_____10	

Circle the days you have your period.

Breast pain diary.

Table 16-5

Treatments for Mastodynia

| MEDICATION | DOSE | RESPONSE RATES† | | SIDE EFFECTS* AND PRECAUTIONS |
		CYCLIC MASTODYNIA	NONCYCLIC MASTODYNIA	
Evening primrose oil (Gamma-linolenic acid)	3 g/d or 1 g tid	44–58%	27%	Nausea,* bloating*
Danazol	100 mg bid x 2 mo, may increase to 200 mg bid if need-ed, then taper to lowest effective dose	70–80%	31%	Alterations of menstrual cycle,* weight gain,* amenorrhea, acne, leg cramps, decreased libido
Oral contraceptive	1/d (28-d pack)	Not studied	Not studied	Nausea,* spotting,* dizziness, headache weight gain, breast tenderness
Bromocriptine	1.25 mg at bedtime, increase over 2 wk up to 2.5 mg bid	47–65%	20%	Nausea,* headache,* dizziness,* seizures, stroke
Tamoxifen	10 mg/d for 3–6 mo	71–90%	Not studied	Increased risk of endometrial cancer and osteoporosis with long-term use
Luteinizing hormone-releasing hormone analogues	Varies depending on product	50–80%	80%	Abrupt onset of menopausal symptoms* (hot flashes, irritability), nausea, headache

*Common side effects.
†Response rates of 20–30% are seen with placebo.

effects of the luteinizing hormone-releasing hormone (LHRH) analogues on bone metabolism limits the use of these medications as well.

Studies have shown that women with benign breast disease are more likely to have lower levels of γ-linolenic acid (an essential fatty acid) than women without breast disease,[32] and several studies have documented the effectiveness of evening primrose oil (9 percent γ-linolenic acid) in decreas-ing breast pain in women with cyclic mastalgia.[33,34] A beneficial effect may not manifest for 3 to 4 months. There are few side effects, so it can be selected as a first-line therapy choice. However, evening primrose oil is expensive, costing up to $2 daily for recommended dosing (see Table 16-5).

Vitamins have commonly been cited in the lay press as a treatment for breast tenderness. Randomized studies looking at vitamins E, B$_1$, and B$_6$ have not shown any effectiveness in the treatment of mastalgia.

PRESCRIPTION MEDICATIONS Several reviews are available that discuss medical therapy in detail.[13,35] Danazol is the only drug approved by the Food and Drug Administration (FDA) for the treatment of mastalgia (see Table 16-5). Controlled trials have shown benefit in 70 to 80 percent of women.[36,37] It is especially effective for cyclic mastalgia in that it suppresses the pituitary-ovarian axis and binds to estrogen and progesterone receptors. Side effects are common at higher doses (see Table 16-5). Once an effective dose is determined, the dose can be tapered gradually to the lowest effective dose for maintenance (100 mg qd or every other day). A course of therapy lasting 2 to 4 months is often sufficient to relieve pain and prevent its recurrence. A recent randomized controlled trial of 200 mg danazol on days 14 to 28 of the menstrual cycle for three cycles demonstrated clinical efficacy during all 3 months of drug administration with a drop-out rate of only 3 percent.[38] Effective nonhormonal contraception is required because danazol is potentially teratogenic.

In general, women using OCs have a decreased incidence of fibrocystic changes and fewer breast biopsies than women who do not use OCs. Although some OCs may cause breast tenderness in some women, they may be considered as a treatment option for women with mastalgia who also need contraception. In one series of 182 patients with a diagnosis of fibrocystic breast disease and associated breast pain, Loestrin 1/20 provided relief of subjective symptoms (pain, tenderness) in about 90 percent of patients within 3 to 6 months.[39] OCs may be used in combination with evening primrose oil. One recent study showed that women using long-acting medroxyprogesterone (Depo-Provera®) had a significantly lower rate of breast pain compared to controls.[40]

Bromocriptine suppresses prolactin secretion. It has been effective in the treatment of women with cyclic mastalgia.[41,42] Although studies have shown this to be effective in cyclic breast pain, side effects with bromocriptine can be severe (see Table 16-5). Side effects, however, can be minimized by gradually increasing the dose over several weeks. Bromocriptine is no longer indicated for lactation suppression because of its potential adverse effects of seizures, stroke, and death. It has not been approved by the FDA for the treatment of mastalgia.

Tamoxifen is an estrogen agonist-antagonist used for both prevention of breast cancer in high-risk women and as an adjunct treatment for breast cancer. Controlled trials have demonstrated success in the treatment of cyclic breast pain[43]; however, relapse rates on discontinuing therapy are reported to be 30 percent.[44] In a small randomized trial of tamoxifen versus danazol or placebo for the treatment of severe cyclic mastalgia, tamoxifen relieved pain in significantly more women (72 percent, 65 percent, 38 percent for tamoxifen, danazol, and placebo, respectively).[45] In addition, more women treated with tamoxifen for the 6-month treatment period remained free of symptoms 1 year after discontinuation of therapy (53 percent, 37 percent, 0 percent for tamoxifen, danazol, and placebo, respectively). Because of the increased risk of endometrial cancer with tamoxifen, however, its use for breast pain should be limited to severe cases that do not respond to other therapies, and the duration of therapy should probably be limited to 2 to 3 months at a time.

The LHRH analogues completely inhibit ovarian production of estrogen and progesterone. Benefit has been reported for women with mastalgia refractory to other therapies, with greater benefit shown with use of injection rather than nasal spray.[46,47] However, these agents have not been evaluated in controlled trials. Side effects are significant, and long-term effects on bone metabolism (due to the hypoestrogenic state induced by these medications) are unknown. Therefore, these agents should be reserved for severe, unresponsive cases.

Investigators from the United Kingdom in a recent case series of 26 women with mastodynia reported that the use of topical NSAIDs (diclofenac or piroxicam) in a gel form applied to the breasts up to four times a day provided satisfactory relief of pain in 81 percent of the women.[48] Although these agents are not available in topical form in the United States, similar products may be compounded by pharmacists.

Diuretics, especially spironolactone, have often been tried for mastodynia. There is no evidence, however, that they are effective.

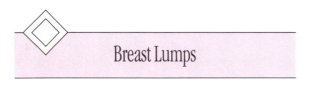

Breast Lumps

Breast lumps are a common problem for women and the second most common breast complaint.[8] Having a breast lump detected is a frightening experience for most women, and it is especially important in these situations to maintain adequate communication throughout the period of workup, problem identification, and management.

Most lumps (67 percent) are discovered by palpation. Of those lumps that are detected, the majority are detected by the woman herself. In one study, 60 percent of women with breast cancer presented with a self-discovered mass.[49]

Types of Breast Lumps

There are four basic types of palpable breast masses that occur in a woman's breast. These are fibroadenomas, cysts, benign breast nodularity (also called fibrocystic breast change), and cancer. The predominant type of breast lump changes with the age of the woman (Table 16-6). Fibroadenomas predominate in younger women (adolescents and women in their twenties and thirties) with 35 to 50 percent occurring in women under age 30.[50] Although solid masses predominate in all age groups, benign lumps are found predominantly in women between the ages of 20 and 55.[34] Masses composed solely of cystic fluid are uncommon in women before the age of 35 and in postmenopausal women but are very common in perimenopausal women. Cysts can also be found in postmenopausal women on HRT. The most common etiology of a breast mass in a postmenopausal woman is carcinoma.

Of all solid lumps biopsied annually in the United States, 25 percent are cancerous.[51] The prevalence of cancer increases with age of the patient; 85 percent of lumps in women over age 55 are found to be cancerous (Fig. 16-5). Although cancer is less common in premenopausal women with lumps, the incidence of the disease in this age group is high enough that every breast symptom requires evaluation. The incidence of cancer among pregnant and lactating women is the same as the incidence among nonpregnant women of the same age.[52]

Diagnosing Breast Lumps

The complete evaluation of a breast mass involves three steps: (1) the history and clinical breast examination; (2) a mammogram before or after aspiration (usually omitted if the woman is less than 30 years old or is pregnant, unless malignancy is strongly suspected); and (3) fine-needle aspiration or referral to a surgeon. Clinicians are encouraged to develop a systematic approach to the assessment and documentation of findings for this complaint. The differential diagnosis of a breast mass is shown in Table 16-6.

HISTORY

Important elements in a focused history for a woman presenting with a breast mass are listed in Table 16-2. The location, characteristics of the mass, and any associated nipple discharge are often helpful in establishing a clinical suspicion for benign versus malignant lesions. However, any persistent breast symptom requires a workup, even if the clinical impression is one of likely benign disease. A breast cancer risk factor assessment should also be obtained as described in the earlier section on breast history.

Table 16-6

Differential Diagnosis of Breast Mass

DIAGNOSIS	AGE GROUP (YEARS)	LIKELIHOOD OF DIAGNOSIS (%)	USUAL CHARACTERISTICS OF THE MASS
Breast cancer	(Common in older women)		Unilateral, hard, and immobile
	<25	<1	
	26–40	5–10	
	41–50	10–20	
	51–70	50–80	
	>70	>80	
Breast cyst	(Somewhat common in perimenopausal women)		Unilateral, soft, and well defined
	<25	1–4	
	26–40	2–5	
	41–50	10–20	
	51–70	7–12	
	>70	<10	
Fibroadenoma	(Common in young women)		Unilateral, smooth, and mobile
	<25	50–75	
	26–40	15–30	
	41–50	10–20	
	51–70	<5	
	>70	<1	
Fibrocystic changes	(Common in young women)		Bilateral, soft, and irregular; change with cycle
	<25	10–25	
	26–40	30–40	
	41–50	Uncommon	
	51–70	Uncommon*	
	>70	Rare	
Duct papilloma		Uncommon for all ages, but most frequent at ages 30–50	Unilateral subareolar mass with discharge

*More frequent in women on hormone replacement therapy.
SOURCE: Reproduced with permission form Schwartz K: Breast problems. In: Sloane PD, Slatt LM, Curtis P, Ebell MH (eds): *Essentials of Family Medicine,* 3rd ed. Baltimore:Williams & Wilkins; 1998;341.

PHYSICAL EXAMINATION

A CBE should be completed on women presenting with a breast mass to further characterize the mass and determine whether any other abnormalities exist. If a mass is palpated on CBE, it is important to document the location and size of the mass and describe its palpable features. The mass should be evaluated to determine its consistency (soft, firm, hard), mobility (mobile or fixed to the skin or chest wall), and contour (well-circumscribed or irregular). A charting diagram for the CBE is often helpful for accurate documentation (Fig. 16-6). If a mass is found, palpate the opposite breast to confirm that it is asymmetrical. If a mirror image mass or thickening is present, the finding can be

Figure 16-5

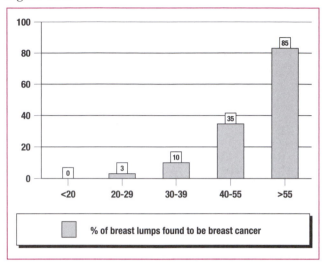

Breast cancer found in breast lumps by age. *(Reproduced with permission from N Love: Primary Care Consideration in Breast Diagnosis. Tampa, FL; American Cancer Society, copyright 1992.)*

considered normal unless the features of the findings differ.

In the progress note, the clinician should carefully document which breast is affected and describe the location in relation to the face of a clock (see Fig. 16-6). Measuring the distance of the mass from the nipple adds to the accuracy of the documentation. If a mass cannot be confirmed on CBE, record the patient's findings and location by history and reexamine the patient in 3 to 6 months.

Next, the clinician needs to determine whether the mass is solid or cystic. A mass that is fluid filled (a cyst) is characteristically well circumscribed, usually round, and sometimes ballotable (able to compress wall), but often firm and indistinguishable from solid lumps. They may be solitary, multiple, or clustered. Solid masses can be any shape, vary in texture from rubbery to firm, can be ballotable, and are typically solitary, although they may present with multiple foci in advanced carcinoma. The typical mass of the past representing a malignancy was immobile and rock hard with irregular borders. It is extremely uncommon to diagnose a malignancy in masses with these

characteristics in today's clinical setting. Physical characteristics alone, however, should not dictate the subsequent evaluation. Malignant masses may

Figure 16-6

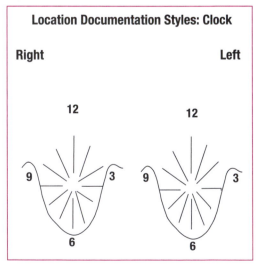

Document for recording physical findings (mass or abnormality is drawn into diagram).

resemble cysts (soft and well defined), fibroadenomas (smooth, mobile, and well defined), or fibrocystic masses (soft and irregular) on physical examination. Overall, the results of physical examination are accurate (true positive + true negative/total patients) in only 60 to 80 percent of cases, and there is often poor agreement among even experienced examiners.[53,54]

If the woman is premenopausal and the mass is vague or questionable, a reexamination of the breasts in a woman who is cycling is recommended within the next month on day 3 to 10 of the menstrual cycle. Any suspicious or persistent breast mass that is identified deserves further evaluation.

DIAGNOSTIC PROCEDURES

OFFICE APPROACH The algorithm presented in Fig. 16-7 outlines the suggested evaluation and management of a breast mass. If the lump is assessed to be cystic by palpation, the clinician could perform an office aspiration procedure of the mass, which can be both diagnostic and therapeutic. Many anxious weeks experienced by women with a palpable abnormality could be eliminated if primary care clinicians became more comfortable with this simple in-office procedure. Ultrasound in women with palpable (as opposed to occult) breast masses is discouraged. It is not cost-effective because, should the ultrasound reveal a cyst, then an aspiration procedure should be performed, and if the ultrasound reveals a solid mass, the finding would not change the clinical management.

Aspiration of a cyst involves placement of a 21- to 23-gauge needle attached to a 5- to 10-mL syringe into the mass, with vacuum aspiration applied manually during the procedure. If the mass is cystic, fluid will fill the barrel of the syringe and the mass will disappear. The color of the fluid removed from a cyst varies greatly, with lighter fluid obtained from cysts of more recent onset and darker fluid found in older cysts. The changes in pigment occur when the epithelial lining of the cyst degenerates and the cells fall into the cystic fluid.

If bloody fluid is obtained on aspiration, curtail the procedure and document the location of the mass so that the consulting physician will know the exact location. The fluid may be sent for cytology, but the patient should be referred for mammography and surgical consultation. Bloody aspirates may represent benign intraductal papillomas, duct ectasia, or carcinoma, with the majority representing intraductal papillomas. Sending nonbloody fluid for cytologic analysis is sometimes done for cyst aspirates from postmenopausal women who are not on HRT, but cysts are uncommon in this clinical setting. Purulent aspirates represent an abscess. In these cases, the fluid obtained should be sent for culture and the abscess treated with incision, drainage, and packing. Other nonbloody aspirates may be discarded. The cytopathologist in the referral laboratory and the clinician should discuss the recommended procedure before sending such samples.

If the aspiration completely collapses the cyst and the fluid is not bloody, the patient may be followed for recurrence. Reaccumulation would require reaspiration, and a second reaccumulation would require referral for surgical excision. It is extremely important to palpate for total mass disappearance and to ensure that there is complete symmetry between one breast and the other at the end of the procedure.

If the aspiration indicates that the mass is solid or residual mass is present after cyst aspiration, most primary care providers would make a prompt referral to a breast surgeon or breast care center, either before or after ordering a mammogram (planned for 2 to 3 weeks after cyst aspiration). Others may choose to pursue the workup with a fine-needle aspiration biopsy (FNAB, see below).

RADIOGRAPHIC EVALUATION If the lump is judged to be solid, either by palpation or diagnostic exclusion from the cyst workup, then further investigation of the lesion should be conducted. A diagnostic mammogram should be performed for women over age 35. It is important to note that diagnostic mammography is not used to rule out breast cancer within the identified mass, but rather is performed to rule out clinically occult lesions in the breasts. An interval of 2 to 3 weeks

Figure 16-7

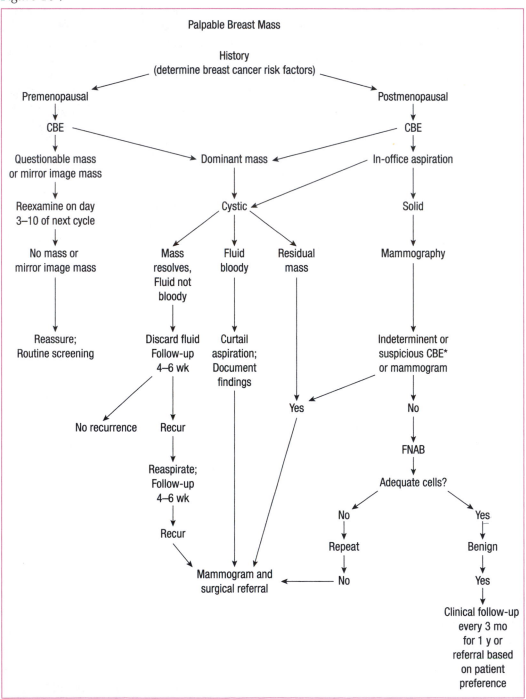

Algorithm for evaluation and management of a breast mass. CBE, clinical breast examination; FNAB, fine-needle aspiration biopsy.

between the mammogram and cyst aspiration is recommended to avoid confusing a possible hematoma with other breast abnormalities. Test characteristics of mammography compared to other diagnostic procedures are shown in Table 16-7.

For women under age 35 with a breast mass, some breast imaging radiologists will recommend ultrasound over mammography to evaluate solid masses because the density of the breast tissue in younger women impedes the reading of a mammogram and the breast tissue is more potentially radiosensitive. The use of mammography for younger women with breast masses can be discussed with the local radiologist specializing in breast imaging. It is important to note that mammograms have both a high false-positive and a high false-negative rate, particularly in younger women. In the BCDDP project, 36 percent of women aged 40 with breast cancer had a normal mammogram compared with 9 percent of women 70 years of age.[55] Therefore, a negative mammogram should not stop the progression of the workup; failure to properly evaluate a breast mass is one of the most common reasons for malpractice litigation.[30]

BIOPSY   Every persistent solid breast mass needs biopsy evaluation. The choice of biopsy technique (open, core, or FNAB) depends on the size and location of the lesion, the size of the breast, the experience and preference of the surgeon/clinician, and the availability of a skilled cytopathologist for cellular interpretation if FNAB is chosen. Although the false-positive rate of FNAB is low, averaging 0.17 percent, the false-negative rate is about 10 percent.[56] Test characteristics of FNAB are shown in Table 16-7. The range of sensitivity and specificity depend on the experience and skill of the person performing the procedure.

Most breast masses in women under age 30 are benign fibroadenomas or other benign conditions, and reevaluation of the abnormality on day 3 to 10 of the next menstrual cycle is suggested before FNAB for premenopausal women. If the mass persists or if the patient is older or at higher risk because of family history, a biopsy should be considered to make a tissue diagnosis. Referral to a breast care center or surgical referral is an additional option.

TRIPLE TEST   If FNAB is chosen as the biopsy technique in evaluating a solid mass, the principles of "triple diagnosis" have been used to increase diagnostic accuracy. This includes CBE, the results of mammography, and the results of FNAB. If one

Table 16-7

Characteristics of Diagnostic Tests Used to Identify Malignancy in a Woman with a Breast Mass

TEST	SENSITIVITY	SPECIFICITY	LR+	LR−
Clinical breast examination	0.92	0.65	2.6	0.12
Mammography	0.89	0.65*	2.5	0.17
Fine-needle aspiration	0.83†	0.90‡	27	0.17
Ultrasound	0.78	0.89	7.1	0.25
CBE + FNA + mammography (one or more individual tests positive is a positive "triple test"; all tests negative is a negative "triple test")	>0.99	0.98	50	0.02

*Range 0.55–0.74.
†Range 0.65–0.99.
‡Range 0.55–0.97, but more recent work suggests a higher specificity.
ABBREVIATIONS: CBE, clinical breast examination; FNA, fine-needle aspiration.
SOURCE: Reproduced with permission from Schwartz K: Breast problems. In: Sloane PD, Slatt LM, Curtis P, Ebell MH (eds): *Essentials of Family Medicine,* 3rd ed. Baltimore:Williams & Wilkins; 1998;342.

or more individual tests are positive or suspicious, the triple test is considered positive and an open biopsy is warranted (see Table 16-7). When all three components of the triple test are interpreted as benign, there is about a 99 percent chance that the lesion is benign. If a woman with a negative triple test chooses to proceed with clinical follow-up, the first follow-up visit should be 3 months later. Subsequent visits should occur at 3-month intervals until the lesion has resolved or has remained stable for 1 year. Using this approach, a 1 percent risk of missing cancer on the initial evaluation must be accepted.

REFERRAL

Some primary care providers prefer to refer women with breast lumps to a breast surgeon or breast care center for workup, diagnosis, and management. In these cases, the provider can assist the patient by providing information about what is likely to happen (or what she may expect) in the process of the workup. Sending copies of any diagnostic tests and previous clinical breast examination findings is helpful to the consultant in making a comprehensive and expedient evaluation.

Management of Breast Lumps

BENIGN DISEASE

FOLLOW-UP Benign breast lesions are usually followed with routine screening (see Chap. 1). Regardless of the outcome of the biopsy, women usually report a heightened fear of breast cancer after being through the process and associated anxiety of a workup for a palpable breast mass. This can lead to improved breast cancer screening behaviors or avoidance of future screening. It is important for clinicians to assess the woman's attitude about future breast cancer screening and ongoing management and monitoring of continuing breast problems.

A tracking system should be developed for follow-up of women with breast abnormalities.

These office recall systems are important for women who need screening or follow-up. For women who seem reluctant to pursue further surveillance, a decision balance exercise may be helpful to analyze her reluctance to comply with screening recommendations and to help her work through some of the barriers to follow-up (Table 16-8).

MALIGNANT DISEASE

REFERRAL The diagnosis of a cancerous lesion will lead to a variety of referrals, including a medical oncologist, surgical oncologist (if not already involved for the biopsy), plastic surgeon, and radiation oncologist. Providing records and reports in a timely fashion will facilitate this process.

ROLE OF THE PRIMARY CARE PROVIDER Although the oncology team will usually assume primary management of the woman's breast cancer, it is important for the primary care provider to maintain good communication with all treatment providers. Often, the primary provider will be relied on to review the options with women and their families and help them through the decision-making process. To assist the patient, a number of informational and self-help materials are available. These breast cancer resources are presented in Table 16-9. Women will usually continue to seek care for non-cancer-related medical problems. Moreover, the primary care provider is an important source of support for the patient and her family during the cancer treatment process.

ALTERNATIVE/COMPLEMENTARY THERAPY

It is important to note that 50 percent of cancer patients seek nontraditional forms of therapy. However, over 80 percent of patients who use complementary healing methods will also use conventional therapies. Because most patients do not discuss their nontraditional methods with their doctor, health providers should regularly question patients about all forms of medications, herbal preparations, and treatments they might be using.

Table 16-8

Decision Balance Exercise for Women Reluctant to Proceed with Screening

	DECISION BALANCE EXERCISE	
	HAVING ANOTHER MAMMOGRAM DESIRED BEHAVIOR	NOT HAVING ANOTHER MAMMOGRAM UNDESIRED BEHAVIOR
Pros	Can find a problem earlier. Make my doctor happy. Gets my family off my case. A negative mammogram would help me worry less.	No pain. Less cost. More convenient. Less stressful. Don't have to deal with it. Doesn't bring up the worry from the last time.
Cons	Painful. Insurance doesn't cover entire cost. Time off from work for appointment. Worry from the minute I make the appointment until I get the result. Embarrassing.	Worry about what might be there. My doctor isn't happy with me. Family gets on my case.

Patient is asked to fill in perceived risks and benefits of each behavior and the clinician discusses this with her. This will identify hidden barriers to the desired behavior and gives the clinician a chance to dispel myths and misconceptions. For example, because pain is a major barrier, the clinician could discuss the option of premedication with an analgesic or narcotic with the patient, as well as discussing the history of pain with the mammogram technician. Low-cost mammograms are often available at certain centers or at certain times of the year (e.g., Breast Cancer Awareness Month). Setting up a speedy appointment with on-site results given could reduce the duration of anxiety.

Fibrocystic Breasts in Context

In the past, the term "fibrocystic disease" was freely used in clinical medicine. In 1982, this term was challenged as being clinically meaningless and frightening to patients,[57] and in 1986, the College of American Pathologists dropped the clinical use of the term in describing pathology findings.[58] Although not recognized as a disease, the term "fibrocystic breasts" continues to be used clinically. Clinicians, however, often have only a vague understanding of its meaning. This has prompted a suggestion for reclassification of benign breast conditions into the ANDI classification (see Table 16-1).

Because "fibrocystic disease or fibrocystic condition" continues to be commonly used, a discussion of its meaning and application is presented here.

The most important aspect to appreciate is that the term can apply to any benign condition of the breast. It is typically used to describe a complex of vague symptoms of breast pain or tenderness, especially if associated with nodularity on CBE. As such, this condition affects up to 80 percent of women of childbearing age and represents a clinical problem of varying degree in about 30 percent of women. It may be defined as cyclic nodularity of the breasts and it is usually bilateral. The nodularity is most often found in the upper, outer quadrant of the breasts. Fibrocystic breasts are often associated with cyclic breast pain. Other terms assigned to this condition are gross cystic disease of the breast,

Table 16-9

Breast Cancer Resources

SUPPORT GROUPS
Local support groups through hospital Local American Cancer Society (ACS) State Department of Public Health Y-ME list of support programs nationwide (1-800-221-2141) Reach to Recovery (ACS office)—visitation service by breast cancer survivor
TELEPHONE HOTLINES
National Cancer Institute (NCI) 1-800-4-CANCER (1-800-422-6237) ACS 1-800-ACS-2345 Y-ME 1-800-221-2141 National Breast Cancer Coalition (202)296-7477 Cancer Care 1-800-813-HOPE (support and counseling) Choice In Dying 1-800-989-WILL (information about living wills, etc.) Corporate Angel Network 1-914-328-1313 (locates free air travel services for people with cancer needing to travel for treatment) National Patient Air Transport Hotline 1-800-296-1212 Mary-Helen Mautner Project for Lesbians with Cancer 1-202-332-5536 National Hospice Organization 1-800-658-8898 National Lymphedema Network 1-800-541-3259 Well Spouse Foundation 1-800-838-0879
WEBSITES

NCI   http://www.nci.nih.gov
        http://rex.nci.nih.gov —news, educational materials, tutorials
        http://cancernet.nci.nih.gov —computerized database of latest treatments, supportive care, screening, prevention, and clinical trials
        http://cancertrials.nci.nih.gov —clinical trials resource center
        www.breastcancerinfo.com —all-purpose website

BOOKLETS
NCI (as above)—Understanding Breast Changes: A Health Guide for All Women; What You Need to Know About Breast Cancer; Chemotherapy and You: A Guide to Self-Help During Treatment; Radiation and You: A Guide to Self-Help During Treatment; Get Relief from Cancer Pain; Understanding Breast Cancer Treatment: A Guide for Patients. Y-ME (as above)—I Still Buy Green Bananas: Living With Hope; Living With Breast Cancer; For Single Women With Breast Cancer.
SELECTED BOOKS
Brack P, Brack B. Moms Don't Get Sick. Aberdeen, SD: Melius Publishing; 1990 Friedewald V, Buzdar A. Ask the Doctor Series–Breast Cancer: Kansas City, KS: Andrews & McNeil; 1997 Lerner M. Choices in Healing: Integrating the Best of Conventional and Complementary Approaches to Cancer. Cambridge, MA: MIT Press; 1994 Love S. Dr. Susan Love's Breast Book. Massachusetts, California: Addison-Wesley Publishing Co.; 1995

mammary dysplasia, and chronic cystic mastitis. For the purposes of this chapter, the term fibrocystic breasts will be used because this is most familiar to patients and physicians.

Pathomorphology

The term "fibrocystic" implies simultaneous progressive and regressive changes that are physiologic and influenced by ovarian hormones. On histologic preparations, the polymorphism of fibrocystic breasts is characterized by fibrosis, cyst formation, epithelial proliferation, and lobular-alveolar atrophy; these processes may coexist in the same biopsy specimen.[59] In 20 to 40 percent of patients with fibrocystic changes, gross palpable cyst formation is observed.[59]

Etiology

Because fibrocystic breasts present in women during the childbearing years and the condition is cyclic in nature, it is believed to be related to hormonal fluctuation. Studies have shown that although estradiol levels are usually normal in women with fibrocystic breast disease, progestin levels tend to be below normal in the luteal phase.[59] Consequently, women with fibrocystic breasts often have irregular ovulation.

Risk of Cancer

Among women who have had a breast nodule biopsied, long-term follow-up studies have shown that the risk of cancer varies based on the histology of the lesion. Women with atypical hyperplasia on breast biopsy are at increased risk of breast cancer as shown in Table 16-3. Women whose biopsies show proliferation without atypia have a slightly increased risk. Nonproliferative breast conditions, which represent the majority of women with fibrocystic breasts who undergo breast biopsy, are not at increased risk for breast cancer.

For women with fibrocystic breasts who have not undergone surgical excision of any masses or cysts, it is harder to estimate cancer risk. Some studies indicate that a woman who has had multiple cysts aspirated may be more apt to have proliferative lesions and therefore be at slightly increased risk for breast cancer, especially if she has a family history of breast cancer.[60] Nodularity alone does not seem to be associated with an increased risk of cancer.

Diagnosis

TYPICAL PRESENTATION

Early signs and symptoms of fibrocystic disease occur between ages 20 and 25 years, but most patients present in their middle thirties and forties. Clinically, three phases of fibrocystic disease have been described.[59] In the early phase, women typically present with breast tenderness about a week before the menstrual cycle, ending with the onset of menses. Menstrual cycles may also be shortened (21 to 24 days). As the woman enters her late thirties, the breasts start to feel more nodular and the pain may worsen. The upper outer quadrants of the breasts are most frequently involved. Breast pain and tenderness may extend to 2 to 3 weeks before menstruation or may be constant. Associated menstrual disorders include irregular menses, dysmenorrhea, or ovarian cysts. In her forties and fifties, the nodularity may increase and present as waxing and waning solitary or multiple lesions, along with the pain. As in the second phase, breast pain and tenderness may extend to 2 to 3 weeks before menstruation or may be constant and debilitating.

HISTORY

The primary symptom is breast pain or tenderness, reported in 40 to 60 percent of women with fibrocystic breasts.[59] Axillary tenderness may also be reported. This is often related to axillary lymph node swelling in reaction to duct ectasia and abacterial inflammatory round cell infiltration. Women also complain of nodularity or the presence of a mass. Nipple discharge is experienced by approximately one-third of women[59]; the discharge is usually expelled following stimulation. The fluid expressed is most often yellow, green, brown, or bluish. Women with watery, serous, serosanguineous, or bloody discharge require thorough investigation (see following section).

PHYSICAL EXAMINATION

A CBE should be performed on all women presenting with symptoms of breast pain or nodularity. Breast nodularity is often verified and the examination itself may be painful. Fibrocystic tissue will feel like irregular plaques and will be symmetrical in a mirror image location. The presence of a dominant mass should prompt evaluation as described in the previous section. Reexamination of the woman on day 3 to 10 of the next menstrual cycle may be helpful if asymmetry is palpated but no suspicious characteristics are found. If an asymmetry persists, it should be evaluated.

Management

INSTRUCTION IN BREAST SELF-EXAMINATION

The initial step in managing fibrocystic breasts is to assist the woman in gaining confidence in performing a BSE. A woman with fibrocystic breasts (as for all women) needs to be carefully instructed in BSE and encouraged to perform this on a monthly basis. Important aspects of the BSE to stress are to palpate the breast using the pads of the fingertips and to observe for any skin changes or spontaneous nipple discharge. Referral to a nurse educator for BSE training, which includes practice sessions on herself and models, may be extremely helpful. In addition, assisting women with behavioral modification techniques to help them remember to perform their BSE, such as shower cards and calendar stickers, should be an integral part of training.

Women should be instructed to report any dominant mass that does not recede with the menstrual cycle for evaluation. Areas of persistent asymmetry, nodularity, or thickening may be a sign of further pathology. Sometimes, comanagement with a local breast surgeon is helpful for the primary care provider and the patient to feel more comfortable in managing fibrocystic breasts.

DIAGNOSTIC TESTS

Mammography often includes descriptions indicating that the breasts are "fibrocystic." This is a vague term that can be applied in a variety of circumstances. In general, however, this description implies that a dense pattern and nonclustered microcalcifications may be present.[59] Unless a dominant mass is identified, breast pain is continuous, or there is unilateral, spontaneous discharge, screening mammography should be performed based on screening guidelines.

Nipple Discharge

Nipple discharge, secretion from the breasts of a nonlactating woman, that is nonspontaneous (requires some manipulation to be expressed) is not uncommon. This type of secretion is considered a normal physiologic process; it arises from multiple ducts, is often bilateral, and is of no clinical importance. In one study of 2685 women undergoing routine health examination including breast compression toward the nipple, nipple discharge was present in 10 percent.[61] In addition, some discharge can be expressed from 50 to 83 percent of healthy women if nipple aspiration by pump expression is performed.[10,62] The symptom of nonspontaneous nipple discharge usually requires no treatment and resolves when nipple compression is avoided.

Overall, nipple discharge accounts for 3 to 10 percent of breast complaints. In primary care practice, this may be an overestimate; the average clinician in a study of 200 general practices in Edinburgh, Scotland saw only 13 women per year with a breast complaint (1.8 percent of women age 45 to 65) and nipple discharge was a rare presentation.[8] The concern about nipple discharge is that 8 to 14 percent of cases are linked to breast cancer.[63,64] Postmenopausal women over age 60 are three times more likely to have breast cancer associated with discharge than younger women[65]; in one study, malignancy was discovered in 7 percent of women less than age 60, but 32 percent of women over age 60 with nipple discharge.[66] Pathologic nipple discharge is typically spontaneous, unilateral, and from a single duct.

Etiology

Women with nipple discharge may be divided into two groups, those with discharge that is physiologic and those whose discharge is caused by breast pathology (Table 16-10). Physiologic discharge is related to hormonal influences on breast tissue; elevated prolactin levels are usually the cause. Increased prolactin may be due to purely physiologic events such as lactation following pregnancy, which may persist for several years after discontinuation of breast feeding, or may result from endocrine causes or medications. The many causes of increased prolactin levels are listed in Table 16-11. Even transient prolactin elevation may result in nipple discharge.

Pathologic nipple discharge can originate from either the nipple/areola region or the ducts. Problems arising from the nipple area associated with discharge include eczema, nipple adenoma, and Paget's disease. These disorders are characterized by erythema and ulceration of the skin with associated bloody discharge. Other causes of "pseudo-discharge" include inverted nipples that have not

Table 16-10

Differential Diagnosis of Nipple Discharge

DIAGNOSIS	FREQUENCY IN OFFICE PRIMARY CARE (% WITHIN PHYSIOLOGIC OR PATHOLOGIC CATEGORY)	TYPICAL PRESENTATION
PHYSIOLOGIC		
Idiopathic	Common (40–45%)	Bilateral, milky or watery
Galactorrhea (prolonged lactation)	Somewhat common (25–30%)	Bilateral, milky
Medication	Uncommon (10–15%)	Bilateral, milky or watery
Anovulatory syndromes	Rare (1–2%)	Bilateral, milky or watery, irregular menses
Sella turcica lesions	Rare (1–2%)	Bilateral, milky or watery, irregular menses
PATHOLOGIC		
Duct papilloma	Common (40–45%)	Unilateral, serous or bloody
Fibrocyst	Uncommon (15–25%)	Usually unilateral, greenish or serous
Duct ectasia	Uncommon (15–20%)	Usually bilateral, multicolored, sticky
Eczema	Rare	Usually unilateral, bloody, crusting
Paget's disease	Rare	Usually unilateral, bloody, crusting
Early ductal carcinoma	Rare (5–10%)	Unilateral, serous or bloody
Infection/inflammation	Rare (5–10%)	Usually unilateral, purulent

SOURCE: Reproduced with permission from Schwartz.K. Breast problems. In: Sloane PD, Slatt LM, Curtis P, Ebell MH (eds): *Essentials of Family Medicine,* 3rd ed. Baltimore:Williams & Wilkins; 1998;337.

Table 16-11
Causes of Elevated Prolactin Levels

PHYSIOLOGIC
Food ingestion
Nipple stimulation (sexual, exercise, sleep)
Pregnancy
Postpartum
Sexual orgasm

ENDOCRINE
Anovulatory syndromes (e.g., polycystic ovaries)
Chest wall trauma
Hypothalamic lesions
Hypothyroidism
Pituitary tumors
Renal failure (decreased prolactin clearance)

MEDICATIONS	
α-Methyldopa	Opiates
Amphetamines	Oral contraceptives
Cocaine	Phenothiazines
Hallucinogens	Reserpine
Haloperidol	Tricyclic
H_2-receptor antagonists	antidepressants
Metoclopramide	Verapamil

been kept clean, herpes simplex infection, Montgomery's gland infection, or an infected sebaceous cyst that points at the border of the areola.

Ductal diseases associated with nipple discharge are listed in Table 16-10. The three most common causes of persistent, unilateral, single duct nipple discharge are intraductal papilloma, duct ectasia, and carcinoma. Duct papilloma, the most common cause, is a benign condition of epithelial hyperplasia when occurring as a single lesion in a central location (retroareolar ducts). Papillomas that occur more peripherally are usually multifocal, more likely to have atypical hyperplastic cells, and are associated with an increased risk of breast cancer.[67]

Duct ectasia, sometimes called periductal mastitis, is caused by glandular involution with terminal ducts becoming obstructed by fibrotic tissue strands, leading to accumulation of secretory mate-

rial. The dilatation of the subareolar ducts with accumulation of stagnant secretions causes an obstruction and subsequent discharge. Sometimes the fluid leaks through the wall of the ducts leading to periductal inflammation, nipple eversion, nipple and areolar thickening, or an abscess. The discharge is usually nonbloody and multicolored (green, brown, gray, yellow, or white). Cultures of the discharge are negative.

Carcinoma, often ductal carcinoma in situ (DCIS), is responsible for about 5 to 10 percent of unilateral nipple discharge.[68–71] The incidence of DCIS has been increasing in recent years, due in part to the increased recognition from the use of screening mammography. DCIS accounts for about 12 percent of newly diagnosed breast cancer cases among white and black women and 30 to 40 percent of mammographically detected breast cancers.[72–74]

Diagnosis of Nipple Discharge

HISTORY

Important elements in a focused history are shown in Table 16-2. To determine whether the discharge is spontaneous, ask the patient if the discharge stains her underclothing or bed sheets. The color of the discharge will help to further establish the likely etiology. Discharges that are milky are galactorrhea and are physiologic. Multicolored, yellow, green, or brownish discharges are often associated with ductal ectasia; clear, watery, or bloody discharges are more worrisome for cancer. The subtleties of color are not as important in the diagnosis and management of nipple discharge as whether the discharge is unilateral or bilateral and whether one or more ducts are involved. Women should also be asked about when the discharge was discovered and whether it is persistent.

Other important factors include recent or current pregnancy or breast trauma or surgery, menstrual patterns, and menopausal status. Information about factors associated with the discharge, such as sexual activity or exercise will assist with treatment plans as well. A history of amenorrhea, headache, visual disturbance, and change in appetite or temperature regulation should raise suspicion about a pituitary or hypothalamic problem. The clinician should also ask about the medications listed in Table 16-11.

PHYSICAL EXAMINATION

A CBE should be performed to determine whether skin retraction, dimpling, or a palpable mass is present, with special attention to the involved breast if the discharge is unilateral. A palpable mass in association with nipple discharge increases the likelihood of cancer. In one surgical series, 87 percent of patients with nipple discharge associated with cancer had a palpable mass.[71]

Careful inspection of the nipple and areola is performed looking for signs of Paget's disease. Associated findings may include redness, crusting, drying, excoriation, or an eczematous appearance. If the areola is involved in an eczematous process and the nipple is not, Paget's disease should not be part of the differential diagnosis. The oozing and weeping from the area of the nipple are not true nipple discharge but may be mistaken for it. Most often, Paget's disease appears as a raw area on the middle of the nipple associated with itching or irritation that gradually increases over time to involve the entire surface of the nipple. Purulent discharge may be produced by an abscess or fistula that points at the border of the areola. This may be recognized as a localized erythema or swelling with tenderness; an infected sebaceous gland may be responsible.

An attempt is made to ascertain whether the discharge is confined to a single duct or multiple ducts. Careful attention is directed to which subareolar areas produce discharge when pressure is applied in a wedge-shaped pattern (see Fig. 16-2). Discharge arising from multiple ducts (see Fig. 16-8) is very unlikely to represent malignancy, particularly if it is bilateral. If the discharge is nonmilky and nonbloody, duct ectasia is the most common etiology. The most common causes of a bloody discharge include intraductal papilloma, duct ectasia,

Figure 16-8

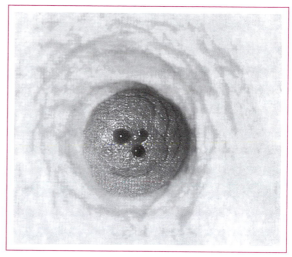

Example of duct ectasia. The discharge is usually of a yellow-green or dark green character. This condition represents a dilatation of the subareolar ducts with accumulation of stagnant secretions that cause an obstruction and subsequent discharge. These symptoms are usually followed, with surgical intervention deferred unless they cause social embarrassment. If surgery is indicated, removal of the subareolar duct system is necessary. This results in inability of the woman to lactate. *(Reproduced with permission from JR Osuch. In: LA Wallis [ed]: Textbook of Women's Health. Philadelphia: Lippincott Raven, copyright 1998.)*

and carcinoma. Watery discharge, although uncommon, has the highest association with carcinoma.

RADIOLOGIC EVALUATION

MAMMOGRAPHY Diagnostic mammography should be ordered for women presenting with spontaneous, unilateral, single duct, nonmilky nipple discharge. The sensitivity of mammography reported in the literature varies greatly (from 13 to 90 percent).[69,71] The specificity, however, is over 95 percent. The most common diagnoses found on mammography in one series of women with nipple discharge were intraductal papilloma (48.1 percent), fibrocystic changes (32.9 percent), precancerous lesions (7.3 percent), and cancer (14.3 percent).[71] Given the potentially high false-negative rate, perhaps the best use of mammography is to determine if other nonpalpable abnormalities are present, increasing the suspicion for cancer. Screening mammography consistent with guidelines should be considered (see Chap. 1).

GALACTOGRAPHY Galactography, also called contrast mammography or ductography, is a technique during which a skilled radiologist passes a catheter or thin probe into the duct and injects a small amount of radiocontrast material into the involved duct to demonstrate a filling defect on mammography. Galactography is helpful under some circumstances, especially when used for surgical localization. It is most often used to identify a lesion requiring biopsy when a woman has significant discharge from a single duct to allow a more conservative surgical excision. Galactography, however, cannot be used to differentiate benign from malignant lesions. Therefore, surgical referral is necessary when a woman has a unilateral persistent discharge from a single duct.

LABORATORY TESTING

The workup for evaluation and management of nipple discharge is shown in Fig. 16-9.

GALACTORRHEA If the history and physical examination are consistent with galactorrhea, and all physiologic and pharmacologic causes have been excluded, a prolactin level should be obtained. For women experiencing amenorrhea, menstrual irregularity, or other symptoms indicating pituitary or hypothalamic dysfunction, both a prolactin and a thyroid-stimulating hormone level should be obtained to rule out hyperprolactinemia and hypothyroidism, respectively. The prolactin level should be drawn fasting and 2 h after awakening because both feeding and sleep can increase the level. If both are normal, a diagnosis of idiopathic galactorrhea can be made and no further testing is indicated. If the prolactin level is elevated, particularly with a level over 200 mg/mL, either computed tomography scanning or magnetic resonance imaging of the brain is warranted to look for pituitary tumor. In

several series, however, normal prolactin levels were found in patients with prolactinomas.[75]

DISCHARGES SUSPICIOUS FOR CANCER Nipple discharge that is unilateral, bloody, serosanguineous, or watery and arising from a single duct should be evaluated with additional tests following mammography. Guaiac testing of the discharge can be useful in determining whether blood is present, but workup will still be necessary regardless of the results. The percent of cancers whose discharges tested positive for the presence of hemoglobin ranges from 53 to 100 percent.[69,70,76]

Cytology of the nipple secretions has a significant false-negative rate and is not generally recommended. Although positive findings are useful and an indication for surgery, negative findings are not diagnostic and surgical referral should not be based on cytology results. In addition, cytology cannot differentiate between in situ and invasive cancer.

DIAGNOSTIC PROCEDURES

A punch biopsy of the involved skin should be obtained when Paget's disease is suspected based on CBE or when an eczematous lesion of the nipple fails to improve after 2 weeks of use of a topical steroid preparation. Once the diagnosis of Paget's disease is made, the patient requires surgical referral.

Microdochectomy, surgical excision of the duct, is the method of choice in determining whether a lesion causing significant discharge is benign or malignant. Several techniques may be used; some surgeons use galactography to localize the lesion before excision; others use suture material introduced into the duct to assist in dissecting down to the lesion, whereas other surgeons use methylene blue dye injected into the identified duct for localization.[77] For lesions that are more than 3 to 4 cm from the nipple, the radiologist can perform a wire localization technique so that the surgeon can excise the area directly over the lesion. The reason for proceeding with duct excision is to attempt to spare the nipple, most of the ducts, and the woman's ability to breast-feed; the procedure

Figure 16-9

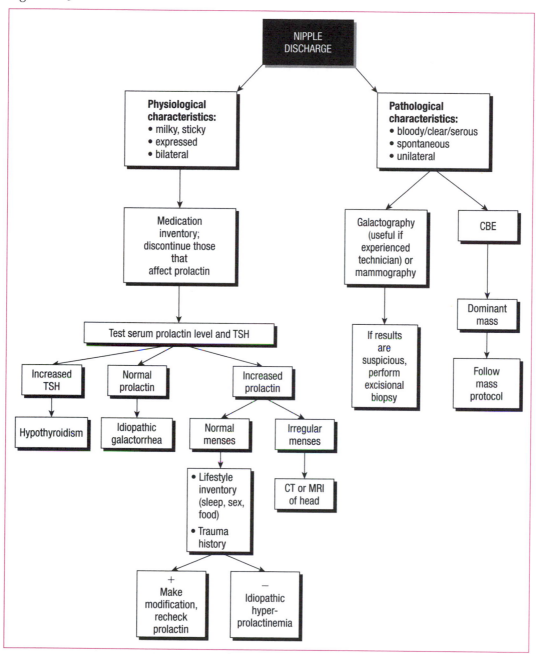

Algorithm for evaluation and management of nipple discharge. *(Reproduced with permission from Schwartz K: Breast problems. In: Sloane PD, Slatt LM, Curtis P, Ebell MH [eds]: Essentials of Family Medicine, 3rd ed. Baltimore: Williams & Wilkins; 1998;340.)*

does not always accomplish these goals. A Japanese group reported on a biopsy method using ductal endoscopy in an effort to decrease the need for surgery and lessen the amount of tissue excised.[78] This method must await further testing.

Management

An algorithm for the diagnosis and management of nipple discharge is shown in Fig. 16-9.

PHYSIOLOGIC NIPPLE DISCHARGE

The management of a physiologic nipple discharge depends on the results of the laboratory testing (see Fig. 16-9). If hypothyroidism is detected, the woman is treated with thyroid replacement. For women with hyperprolactinemia, a cause should be sought and steps taken to remedy the hyperprolactinemic state. Management may include changes in medication or lifestyle and evaluation for a pituitary tumor. Pituitary tumors are usually treated surgically, although radiation therapy and bromocriptine are sometimes used. If the only abnormal result from the evaluation and imaging study is an elevated prolactin level, a diagnosis of idiopathic hyperprolactinemia can be made and reassurance given. The patient should be followed, however, for further increases in prolactin level or signs and symptoms of pituitary tumor.

For women whose laboratory testing is normal, a diagnosis of idiopathic galactorrhea can be made and reassurance given. If she has recently stopped breast-feeding, she should be advised that it may take several years for the secretions to stop. Women should be cautioned against manual expression to check for continued discharge because this may promote continued milk production.

SPONTANEOUS, NONMILKY DISCHARGE FROM MULTIPLE DUCTS

Women with spontaneous, nonmilky discharge from multiple ducts do not require treatment. The usual cause is duct ectasia. If pain is associated with

the discharge, treatment may include ice packs and NSAIDs. Women with unilateral discharge, in particular, should be followed closely to determine whether the discharge has changed to bloody; further evaluation may be needed. If discharge traceable to a benign lesion in the duct is troubling to the patient, removal of the discharging duct may be considered with the understanding that this procedure may change the sensation of the nipple and areola and destroy her ability to breast-feed from that breast. According to one author, approximately 10 percent of women elect further treatment.[77]

UNILATERAL DISCHARGE FROM A SINGLE DUCT

Women with unilateral discharge from a single duct require surgical referral. Mammography or galactography, along with cytology of the discharge, may be ordered before referral. If a mass is detected, the protocol in the previous section should be followed.

Breast Augmentation

There were nearly 900,000 augmentation mammaplasty procedures performed in the United States between 1963 and 1989.[79] Although this number is lower than previous reports, it still reveals a high rate of women's dissatisfaction with their breast size.

Silicone breast implants first became available in 1963 and saline implants shortly thereafter, totaling 35 years of cumulative experience with augmentation mammaplasty. Despite a high rate of overall patient satisfaction with their augmentation procedures, silicone breast implants were removed from the market in 1992 because of anecdotal reports about a causal relationship of silicone implants to autoimmune disorders. Since then, silicone breast implants have been available only for reconstruction mammaplasty and then only when the patient is deemed unsuitable for a saline implant and the patient agrees to join a study looking prospectively for any adverse health effects of the implants.

Because of the wide coverage of this controversy in the lay press and a resulting class action lawsuit against pharmaceutical companies who made silicone breast implants, many women with these implants are concerned about potential health risks. They may present for an opinion about the risks and the possible relationship of symptoms they have experienced with the implant. These concerns should be elicited and discussed, and the patient given information about the lack of scientific evidence about the health risks of implants. Any reported symptoms or complaints should be assessed and evaluated as deemed appropriate. Many women have elected to have the implants removed because of their concerns. Unfortunately, the cosmetic result following removal is often unfavorable and sometimes necessitates subsequent reconstruction procedures, including insertion of a saline implant or autologous flap reconstruction. Women who are considering replacement should be counseled that saline implants may result in a breast texture that is not as realistic as the silicone.

Health Risks

Before 1992, most implants were polyurethane shells filled with silicone gel; only 10 percent of the implants used contained saline. Today, almost all breast implants are silicone shells filled with saline. The polyurethane/silicone implant, used in about 110,000 women before 1991, was selected because it reduced the incidence of capsular contraction. This implant was removed from the market when it was found that polyurethane foam could break down in vivo into toluenediamine, a known carcinogen. Subsequent investigation revealed a negligible risk of cancer as a result of these implants, and implant removal is currently not recommended for this reason alone.

Although there is currently no documentation of an increased risk of breast cancer with the presence of implants, breast implants have only been used for 25 years and are most often inserted in younger women. Even the earliest recipients are only now approaching an age where their breast cancer risks are increasing. Moreover, women with implants may actually engage in breast cancer screening more frequently than controls. The controversy about the relationship of silicone and autoimmune disorders continues today, despite multiple scientific studies concluding there is no evidence for concern.[80]

Both saline and silicone implants are known to rupture over time. Nearly half of the implants will rupture within 15 years, and the risk increases with the age of the implant. Implant rupture results in deflation and, therefore, obvious asymmetry of the breasts. Silicone implants usually rupture more slowly, releasing silicone into the surrounding tissue. Besides breast asymmetry, this can also cause other lumps in surrounding tissue. This leakage of silicone led to the concern about autoimmune disorders. Saline implants usually rupture suddenly, resulting in deflation that necessitates immediate removal and replacement. Health risks and side effects associated with breast implants are listed in Table 16-12. These risks should be discussed with women who are considering this procedure.

Procedure

Implants are now typically inserted under the pectoralis muscles. This results in a better and more stable cosmetic effect. The size of the augmentation can be initially adjusted somewhat with the saline implant by adding or removing fluid through a subcutaneous port, until the desired cosmetic result is achieved. Once satisfied with the size, the port is removed, requiring another brief procedure. The cost of the procedure ranges greatly from $4000 to $7000.

Side Effects

Capsular contraction may be the most common complication from breast augmentation, occurring

Table 16-12

Risks of Breast Implants

RISK	OUTCOME	RATE OF OCCURRENCE
Capsular contracture	Hardening of the breast Pain Unfavorable cosmetic result	20%
Leak or rupture	Silicone—usually occurs slowly, releasing silicone into surrounding tissues (10–23%) (this led to concern about relationship to autoimmune disorders)	At 5–10 years: 10–20%
	Saline—usually occurs suddenly, resulting in deflation and may require immediate removal and/or replacement	At 12–15 years: 10–49%
Nipple hypesthesia or anesthesia	Altered sensation of breast tissue and/or nipple	33–49%
Shifting of placement	Unfavorable cosmetic result	
Breast pain	Chronic discomfort	
Interference with mammographic readings	More with silicone—can obscure breast tissue visualization	
Insufficient lactation	Delayed or inadequate lactogenesis after birth and inadequate infant growth with exclusive breast-feeding	64%

in up to 50 percent of women. This may result in hardening of the breast, chronic breast pain, and an unfavorable cosmetic result. There are no reliable data on the frequency of complications from augmentation mammaplasty, and those reports available vary widely in frequency.[81–83] Side effects of augmentation mammaplasty include surgical risks of infection (1 to 4 percent), hematoma (1 to 6 percent), anesthesia complications, and skin necrosis as well as many risks specific to that procedure. Nipple anesthesia or hypesthesia is common, depending on the technique used. One study showed an overall complication rate of 24 percent.[84] In addition, there is a 1 in 8 chance of needing a second surgery within 5 years.

Breast-Feeding

Breast-feeding is often adequate after augmentation mammaplasty; however, there is a higher rate of insufficient lactation for women with implants compared to women without implants (64 versus 7 percent).[85]

Alternative Therapy

Many comfortable and realistic nonsurgical options for breast enhancement are available for women unhappy with their breast size. Many women have found satisfaction with push-up bras, silicone bra inserts, and bras with a silicone gel or oil filling, all of which enhance breast size and accentuate natural breast contour. These options are cheaper and safer, but of course only enhance the breasts while the woman is clothed. Because much of the drive for surgical augmentation comes from feeling unfeminine in a sexual setting, this may not be a satisfactory option for all women.

Patient Education

Women will often see their primary care provider for advice before consulting a plastic surgeon regarding augmentation mammaplasty. Because the primary provider often has an established relationship with the patient, a thorough discussion should take place with the woman about why she wants the procedure, the potential advantages and side effects of the procedure, and alternatives to surgical breast augmentation. Women most commonly cite being unhappy with the size of their breasts as the reason for seeking breast augmentation: feeling sexually inhibited because of it, feeling uncomfortable undressing in front of their spouse and even other women, and feeling unfeminine. A woman's desire for larger breasts is a complex one, involving personal, sociological, cultural, and psychosexual issues. As with any cosmetic procedure, if there seems to be underlying psychological pathology that the woman seeks to compensate for with surgery, she should be encouraged to consider counseling before the procedure to address those issues.

It is essential that a woman understands that breast implants are not a lifetime device. The risk of rupture is high, and the implants will require replacement in 8 to 15 years. After augmentation mammaplasty, women should be instructed in BSE and should engage in regular CBEs with the same frequency of any other woman, based on recommended screening protocols and personal risk factors for breast cancer. Mammography, however, can be challenging with implants and should be performed at a breast imaging center familiar with the procedure. Magnetic resonance imaging has become an important tool for identifying rupture of silicone implants, although inspection of the implant remains the gold standard for diagnosing rupture.

Breast Reduction

Macromastia is a condition of large breasts, also termed breast hyperplasia or breast hypertrophy. The condition exists when the breast size exceeds the woman's proportions and she feels that it causes her physical and emotional consequences. Macromastia is associated with a wide range of both physical and emotional consequences. Physical symptoms associated with macromastia include neck pain, back pain, headache, and shoulder grooving from the bra strap. Another health effect, harder to quantify but also important to consider, is that women with large breasts often avoid exercise. This is partly because of the physical discomfort associated with exercise and a wish to avoid social exposure in skimpier exercise clothing, especially bathing suits and leotards.

Emotional consequences include embarrassment about breast size, often to the extent of limiting social exposure to avoid ridicule, teasing, and ogling. Women with macromastia usually have difficulty in finding clothes to fit because their breast size is out of proportion to their body. Larger clothes that accommodate their breast size may make them appear heavier than they really are and further affect self-image. These psychological effects should not be minimized with a woman seeking advice about her large breasts. Breast reduction mammaplasty is considered when a woman has significant symptoms.

Health Risks

There is no known increase in breast cancer with reduction mammaplasty. Surgical alteration of the breasts will result in distortions of the breast tissue and may make screening and diagnosis of breast lumps more challenging. Some plastic surgeons recommend mammography 3 months following reduction mammaplasty to document the baseline postoperative breast parenchyma.

Procedure

With reduction mammaplasty, sections of the breast tissue are removed bilaterally, preserving the nipple-areolar complex. Many insurance companies will only cover this procedure if the woman has documented chronic neck or back pain and shoulder grooving as indicators of medical necessity. Furthermore, they often require a minimum of 500 g breast tissue removed on each side to satisfy medical necessity.

Side Effects

Side effects of this procedure include fat necrosis, infection, skin separation at suture line, unsatisfactory scar, and hematoma. In one study, 45 percent of 185 patients experienced some complication, the most common being fat necrosis or infection (22 percent of the women).[86] The complication rate increased with the amount of breast tissue removed. Only 9 percent of women required an additional procedure because of the complication. Although complication rates can be high with this procedure, it is interesting to note that the postoperative patient satisfaction with this procedure is extremely high (86 to 97 percent).[86–88] In fact, two studies showed that 98 percent of women who have breast reduction mammaplasty would recommend the procedure to others.[86,87]

Breast-Feeding

Although the nipple-areola complex is maintained with reduction mammaplasty, the ducts are often disrupted with surgery and therefore breast-feeding may not be possible. In procedures, such as the inferior pedicle technique, where the connection of the nipple to some breast tissue is preserved, breast-feeding may be possible. In one small series of 20 women who had pregnancies following reduction mammaplasty using the inferior pedicle technique, 100 percent of the women lactated and 35 percent breast-fed successfully.[89] Women considering reduction mammaplasty should be warned that breast-feeding may not be possible, and they may wish to delay the procedure until after pregnancy. Furthermore, the breast changes associated with pregnancy may distort the cosmetic result of the reduction mammaplasty.

Alternative Therapy

Women will most often seek advice about the physical symptoms of macromastia. Care should be taken to also include questions that assess the psychological impact of the condition and offer support and referral if indicated. Many women are not wearing bras that give adequate support. Referral to a local or regional foundation shop is often helpful as a first step. These shops have specially trained saleswomen who can assist the woman in selecting a proper fitting and supportive brassiere for her size. Although brassieres at these shops are often more expensive, patients can be advised to view this as a consultation where they can learn proper fitting techniques.

Patient Education

Despite the risks and side effects noted above, several studies have shown a drastic reduction in symptoms following reduction mammaplasty. In one series, 97 percent of women experienced improvement and 59 percent were asymptomatic after surgery.[86] Considering the significant rates of improvement of symptoms and the substantial psychological and physical burden from macromastia, clinicians should be supportive of a woman's request for reduction mammaplasty and counsel her about her options. Many proponents of the procedure (especially women who have had reduction mammaplasty) feel that the procedure is significantly underutilized.

Women over 40 should be fully evaluated for breast cancer before surgery is performed, with a careful CBE and baseline mammography.

References

1. The breast. In: Sperhoff L, Glass RH, Kase NG (eds): *Clinical Gynecologic Endocrinology and Infertility*, 5th ed. Baltimore: Williams & Wilkins; 1994:547.

2. Going JJ, Anderson TJ, Battersby S, MacIntyre CC: Proliferative and secretory activity in human breast during natural and artificial menstrual cycles. *Am J Pathol* 130:193, 1998.

3. Hughes LE: A unifying concept for benign disorder of the breast: ANDI. In: Donegan WL, Spratt JS (eds): *Diseases of the Breast*. Philadelphia: Saunders; 1995.

4. Pahroah PDP, Day NE, Duffy S, et al: Family history and the risk of breast cancer: a systematic review and meta-analysis. *Int J Cancer* 71:800, 1997.

5. Anderson DE, Badzioch MD: Risk of familial breast cancer. *Cancer* 56:383, 1985.

6. Burke W, Daly M, Garber J, et al: Recommendations for follow-up care for individuals with an inherited predisposition to cancer: II. BRCA1 and BRCA2. Cancer Genetics Consortium. *JAMA* 277:997, 1997.

7. Newman B, Mu H, Butler LM, et al: Frequency of breast cancer attributable to BRCA1 in a population-based series of American women. *JAMA* 279:915, 1998.

8. Hislop TG, Elwood JM, Coldman AJ, et al: Second primary cancers of the breast: incidence and risk factors. *Br J Cancer* 49:79, 1985.

9. Cancer Committee, College of American Pathologists: Is 'fibrocystic disease' of the breast precancerous? *Arch Pathol Lab Med* 110:171, 1986.

10. Byrne C: Breast. In: Harris A, Edwards BK, Blot WJ, Ries LAG (eds): *Cancer Rates and Risk*. NIH Publication no. 96–691. National Cancer Institute; May 1996:120.

11. Michels KB, Willett WC, Rosner BA, et al: Prospective assessment of breast feeding and breast cancer incidence among 89,887 women. *Lancet* 347:431, 1996.

12. Melbye M, Wohlfahrt J, Olsen JH, et al: Induced abortion and risk of breast cancer. *JAMA* 336:81, 1997.

13. Smith-Warner SA, Spiegelman D, Yaun S-S, et al: Alcohol and breast cancer in women: a pooled analysis of cohort studies. *JAMA* 279:535, 1998.

14. Collaborative Group on Hormonal Factors in Breast Cancer: Breast cancer and hormonal contraceptives: collaborative reanalysis of individual data on 53,297 women with breast cancer and 100,239 women without breast cancer from 54 epidemiological studies. *Lancet* 347:1713, 1996.

15. Collaborative Group on Hormonal Factors in Breast Cancer: Breast cancer and hormone replacement therapy: collaborative reanalysis of data from 51 epidemiological studies involving 52,705 women with breast cancer and 108,411 women without breast cancer. *Lancet* 350:1047, 1997.

16. Gail MH, Brinton LA, Byar DP, et al: Projecting individualized probabilities of developing breast cancer for white females who are being examined annually. *J Natl Cancer Inst* 81:1879, 1989.

17. Spiegelman D, Colditz GA, Hunter D, Hertzmark E: Validating the Gail et al. model for predicting individual breast cancer risk. *J Natl Cancer Inst* 86:600, 1994.

18. Saunders KJ, Pilgrim CA, Pennypacker HS: Increased proficiency of search in breast self-examination. *Cancer* 58:2531, 1986.

19. Mann LC: Physical examination of the augmented breast: description of a displacement technique. *Obstet Gynecol* 85:290, 1995.

20. Fletcher SW, O'Malley MS, Bunce LA: Physicians' abilities to detect lumps in silicone breast models. *JAMA* 253:2224, 1985.

21. Osuch JR, Bonham VL, Morris LL: Primary care guide to managing a breast mass: step-by-step workup. *www.medscape/Medscape/Womenshealth/journal/1998/vo3.n05/wh3026.osuc/wh3026.osuc-01.html.*

22. Campbell BG, Trachtenbarg DE, Barclay A: Cyclic breast pain. *J Fam Pract* 19:549, 1984.

23. Roberts MM, Elton RA, Robinson SE, French K: Consultations for breast disease in general practice and hospital referral patterns. *Br J Surg* 74:1020, 1987.

24. Preece PE, Baum M, Mansel RE, et al: The importance of mastalgia in operable breast cancer. *BMJ* 284:1299, 1982.

25. DeVane GW: Breast dysfunction: galactorrhea and mastalgia. In: Blackwell RE, Grotting JC (eds): *Diseases of the Breast*. Cambridge, MA: Blackwell Science; 1996:19.

26. Klimberg VS: Etiology and management of breast pain. In: Bland KI, Copeland EM (eds): *The Breast: Comprehensive Management of Benign and Malignant Disease*. Philadelphia: Saunders; 1998:247.

27. Maddox PR, Mansel RE: Management of breast pain and nodularity. *World J Surg* 13:699, 1989.

28. Wisbey JR, Kumar S, Mansel RE, et al: Natural history of breast pain. *Lancet* 2:672, 1983.

29. Davies EL, Gateley CA, Miers M, Mansel RE: The long-term course of mastalgia. *J R Soc Med* 91:462, 1998.

30. Wilson MC, Sillwood RA: Therapeutic value of a supporting brassiere in mastodynia. *BMJ* 2:90, 1976.

31. Boyd NF, McGuire V, Shannon P, et al: Effect of a low-fat high-carbohydrate diet on symptoms of cyclic mastopathy. *Lancet* 2:128, 1988.

32. Gateley CA, Maddox PR, Pritchard GA, et al: Plasma fatty acid profiles in benign breast disorders. *Br J Surg* 79:407, 1992.

33. Gateley CA, Maddox PR, Mansel RE, et al: Mastalgia refractory to drug treatment. *Br J Surg* 77:1110, 1990.

34. Holland PA, Gateley CA: Drug therapy of mastalgia: what are the options. *Drugs* 48:709, 1994.

35. Steinbrunn BS, Zera RT, Rodrigue JL: Mastalgia. *Postgrad Med* 102:183, 1997.

36. Hinton CP, Bishop HM, Holliday HW, et al: A double-blind controlled trial of danazol and bromocriptine in the management of severe cyclical breast pain. *Br J Clin Pract* 40:326, 1986.

37. Mansel RE, Wisbey JR, Hughes LE: Controlled trial of the antigonadotropin danazol in painful nodular breast disease. *Lancet* 1(8278):928, 1982.

38. O'Brien PMS, Abukhalil IEH: Randomized controlled trial of the management of premenstrual syndrome and premenstrual mastalgia using luteal phase-only danazol. *Am J Obstet Gynecol* 180:18, 1999.

39. Vorherr H: Fibrocystic breast disease: pathophysiology, pathomorphology, clinical picture, and management. *Am J Obstet Gynecol* 154:161, 1986.

40. Euhus DM, Uyehara C: Influence of parenteral progesterones on the prevalence and severity of mastalgia in premenopausal women: a multi-institutional cross-sectional study. *J Am Coll Surg* 184:596, 1997.

41. Nazli K, Syed S, Mahmood MR, et al: Controlled trial of prolactin inhibitor bromocriptine (Parlodel) in the treatment of severe cyclical mastalgia. *Br J Clin Pract Symp* (suppl) 68:43, 1989.

42. Mansel RE, Dogliotti L: European multicentre trial of bromocriptine in cyclic mastalgia. *Lancet* 335 (8683):190, 1990.

43. Fentiman IS, Caleffi M, Hamed H, et al: Studies of tamoxifen in women with mastalgia. *Br J Clin Pract Symp* (suppl) 68:34, 1989.

44. Fentimen IS: Tamoxifen and mastalgia: an emerging indication. *Drugs* 32:477, 1986

45. Kontostolis E, Stefanidis K, Navrozoglou I, Lolis D: Comparison of tamoxifen with danazol for treatment of cyclical mastalgia. *Gynecol Endocrinol* 11:393, 1997.

46. Hamed H, Caleffi M, Chaudary MA, et al: LHRH analogue for treatment of recurrent and refractory mastalgia. *Ann R Coll Surg Engl* 72:221, 1990.

47. Roberts JV: Experience in the use of nafarelin for treatment of benign breast disease. *Br J Clin Pract Symp* (suppl) 68:37, 1989.

48. Irving AD, Morrison SL: Effectiveness of topical non-steroidal anti-inflammatory drugs in the management of breast pain. *J R Coll Surg Edinb* 43:158, 1998.

49. Physician Insurers Association of America: *Breast Cancer Study*. Lawrenceville, NJ: Author; 1995.

50. Love N: *Primary Care Considerations in Breast Diagnosis*. Tampa, FL: American Cancer Society, Florida Division; 1992.

51. Donegan WL: Diagnosis. In: Donegan WL, Spratt JS (eds): *Cancer of the Breast*. Philadelphia: Saunders; 1995:198.

52. Byrd BF, Bayer DS, Robertson JC, et al: Treatment of breast tumors associated with pregnancy and lactation. *Ann Surg* 155:940, 1962.

53. VanDam PA, Van Goethem MLA, Kersschot E, et al: Palpable solid breast masses: retrospective single- and multimodality evaluation of 201 lesions. *Radiology* 166:435, 1988.

54. Donegan WL. Evaluation of a palpable breast mass. *N Engl J Med* 327:942, 1992.

55. Kern KA: The delayed diagnosis of symptomatic breast cancer. In: Bland KI, Copeland EM (eds): *The Breast: Comprehensive Management of Benign and Malignant Disease*. Philadelphia: Saunders; 1998:1588.

56. Layfield LJ, Glasgow BJ, Cramer H: Fine needle aspiration in the management of breast masses. *Pathol Annu* 24:23, 1989.

57. Love SM, Gelman RS, Silen WS: Fibrocystic "disease" of the breast: a nondisease. *N Engl J Med* 307:1010, 1982.

58. The Cancer Committee of the College of American Pathologists: Is "fibrocystic disease" of the breast precancerous? *Arch Pathol Lab Med* 110:173, 1986.

59. Vorherr H: Fibrocystic breast disease: pathophysiology, pathomorphology, clinical picture, and management. *Am J Obstet Gynecol* 154:161, 1986.

60. Dupont WD, Page DL: Risk factors in women with proliferative breast disease. *N Engl J Med* 312:146, 1985.

61. Newman HF, Klein M, Northrup JD, et al: Nipple discharge: frequency and pathogenesis in an ambulatory population. *N Y State J Med* 83:928, 1983.

62. Love SM, Schnitt SJ, Connolly JL, et al: Benign breast disorders. In: Harris JR, Hellman S, Henderson IC, et al (eds): *Breast Diseases*. Philadelphia: Lippincott; 1987:15.

63. Conry C: Evaluation of breast complaint: is it cancer? *Am Fam Physician* 49:445, 1994.

64. Paterok EM, Rosenthal H, Sabel M: Nipple discharge and abnormal galactogram: results of a

long-term study (1964–1990). *Eur J Obstet Gynecol Reprod Biol* 50:227, 1993.

65. Sletzer MH, Perloff LJ, Kelley RI, Fitts WT: The significance of age in patients with nipple discharge. *Surg Gynecol Obstet* 131:519, 1970.

66. Fisher B, Costatino J, Redman C, et al: Lumpectomy compared with lumpectomy and radiation therapy for the treatment of intraductal breast cancer. *N Engl J Med* 328:1581, 1993.

67. Raju U, Vertes D: Breast papillomas with atypical ductal hyperplasia: a clinicopathologic study. *Hum Pathol* 27:1231, 1991.

68. Paterok EM, Rosenthal H, Sabel M: Nipple discharge and abnormal galactogram. Results of a long-term study (1964–1990). *J Obstet Gynecol Reprod Biol* 50:227, 1993.

69. Fung A, Rayter Z, Fisher C, et al: Preoperative cytology and mammography in patients with single-duct nipple discharge treated by surgery. *Br J Surg* 77:1211, 1990.

70. Chaudary MA, Millis RR, Davies GC, Haywood JL: Nipple discharge: the diagnostic value of testing for occult blood. *Ann Surg* 196:651, 1982.

71. Leis HP: Management of nipple discharge. *World J Surg* 13:736, 1989.

72. Surveillance, Epidemiology, and End Results (SEER) Program public use CD-ROM (1973–1992). Bethesda, MD: National Cancer Institute, DCPC, Surveillance Program, Cancer Statistics Branch; 1995.

73. Lynde JI: Low-cost screening mammography: results of 21,141 consecutive examinations in a community program. *South Med J* 86:338, 1993.

74. Rebner M: Noninvasive breast cancer. *Radiology* 190:623, 1994.

75. Blackwell RE: Diagnosis and management of prolactinomas. *Fertil Steril* 43:5, 1985.

76. Gupta Rk, Pant CS, Tandon US, Singh B: Diagnostic value of galactography in patients with nipple discharge. *Indian J Cancer* 24:22, 1987.

77. Donegan WL, Greene FL, Love SM: Nipple discharge: Is it cancer? *Patient Care* January 30:79, 1990.

78. Makita M, Sakamoto G, Akiyama F, et al: Duct endoscopy and endoscopic biopsy in the evaluation of nipple discharge. *Breast Cancer Res Treat* 18:179, 1991.

79. Terry MB, Skovron ML, Garbers S, et al: The estimated frequency of cosmetic breast augmentation among US women, 1963 through 1988. *Am J Public Health* 85(Part 1):1122, 1995.

80. Brown SL. Langone JJ. Brinton LA: Silicone breast implants and autoimmune disease. *J Am Med Womens Assoc* 53:21, 1998.

81. *Breast Implants: An Information Update*, 1998. U.S. Food and Drug Administration.

82. Silverman BG: Reported complications of silicone breast implants. *Ann Intern Med* 124:744, 1996.

83. Brown SL, Silverman BG, Berg WA: Rupture of silicone-gel breast implants: causes, sequelae, and diagnosis. *Lancet* 350:1531, 1997.

84. Gabriel SE, Woods JE, O'Fallon WM, et al: Complications leading to surgery after breast implantation. *N Engl J Med* 336:677, 1997.

85. Hurst N: Lactation after augmentation mammaplasty. *Obstet Gynecol* 87:30, 1996.

86. Dabbah A, Lehman JA, Parker MG, et al: Reduction mammaplasty: an outcome analysis. *Ann Plast Surg* 35:337, 1995.

87. Raipis T, Zehring RD, Downey D: Long-term functional results after reduction mammaplasty. *Ann Plas Surg* 34(2):113, 1995.

88. Klassen A, Fitzpatrick R, Jenkinson C, et al: Should breast reduction surgery be rationed? A comparison of the health status of patients before and after treatment: postal questionnaire survey. *BMJ* 313:454, 1996.

89. Harris L, Morris SF, Freiberg A: Is breast feeding possible after reduction mammaplasty? *Plast Reconstruct Surg* 89:836, 1992.

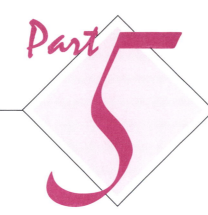

Other Common Health Concerns

James P. Olson
Duane Warren

Hypertension and Ischemic Heart Disease

Anticoagulant Therapy	Noninvasive Cardiac Testing
Beta Blockers	Summary
Angiotensin-Converting Enzyme Inhibitors	

Overview

Hypertension and ischemic heart disease (IHD) transcend gender and take an enormous toll in morbidity and mortality of women. Unfortunately studies show that women often do not realize the extent of their cardiovascular risk.

To get a statistical perspective, Table 17-1 contains data from the *Health U.S. 1998 Report*[1] comparing the impact of IHD, stroke, and breast cancer on the death rate and years of potential life lost (YPLL) for women. Despite the fact that many women believe that breast cancer poses a greater risk to their health, the mortality rates of stroke and IHD are two and five times higher, respectively, than the breast cancer mortality rate. Although this belief may be due to a fear of premature death, data on YPLL show that cardiovascular disease also causes more years of life to be lost prematurely than breast cancer (see Table 17-1). These misconceptions may harm women by undermining primary prevention efforts (e.g., avoiding hormone replacement therapy [HRT]) and causing delays in seeking care (e.g., not recognizing symptoms of a myocardial infarction [MI]).

Hypertension

Hypertension[2–4] affects approximately 50 million Americans; 60 percent are women. High blood pressure accounts for more visits to and prescriptions from primary care providers than any other con-

dition. Yet, only about half the persons with hypertension are under treatment. Equally concerning is that, of those treated, only half have controlled blood pressure. This represents an opportunity for improvement in women's health through identification and adequate medical treatment of hypertension in this large group at risk for stroke, IHD, renal disease, and congestive heart failure (CHF).

Joint National Committee-VI

In 1972, the National High Blood Pressure Education Program (NHBPEP) was created as a cooperative group involving professional, governmental, and public organizations. The NHBPEP is administered and coordinated by the National Heart, Lung and Blood Institute of the National Institutes of Health. The mission of the NHBPEP is to reduce the morbidity and mortality associated with hypertension through educational programs for professionals, patients, and the general public. Among its many efforts is the *Report of the Joint National Committee on Prevention, Detection, Evaluation and Treatment of High Blood Pressure*. In the fall of 1997, the Joint National Committee (JNC) released its sixth report (the JNC-VI)[5] with the next update scheduled for 2001.

The JNC is concerned with recent trends of hypertension-related disease. After dropping for many years, the rate of coronary artery disease is leveling off. The rates for CHF, stroke, and renal failure are increasing. Selected goals of the report that target these concerns are (1) to improve primary prevention of hypertension, (2) to improve lowering of blood pressure to the goal of 140/90 mmHg, (3) to increase the recognition of the need to control isolated systolic hypertension, and (4) to improve the recognition of the implications of

Table 17-1

Statistical Comparisons of Conditions Involving Women

	ALL CAUSES OF DEATH		DISEASE OF THE HEART		ISCHEMIC HEART DISEASE		CEREBROVASCULAR DISEASE		MALIGNANT NEOPLASM BREAST	
	1985	1996	1985	1996	1985	1996	1985	1996	1985	1996
Age-Adjusted Death Rate	410.3	381.0	127.4	98.2	84.2	60.4	30.0	24.6	12.6	10.2
YPLL White Female	5607	4900	832	637	501	352	189	157	388	309
YPLL Black Female	10,631	10,013	1993	1636	918	682	545	423	479	484

NOTES: Age-adjusted death rate—in deaths per 100,000 women in the population.
YPLL is age-adjusted years of potential life lost before the age of 75 per 100,000 women in the population under 75 years of age.
SOURCE: National Center for Health Statistics: *Health*, United States, Copyright 1998.

high-normal blood pressure. Important proposed management strategies in the report are (1) to stratify patients with hypertension based on blood pressure stage and risk factors to guide treatment decisions, (2) to identify compelling "reasons" for selecting specific treatments, and (3) to apply population-based strategies such as primary prevention through lifestyle changes.

The JNC-VI is intended to be a tool for primary care providers to adapt to individual patients and local situations. It is not meant to preempt a clinician's judgment, which remains critical in assessing and treating patients. Some strengths of the report are that it includes perspectives from diverse groups concerned with blood pressure control and that it clearly cites and rates the evidence for its recommendations.

Blood Pressure Measurement and Classification

MEASUREMENT

To correctly diagnose and treat hypertension, accurate blood pressure measurement is manda-tory. A summary of the technique for properly determining blood pressure is outlined in Table 17-2.[6] Failing to perform the technique properly will diminish measurement accuracy. Factors that can confound results and the effects and remedies are summarized in Table 17-3.[6]

CLASSIFICATION

It has long been recognized that there is a strong, positive, independent, continuous, and consistent relationship between blood pressure and cardiovascular disease. Due to the continuous relationship between the blood pressure and outcomes, classification of blood pressure is somewhat arbitrary. The JNC-VI defines hypertension as a systolic blood pressure (SBP) of 140 mmHg and above, or a diastolic blood pressure (DBP) of 90 mmHg and above. Further classification is useful to identify risk groups, guide treatment, and assist in trial design (Table 17-4).[5]

OPTIMAL BLOOD PRESSURE

Epidemiologic studies show that blood pressures below 120/80 mmHg are optimal with

Table 17-2

Recommendations for Determining Blood Pressure by Sphygmomanometry

1. The patient should refrain from smoking or caffeine intake for the 30 min prior to testing.
2. The patient's arm should be supported at heart level.
3. The patient should be sitting with back support.
4. The manometer should be at eye level, easy to read, and deflated to zero before measurement begins.
5. The proper size bladder should be selected. (When in doubt, select the large size. Some physicians use a large cuff for most adults as long as the bladder does not overlap itself.)
6. The bladder center, located by folding the cuff in half, is aligned with the brachial artery, and the cuff should be affixed so that its inferior edge lies 2.5–3.0 cm above the antecubital fossa.
7. The point of maximal inflation should be identified by palpation of the radial artery and inflating the cuff to 30 mmHg above the pressure where the pulse is last palpated. If the radial artery cannot be palpated, inflate cuff to 230 mmHg.
8. The bell or diaphragm of the stethoscope can be used but must be pressed lightly over the brachial artery.
9. The cuff is rapidly inflated to the predetermined point of maximal inflation and then deflated slowly at 2–3 mmHg/s.
10. The systolic blood pressure, the point at which at least two consecutive faint tapping beats are heard, is noted and recorded in even numbers.
11. The diastolic blood pressure is the point at which the last muffled sound is heard. It also is recorded in even numbers.
12. Record the pressures, cuff size, patient's position, and arm used for measurement.
13. No talking should occur between technician and patient during the measurement.
14. Repeat measurements should be delayed 1–2 min before retesting the same arm.

SOURCE: Modified with permission from LE Kay, *J Am Board Fam Pract* 11:252, Copyright 1998.[6]

respect to minimizing cardiovascular risk.[5] As blood pressure increases from this level, morbidity and mortality increase. Therefore, women with blood pressure in what is now considered the "high-normal" range are candidates for lifestyle modification intervention. If blood pressure is not lowered in these women, they are at increased risk of developing frank hypertension (RR = 1.89 for women, 95 percent CI = 1.5 to 2.3).[7]

There is concern that lowering blood pressure goals too much will, at some point, result in an increase in mortality (e.g., the "J point" phenomenon). The reasoning is that as the DBP is lowered, coronary circulation (which is dependent on DBP) will fall, potentially leading to myocardial ischemia and an increase in cardiac events. Study results have been contradictory as to the blood pressure levels at which this may occur. The recently published Hypertension Optimal Treatment (HOT)[8] study concluded that, for most patients, the majority of the benefit of treatment occurred in reaching a goal blood pressure of 140/85 mmHg; no significant additional gain was derived in most patients from further lowering the blood pressure. However, there was no adverse effect of lowering blood pressures down to a SBP of 120 mmHg and a DBP of 70 mmHg. For some subgroups, such as patients with diabetes, a lower DBP of 80 mmHg was associated with a decreased risk of cardiovascular events.

There is interest among both patients and providers in the use of ambulatory blood pressure measurements in managing hypertension. Research has shown that these measurements are lower than

Table 17-3

Factors Confounding the Accuracy of Auscultatory Blood Pressure Measurements

FACTOR/ERROR	EFFECT (AND DEGREE OF EFFECT)	REMEDY
Body posture		
Sitting without back support	Increased DBP & SBP (5–10 mmHg)	Use standard seated position with back support.
Standing	Increased DBP & SBP	
Lying	Decreased DBP & SBP	
Arm support—patient supporting	Increased DBP & SBP (4+ mmHg)	Examiner support arm.
Arm position		
At level of sternomanubrial junction	Decrease in DBP & SBP (5 mmHg)	Use standard arm position at fourth intercostal space.
At level of xiphoid process	Increase in DBP & SBP (5 mmHg)	
Rate of deflation too fast	Underestimate SBP	Deflate cuff at 2–3 mmHg/s.
Auscultatory gap missed	Overestimate DBP	Determine point of maximal inflation by palpation first, then inflate 30 mmHg above this or inflate to 230 mmHg.
	Underestimate SBP	
Pressure on head of stethoscope		
10 mmHg	Decrease DBP (10 mmHg)	Apply only enough pressure to seal stethoscope to skin.
Firm pressure	Sounds may persist to 0 mmHg	
Size of cuff		
Too small	Overestimate SBP (5–9.5 mmHg)	Always choose proper-sized cuffs. Bladder cuff should encircle at least 80% of arm.
	Overestimate DBP (4–7 mmHg)	
Too large	Underestimate SBP (0–4 mmHg)	
No delay between readings	Variable effect on SBP & DBP	Allow 1–2 min between reading.
Only measuring in one arm	Up to 10 mmHg difference between arms in up to 6% of patients	Take measurements in both arms and use the higher number. Document which arm used.
Using the wrong Korotkoff sound to determine DBP	Overestimate DBP (5–10 mmHg)	Use the fifth Korotkoff sound, the last sound heard.
Digit preference (rounding to nearest 5 or 10 mmHg)	0–5 mmHg inaccuracy	Round to nearest 2 mmHg.
Equipment errors		
Aneroid sphygmomanometers	22–60% inaccuracy	Regular inspection and calibration.
Mercury column manometers	2–8% inaccuracy	
Environmental		
Cold room	Increase in DBP (up to 15 mmHg)	Use warm rooms.
Talking during measurement	Increase in DBP (8–15 mmHg)	Do not talk during measurement.

ABBREVIATIONS: DBP, diastolic blood pressure; SBP, systolic blood pressure.

SOURCE: Modified with permission from LE Kay; *J Am Board Fam Praci* 11:252, Copyright 1998.[6]

Table 17-4

Classification of Blood Pressures for Adults*

	BLOOD PRESSURE, mmHg		
CATEGORY	SYSTOLIC		DIASTOLIC
Optimal[†]	<120	and	<80
Normal	<130	and	<85
High-Normal	130–139	or	85–89
Hypertension[‡]			
Stage 1	140–159	or	90–99
Stage 2	160–179	or	100–109
Stage 3	≥180	or	≥110

*Not taking antihypertensive drugs and not acutely ill. When diastolic and systolic blood pressures fall into different categories, the higher category should be selected to classify blood pressure.
[†]Optimal blood pressure with respect to cardiovascular risks is less than 120/80.
[‡]Based on the average of 2 or more readings taken at each of 2 or more visits.
SOURCE: The Joint National Committee on Prevention, Detection, Evaluation and Treatment of High Blood Pressure, NIH Pub No. 98-4080, Nov, 1997.[5]

measurements obtained in the office.[9] Based on a prospective study of mortality and home blood pressure values,[10] the JNC-VI recommends using an ambulatory home blood pressure goal of 135/85 mmHg. A helpful role for home blood pressure monitoring is in evaluating early morning blood pressures to ensure that the morning hypertensive surge is controlled. This can especially be a problem with once-daily dosing formulations, which are at the end of their 24-h dosing interval.

Table 17-5 contains information on personal blood pressure monitors.[11]

Pathophysiology and Gender[12]

Blood pressure represents the summation of complex interactions of many systems—peripheral and central adrenergic, endocrine, renal, hemodynamic, and vascular. When a specific cause for

Table 17-5

Home Blood Pressure Monitors

MODEL TYPE	COMMENTS	COST
Electronic arm	Brands show a wide range of accuracy. Highly rated brands for ease of use, accuracy, and instructions include AND UA-767 or UA-702 and Omron HEM-711 or HEM-712C.	$40–100
Electronic wrist	Easier to use but less accurate and more expensive than arm models. Highly rated brands were Omron HEM-605 or HEM-601.	$100–125
Electronic finger	These are unacceptable due to inaccuracy and inconsistency.	
Manual arm	More difficult to use and requires the ability to listen with a stethoscope. Accuracy is good with practice. Inexpensive.	$20–25

SOURCE: Modified with permission from Consumer Reports, *Consumer Rep* 61:50, Copyright 1996.[11]

hypertension can be identified, it is classified as secondary hypertension. However, about 95 percent of individuals with hypertension have primary or essential hypertension. In these patients, we are not yet able to determine which specific systems are responsible.

When women develop hypertension, they are protected to a greater degree than men against stroke and heart disease at equivalent blood pressure elevations. However, hypertension still increases a woman's relative risk of cardiovascular events up to five times above the level of women with normal blood pressure.

As a group, women not only display different physiologic patterns of blood pressure from men, but the pattern varies by age and race. The effect of aging on blood pressure is more pronounced in women than in men. Although with aging SBP increases for both genders, men experience a gradual increase in SBP throughout adulthood, whereas for women the rate of increase is much slower throughout younger adulthood and more rapid after menopause. At equivalent ages before menopause, women are less likely than men to be hypertensive. By age 60, the average female SBP exceeds the average male SBP. Above 65 years of age, it is estimated that about one-half of white women and three-fourths of black women are hypertensive.[13]

Hypertension in younger women is characterized by a higher heart rate, cardiac index, and pulse pressure but a lower peripheral vascular resistance. Therefore, beta blockers and diuretics may be more effective drug classes than vasodilators for these patients.[5] In addition, premenopausal women tend to have low plasma renin activity, which increases during the luteal phase and is associated with increased plasma volume.

PERIPHERAL VASCULAR RESISTANCE

As women age, their hypertension is associated with increased peripheral resistance, low or normal plasma volume, and low plasma renin levels. Women have a lower total peripheral vascular resistance than men for equivalent levels of arterial pressure.[4]

BLOOD PRESSURE LABILITY

Women also appear to have a higher rate of labile/episodic elevation of blood pressure (such as "white coat hypertension"). For example, a study of elevated incidental DBPs obtained in an office setting subsequently led to a diagnosis of hypertension in 69 percent of men but only 49 percent of women.[14]

CARDIAC HYPERTROPHY

The heart's hypertrophic response to elevated blood pressure also varies by gender. For women, an increased body weight is a greater cocontributor to left ventricular hypertrophy (LVH) than for men. In women, LVH tends to develop concentrically, leading to increased wall thickness.[15] In men, the response tends to occur eccentrically, leading to ventricular dilation. The concentric hypertrophy in women is reported to increase cardiovascular morbidity and mortality to a greater degree than the eccentric pattern; if concentric LVH occurs in response to hypertension, it nearly abolishes the risk advantage that women have in general.[16]

ETHNIC VARIATION

Hypertension in African American women is especially dangerous. As shown in Table 17-1, African American women have rates of YPLL that are two to three times higher than white women for both heart disease and stroke.[1] As a group, black women tend to have low plasma renin levels and respond poorly to angiotensin-converting enzyme (ACE) inhibitors.

Clinical Evaluation

The evaluation of a patient with elevated blood pressure involves answering a number of questions. Are there other cardiac risk factors that need attention? Is there evidence of a secondary cause for the hypertension? Is there end organ damage or clinical cardiovascular disease? Are there any medical conditions that might provide compelling indications or contraindications to selecting a specific therapy? Table 17-6 contains a summary of the clinical evaluation built on JNC-VI recommendations.

RISK STRATIFICATION

The JNC-VI approaches treatment decisions through a risk stratification process. A patient's risk from hypertension is greater when she has other major cardiovascular risk factors, end organ damage, clinical cardiovascular disease, or a high stage of blood pressure (see Table 17-4). The JNC-VI risk stratifying recommendations are summarized in Table 17-7. For patients with CHF, diabetes, or renal disease, the JNC suggests a more aggressive approach; medications are started sooner and the

Table 17-6

Clinical Evaluation of a Woman with Newly Diagnosed Hypertension

HISTORY
Length of time of blood pressure (BP) elevation
Prior treatments, efficacy, and side effects
Menstrual history/menopausal status
Symptoms of coronary artery disease (CAD) or cerebrovascular disease
Smoking
Diet including salt, fat, alcohol, and caffeine intake
Exercise
Weight changes
Work and hobbies
Family dynamics
Medications including oral contraceptives, nonprescription drugs, "natural" treatments, vitamins, and illicit drugs
Personal past history of CAD, stroke, renal disease, hyperlipidemia, congestive heart failure, diabetes mellitus (DM), peripheral vascular disease, asthma, gout
Family history of hypertension, early CAD, stroke, DM, renal disease
Symptoms that suggest a secondary cause (see Table 17–8)
PHYSICAL EXAMINATION
Two or more BP readings to include both arms and a standing BP
Height, weight, abdominal circumference
Ophthalmic exam to assess for retinopathy
Ear-nose-throat including thyroid and stigmata of obstructive sleep apnea
Vascular exam including peripheral pulses, carotid bruits, jugular vein distention, hepatojugular reflux, edema
Pulmonary exam including rales, wheezes, signs of chronic obstructive pulmonary disease
Cardiac exam including murmurs, gallops, heart rate
Abdominal exam including bruits, aortic size, renal masses
TESTING
Complete blood count
Chemistry profile to include electrolytes, fasting blood sugar, blood urea nitrogen, creatinine, uric acid
Lipid profile
Electrocardiogram

Table 17-7

Risk Stratification and Treatment

BLOOD PRESSURE STAGE	RISK GROUP A (NO MRF/EOD/CCD)	RISK GROUP B (AT LEAST 1 MRF BUT NOT DIABETES AND NO EOD/CCD)	RISK GROUP C (ANY EOD, CCD, OR DIABETES)
High-normal	Lifestyle modification	Lifestyle modification	Drug therapy[†]
Stage 1	Lifestyle modification for up to 12 mo	Lifestyle modification for up to 6 mo*	Drug therapy
Stages 2 and 3	Drug therapy	Drug therapy	Drug therapy

NOTES: Lifestyle modification should be included for all patients receiving drug therapy.
*For patients with multiple risk factors, drug therapy should be started initially.
[†]Those with heart failure, renal insufficiency, or diabetes require drug treatment and lower goal blood pressure.
ABBREVIATIONS: Major risk factors (MRF)—Smoking, dyslipidemia, diabetes, age >60 y, sex (male or postmenopausal female), family history of cardiovascular disease in a first-degree relative who is a male < 55 y or a female < 65 y.
End organ disease/clinical cardiovascular disease (EOD/CCD)—Heart diseases (left ventricular hypertrophy, coronary artery disease—angina or myocardial infarction, prior coronary revascularization, congestive heart failure), stroke or transient ischemic attack, nephropathy, peripheral artery disease, retinopathy.
SOURCE: Modified from The Joint National Committee on Prevention, Detection, Evaluation and Treatment of High Blood Pressure, NIH Pub No. 98-4080, Nov, 1997.[5]

goal blood pressure is lowered to less than 130/85 mmHg.

SECONDARY HYPERTENSION

Although secondary hypertension is uncommon, the clinician needs to be alert to the findings that suggest it. Selected causes are summarized in Table 17-8. For women, oral contraceptive (OC) use and renovascular disease deserve special comment.

ORAL CONTRACEPTIVES   The JNC points out that OCs can induce a small but consistent increase in SBP and DBP. The older formulations containing at

Table 17-8

Selected Causes of Secondary Hypertension

CAUSE	CLUES
Cushing's syndrome/disease	Truncal obesity, striae
Coarctation of the aorta	Delayed or absent femoral pulses
Hyperparathyroidism	Elevated serum calcium, low phosphorus
Pheochromocytoma	Labile hypertension, paroxysms of marked hypertension associated with headaches, pallor, palpitations, perspiration
Polycystic kidneys	Abdominal or flank masses, family history
Primary aldosteronism	Unprovoked hypokalemia
Renal parenchymal disease	Abnormal urinalysis, elevated serum creatinine
Renovascular disease	Age <30 and female or >55 and new onset with other signs of vascular disease, abdominal bruit that lateralizes and extends into diastole, acute renal failure precipitated by an angiotensin-converting enzyme inhibitor

least 50 μg estrogen and 1 to 4 mg progestin have been associated with about a 5 percent incidence of hypertension. The newer lower-dose OC formulations, however, rarely produce an elevated blood pressure. If hypertension occurs (BP > 140/90), the JNC-VI recommends discontinuing OCs. Another option would be switching to a progestin-only pill. The JNC-VI states for select patients for whom the risks associated with pregnancy are great enough, and other birth control options are not acceptable, OCs may be used despite producing an increase in blood pressure. In these women, an antihypertensive agent could be added to the treatment. When OCs are discontinued, blood pressure should normalize over the course of 3 months.

HORMONE REPLACEMENT THERAPY   A closely related issue is the effect that HRT has on blood pressure. In the Postmenopausal Estrogen/Progestin Interventions (PEPI) trial,[17] SBP was one of the primary outcomes of interest because it had previously been speculated that estrogen may be relatively contraindicated for patients with hypertension. Various HRT regimens involving estrogen had no effect on SBP compared to placebo at the end of the 3-year trial period. Numerous other studies have also shown that HRT does not significantly raise blood pressure in normotensive or hypertensive women. In fact, transdermal estrogen has been reported to actually decrease blood pressure slightly in a group of postmenopausal women.[18]

RENOVASCULAR HYPERTENSION   Renovascular hypertension has two typical profiles. The first is renal artery narrowing due to atherosclerotic disease that is associated with the same risk factors as atherosclerotic changes elsewhere—older age, smoking, hyperlipidemia, and so on. The second form is fibromuscular dysplasia that typically affects women 20 to 50 years old. Additional diagnostic clues that suggest fibromuscular dysplasia are abdominal bruits (especially if they lateralize and extend into diastole) and hypertension resistant to treatment. A captopril renal scan, a radionuclide study where angiotensin-mediated compensatory blood flow to the affected kidney is temporarily blocked by captopril, is a useful test in evaluating possible renovascular disease.[19]

Treatment [20]

PRIMARY PREVENTION

Primary prevention is critical to controlling the morbidity and financial and personal costs of hypertension. Primary prevention, in a population-based manner, addresses the cardiovascular disease that may develop in patients with blood pressures above the "optimal" range but not high enough to be labeled hypertensive. The blood pressure rise that develops as Americans age is not inevitable and can be minimized with primary prevention strategies. These lifestyle modifications, which are the same as those described below for treating established hypertension, are thought to be helpful in primary prevention of hypertension.

TREATMENT OF ESTABLISHED HYPERTENSION

NONPHARMACOLOGIC INTERVENTIONS   Many lifestyle changes have been shown to lower blood pressure (Table 17-9). They have the additional benefit of positively affecting other major risk factors such as diabetes and dyslipidemia, which add to the end organ damage of hypertension.

Weight Reduction.   An increase in blood pressure is closely correlated with an increase in body mass index (BMI). Even the loss of as little as 10 lb can reduce blood pressure.[21] The association between weight change and hypertension is strongest in women less than 45 years old.[22] Lowering a woman's BMI has also been shown to decrease insulin resistance, aid in dyslipidemia control, and help reverse LVH. It will also augment the effects of antihypertensive medication. Women who display central or truncal obesity (a waist circumference of 40 inches [100 cm] or above) are at increased cardiovascular risk compared to those with obesity of the lower body.[23]

Table 17-9

Lifestyle Modifications for Women with Hypertension

WEIGHT CONTROL
Risk increase for body mass index >30 and waist circumference >40 in. (100 cm)

LIMIT ALCOHOL
No more than 0.5 oz (15 mL) ethanol per day. This is 12 oz of beer, 5 oz of wine, or 1 oz of 100 proof "hard liquor"

EXERCISE
Aerobic activity of 3–4 h/w divided over 3 to 6 d

DIET	
Sodium	Limit sodium intake to 2.4 g (6 g sodium chloride)
Potassium	Potassium-rich foods are fruits and vegetables (at least 90 mmol/d)
Fiber	Fruit fiber may be better
Calcium	Women are advised to consume 1000–1500 mg Ca/d; this is equal to 3–4 glasses of milk/d

SMOKING
Although not a cause of hypertension, it should be addressed for its effect on ischemic heart disease risk

SOURCE: Modified from The Joint National Committee on Prevention, Detection, Evaluation and Treatment of High Blood Pressure, NIH Pub No. 98-4080, Nov, 1997.[5]

Alcohol Consumption. Heavy alcohol consumption (> 2 to 3 oz of alcohol daily) is a risk factor for hypertension and can cause resistance to antihypertensive therapy. Women absorb alcohol more efficiently than men, due to reduced alcohol dehydrogenase in the gastric mucosa, and are generally smaller, so the amount of alcohol needed to cause adverse effects is less than for men.[24] Therefore, the JNC-VI recommendation is that women limit their intake to 0.5 oz ethanol per day (see Table 17-9). At this lower level, alcohol does not elevate blood pressure.[25]

Exercise. Exercise has been shown to lower blood pressure independent of changes in weight, dietary changes, and aerobic capacity in sedentary adults[26] and postmenopausal women.[27] A program of brisk walking (at 60 to 70 percent of maximal effort) for 3 to 4 h a week divided over 3 to 6 days can produce SBP and DBP drops averaging in the range of 5 to 10 mmHg within 3 months in women.[28] Again, this behavioral change will also help to control other risk factors.

Diet. Many different dietary components are associated with hypertension. Sodium is the most common dietary factor considered. To elevate BP, sodium requires concomitant chloride intake to fully affect responders. Nonchloride sodium salts are less likely to increase blood pressure.

About 30 to 50 percent of all individuals with hypertension, and up to 75 percent of African Americans with hypertension, are salt sensitive. African Americans, the elderly, and patients with hypertension or diabetes, are most likely to respond to sodium restriction. Women are also more likely than men to be sensitive to sodium. Dietary sodium reduction of 100 mmol (2.3 g)/d will lower blood pressure, over a period of 1 to 2 months, on average 6/2 mmHg in elderly individuals with hypertension.[29] In addition, limiting salt can improve the efficacy of diuretics and ACE inhibitors[30] and help limit potassium wasting with diuretics.[31] The most common source of dietary sodium is processed foods. Patients need to be instructed about how to identify foods high in sodium chloride.

Low dietary potassium, calcium, and magnesium intake have also been implicated in elevating blood pressure.[5,32] Evidence supports the role of oral potassium intake (60 to 120 mEq/d) in lowering blood pressure, but this benefit mainly occurs among patients with chronically low potassium intake.[33] Clinically important reductions in blood pressure have not been demonstrated with calcium supplementation.[34] Certain subgroups of women may be more responsive to calcium supplementation, but specific information is lacking. Women's diets should contain adequate calcium for osteoporosis prevention, and this will meet the quantity claimed to have an antihypertensive effect. For magnesium, data are again inconclusive and specific recommendations cannot be made. Caffeine can raise blood pressure transiently, but tolerance to this effect usually develops.[35] Diets high in fruit fiber (24 g/d) have been shown to lower blood pressure.[36]

These dietary recommendations were incorporated into the Dietary Approaches to Stop Hypertension (DASH) trial[36] and found to lower blood pressure in patients with hypertension on average by 11/5 mmHg. This diet, which is rich in fruits, vegetables, and low-fat dairy foods, while restricting saturated and total fat, is outlined in Table 17-10.

PHARMACOLOGIC TREATMENT   Although it is estimated that 60 percent of the hypertensive population is female, most of the information regarding treatment was obtained in study populations that were either totally, or at least predominantly, male. It was assumed that there were no gender-related differences in the treatment of hypertension. In a

Table 17-10
Dietary Approaches to Stop Hypertension (DASH) Diet

FOOD GROUP	DAILY SERVINGS	EXAMPLES AND COMMENTS	SIGNIFICANCE IN THE DIET
Grains and grain products	7–8	Whole wheat bread, pita bread, cereals, oatmeal	Major source of energy and fiber
Vegetables	4–5	Tomatoes, potatoes, carrots, peas, squash, broccoli, beans	Important sources of potassium, magnesium, and fiber
Fruits	4–5	Bananas, dates, grapes, oranges, apples, fruit juices, raisins, strawberries	Important sources of potassium, magnesium, and fiber
Low-fat or nonfat dairy	2–3	Skim or 1% milk, nonfat or low-fat yogurt, nonfat cheeses	Major sources of protein and calcium
Meat, poultry, and fish	2 or less	Select lean meats, trim away visible fat, broil or roast instead of frying, cut away skin from poultry	Rich sources of protein and magnesium
Nuts, seeds, and legumes	4–5/wk	Almonds, peanuts, sunflower seeds, lentils	Rich sources of energy, magnesium, potassium, and fiber

SOURCE: Modified from The Joint Committee on Prevention, Detection, Evaluation and Tratment of High Blood Pressure, NIH Pub No. 98-4080, Nov, 1997.[5]

review[12] of 10 major clinical trials evaluating the pharmacotherapy of hypertension, it was noted that 3 of the trials specifically excluded women from the study,[37–39] 3 others only studied elderly populations,[40–42] and the rest were not designed to detect gender differences due to design factors or lack of statistical power.[43–46] Even the JNC-VI issued a single set of guidelines for diagnosis and treatment intended for use for both men and women.

Figure 17-1

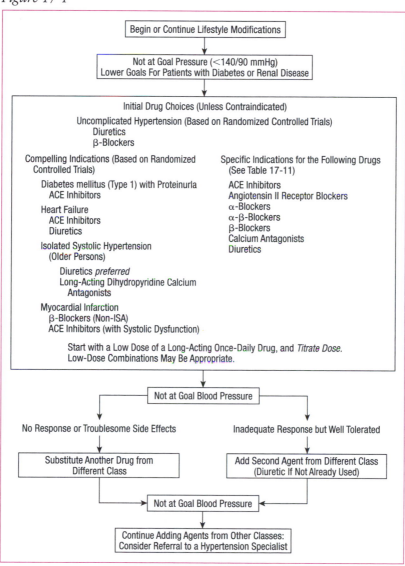

Algorithm for the treatment of hypertension.
ABBREVIATIONS: ACE, angiotensin-converting enzyme; ISA, intrinsic sympathomimetic activity.
SOURCE: Modified from The Joint National Committee on Prevention, Detection, Evaluation and Treatment of High Blood Pressure, NIH Pub No. 98-4080, Nov, 1997.[5]

JNC-VI Overview.   The treatment algorithm offered by the JNC is presented in Fig. 17-1. As a general rule, most patients should be started on a single agent in a low dose, with gradual increases as needed for blood pressure control. Consideration should be given early to combination therapy because it can often be effective with lower doses of each agent; therefore, fewer side effects will result.[47]

The JNC-VI recognizes that there will be times when patients may be started on antihypertensive agents that will also benefit comorbid conditions. Some treatments have such strong benefits in certain comorbid conditions that they should be used unless a contraindication to their use exists. Conversely, some agents may have a negative effect on comorbid conditions and should be avoided. A list of conditions that can affect drug selection is contained in Table 17-11.

According to JNC-VI, a thiazide diuretic or a beta blocker is the preferred initial drug choice for the pharmacotherapy of hypertension in men and women, unless there are "compelling reasons" to choose another agent. This is based on the findings that, of all the antihypertensive agents, only these two classes have consistently been shown to decrease morbidity and mortality from hypertension. Beta blockers can be used as initial therapy in women who do not have "compelling indications" to the contrary (i.e., type 1 diabetes mellitus with proteinuria or isolated systolic hypertension [ISH]) and are strongly indicated in patients after MI.

Isolated systolic hypertension is recognized as a "compelling indication" for choosing a diuretic or a long-acting calcium channel blocker as initial drug therapy, because of demonstrated efficacy in reducing long-term morbidity and mortality. Controversy has surrounded calcium channel blockers in recent years. Initial concerns were raised when early calcium channel blockers were found to be associated with adverse outcomes in patients who had a history of MI and in those with LVH.[48] When retrospective studies suggested that short half-life calcium channel blockers were associated with an increased risk of MIs in a less select group of patients, the controversy accelerated. This cardiovascular risk was recently demonstrated in the prospective randomized Multicenter Isradipine

Diuretic Atherosclerosis Study (MIDAS) that compared isradipine, a short-acting drug (a member of the dihydropyridine subclass of calcium channel blockers), to hydrochlorothiazide.[49] Some researchers have argued that the risk of mortality from calcium channel blockers is confined to the short-acting dihydropyridines. However, an increased risk was also present in the Appropriate Blood Pressure Control in Diabetes (ABCD) trial that compared nisoldipine, a long-acting dihydropyridine calcium channel blocker, to enalapril in patients with diabetes; the nisoldipine-treated group had a fivefold greater risk of MI.[50] Given this information, it would be prudent to avoid dihydropyridine calcium channel blockers and to select other agents for patients with diabetes. It should be noted, however, that only the dihydropyridines have been associated with this risk, and thus far, verapamil and diltiazem have not been implicated.

The JNC-VI guidelines recommend using ACE inhibitors as first-line therapy for hypertension in patients with diabetes mellitus and proteinuria, in patients with CHF, or, by itself or in conjunction with a beta blocker, in a patient after MI.

Other drug classes used to treat hypertension are angiotensin receptor blockers, alpha-1 blockers, vasodilators, and centrally acting agents. Although many claims are made for the advantages of different agents, they are based on surrogate markers and not the results of ultimate mortality and morbidity reduction in clinical trials. The angiotensin receptor blocker class is hoped to work like the ACE inhibitors without the side effect of cough. The alpha-1 blockers have favorable effects on lipid parameters (reducing total and low-density lipoprotein cholesterol [LDL-C] and slightly increasing high-density lipoprotein cholesterol [HDL-C]).[51] However, clinical outcome trials have not been done to demonstrate whether these classes truly have advantages over diuretics or beta blockers.

Diuretics.   Diuretics (Table 17-12) act to increase urine volume by inhibiting electrolyte reabsorption (including sodium) at various sites in the nephron. Numerous long-term randomized controlled trials have demonstrated the effectiveness of thiazide diuretics in reducing cerebrovascular and cardio-

Table 17-11

Considerations in Selecting Antihypertensive Medications

CONDITION	DRUG THERAPY
COMPELLING INDICATIONS TO USE THIS THERAPY UNLESS OTHERWISE CONTRAINDICATED	
Diabetes (type 1) with proteinuria	ACEI
Heart failure	ACEI, diuretic
Isolated systolic hypertension (elderly)	Diuretic, CCB (long-acting dihydropyridine)
Myocardial infarction	BB without ISA, ACEI (with LV dysfunction)
CONDITIONS WHERE SPECIFIC THERAPIES MAY BE MORE EFFECTIVE	
African-Americans	Diuretic, CCB, labetalol
Financial restrictions	Diuretic, BB, reserpine
CONDITIONS WHERE DRUG THERAPY MAY POSITIVELY EFFECT COMORBID CONDITIONS	
Angina	BB
Atrial tachycardia and fibrillation	BB, CCB (non-dihydropyridine)
Cyclosporine-induced hypertension	CCB
Diabetes (type 2) with proteinuria	ACEI
Diabetes (type 2)	Diuretic
Dyslipidemia	α-1 blocker
Essential tremor	BB (non-cardioselective)
Heart failure	Carvedilol, ARB
Hyperthyroidism	BB
Migraine	BB (non-cardioselective), CCB ([non-dihydropyridine] with non-Q-wave infarction)
Myocardial infarction	Diltiazem, verapamil
Osteoporosis	Thiazide diuretic
Preoperative hypertension	BB
Renal insufficiency (caution in renovascular hypertension and creatinine level ≥ 265.2 μmd/L [≥ 3 mg/dL])	ACEI
CONDITIONS WHERE DRUGS MAY WORSEN COMORBID CONDITIONS (*CONTRAINDICATED)	
Bronchospastic disease	BB*
Depression	BB, central alpha agents, reserpine*
Diabetes (types 1 and 2)	BB, high-dose diuretics
Dyslipidemia	BB (non-ISA), high-dose diuretic
Gout	Diuretic
2nd- or 3rd-degree heart block	BB,* CCB (non-dihydropyridine)
Heart failure	BB, CCB (except amlodipine and felodipine)
Liver disease	Labetalol, methyldopa*
Peripheral vascular disease	BB
Pregnancy	ACEI,* ARB*
Renal insufficiency	Potassium-sparing agents

ABBREVIATIONS: ACEI, angiotensin-converting enzyme inhibitors; ARB, angiotensin II receptor blockers; BB, beta blockers; CCB, calcium channel blockers; ISA, intrinsic sympathomimetic activity; LV, left ventricular.
SOURCE: From The Joint National Committee on Prevention, Detection, Evaluation and Treatment of High Blood Pressure, NIH Pub. No. 98-4080, Nov, 1997.[5]

Table 17-12

Selected Diuretics

GENERIC NAME	TRADE NAME	USUAL DOSE (MG/D)	COMMENTS
THIAZIDES*			
Benzthiazide	Exna	12.5–25 mg qd	
Chlorothiazide	Diuril	125–1000 mg qd	
Chlorthalidone	Hygroton	12.5–25 mg bid	
Hydrochloro-thiazide (HCTZ)	HydroDIURIL	12.5–25 mg qd	The most commonly used thiazide
Indapamide	Lozol	1.25–5 mg qd	Not strictly a thiazide but an indole derivative. Slow onset of action up to 1–2 mo.
Metolazone	Zaroxolyn	2.5 mg qd	Behaves like a loop agent and can be used in patients with low glomerular filtration rates. If combined with a loop agent can create spectacular diuresis and severe electrolyte alterations.
LOOP†			
Bumetanide	Bumex	0.5–2.0 mg qd	The dose can be increased greatly.
Furosemide	Lasix	20–80 mg bid	The dose can be increased greatly.
Torsemide	Demadex	5–10 mg qd	The dose can be increased greatly.
POTASSIUM SPARING‡			
Amiloride	Midamor	5–20 mg qd	Usually combined with a thiazide. Ratio of HCTZ/amiloride of 10:1. Alone it can produce a mild diuresis.
Spironolactone	Aldactone	25–100 mg bid	Acts as an aldosterone antagonist only. Antiandrogenic side effect can sometimes be useful.
Triamterene	Dyrenium	50–100 mg qd	Usually combined with a thiazide because of little intrinsic antihypertensive effect. Ratio of HCTZ/triamterene 0.5:1.

*Thiazide diuretics are ineffective in severe renal impairment, Cr clearance less than 30 mL/min (a serum creatinine < 2.5 mg/dL). Higher doses above those listed are associated with increasing metabolic side effects and very little additional therapeutic benefit. Antihypertensive effect may take 3–4 wk.

†Loop diuretics act in the ascending limb of the loop of Henle. They can be effective even in severe renal impairment. Useful in edematous states associated with hypertension. Potassium loss is a concern.

‡Potassium-sparing agents are most frequently used in fixed-ratio doses with other diuretics to prevent potassium wasting.

vascular mortality. For this reason, the JNC-VI reasserted its prior recommendations to include thiazide diuretics as first-line agents. Despite the JNC's past endorsements, diuretic use has fallen in recent years. One reason for this has been a concern about the side effects of diuretics. Early studies revealed that significant metabolic abnormalities were induced in women receiving more than 50 mg hydrochlorothiazide or the equivalent.[52] Newer studies, however, using smaller doses of the thiazides (6.25 to 25 mg/d) have shown similar morbidity and mortality reduction, without inducing significant hypokalemia, hyperglycemia, hyperlipidemia, or hyperuricemia.[53] Studies show that thiazides work best in low-renin hypertension (most common in African Americans) and in the elderly.[54]

Hypercholesterolemia, induced by high-dose thiazides, particularly in postmenopausal women, has been a concern. This increase was speculated to be due to decreased levels of estrogen, which normally enhances hepatic clearance of LDL-C through increased lipoprotein lipase activity. Studies using currently recommended doses of chlorthalidone (15 to 25 mg/d) or hydrochlorothiazide (see Table 17-12) reveal that any hypercholesterolemia induced by low-dose diuretics is of a small magnitude and usually returns to baseline within several months of continued therapy.[55]

A potential benefit of thiazide diuretics is the possibility of conferring some protection from osteoporosis in postmenopausal women due to the drug's ability to decrease the urinary excretion of calcium. Several studies have examined the long-term effects of thiazides on bone.[56] In general, bone density is increased in the group treated with the diuretic, although variable changes were reported depending on the site measured. One meta-analysis revealed that current thiazide users (men and women) experienced an 18 percent reduction in the incidence of hip fractures.[56]

In animal models, the reduction of calcium excretion caused by thiazides is potentiated further by the presence of estrogen.[57] If the findings of estrogen augmentation of the anticalciuric effect of thiazides are confirmed in humans, there could be significant clinical implications regarding the initial choice for treatment of hypertension in women.

Beta Blockers. Beta blockers (Table 17-13) act by inhibiting catecholamines from binding to β-adrenergic receptors. This class of drugs has been equally effective at controlling hypertension in both genders. Beta blockers can be subgrouped,

Table 17-13

β-Adrenergic Blocking Drugs

GENERIC NAME	TRADE NAME	USUAL DOSE (MG/D)	DOSING FREQUENCY	CARDIO-SELECTIVITY	INTRINSIC SYMPATHOMIMETIC ACTIVITY	LIPID SOLUBILITY	MONTHLY COST*
Acebutolol	Sectral	200–1200	bid	++	+	Moderate	$47
Atenolol	Tenormin	25–100	qd	++	0	Low	$2**
Betaxolol	Kerlone	5–40	qd	++	0	Low	$39
Bisoprolol	Zebeta	5–20	qd	++	0	Low	$33
Carteolol	Cartrol	2.5–10	qd	0	++	Low	$32
Labetalol[†]	Trandate, Normodyne	200–800	bid	0	0	Moderate	$15**
Metoprolol	Lopressor, Toprol	50–200	qd–bid	+	0	Moderate	$3**
Nadolol	Corgard	20–240	qd	0	0	Low	$11**
Penbutolol	Levatol	20–80	qd	0	+	High	$78
Pindolol	Visken	10–60	bid	0	+++	Moderate	$6**
Propranolol	Inderal	40–240	bid	0	0	High	$2**
Sotalol[‡]	Betapace	160–640	qd–bid	0	0	Low	$219
Timolol	Blocadren	20–40	bid	0	0	Moderate	$20**

*Monthly cost to pharmacy based on average wholesale price of usual regimen.
**Generic drug is available. Generic cost based on typical contract pricing.
[†]Labetalol has both α-blocking (vasodilation) and β-blocking actions.
[‡]Sotalol is more toxic than other beta-blockers and is only used for life-threatening ventricular arrhythmias.

based on cardioselectivity, intrinsic sympathomimetic activity, and lipid solubility. Lipophilic agents that do not contain intrinsic sympathomimetic activity are indicated for use in patients following MI. Beta blockers may be less effective than diuretics in reducing cardiac events in elderly patients who have not had an MI.[54] In this systemic review, diuretics were found to produce an absolute risk reduction of 3.3 percent over 5 years in all-cause mortality compared to beta blockers. The number needed to treat (NNT) to prevent one death over 5 years is 33.

Estrogens have shown an interaction with intracellular formation of cyclic adenosine monophosphate after β-adrenoreceptor stimulation.[58] Such an interaction would be expected to increase the pharmacologic activity of beta blockers. Although such an interaction has been shown in animal models, it is unclear whether it has any relevance in humans.[59]

Angiotensin-Converting Enzyme Inhibitors. The ACE inhibitors (Table 17-14) exert their main effect by blocking the conversion of angiotensin I to angiotensin II, thereby preventing vasoconstriction and decreasing aldosterone levels. The ACE inhibitors are more effective in reducing blood pressure in whites than in African Americans, but there have been no studies of gender differences with these drugs. Animal studies do show a role for estrogen-mediated attenuation of the renin-angiotensin-aldosterone system.[60] One might predict that in the presence of estrogen smaller doses of ACE inhibitors might be sufficient to achieve a therapeutic effect on blood pressure, but this is an untested hypothesis in humans.

A major class-specific side effect is cough. It occurs in 10 to 25 percent of patients; women are twice as likely as men to develop cough.[61] Cough is thought to be due to the effect of the ACE inhibitor on the kinin system and the accumulation of kinins, substance P, and prostaglandins. To determine whether cough is related to the drug, improvement should be noted if the medication is withheld for 4 to 5 days. If a cough develops, cromolyn (2 puff qid, standard asthma doses)[62] or baclofen (5 to 10

Table 17-14

Angiotensin-Converting Enzyme Inhibitors (ACEI) and Angiotensin Receptor Antagonists (ARA)

GENERIC NAME	TRADE NAME	USUAL DOSE (MG/D)	DOSING FREQUENCY	ACE / ARA	MONTHLY COST*
Benazepril	Lotensin	5–80	qd–bid	ACE	$24
Candesartan	Atacand	8–32	qd–bid	ARA	$36
Captopril	Capoten	12.5–450	bid–tid	ACE	$6**
Enalapril	Vasotec	2.5–40	qd–bid	ACE	$38
Fosinopril	Monopril	10–80	qd–bid	ACE	$23
Irbesartan	Avapro	150–300	qd	ARA	$32
Lisinopril	Zestril, Prinivil	5–80	qd	ACE	$42
Losartan	Cozaar	25–200	bid	ARA	$75
Moexipril	Univasc	3.75–15	qd–bid	ACE	$18
Quinapril	Accupril	2.5–80	qd–bid	ACE	$29
Ramipril	Altace	1.25–20	qd–bid	ACE	$32
Trandolapril	Mavik	0.5–4	qd	ACE	$20
Valsartan	Diovan	80–320	qd	ARA	$36

*Monthly cost to pharmacy based on average wholesale price of usual regimen.
**Generic drug is available. Generic cost based on typical contract pricing.
NOTE: The only major differences between the ACEs is their duration of action. Most managed care organizations will only pay for a couple of them. ARAs may be reserved for patients who develop chronic cough on one of the older ACEs.

mg tid)[63] have been shown to minimize cough due to the ACE inhibitor. Another strategy would be to substitute an angiotensin receptor blocker. These agents may have similar benefits without the kinin system interference, but this has yet to be proven in clinical trials.

For women in their childbearing years it must be remembered that the ACE inhibitors are Pregnancy Category X drugs and should be avoided if pregnancy is being considered. These agents may cause fetal skull hypoplasia and serious neonatal problems including hypotension, renal failure, and even death if exposure occurs during the last two trimesters of pregnancy.

Calcium Channel Blockers. The calcium channel blockers (Table 17-15) are a diverse group of agents that exert most of their antihypertensive action through vasodilatory properties. Early clinical trials of the calcium antagonists did not stratify for gender responses. The Amlodipine Cardiovascular Community Trial,[64] however, did examine differential responses by gender in the treatment of hypertension. The investigators demonstrated that women had significantly greater blood pressure decreases than men from baseline systolic and diastolic pressures, after adjusting for age, weight, and dose (in mg/kg). From other trials, however, there have been no indications that calcium antagonists are more or less effective for the treatment of hypertension in either gender. The JNC-VI recommends that for isolated systolic hypertension in the elderly, a thiazide diuretic or a calcium antagonist should be the initial choice. In other situations,

Table 17-15

Calcium Channel Blocking Agents (CCB)

GENERIC NAME	TRADE NAME	USUAL DOSE (MG/D)	DOSING FREQUENCY	VASO-DILATION	DECREASED CONTRACTILITY	HEART RATE	MONTHLY COST*
DIHYDROPYRIDINES							
Amlodipine	Norvasc	2.5–10	qd	++	0	↔	$40
Felodipine	Plendil	5–20	qd	++	0	↔	$52
Isradipine	Dynacirc	2.5–10	bid	++	0	0/↑	$31
Nicardipine	Cardene	60–120	bid-tid	++	0/+	↔	$33
Nifedipine	Adalat	30–120	tid,	++	0/+	↑	$6**
	Procardia		qd (SR)				$72
Nisoldipine	Sular	10–60	qd	++	0	↔	$28
DIPHENYLALKYLAMINES							
Verapamil	Calan,	80–480	qid,	+	++	↓	$3**
	Isoptin,		qd (SR)				$4**
	Covera,						
	Verelan						
BENZOTHIAZEPINES							
Diltiazem	Cardizem	90–360	tid,	+	++	↓	$5**
	Dilacor		qd (SR)				$20

*Monthly cost to pharmacy based on average wholesale price of usual regimen.
**Generic drug is available. Generic cost based on typical contract pricing.

calcium antagonists are effective alternatives for the treatment of hypertension in women, but play no special role.

Other Agents. Other commonly prescribed antihypertensive agents are summarized in Table 17-16.

RESISTANT HYPERTENSION[65,66]

Although most patients will be controlled with mono- or dual therapy, in some patients blood pressure is difficult to control. To be considered resistant, a patient must be on a triple-drug regimen that includes a diuretic and still not be at goal blood pressure. Table 17-17 contains a list of conditions that need to be considered in these cases.

Among elderly patients, "pseudohypertension" is one consideration. This should be considered when there is marked hypertension without evidence of end organ damage, and treatment of hypertension is producing symptoms of hypotension. These patients have arteries that are difficult to compress due to atherosclerotic changes. When inflating the sphygmomanometer, cuff pressure needs to overcome the arterial stiffness along with the intraarterial blood pressure, leading to a falsely elevated reading. In these cases, the only way to get a truly accurate result is to obtain intraarterial readings. It has been suggested that the "Osler test" could help distinguish this condition. This test is performed by locating the patient's radial pulse, inflating the sphygmomanometer cuff to a level that terminates pulsation, and noting if the radial artery is still palpable. Unfortunately, this test is not considered reliable.[67]

Table 17-16

Other Selected Antihypertensives

GENERIC NAME	BRAND NAME	DAILY DOSAGE	FREQUENCY	COMMENTS
ALPHA-1 BLOCKERS*				
Doxazosin	Cardura	1–16 mg	daily	
Prazoxin	Minipress	2–15 mg	bid or tid	Shows tendency for tachyphylaxis
Terazosin	Hytrin	1–20 mg	daily or bid	
CENTRALLY ACTING AGENTS†				
Clonidine	Catapres	0.1–2.4 mg	bid or tid	Available as a once-a-week patch
Guanabenz	Wytensin	4–32 mg	bid	
Guanfacine	Tenex	1–3 mg	daily or bid	
Methyldopa	Aldomet	500–3000 mg	bid or tid	A drug of choice in pregnancy
VASODILATORS‡				
Hydralazine	Apresoline	40–300 mg	bid to qid	
NEURONAL AND GANGLIONIC BLOCKER				
Reserpine		0.1–0.2 mg	daily	

*As a group these agents tend to reduce total and LDL cholesterol and increase HDL cholesterol. They also have a risk of first-dose hypotension.
†This group appears to work by stimulating alpha-2 adrenoreceptors in the central nervous system. A major side effect of these agents is sedation. First three agents can produce severe rebound hypertension if discontinued abruptly.
‡This class of drugs tends to produce reflex tachycardia and water/salt retention and therefore is usually used in combination with beta-blockers and a diuretic.
SOURCE: Reproduced with permission from WH Frishman, *Current Cardiovascular Drugs,* 2nd ed. Philadelphia: Current Medicine, Copyright 1995.[51]

Table 17-17

Causes of Inadequate Hypertension Control

Pseudohypertension	"White coat hypertension," pseudohypertension in the elderly, poor measurement technique
Noncompliance with treatment	
Volume overload	Excess salt intake, progressive renal insufficiency
Drug-related causes	Doses inadequate, wrong type of diuretic, tachyphylaxis
Drug-induced	Sympathomimetics, (including nasal decongestants), appetite suppressants, cocaine and other illicit drug use, oral contraceptives, adrenal steroids, licorice, chewing tobacco, cyclosporine, erythropoietin, antidepressants, nonsteroidal anti-inflammatory drugs
Comorbid conditions	Smoking, obesity, sleep apnea, insulin resistance, alcohol intake, anxiety conditions, chronic pain
Secondary hypertension	See Table 17-8

SIDE EFFECTS OF ANTIHYPERTENSIVE AGENTS

Although some studies have shown that women may experience more side effects from individual antihypertensive agents than men, no well-designed trials have confirmed this hypothesis. Quality of life measures used in several well-designed studies show no significant differences in quality of life parameters between women treated with antihypertensive drugs or placebo.[68]

Some studies show that most reports of sexual dysfunction induced by antihypertensives occur in men, yet the questionnaires used were not well designed to detect sexual dysfunction in women. These reports contained a gender bias in both interviews and written queries, and their results cannot be considered definitive.

Summary

Hypertension has different characteristics in women, with a later average age at onset, a more rapid progression to higher systolic pressures, and a more malignant pattern of LVH than in men. From these data, one would anticipate that there would be significant gender differences in the optimal pharmacotherapy of elevated blood pressure.

Although studies clearly show that women benefit from aggressive treatment of hypertension, it is unclear whether there are significant advantages from any specific drug regimen. The best evidence, although not yet conclusive, suggests that low doses of thiazide diuretics, which have been shown to decrease long-term morbidity and mortality, are a good first choice in women, both because of their antihypertensive effects and their effects on helping to maintain bone density in the postmenopausal state. Antihypertensive effects of diuretics in postmenopausal women might be optimized by including estrogen replacement therapy (see Chap. 4).

Beta blockers may be preferred initial agents in women who have documented coronary artery disease or have had an MI, due to the antianginal and antiarrhythmic effects of beta blockers and a well-documented improvement in morbidity and mortality. The ACE inhibitors are indicated as first-line agents for women with diabetes mellitus and proteinuria or heart failure.

The current JNC-VI guidelines do not offer gender-specific recommendations for initial antihypertension regimens. The initial choices of small doses of a thiazide diuretic or a beta blocker are consistent with the current state of knowledge on gender differences.

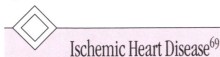

Ischemic Heart Disease[69]

Heart disease is the leading cause of death in the United States. At all ages, men have a higher death rate from IHD than women. However, IHD is not a "male problem." Equivalent death rates for women are just delayed about 10 years compared to men, and women who develop IHD appear to have worse outcomes than men.[70] Each year about 240,000 women die from heart disease.

Gender Issues[70]

As in hypertension, early studies on IHD excluded women or enrolled few women. Many researchers assumed that women would respond to treatment in the same way as men. This supposition has proven to be incorrect, and future studies need to include adequate numbers of women to identify differences in outcomes and responses to treatments.

TREATMENT

There is concern that, in the United States, medications and other therapies for IHD are underused in the treatment of women.[71] One multicenter study showed that women presenting to an emergency room with chest pain were significantly less likely to be treated acutely with aspirin than men, even after adjusting for patient age and hospital type.[72] There was also a trend toward lower rates of beta blocker and thrombolytic use among eligible women, despite evidence that these therapies are equally beneficial to both sexes.[72] Women experience MIs at an average age 8 to 10 years later than men. Women more often have a history of CHF, hypertension, or diabetes mellitus, which may lead to poorer outcomes and altered therapy. Studies also suggest that women are significantly less likely to receive coronary angiography, percutaneous transluminal coronary angioplasty (PTCA), or coronary artery bypass grafting (CABG). Part of the lower rate of thrombolytic use in women may be due to the fact that women seek medical

attention an average of 2 h later than men. Stroke, major bleeding, and recurrent MIs complicating thrombolytic therapy are more common in women. The bleeding problems may in part be due to fixed dosing schedules for thrombolytics, developed in men, being applied to all patients regardless of their weight and size.

OUTCOMES

Complications during acute MI that are more common in women compared to men include prolonged angina (34 versus 28 percent), reinfarction (5.2 versus 3.7 percent), CHF (37 versus 26 percent), and stroke (2.5 versus 1.6 percent). Mortality occurring during the hospital stay is also higher for women (13.7 versus 7.8 percent for men). The 30-day mortality rate in the Global Utilization of Streptokinase and t-PA for Occluded Coronary Arteries (GUSTO-1) study was twice as high for women as for men.[73] Some of the difference can be explained by the fact that women present at an older age, have more advanced disease at presentation, and have a higher rate of comorbid diseases. Yet, even after adjusting for age and coexisting illness, studies show women are still up to 20 percent more likely to die than men during an acute hospitalization for IHD. An important part of the increased mortality is due to the high mortality rate for African American women. The Multicenter Investigation of the Limitation of Infarct Size (MILIS) study showed a cumulative 48-month mortality rate of 21 percent for all men, 36 percent for all women, and 48 percent for black women.[74]

Women have higher mortality and complication rates with angioplasty and CABG. Again, some of the increased risk is due to older age and greater rate of comorbid conditions, which increase procedural risk. Some of this disadvantage has decreased in recent years as improved techniques and equipment have been used that compensate for the smaller coronary vessels in women.

In the postdischarge period following hospitalization for IHD, women fare better than they do in the hospital and the age-adjusted death rate was similar for women and men.[75] If in-hospital deaths for women are excluded, long-term survival for women was actually better than for men.

Risk Factors and Their Treatment

Many of the risk factors for IHD are the same in women and men. The major risk factors are dyslipidemia, family history of IHD, diabetes mellitus, smoking, hypertension, postmenopausal status, obesity, and sedentary lifestyle. Nutritional factors such as vitamin E and other antioxidant consumption and homocysteine metabolism are also being studied.

LIPIDS

Dyslipidemia continues to gain attention as an important and modifiable risk factor for IHD. Elevated total cholesterol (TC) and LDL-C and a low HDL-C are the common clinically useful measurements for guiding treatment decisions. An elevated triglyceride level is now increasingly considered as an independent risk factor. For women, low HDL levels and elevated triglycerides are stronger risk predictors than in men. In addition, lipid levels have a higher predictive value in postmenopausal women than in premenopausal women.

Metabolism of lipids in women follows a well-described pattern. Based on a number of studies, HDL-C level is inversely correlated with coronary heart disease risk and is normally higher throughout life for women than men. After menopause, HDL-C levels decrease somewhat, but still remain higher than in men. The risk for IHD in women increases when HDL levels are less than 45 mg/dL, compared to less than 35 mg/dL for men. A level greater than 60 mg/dL is more likely to occur in women and is reported to reduce the risk of IHD by 2 to 3 percent for each 1 mg/dL over 60 mg/dL. High levels of very-low-density lipoprotein confer a significant risk to both genders, but appear to be a more important risk factor for women.

The current National Cholesterol Education Program (NCEPII) guidelines,[76] issued in 1993, call for periodic total serum cholesterol measurements in all adults over 20 years of age. Evidence-based guidelines, however, like the Preventive Service Task Force, do not agree with nonselective periodic screening for hyperlipidemia. Rather, they suggest screening only for those with risk factors. Risk factors for determining the need for cholesterol-lowering treatment in women are listed in Table 17-18.

Cholesterol-lowering treatment is recommended for women with zero or one risk factor and an LDL-C level of 160 mg/dL or greater. For women with two or more risk factors, whose LDL-C levels are 130 mg/dL or greater, treatment is also recommended. For women who have IHD or diabetes, a goal LDL-C of 100 mg/dL or less is recommended (Table 17-19). The newer version of the guidelines call for less intensive treatment of premenopausal women with LDL levels in the range of 160 to 220 mg/dL and suggest a more aggressive approach to treatment of high-risk postmenopausal women and asymptomatic elderly patients.

Although clinical study data demonstrate that an increase in HDL-C is effective in reducing coronary heart disease in men, there are little trial data to document the benefit of increasing HDL-C in women.

DIETARY MODIFICATION　The American Heart Association (AHA) dietary guidelines for the general

Table 17-18

Risk Factors for Determining the Need for Cholesterol-Lowering Medication for Women

HISTORY
Age >55
Premature menopause without estrogen replacement
Family history of premature ischemic heart disease (before age 55 in a male or before age 65 in a female first-degree relative)
Current cigarette smoking
Hypertension (uncontrolled or controlled by medication)
Low HDL-C (<35 mg/dL was adopted for both men and women by NCEP)
Diabetes mellitus

ABBREVIATIONS: HDL-C, high-density lipoprotein cholesterol; NCEP, National Cholesterol Education Program.

Table 17-19

NCEP Treatment Guidelines for Women

	DRUG TREATMENT	**DIETARY TREATMENT**	**GOAL**
Known IHD or diabetes	LDL-C≥130 mg/dL	LDL-C≥100 mg/dL but <130 mg/dL	LDL-C<100 mg/dL
2 or more risk factors	LDL-C≥160 mg/dL	LDL-C≥130 mg/dL but <160 mg/dL	LDL-C<130 mg/dL
0 or 1 risk factor	LDL-C≥190 mg/dL	LDL-C≥160 mg/dL but <190 mg/dL	LDL-C<160 mg/dL

NOTES: Risk factors are age >55 or premature menopause without ERT, family history of first-degree relative with IHD before 55 in a male and 65 in a female, smoking, hypertension, and low LDL-C (<35 mg/dL).
ABBREVIATIONS: ERT, estrogen replacement therapy; IHD, ischemic heart disease; LDL-C, low-density lipoprotein cholesterol; NCEP, National Cholesterol Education Program.

public are recommended if a patient has hyperlipidemia and is not following a low-fat diet. If patients are unable to lower their lipid levels on this initial diet, the Step I diet, then the AHA recommends the Step II diet. These dietary recommendations are summarized in Table 17-20.

MEDICATIONS There are no convincing data that antihyperlipidemic agents other than the statins lower cardiovascular morbidity and mortality in the female population, whether used for primary or secondary prevention. However, it is common practice to use bile acid–binding agents, niacin and fibrates, in women because they have been shown to be effective in producing lipid changes that are favorable. As discussed below, however, available long-term data are primarily from studies with the statins, not for other agents.

The statins (hydroxymethylglutaryl-coenzyme A reductase inhibitors) lower cholesterol by inhibiting the rate-limiting enzyme responsible for cholesterol synthesis in the liver. They are important agents in the NCEPII recommendations. There are currently five statins available in the United States. These agents all work by a common mechanism, but differ in their pharmacokinetic profiles, potencies, and cost. As a class they reduce both LDL-C and TC significantly, and at the same time produce mild elevations of HDL-C. Table 17-21 contains a summary of lipid-lowering agents.

Primary Prevention with Statins. Most studies involving drug treatment in primary prevention strategies have demonstrated benefit primarily to men, with little or no benefit being observed among low-risk women. One recent study that did demon-

Table 17-20

American Heart Association Dietary Guidelines*

DIETARY COMPONENT	GENERAL PUBLIC AND STEP I	STEP II
Total fat	≤ 30%	≤ 30%
Saturated fatty acids	8–10%	≤ 7%
Polyunsaturated fatty acids	up to 10%	up to 10%
Monounsaturated fatty acids	up to 15%	up to 15%
Cholesterol	<300 mg/d	<200 mg/d
Carbohydrates	≥ 55%	≥ 55%
Protein	Approximately 15%	Approximately 15%

*Expressed as a percentage of total calorie intake unless otherwise stated.

Table 17-21

Antihyperlipidemic Agents

Generic Name	Trade Name	Bioavailability	Excretion	Half-Life	Effects on Cholesterol	Effects on Tryglycerides	Effects on LDL	Effects on HDL
Atorvastatin	Lipitor	12%	<2% urine	14 h	↓	↓	↓	↑
Cerivastatin	Baycol	60%	24% urine, 70% feces	2–3 h	↓	↓	↓	↑
Cholestyramine	Questran	Nonabsorbable resin	100% feces		↓	↑/→	↓	↑/→
Colestipol	Cuemid	Nonabsorbable resin	100% feces		↓	↑/→	↓	↑/→
Fenofibrate	Tricor	60%	60% urine	20 h	↓	↓	↑	↑
Fluvastatin	Lescol	>90%	5% urine, 90% feces	<1 h	↓	↓	↓	↑
Gemfibrozil	Lopid	97%	2% urine, 6% feces	1.5 h	↓	↓	↓/→	↑
Lovastatin	Mevacor	35%, first-pass metabolized	10% urine, 85% feces	3–4 h	↓	↓	↓	↑
Nicotinic acid	various	~100%	Primary urine		↓	↓	↓	↑
Pravastatin	Pravachol	35%, first-pass metabolized	20% urine, 70% feces	1.8 h	↓	↓	↓	↑
Simvastatin	Zocor	60–80%, extensive first-pass metabolism	13% urine, 60% feces	3 h	↓	↓	↓	↑

ABBREVIATIONS: HDL, high-density lipoprotein; LDL, low-density lipoprotein.

strate some primary prevention benefit in women was the Air Force/Texas Coronary Atherosclerosis Prevention Study (AFCAPS/TexCAPS) of lovastatin.[77] This study investigated whether long-term lipid-lowering with lovastatin would decrease the rate of first acute major coronary events compared with placebo during at least 5 years of follow-up in a cohort without clinical evidence of atherosclerotic cardiovascular disease and had average TC and LDL-C levels and below-average HDL-C levels. Of the 6605 patients involved, 997 were postmenopausal women. Among women treated with lovastatin (20 to 40 mg/d), the TC level was reduced from 240 mg/dL to 192 mg/dL, LDL-C was reduced from 161 mg/dL to 116 mg/dL, and HDL-C was raised from 41 mg/dL to 43 mg/dL. The primary endpoint was onset of first major coronary event. For women, the rate of first coronary events in the placebo group was 13/1000 patient-years at risk; in the lovastatin group it was 7/1000 (RR = 0.54, CI not calculable from data given). However, the incidence of first events in the placebo group was sufficiently low (13 compared to 170 in the male group) that the NNT was 167 (i.e., 167 women treated for 5 years to prevent one major coronary event). This is compared with an NNT for men of 16.4. This number is sufficiently high that many physicians consider it inappropriate to use medication for premenopausal low-risk women, considering the potential side effects, cost, and inconvenience of therapy.

Secondary Prevention with Statins. Two major studies have shown decreased morbidity and mortality from IHD in secondary prevention trials using the statins. The Cholesterol and Recurrent Events (CARE) trial[78] studied the use of pravastatin (40 mg/d) or placebo on more than 4000 patients following an MI (576 were female) with average baseline TC level of 209 mg/dL and LDL-C concentrations of 139 mg/dL. Primary endpoints were combined incidence of nonfatal MI or death from IHD. In the 5 years of the study, 10.2 percent of the patients taking pravastatin experienced a primary endpoint compared to 13.2 percent of the placebo group, yielding a NNT of 33 for 5 years to prevent one primary event. Subgroup analysis of

women in the study confirmed significant reductions in cardiovascular events.[79] Current NCEP guidelines call for aggressively treating patients with previous IHD until the LDL level is less than 100 mg/dL. The CARE data did not support this recommendation because patients with LDL less than 100 mg/dL did not fare any better than patients with LDL less than 125mg/dL.

The 4S trial (Scandinavian Simvastatin Survival Study)[80] used simvastatin 20 to 40 mg daily in approximately 4400 patients (871 female) with a previous MI or angina. Baseline mean TC level was 261 mg/dL, and mean LDL-C was 188 mg/dL (much higher mean levels than in the CARE study). This trial was also a 5-year study, and the goal was to reduce TC concentrations to 116 to 201 mg/dL; the primary endpoint was overall mortality. There was a significant reduction in the number of people dying in the simvastatin group, 8.2 percent compared to 11.5 percent in the placebo group, with a NNT of 30 for 5 years to prevent one death. Acute MIs were also significantly reduced in the treated group, 7.4 percent versus 12.1 percent (NNT = 21).

Most trials of secondary prevention through treatment of elevated TC levels with statins have required at least 2 years of continuous drug treatment before any differences in outcome have been observed. Therefore, some practitioners limit secondary prevention treatment to patients who have a life expectancy of more than 2 years because no benefit is likely to be seen before that time period.

The cost-effectiveness of statins in the secondary prevention 4S trial is estimated at $10,300 per year of life saved (YOLS) for women ($5,500 per YOLS for men). This would fit in the category of "highly cost effective" (< $20,000 per Quality Adjusted Life Year).

INSULIN RESISTANCE AND DIABETES

Diabetes increases the risk for IHD in women threefold to sevenfold over the risk in men.[69] Diabetes exerts a strong effect both directly and via lipid abnormalities. When diabetes is present it negates the general protective benefit that gender usually confers to women, so that women with diabetes experience cardiovascular events at the same rate and age as men with diabetes.

It has been recommended by the American Diabetes Association (ADA) that all individuals with diabetes, even those without established IHD, be treated according to NCEP guidelines for secondary prevention of IHD. This is based on the fact that diabetes confers an increased risk for and rate of atherosclerotic changes. Approximately half the patients with diabetes who have a fatal MI will not show any previous warning signs of IHD. The ADA acknowledges that their recommendations are based on subgroup analyses of several major studies, none of which were specifically designed to show that more aggressive treatment of diabetes is beneficial. The results of those trials, however, show trends that support aggressive screening and treatment of all individuals with diabetes.

Pending more conclusive information, it seems reasonable for patients with diabetes to be screened and treated to more stringent lipid goals. These patients in particular have a twofold greater risk of mortality from MI, CHF, and all other causes than men with diabetes.

Similar to women with diabetes, women with polycystic ovary syndrome (PCOS) are a group with insulin resistance. These women have a number of endocrine abnormalities—insulin resistance, increased testosterone, and lowered estradiol—that can produce elevated triglyceride and lowered HDL-C levels. In one study of women being evaluated for chest pain, those with polycystic ovaries were more likely to have extensive coronary disease on angiography than women with normal ovaries.[81] Finally, PCOS is associated with hypertension and central obesity, two additional cardiac risk factors. Although there is no definitive treatment for PCOS, women with this syndrome should be screened for these cardiac risk factors and treated appropriately.

Cigarette Smoking

Smoking is the leading cause of preventable IHD in women. Smoking cessation is the single most important change that a smoker can make to decrease the risk of IHD. Fifty percent of all MIs in middle-aged women are attributed to tobacco smoking,[82] and 84 percent of women who develop IHD before 50 years of age are smokers.[83] Smoking can lead to vascular plaque erosion, an important mechanism for sudden death in young women. For young women taking OCs, smoking is the major risk factor for MI, and OCs are not recommended for women over age 35 who smoke 20 or more cigarettes per day.[84]

The goal for smokers should be complete abstinence. Firm, direct, and compassionate advice from health care providers is important in smoking cessation. Formal cessation programs, nicotine replacement, and bupropion (Zyban®) can help in the process. Chapter 8 provides detailed information for providers to assist women in quitting smoking. After quitting, a smoker's risk of IHD drops quickly; the increased risk drops 50 percent after 1 year and 90 percent after 2 years.

Hypertension

Either an elevated SBP or DBP puts women at increased risk for IHD. Treatment with diuretics and beta blockers has been shown to decrease IHD (25 percent in the Systolic Hypertension in the Elderly Program [SHEP][40]), although not to the same extent as stroke reduction (36 percent in SHEP[40]). Isolated systolic hypertension, which is prevalent among elderly women, is an important risk factor that requires treatment. The treatment of hypertension was outlined earlier in this chapter.

Menopausal Status

Women who are postmenopausal, either naturally or surgically, have an increased risk of IHD. This is due in part to an increase in LDL-C and a decrease in HDL-C that occurs following menopause. Lipid changes can be reversed through the use of hormone replacement strategies, and observational studies have suggested that estrogen replacement therapy can decrease IHD up to 50 percent.[85]

Hormone replacement therapy has favorable effects on the lipid profile; it raises HDL-C and lowers LDL-C by an average of 15 percent. The PEPI trial was one of the first long-term studies to specifically look at heart disease risk factors in postmenopausal women.[17] This study of 875 post-menopausal women demonstrated that unopposed conjugated equine estrogen (CEE) replacement increased the HDL-C to a significantly greater degree than any regimen that included a non-micronized progestin. Women who received cycled micronized progesterone in addition to CEE also had a significant increase in HDL-C compared to the placebo group as well as the groups receiving cycled or continuous medroxyprogesterone acetate (MPA) with the estrogen.

Levels of LDL and TC were reduced significantly in all groups taking estrogen and seemed to be independent of which progestin or regimen was used in the PEPI trial. The LDL reduction (average 15.9 mg/dL) with estrogen is large, but LDL is less closely correlated with IHD development in women, and the clinical importance of this reduction has not yet been demonstrated.

However, all treatment groups receiving oral estrogen in the PEPI study developed substantial increases in serum triglycerides, probably through increased production of triglycerides. This increase could be particularly detrimental in women with diabetes, in whom triglyceride levels may already be elevated (a population excluded from the PEPI trial).

Although the PEPI trial answered many questions about the effect of HRT on lipids in women, all of the endpoints (i.e., lipid, fibrinogen, and insulin levels) were surrogate markers and not morbidity and mortality outcomes. The more important question of whether HRT, as primary prevention, will reduce overall IHD mortality in a long-term controlled trial to the degree of that seen in some observational studies (up to 50 percent) remains to be answered. The NIH-sponsored Women's Health Initiative is conducting such a trial, but the results are at least 2 years away.

HORMONE REPLACEMENT Observational surveys and studies have consistently shown that estrogen replacement is particularly beneficial for secondary prevention of cardiac events in women with an IHD history, reducing events from 35 to 80 percent.

However, the results of the Heart and Estrogen-Progestin Replacement Study (HERS), a large randomized placebo-controlled trial of HRT in more than 2700 postmenopausal women with confirmed IHD,[86] showed that after 1 year of treatment, the HRT group (0.625 mg CEE + 2.5 mg MPA/d) had a higher risk of venous thromboembolic events (RR = 3.29, 95 percent CI =1.07 to 10.08) and a trend toward more IHD events and sudden death than the placebo group (IHD death RR = 1.56, 95 percent CI = 0.73 to 3.32). During the fourth and fifth years of the study the trend had reversed, and the RR of nonfatal MI for women on HRT was 0.58 (95 percent CI = 0.34 to 1.02) and 0.95 for IHD death (95 percent CI = 0.49 to 1.84). The authors theorize that the increase in thromboembolic events seen in the first year was due to the thrombogenic potential of estrogens, causing increases in clot formation and cardiac events. As treatment continued over time, they believe that the hematologic system adapted, and the positive effects of estrogen predominated, reducing the progression of IHD.

Although the HERS findings need confirmation and clarification, they have significant implications for hormonal therapy in postmenopausal women with IHD. For now, it appears that HRT should not be used as a specific therapy for secondary prevention in women with established IHD because of the inverse trend to more IHD events during the early years of therapy. If a woman with IHD is already receiving HRT, she may continue; the use of HRT for other women with IHD should be determined on an individual basis. Chapter 4 reviews decision-making for HRT.

OBESITY

The AHA recently issued a call to action on obesity as a major cardiac risk factor.[87] In the United States, the prevalence of obesity is growing. The AHA defines a desirable weight as a BMI of 21 to 25 kg/m², overweight as a BMI of 25 to 30 (RR for IHD of 2.5), and obesity as a BMI of 30 (RR for IHD of 3.5). For women, the BMI, as a risk factor, should be qualified by the distribution type of the obesity. Truncal obesity, a waist/hip ratio greater than 0.88 in women, conveys a greater risk than hip and thigh obesity (RR = 3.06, 95 percent CI = 1.78 to 5.95, adjusted for BMI).[88]

Weight reduction programs should include adequate activity levels, dietary advice, and strategies for lifetime weight control. The diet should contain less than 30 percent of total calories from fat, less than 10 percent of total calories from saturated fat, and emphasize adequate servings of fruits and vegetables each day. Management strategies for weight control are discussed in Chap. 6. A decrease in body weight of 5 to 10 percent can produce metabolic changes that decrease blood pressure, improve glucose tolerance, and improve lipid profiles.

ACTIVITY LEVEL

Physical fitness programs have a benefit in modifying many cardiac risk factors including hypertension, glucose intolerance, hyperlipidemia, and obesity. An exercise program of 30 min of moderate activity three to four times a week is the minimum amount that will provide cardiovascular benefit. A maximal benefit is reached at 5 to 6 h of moderate activity per week. The exercise can be obtained in a single 30-min session or can be apportioned out to three 10-min sessions a day. Also daily activities can be altered to increase activity: use of stairs instead of elevators, selecting distant parking spaces, and altering recreational activities (e.g., walking a golf course instead of using a cart) (see Chap. 6). Some patients may need a rehabilitation program to assist in implementing an exercise program. Although most women can safely increase their physical activity without a medical evaluation, women with cardiac or other serious health problems should first undergo a medical evaluation, often including a cardiac stress test, and may need referral to a medically supervised exercise program.

HOMOCYSTEINE AND VITAMIN E

Studies show a correlation between high homocysteine levels and IHD.[89] However, controversy exists as to whether homocysteine is a marker for other factors that cause IHD or is itself a causal factor. If homocysteine is found to be a causal factor, then folic acid, vitamin B_{12}, and vitamin B_6, which lower homocysteine, levels may be used to positively affect the atherosclerotic process. At this time there is incomplete evidence to support this treatment.[90,91] Recommendations may be generated when randomized trials testing this association are completed.

Vitamin E is another "natural product" that has been promoted as a cardioprotectant due to its antioxidant capabilities. A large randomized study in 2002 patients (including 312 women) with angiographically proven IHD showed a reduction (RR = 0.23, 98 percent CI = 0.11 to 0.47) in nonfatal MIs after 1 year of treatment with vitamin E (400 to 800 IU/d).[92]

Presentations of Ischemic Heart Disease

Although chest pain is a common symptom of IHD, women with IHD are more likely than men to have atypical chest pain. Symptoms that are more common in women are so-called atypical symptoms including chest pain at rest or sleep, neck and shoulder pain, chest pain precipitated by mental stress, nausea and vomiting, fatigue, and dyspnea.[93] Nonetheless, classic symptoms are still more frequent in women than atypical symptoms. Women are more likely than men to delay seeking treatment, however, because either they do not adequately appreciate their risk of IHD[94] or they do not recognize their symptoms as indicative of IHD.[93]

Sudden death, while more common in men, is also an important component of IHD in women. It accounts for about one-third of IHD deaths in women. Two-thirds of women with sudden death had no prior signs or symptoms to warn them of IHD; for men the figure is 50 percent. Women are also more likely to present with atypical cardiac syndromes like vasospastic angina and microvascular disease. Postmenopausal women are the largest group with exertional angina, a positive exercise test but a normal coronary angiography (sometimes called syndrome X). Framingham data show a higher rate of silent MIs in women (35 percent of MIs detected by surveillance electrocardiograms [ECGs]) compared with men (25 percent).[95]

EVALUATION[96]

In evaluating chest pain, it is important to determine the pretest probability for disease based on the type of pain and the number of risk factors present. This will guide the selection and interpretation of test results. A positive test result in a patient with a low pretest probability is most likely a false-positive. Conversely, a negative result in a patient with a high pretest probability of disease is most likely a false-negative.

There have been a number of attempts to develop assessment guidelines for stratifying patients based on their pretest likelihood of having IHD as a cause for chest pain. One method for determining pretest probability is based on the age of the patient and the pattern of chest pain, using the results of a study correlating presenting symptoms and angiographic findings in almost 5000 patients.[97] "Typical chest pain" is retrosternal, precipitated by exertion or emotion, and relieved with rest or nitroglycerin. "Atypical chest pain" is described as sharp, prolonged, not associated with exercise, and in an atypical location. Finally there is "nonanginal chest pain." The results of using this symptom classification as a means to identify IHD are summarized in Table 17-22.

Table 17-22

Pretest Likelihood of Ischemic Heart Disease in Women

AGE	TYPICAL CHEST PAIN	ATYPICAL CHEST PAIN	NONANGINAL CHEST PAIN
30–39	26%	4%	1%
40–49	55%	13%	3%
50–59	80%	32%	8%
60–69	91%	54%	19%

SOURCE: Adapted with permission from GA Diamond, JS Forrester, *N Engl J Med* 300:1350, Copyright 1979.[97]

A second approach, summarized in Tables 17-23 and 17-24, can also give a clinician guidance in approaching a woman with chest pain.[98] This method, though based on research, has not yet been verified in a prospective trial.

The evaluation of chest pain for a possible acute MI is based on symptom description, the ECG, and cardiac enzymes. Although there are some gender differences in the presenting symptoms, with women more likely to present with atypical symptoms, studies have not shown any significant differences in the ECG manifestations of ischemia by gender. Enzymes used to evaluate acute chest pain include creatine phosphokinase (CPK), CPK-MB fraction, aspartate transaminase, lactic dehydrogenase, troponin T and I, and myoglobin. The individual characteristics of each test determines its

Table 17-23

Determinants of Coronary Heart Disease in Women with Chest Pain

Major determinants	Typical angina pain
	Postmenopausal status without hormone replacement therapy
	Diabetes
	Peripheral vascular disease
Intermediate determinants	Hypertension
	Smoking
	Lipoprotein abnormalities, especially low high-density lipoprotein levels
Minor determinants	Age > 65 y
	Obesity, especially central
	Sedentary lifestyle
	Family history of ischemic heart disease

SOURCE: Adapted with permission from PS Douglas and GS Ginsburg, *N Engl J Med* 334:1131, Copyright 1996.[98]

Table 17-24

Use of Diagnostic Tests in Women with Chest Pain

LIKELIHOOD OF IHD	INITIAL TEST	SUBSEQUENT TEST
Low (<20%) No major and ≤ 1 intermediate or ≤ 2 minor determinants	None indicated	None indicated
Moderate (20–80%) 1 major or multiple intermediate and minor determinants	Routine ETT Negative *Inconclusive* Positive Imaging ETT Negative *Inconclusive* Positive	 None indicated *Further testing indicated;* *selection must be individualized* Imaging test or catheterization None indicated *Catheterization* Catheterization
High (>80%) ≥2 major or 1 major plus >1 intermediate and minor determinants	Routine ETT Negative *Inconclusive* Positive	 None indicated; observe closely *Catheterization* Catheterization

ABBREVIATION: ETT, exercise tolerance test.
SOURCE: Adapted with permission from PS Douglas and GS Ginsburg, *N Engl J Med* 334:1311, Copyright 1996.[98]

role and usefulness in the evaluation of patients with suspected MI (Table 17-25). Many studies are being conducted to determine optimal use of these tests in evaluating acute chest pain syndromes. Emergent radionuclide imaging is advocated by some when the diagnosis is still in question following standard testing.

Noninvasive cardiac testing is the next step in the evaluation of chest pain for women who have a negative evaluation in the emergency setting and for those who present for care in the office. The most widely used tests are the traditional exercise stress test, stress radionuclide studies using thallium-201 or technetium 99m (sestamibi),

Table 17-25

Characteristics of Cardiac Enzyme Markers

TEST	RISE OCCURS IN	PEAK LEVELS AT	NORMALIZES IN	COMMENTS
CK-MB	3–8 h	10–24 h	3–4 d	Fairly specific, value often reported as percentage of total CK with normal 3–6%
Troponin I and T	3–4 h	12–24 h	10–15 d	The cardiac isoenzymes are very specific
Myoglobin	2–4 h	6–8 h	20–36 h	Nonspecific but rises early
LDH	24 h	3 d	8–9 d	Can fractionate isoenzymes to increase specificity

ABBREVIATIONS: CK-MB, creatine kinase-muscle, brain; LDH, lactic dehydrogenase.

and stress echocardiography. For traditional exercise stress testing to give valid results the patient should have a normal baseline ECG (no bundle branch block patterns or repolarization abnormalities that interfere with interpretation) and be able to exercise enough to elevate the heart rate to 85 percent of predicted maximum. Pharmacologic cardiac stressors (dipyridamole, adenosine, and dobutamine) are used with patients who are unable, via exercise, to reach an adequate heart rate.

There are gender effects on the sensitivity and specificity of these tests. Young women are more likely to have false-positive exercise stress tests due in part to their low pretest probability and the fact that estrogen can induce false-positive ST-segment depression. In addition, women are more likely to have inconclusive testing because they more frequently fail to reach an adequate exertion level. When using dobutamine as a cardiac stimulant, women respond with an elevated heart rate more quickly than men, leading to premature ending of the testing. Finally, breast tissue can attenuate the signals in radionuclide testing, especially with thallium, producing a false-positive result. The sestamibi scan is a higher energy technique and may be able to overcome this limitation. The decision of which test to use must be individualized based on patient characteristics. Table 17-26 summarizes some factors to be considered.

Treatment of Myocardial Infarction

In 1996, the American College of Cardiology (ACC) and the AHA released guidelines for the management of acute MI.[99] In these guidelines, recommendations are stratified based on the level of evidence that supports each intervention. Those recommendations that are rated "Class I" have "evidence for and/or general agreement that a given procedure or treatment is beneficial, useful, and effec-

Table 17-26

Noninvasive Cardiac Testing

TEST	ADVANTAGES	DISADVANTAGES
Standard stress testing (SXT)	Relatively inexpensive	Need normal baseline
	Widely available	electrocardiogram (ECG)
	Best results with intermediate-risk patients	More false-positives, especially in young women
Thallium 201	Can use with abnormal ECGs	Increased expense
	Greater sensitivity and specificity than SXT	Need to have radioisotopes, which are often not available on an emergent basis
		Lower energy levels prone to attenuation artifact from soft tissue with obesity and breasts
Technetium 99–sestamibi	Can use with abnormal ECGs	Increased expense
	Greater sensitivity and specificity than SXT	Need to have radioisotopes, which are often not available on an emergent basis
	Higher energy levels reduce signal attenuation from soft tissue	
Stress echocardiography	Can get structural information on the heart	Increased expense
	Can be done on an emergent basis	Need good echocardiographic windows

tive" and are the foundation of the therapies described below.

REPERFUSION THERAPY

It is critical that patients present early in the course of an MI to gain the greatest benefit from reperfusion therapies (e.g., PTCA and thrombolysis). There has been controversy over which therapy is best. Recent studies indicate that when PTCA, rather than thrombolytic therapy, can be performed within 60 to 90 min of presentation better outcomes are achieved. This benefit is best seen in high-risk patients with advanced age (over 70), anterior MIs, and left ventricular dysfunction. These results, however, were obtained in high-volume institutions, and the same benefits may not be seen in low-volume centers. In addition, only about 20 percent of hospitals have the capability of performing emergency angioplasty; therefore, thrombolysis remains an important early treatment option. None of these studies compared outcomes in men versus women.

A woman with an initial ECG that shows ST-segment elevation of 0.1 mV or more in two contiguous leads, or left bundle branch block with typical MI symptoms, would be a candidate for thrombolytic therapy. If thrombolytic agents are given in the first 7 to 12 h of symptoms, 16 lives can be saved per 1000 patients treated. If thrombolytic agents are given within the first hour, the number increases to 35/1000 patients treated. The most serious complication from thrombolysis is intracerebral hemorrhage; this occurs in fewer than 1 percent of low-risk patients. Factors that increase the risk for intracerebral hemorrhage include age over 65 (RR = 2.2, 95 percent CI = 1.4 to 3.5), a body weight less than 70 kg (RR = 2.1, 95 percent CI = 1.3 to 3.2), and hypertension on presentation (RR = 2.0, 95 percent CI = 1.2 to 3.2).

OXYGEN, ANALGESICS, AND ASPIRIN

Supplemental oxygen should be started as soon as possible. Analgesics (morphine or meperidine) are administered as needed. A dose of 160 to 325 mg aspirin to chew is given promptly, unless the patient is allergic to aspirin. Aspirin should be continued as a daily medication indefinitely. Sublingual nitroglycerin can be given if the patient has stable vital signs (SBP > 90 and heart rate between 50 and 100). If the patient continues to have chest pain, despite these interventions, a nitroglycerin infusion can be started. For patients whose pain is easily controlled, topical nitroglycerin may be considered. The guidelines also recommend intravenous nitroglycerin for 24 to 48 h in patients with CHF, large anterior infarcts, persistent ischemia, or hypertension.

ANTIARRHYTHMIC THERAPY

Prophylactic antiarrhythmic therapy has not been shown to improve outcomes.[100] However, treatment of an arrhythmia is indicated if it develops. Studies have not confirmed a role for the routine administration of magnesium in the prevention of rhythm disturbances. It is reasonable to examine magnesium levels and treat if the level is low. Normal magnesium levels are 1.5 to 1.9 mEq/L (0.75 to 1.0 mmol/L or 1.7 to 2.2 mg/dL). A dosing of 2 g over 15 min, followed by 18 g over the next 18 to 24 h has been used successfully in past studies.[99]

ANTICOAGULANT THERAPY

Heparin therapy with full doses of unfractionated heparin is indicated for the first 48 h after MI in patients who have received alteplase or reteplase thrombolysis. In patients with a high risk of systemic or venous thromboembolism (anterior MI, CHF, prior embolism, atrial fibrillation), heparin therapy may be continued, or conversion to warfarin may be considered. In patients not receiving thrombolysis, the Fifth American College of Chest Physicians Consensus Conference on Antithrombotic Therapy recommends that all patients receive not less than low-dose therapy (7500 units heparin every 12 h subcutaneously) until ambulatory, unless there is a specific contraindication.[101]

BETA BLOCKERS

Lipophilic beta blockers without intrinsic sympathomimetic activity have been shown to decrease mortality in patients after MI.[102] They can be started within the first 12 h of infarction and are continued indefinitely. Dosing for metoprolol is 5 mg intravenously every 2 to 5 min as tolerated up to a total dose of 15 mg, followed by a maintenance dose of 25 to 100 mg bid.

ANGIOTENSIN-CONVERTING ENZYME INHIBITORS

Evidence also indicates that ACE inhibitors can improve outcomes after MI. These agents are started within the first 24 h and continued for at least 6 weeks. The NNT to prevent 1 death over 4 to 6 weeks, when ACE inhibitors are begun in the first 24 to 36 h, is 200.[103] Patients with anterior MIs, poor left ventricular function (ejection fraction < 40 percent), and those with clinical signs of CHF especially benefit from this intervention. Patients taking ACE inhibitors are at risk for prolonged hypotension, cardiogenic shock, and renal dysfunction. Regimens that can be used are: captopril, 6.25 to 25 mg tid with titration to 50 mg tid; lisinopril, 5 mg daily titrated to 20 mg; or enalapril, 2.5 to 5 mg bid titrated to 15 mg bid.

Noninvasive Cardiac Testing

Exercise testing after an MI is used to identify any remaining regions of ischemic myocardium and to risk stratify patients to guide further treatment. A submaximal symptom-limited treadmill test can be done prior to discharge or within the first month after discharge. These results can be used to guide cardiac rehabilitation. Left ventricular function should also be assessed. This is most often done with an echocardiogram, but can also be determined with radionuclide studies.

Summary

Clinical trials do not provide sufficient evidence that lowering lipids pharmacologically, as primary prevention of IHD in women, is cost-effective. Although there are few clinical trial data support-

ing the efficacy of lowering lipid levels in women with IHD, the information available would support the use of lipid-lowering agents to slow progression of the atherosclerotic process. For secondary prevention, the only drugs that have been shown to decrease mortality for women are simvastatin and pravastatin.

Diabetes increases the risk for IHD in women to a greater degree than it does for men. It has been recommended by the ADA that women with diabetes be treated according to the NCEP guidelines for secondary prevention of IHD. Smoking is the leading cause of preventable IHD in women. Ideally, the goal should be complete abstinence. After quitting, a smoker's risk of IHD drops quickly to that of nonsmokers after approximately 2 years.

Use of HRT has favorable effects on lipids, raising HDL-C and lowering LDL-C. Observational studies have shown that HRT is beneficial for secondary prevention of cardiac events in women with IHD. However, the recent HERS results raise concerns after finding more IHD events and sudden death for women in the HRT group versus placebo group early in therapy, although some protective effect was noted by years 4 and 5. Finally, obesity and a sedentary lifestyle are additional modifiable risk factors for women; improving these factors can reduce the risk of IHD.

References

1. National Center for Health Statistics: *Health*, United States, 1998 with socioeconomic status and health chartbook, 1998.
2. Gifford RW: New hypertension guidelines set aggressive goals based on risk factors. *Cleve Clin J Med* 65:18, 1998.
3. Lewis CE: Characteristics and treatment of hypertension in women: a review of the literature. *Am J Med Sci* 311:193, 1996.
4. Legato MJ: Cardiovascular disease in women: gender-specific aspects of hypertension and the consequences of treatment. *J Womens Health* 7:199, 1998.
5. The Joint National Committee on Prevention, Detection, Evaluation and Treatment of High Blood Pressure: The Sixth Report of the Joint National Committee of Prevention, Detection, Evaluation and

Treatment of High Blood Pressure. National Institutes of Health. NIH Pub No. 98-4080, Nov, 1997.

6. Kay LE: Accuracy of blood pressure measurement in the family practice center. *J Am Board Fam Pract* 11:252, 1998.

7. Leitschuh M, Cupples LA, Kannel W, et al: High-normal blood pressure progression to hypertension in the Framingham Heart Study. *Hypertension* 17:22, 1991.

8. Hansson L, Zanchetti S, Carruthers SG, et al: Effects of intensive blood-pressure lowering and low-dose aspirin in patients with hypertension: principal results of the Hypertension Optimal Treatment (HOT) randomised trial. *Lancet* 351:1755, 1998.

9. Pickering TJ: Recommendations for the use of home (self) and ambulatory blood pressure monitoring. American Society of Hypertension Ad Hoc Panel. *Am J Hypertens* 9:1, 1996.

10. Tsuji I, Imai Y, Ohkubo T, et al: Proposal of reference values for home blood pressure measurement: prognostic criteria based on a prospective observation of the general population on Ohasama, Japan. *Am J Hypertens* 10:409, 1997.

11. Consumer Reports: Blood-pressure monitors: convenience doesn't equal accuracy. *Consumer Rep* 61:50, 1996.

12. Hayes SN, Taler SJ: Hypertension in women: current understanding of gender differences. *Mayo Clin Proc* 73:157, 1998.

13. Anastos K, Charney P, Charon RA: Hypertension in women: what is really known? The Women's Caucus, Working Group on Women's Health of the Society of General Internal Medicine. *Ann Intern Med* 115:287, 1991.

14. Trembath CR, Hickner JM, Bishop SW: Incidental blood pressure elevations: A MIRNET Project. *J Fam Prac* 32:378, 1991.

15. Krumholz HM, Larson M, Levy D: Sex differences in cardiac adaptation to isolated systolic hypertension. *Am J Cardiol* 72:310, 1993.

16. Liao Y, Cooper RS, Mensah GA, et al: Left ventricular hypertrophy has a greater impact on survival in women than in men. *Circulation* 92:805, 1995.

17. Writing Group for the PEPI Trial: Effects of estrogen or estrogen/progestin regimens on heart disease risk factors in postmenopausal women: the postmenopausal estrogen/progestin interventions trial. *JAMA* 273:199, 1995.

18. Mercuro G, Zoncu S, Pilia I, et al: Effects of acute administration of transdermal estrogen on post-menopausal women with systemic hypertension. *Am J Cardiol* 80:652, 1997.

19. Khairullah QT, Somers DL, Aktay R: Captopril renal scintigraphy in renovascular hypertension. *Am Fam Physician* 55:2240, 1997.

20. Reynolds E, Baron RB: Hypertension in women and the elderly. *Postgrad Med* 100:58, 1996.

21. Trials of Hypertension Prevention Collaborative Research Group: effects of weight loss and sodium reduction intervention on blood pressure and hypertension in overweight people with high-normal blood pressure: the Trials of Hypertension Prevention, phase I. *Arch Intern Med* 157:657, 1997.

22. Huang Z, Willett WC, Manson JE, et al: Body weight, weight change and risk for hypertension in women. *Ann Intern Med* 128:81, 1998.

23. Pouliot MC, Despres JP, Lemieux S, et al: Waist circumference and abdominal sagittal diameter: best simple anthropometric indexes of abdominal visceral adipose tissue accumulation and related cardiovascular risk in men and women. *Am J Cardiol* 73:460, 1994.

24. Frezza M, di Padova C, Pozzato G, et al: High blood alcohol levels in women: the role of decreased gastric alcohol dehydrogenase activity and first-pass metabolism. *N Engl J Med* 322:95, 1990.

25. Rabbia F, Veglio F, Russo R, et al: Role of alcoholic beverages in essential hypertensive patients. *Alcohol Alcohol* 30:433, 1995.

26. Braith RW, Pollock ML, Lowenthal DT, et al: Moderate- and high-intensity exercise lowers blood pressure in normotensive subjects 60 to 79 years of age. *Am J Cardiol* 73:1124, 1994.

27. Seals DR, Silverman HG, Reiling MJ, et al: Effect of regular aerobic exercise on elevated blood pressure in postmenopausal women. *Am J Cardiol* 80:49, 1997.

28. Fish AF, Smith BA, Frid DJ, et al: Step treadmill exercise training and blood pressure reduction in women with mild hypertension. *Prog Cardiovasc Nurs* 12:4, 1997.

29. Midgley JP, Matthew AG, Greenwood CMT, et al: Effect of reduced dietary sodium on blood pressure. A meta-analysis of randomized controlled trials. *JAMA* 275:1590, 1996.

30. Singer DR, Markandu ND, Cappuccio FP, et al: Reduction of salt intake during converting enzyme inhibitor treatment compared with addition of a thiazide. *Hypertension* 24:1042, 1995.

31. Ram CV, Garrett BN, Kaplan NM: Moderate sodium restriction and various diuretics in the treatment of

hypertension: effects of potassium wastage and blood pressure control. *Arch Intern Med* 141:1015, 1981.

32. Kotchen TA, Kotchen JM: Dietary sodium and blood pressure: interactions with other nutrients. *Am J Clin Nutr* 65:708S, 1997.

33. Whelton PK, He J, Cutler JA, et al: Effects of oral potassium on blood pressure: meta-analysis of randomized controlled clinical trials. *JAMA* 277:1624, 1997.

34. Allender PS, Cutler JA, Follman D, et al: Dietary calcium and blood pressure: a meta-analysis of randomized clinical trials. *Ann Intern Med* 124:825, 1996.

35. Myers MG: Effects of caffeine on blood pressure. *Arch Intern Med* 148:1189, 1988.

36. Appel LJ, Moore TJ, Obarzanek E, et al: A clinical trial of the effects of dietary patterns on blood pressure. *N Engl J Med* 336:1117, 1997.

37. Veterans Administration Cooperative Study Group: Effects of treatment on morbidity in hypertension: II. Results in patients with diastolic blood pressure averaging 90 through 114 mmHg. *JAMA* 213:1143, 1970.

38. Multiple Risk Factor Intervention Trial Research Group: Multiple Risk Factor Intervention Trial: risk factor changes and mortality results. *JAMA* 248:1465, 1982.

39. Helgeland A: Treatment of mild hypertension: a five-year controlled drug trial: the Oslo Study. *Am J Med* 69:725, 1980.

40. SHEP Cooperative Research Group: Prevention of stroke by antihypertensive drug treatment in older persons with isolated systolic hypertension: final results of the Systolic Hypertension in the Elderly Program (SHEP). *JAMA* 265:3255, 1991.

41. Amery A, Birkenhager W, Brixko P, et al: Mortality and morbidity results from the European Working Party on High Blood Pressure in the Elderly trial. *Lancet* 1:1349, 1985.

42. Dahlof B, Hansson L, Lindholm LH, et al: Swedish Trial in Old Patients with Hypertension (STOP–Hypertension) analyses performed up to 1992. *Clin Exp Hyperten* 15:925, 1993.

43. Neaton JD, Grimm RH, Prineas RJ, et al: Treatment of Mild Hypertension Study: final results. *JAMA* 270:713, 1993.

44. Hypertension Detection and Follow-Up Program Cooperative Group: Five-year findings of the hypertension detection and follow-up program: II. Mortality by race, sex and age. *JAMA* 242:2572, 1979.

45. The Australian therapeutic trial in mild hypertension: report by the management committee. *Lancet* 1:1261, 1980.

46. Medical Research Council Working Party: MRC trial of treatment of mild hypertension: principal results. *BMJ* 291:97, 1985.

47. Rodgers PT: Combination drug therapy in hypertension: a rational approach for the pharmacist. *J Am Pharm Assoc* (Wash) 38:469, 1998.

48. Califf RM, Kramer JM: What have we learned from the calcium channel blocker controversy? *Circulation* 97:1529, 1998.

49. Borhani NO, Mercuri M, Borhani PA, et al: Final outcome results of the Multicenter Isradipine Diuretic Atherosclerosis Study. *JAMA* 276:785, 1996.

50. Estacio RO, Barrett WJ, Hiatt WR, et al: The effect of nisoldipine as compared with enalapril on cardiovascular outcomes in patients with non-insulin-dependent diabetes and hypertension. *N Engl J Med* 338:645, 1998.

51. Frishman WH: *Current Cardiovascular Drugs,* 2nd ed. Philadelphia: Current Medicine; 1995.

52. Boehringer K, Weidmann P, Mordasini R, et al: Menopause-dependent plasma lipoprotein alterations in diuretic-treated women. *Ann Intern Med* 97:206, 1982.

53. Moser M: Why are physicians not prescribing diuretics more frequently in the management of hypertension? *JAMA* 279:1813, 1998.

54. Messerli FH, Grossman E, Goldbourt U: Are beta-blockers efficacious as first-line therapy in the elderly?: a systematic review. *JAMA* 279:1903, 1998.

55. Neutel JM: Metabolic manifestations of low-dose diuretics. *Am J Med* 101(suppl 3A):71, 1996.

56. Jones G, Nguyen T, Sambrook PN, et al: Thiazide diuretics and fractures: can meta-analysis help? *J Bone Min Res* 10:106, 1995.

57. Chen Z, Vaughn DA, Faneshi DD: Influence of gender on renal thiazide diuretic receptor density and response. *J Am Soc Nephrol* 5:1112, 1994.

58. Petitti N, Etgen A: Alpha-1 adrenoreceptor augmentation of beta-stimulated cAMP formation is enhanced by estrogen and reduced by progesterone in rat hypothalamic slices. *J Neurosci* 10:2842, 1990.

59. Hanes DS, Weir MR: Gender considerations in hypertension pathophysiology and treatment. *Am J Med* 101(suppl 3A):10S, 1996.

60. Seltzer A, Pinto JI, Vigione PN, et al: Estrogens regulate angiotensin-converting enzyme and angio-

tensin receptors in female rat anterior pituitary. *Neuroendocrinology* 55:460, 1992.

61. Os I, Bratland B, Dahlof B, et al: Female preponderance for lisinopril-induced cough in hypertension. *Am J Hypertens* 7:1012, 1994.

62. Hargreaves MR, Benson MK: Inhaled sodium cromoglycate in angiotensin-converting enzyme inhibitor cough. *Lancet* 345:13, 1995.

63. Dicpinigaitis PV: Use of baclofen to suppress cough induced by angiotensin-converting enzyme inhibitors. *Ann Pharmacother* 30:1242, 1996.

64. Kloner RA, Sowers JR, DiBona GF, et al: Sex and age-related antihypertensive effects of amlodipine. *Am J Cardiol* 77:713, 1996.

65. Gandhi S, Sntiesteban H: Resistant hypertension. *Postgrad Med* 100:97,1996.

66. Grauer K, Curry CL, Gums J: Management of uncontrolled hypertension. *AFP Monograph No. 2*, 1998.

67. Blemin J, Visitin JM, Salvatore R, et al: Osler's maneuver: absence of usefulness for the detection of pseudohypertension in an elderly population. *Am J Med* 98:42, 1995.

68. Leonetti G, Gomerio G, Cuspidi C: Evaluating quality of life in hypertensive patients. *J Cardiovasc Pharmacol* 23(suppl 5):554, 1994.

69. Mosca LM, Manson JE, Sutherland SE, et al: Cardiovascular disease in women: a statement for healthcare professionals from the American Heart Association. *Circulation* 96:2468, 1997.

70. Chandra NC, Ziegelstein RC, Rogers WJ, et al: Observations of the treatment of women in the United States with myocardial infarction: a report from the National Registry of Myocardial Infarction-I. *Arch Intern Med* 158:981, 1998.

71. Maynard C, Every NR, Martin JS, et al: Association of gender and survival in patients with acute myocardial infarction. *Arch Intern Med* 157:1379, 1997.

72. McLaughlin TJ, Soumerai SB, Willison DJ, et al: Adherence to national guidelines for drug treatment of suspected acute myocardial infarction: evidence for undertreatment in women and the elderly. *Arch Intern Med* 156:799, 1996.

73. The Global Utilization of Streptokinase & t-PA for Occluded Coronary Arteries (GUSTO) Investigators: An international randomized trial comparing four thrombolytic strategies for acute myocardial infarction. *N Engl J Med* 329:673, 1993.

74. Tofler GH, Stone PH, Muller JE, et al: Effects of gender and race on prognosis after myocardial infarction: adverse prognosis for women, particularly black women. *J Am Coll Cardiol* 9:473, 1987.

75. Vaccarino V, Krumholz HM, Berkman LF, et al: Sex differences after myocardial infarction: is there evidence for an increased risk for women? *Circulation* 91:1861, 1995.

76. Expert panel on detection, evaluation, and treatment of high blood cholesterol in adults. Summary of the second report of the National Cholesterol Education Program (NCEP) expert panel on detection, evaluation, and treatment of high blood cholesterol in adults (adult treatment panel II). *JAMA* 269:3015, 1993.

77. Downs JR, Clearfield M, Whitney E, et al: Primary prevention of acute coronary events with lovastatin in men and women with average cholesterol levels: results of AFCAPS/TexCAPS. Air Force/Texas Coronary Atherosclerosis Prevention Study. *JAMA* 279: 1615, 1998.

78. Sacks FM, Pfeffer MA, Moye LA, et al: The effect of pravastatin on coronary events after myocardial infarction in patients with average cholesterol levels. *N Engl J Med* 335:1001, 1996.

79. Lewis SJ, Sacks FM, Mitchell JS, et al: Effect of pravastatin on cardiovascular events in women after myocardial infarction: the Cholesterol and Recurrent Events (CARE) trial. *J Am Coll Cardiol* 32:140, 1998.

80. Scandinavian Simvastatin Survival Study Group: Randomised trial of cholesterol lowering in 4444 patients with coronary heart disease: the Scandinavian Simvastatin Survival Study (4S). *Lancet* 344: 1383, 1994.

81. Birdsall MA, Farquhar CM, White HD: Association between polycystic ovaries and extent of coronary artery disease in women having cardiac catheterization. *Ann Intern Med* 126:32, 1997.

82. Willett WC, Green A, Stampfer MJ, et al: Relative and absolute excess risks of coronary heart disease among women who smoke cigarettes. *N Engl J Med* 317:1303, 1987.

83. Rosenberg L, Miller DR, Kaufman DW, et al: Myocardial infarction in women under 50 years of age. *JAMA* 250:2801, 1983.

84. Hatcher RA, Trussell J, Stewart F, et al: *Contraceptive Technology*, 17th ed. New York: Ardent Media; 1998;420.

85. Stampfer MF, Colditz GA, Willett WC, et al: Postmenopausal estrogen treatment and cardiovascular disease: 10-year follow-up from the Nurses Health Study. *N Engl J Med* 325:756, 1991.

86. Hulley S, Grady D, Bush T, et al: Randomized trial of estrogen plus progestin for secondary preven-

tion of coronary heart disease in postmenopausal women. *JAMA* 280:605, 1998.

87. Eckel RH, Krauss RM: American Heart Association call to action: obesity as a major risk factor for coronary heart disease. *Circulation* 97:2099, 1998.

88. Rexrode KM, Carey VJ, Hennekens CH, et al: Abdominal adiposity and coronary heart disease in women. *JAMA* 280:1843, 1998.

89. Alftha G, Aro A, Gey KF, et al: Plasma homocysteine and cardiovascular disease mortality. *Lancet* 349:397, 1997.

90. Kuller LH, Evans RW: Homocysteine, vitamins and cardiovascular disease. *Circulation* 98:196, 1998.

91. Folsom AR, Nieto FJ, McGovern PG, et al: Prospective study of coronary heart disease incidence in relation to fasting total homocysteine, related genetic polymorphisms and B vitamins. *Circulation* 98:204, 1998.

92. Stephens NG, Parsons A, Schofield PM, et al: Randomised controlled trial of vitamin E in patients with coronary disease: Cambridge Heart Antioxidant Study. *Lancet* 347:781, 1996.

93. Goldberg RJ, O'Donnell C, Yarzebski J, et al: Sex differences in symptom presentation associated with acute myocardial infarction: a population-based perspective. *Am Heart J* 136:189, 1998.

94. Legato MJ, Padus E, Slaughter E: Women's perceptions of their general health, with special reference to their risk of coronary artery disease: Results of a national telephone survey. *J Womens Health* 6:189, 1997.

95. Kannel WB: Silent myocardial ischemia and infarction: insights from the Framingham Study. *Cardiol Clin* 4:583, 1986.

96. Kerr J, Ramamurthy G, Botros E, et al: Diagnostic approach to chest pain syndrome in women. *Journal of Clinical Outcomes Management* 5:57, 1998.

97. Diamond GA, Forrester JS: Analysis of probability as an aid in the diagnosis of coronary-artery disease. *N Engl J Med* 300:1350, 1979.

98. Douglas PS, Ginsburg GS: The evaluation of chest pain in women. *N Engl J Med* 334:1311, 1996.

99. Ryan TJ, Anderson JL, Antman EM, et al: ACC/AHA guidelines for the management of patients with acute myocardial infarction: a report of the American College of Cardiology/American Heart Association Task Force on Practice Guidelines (Committee on Management of Acute Myocardial Infarction). *J Am Coll Cardiol* 28:1328, 1996.

100. Pharand C, Kluger J, O'Rangers E, et al: Lidocaine prophylaxis for fatal ventricular arrhythmias after acute myocardial infarction. *Clin Pharmacol Ther* 57:471, 1995.

101. Cairns JA, Kennedy JW, Fuster V: Coronary thrombolysis in the Fifth ACCP Consensus Conference on Antithrombotic therapy. *Chest* 114:634S, 1998.

102. Hjlmarson A: Effects of beta blockade on sudden cardiac death during acute myocardial infarction and the postinfarction period. *Am J Cardiol* 80(9B):35J, 1997.

103. ACE Inhibitor Myocardial Infarction Collaborative Group: Indication for ACE inhibitors in the early treatment of acute myocardial infarction. Systematic overview of individual data from 100,000 patients in randomized trials. *Circulation* 97:2202, 1998.

Rosemary R. Berardi
Juliana Chan
Ellen M. Zimmermann

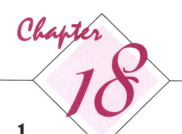

Chapter

18

Gastrointestinal Disorders

Overview

Gastroesophageal reflux disease (GERD), non-steroidal anti-inflammatory drug (NSAID)-induced ulcers, constipation, and irritable bowel syndrome (IBS) are common disorders of the gastrointestinal (GI) tract that are either more prevalent in women or exacerbated during pregnancy. This chapter reviews the pathophysiology, clinical presentation, diagnosis, and management of these disorders in primary care and focuses on special health care issues related to women. The efficacy, safety, and pharmacoeconomics of drug therapy are highlighted.

Gastroesophageal Reflux Disease

Gastroesophageal reflux disease is a chronic disorder characterized by symptoms, esophageal tissue damage, or both, resulting from reflux of acidic gastric contents into the esophagus. Reflux esophagitis is diagnosed in a subset of patients with demonstrable changes in the esophageal mucosa. Endoscopic findings range from a normal-appearing mucosa, to mild erythema, erosions, ulcers, strictures, or Barrett's epithelium. Hiatal hernia, an anatomic abnormality resulting in displacement of the gastroesophageal (GE) junction and a portion of the stomach above the diaphragm, may predispose patients to GERD. Drug treatment provides symptomatic relief and mucosal healing. However, symptomatic relapse of GERD is reported in up to 80 percent of patients within 6 to 8 months of discontinuing esophageal healing therapy.[1] Most patients with moderate to severe symptoms will likely require long-term maintenance therapy.

Epidemiology

Gastroesophageal reflux disease represents one of the most common clinical problems for primary care practitioners. It is estimated that roughly 40 percent of adults in the United States have heartburn at least once a month and that 10 percent experience heartburn daily.[1] Men and women are equally affected, but there is a male preponderance of esophagitis (2:1) and of Barrett's esophagus (10:1).[2] About 48 to 79 percent of patients with symptomatic GERD have esophagitis, with the prevalence of esophagitis being higher in patients older than 55 years of age (5 percent) than in the general population (3 percent).[2] The highest incidence of heartburn occurs in pregnant women (30 to 50 percent) with 48 to 79 percent experiencing daily heartburn.[2] The increased frequency with which GERD is being diagnosed in the United States is attributed to a greater awareness of the underlying pathogenic mechanisms as well as the availability of effective pharmacologic therapy.

Pathophysiology

Gastroesophageal reflux (GER) is the movement of gastric contents from the stomach into the esophagus. Under normal circumstances, GER is prevented by an antireflux barrier located at the GE junction. The functional integrity of this complex zone is attributed primarily to the crural diaphragm and the integrity of the lower esophageal sphincter (LES), which remains contracted in the resting state. This high-pressure zone creates a barrier that acts to decrease the frequency of reflux.[2] Spontaneous transient LES relaxation and associated reflux, however, occur in healthy individuals without symptoms or signs of esophageal damage.

The normal physiologic process becomes pathologic when noxious refluxate (acid and other substances, e.g., pepsin, bile salts, pancreatic enzymes) overcomes the esophageal protective mechanisms, producing symptoms and signs of esophageal injury. Acid is the primary injurious agent in the refluxate, and its ability to damage esophageal epithelium depends on the duration of time the esophageal mucosa remains acidified to a pH of less than 4. Because most patients with GERD have acid secretory rates similar to those observed in healthy individuals, it is likely that many other factors contribute to the development of GERD.[1,2]

Incompetence of the GE junction has been attributed to three primary mechanisms: transient LES relaxation, disruption of the GE junction associated with hiatal hernia, or a hypotensive LES without anatomic abnormality.[2] It is likely that the

dominant mechanism varies with disease severity, with transient LES relaxation associated with mild disease and a hypotensive LES more dominant in severe disease.[2] Agents that decrease LES pressure are listed in Table 18-1.

After GER, esophageal acid-clearing mechanisms (e.g., gravity, saliva, and peristalsis) reduce the duration of mucosal contact with the refluxate, but these mechanisms are less effective when the patient is in the recumbent position. Diseases such as diabetes can decrease esophageal peristalsis, and medications such as anticholinergics can impair

Table 18-1

Agents That Affect Lower Esophageal Sphincter (LES) Pressure

DECREASES LES PRESSURE	INCREASES LES PRESSURE
HORMONES AND PHYSIOLOGIC FACTORS	
Cholecystokinin	Motilin
Gastric acidification	Gastrin
Glucagon	Substance P
Progesterone	
Prostaglandins (E_2, I_2)	
Secretin	
Serotonin	
Somatostatin	
DIETARY FACTORS	
Chocolate	Protein
Alcohol	
Fat	
Peppermint	
MEDICATIONS	
α-Adrenergic antagonists, e.g., phentolamine	Antacids
β-Adrenergic agonists, e.g., isoproterenol	Prokinetic agents, e.g., cisapride
Anticholinergics, e.g., atropine	
Barbiturates, e.g., phenobarbital	
Benzodiazepines, e.g., diazepam	
Calcium channel blockers, e.g., nifedipine	
Narcotics, e.g., morphine, meperidine	
Nicotine, e.g., smoking, transdermal patch	
Progesterone, e.g., contraceptives	
Theophylline	
Tricyclic antidepressants, e.g., imipramine	

saliva production. The esophagus, unlike the stomach, does not have a well-defined premucosal barrier to minimize mucosal epithelial contact with the refluxate.[2] An incompetent pylorus or delayed gastric emptying may contribute to disease severity. The role of *Helicobacter pylori* in GERD is unclear, but it does not appear to be pathogenic.[3]

PREGNANCY

The pathophysiology of GERD in pregnancy is also multifactorial and includes hormonal effects on LES function and mechanical factors. It appears that LES competence is impaired early in pregnancy before GERD symptoms develop and that the pressure progressively falls, reaching a nadir at 36 weeks' gestation, with subsequent return of normal LES pressure after delivery.[4,5] Animal and human studies suggest that a combination of estrogen and progesterone is necessary to lower LES pressure.[4,5] Although progesterone is considered the primary hormone responsible for relaxation of the LES, the reaction may be sequential with estrogen serving as a "primer." Mechanical factors, resulting from an enlarging gravid uterus with accompanying increases in intraabdominal pressure, have also been implicated. However, studies in cirrhotic men with tense ascites, not all of whom had GERD, appear to disprove the theory that intraabdominal pressure alone is associated with heartburn.[5] Delayed gastric emptying, in response to either hormonal effects or mechanical factors, may contribute to the pathogenesis of GERD in pregnancy.

Clinical Presentation

HEARTBURN

Heartburn, often described as retrosternal burning or a discomfort that moves from the xiphoid region upward toward the neck, is reported by more than 80 percent of persons with GERD.[1,6] Patients with mild disease usually report heartburn 1 to 3 h after meals or on reclining, whereas nocturnal heartburn increases with disease severity. Although most patients with reflux esophagitis complain of heartburn, neither the frequency nor the severity of heartburn are of value in predicting the degree of mucosal damage.[2] Patients with normal esophageal mucosa may complain of frequent and severe heartburn, whereas others with severe esophagitis or Barrett's esophagus may be asymptomatic.

Regurgitation, or a bitter or acid taste in the mouth, occurs in about 70 percent of patients and is related to the reflux of gastric contents.[1,2] Bilious stains on the pillowcase in the morning may suggest regurgitation during sleep. Heartburn is a serious symptom that requires careful evaluation because it is the hallmark of esophagitis, which can lead to Barrett's esophagus and ultimately adenocarcinoma of the esophagus.[7,8]

DYSPHAGIA

Dysphagia (impaired or difficult swallowing) is reported in 30 percent of patients and occurs primarily with the ingestion of solids.[2] Patients with dysphagia initially complain of difficulty in swallowing dry substances such as toast or crackers. Dysphagia may be caused by esophageal stricture, peristaltic dysfunction, or esophageal carcinoma.

OTHER GERD SYMPTOMS

Other GERD symptoms include anginal-type chest pain, water brash, globus sensation, and odynophagia.[2,6] Patients with reflux esophagitis sometimes complain of chest pain that more closely resembles cardiac disease than heartburn. The cause of chest pain in GERD is unclear, and additional tests are required to determine the origin of the pain. Water brash is an unusual GERD symptom characterized by hypersalivation. The globus sensation is described as constant lump in the throat. Odynophagia, a sharp pain on swallowing, is a rare symptom of typical GERD and is most often associated with deep erosions and ulcers related to drug-induced or infectious esophagitis. Patients with odynophagia are often unable or afraid to eat.

GERD-Related Conditions

Mounting evidence suggests that GERD, accompanied by regurgitation and aspiration, may be implicated in the development of extraesophageal conditions such as nonseasonal asthma, pneumonitis, posterior laryngitis, chronic coughing, wheezing, nocturnal choking, chronic hoarseness, and dental disease.[2,6] Epidemiologic studies indicate that up to 80 percent of asthmatics have GERD and up to 40 percent have peptic esophagitis.[2] Although the cause and effect relationship between reflux and asthma is difficult to establish, it has been hypothesized that reflux-induced asthma may result from either aspiration of gastric contents into the lung or activation of a vagal reflex from the esophagus to the lung, both of which result in bronchoconstriction.[2] The effectiveness of antireflux drug therapy in asthmatics is uncertain. Case reports and uncontrolled trials suggest that acid blockade is of benefit in a subset of asthmatic patients, but these studies evaluated symptomatic improvement rather than improved pulmonary function.[2]

Complications

The major complications of GERD include esophageal stricture formation, bleeding, Barrett's esophagus, and adenocarcinoma of the esophagus. Esophageal stricture develops in up to 20 percent of patients with esophagitis.[2] About 2 percent of patients with esophagitis develop clinically important GI bleeding.[2] Barrett's esophagus is a premalignant condition in which the normal squamous mucosa of the esophagus is replaced by specialized columnar epithelium (i.e., intestinal metaplasia).[7–9] It occurs as a consequence of chronic GERD and is more common in men and whites.[2,8] Barrett's esophagus has been reported in 8 to 20 percent of patients with esophagitis and in 44 percent of patients with esophageal stricture.[2] The presence of Barrett's epithelium is related to long-standing (> 5 years) severe esophagitis and is associated with an increased risk (about 1 percent per year) for esophageal adenocarcinoma.[7–9] Because medications do not reverse Barrett's epithelium, early

recognition is important.[10] Several excellent articles provide an update on the screening, surveillance, and treatment of Barrett's esophagus.[8,9]

Conditions Associated with GERD

Other conditions associated with GERD include diseases with altered GI motility (e.g., diabetes mellitus), connective tissue disorders (e.g., scleroderma), hypersecretory states (e.g., Zollinger-Ellison syndrome), and pregnancy.[2]

Pregnancy

The clinical presentation of GERD in pregnancy is similar to that in the general population, with heartburn and regurgitation being the most common symptoms.[2,6] Esophagitis (with or without bleeding) and esophageal stricture are rare. In most women, GERD symptoms are limited to pregnancy and resolve upon delivery.

Diagnosis

In most patients, characteristic symptoms provide adequate support for the diagnosis of GERD. Diagnostic studies (Table 18-2) should be considered for GERD patients with signs and symptoms of esophageal injury (e.g., dysphagia, odynophagia, guaiac-positive stool, hematemesis, anemia), symptoms unresponsive to drug therapy, chronic symptoms (raising the possibility of Barrett's esophagus), chest pain, and extraintestinal manifestations (e.g., wheezing, nonseasonal asthma, nocturnal choking, chronic hoarseness). The distinction between peptic esophagitis, infectious esophagitis (e.g., candidal esophagitis), and pill-induced esophagitis can usually be made by endoscopy.

History

A history of typical postprandial or nocturnal heartburn is sufficient for the diagnosis of GERD and provides adequate rationale to initiate therapy. The complete resolution of symptoms with

Table 18-2

Diagnostic Tests and Procedures Used to Evaluate Patients with Gastroesophageal Reflux Disease (GERD)

UPPER GI RADIOGRAPHY/BARIUM SWALLOW
Upper GI radiography/barium swallow is the most sensitive test for detecting esophageal webs. Radiography can also be used to calibrate the esophageal lumen and to detect the presence or absence of hiatus hernia. However, these tests are insensitive in their ability to detect mucosal inflammation or the presence of Barrett's esophagus. Widely available; relatively inexpensive.
UPPER GI ENDOSCOPY/BIOPSY
Upper GI endoscopy is the gold standard for documenting esophageal injury, esophageal healing, and Barrett's esophagus. Also used to document hiatus hernia and most types of esophageal strictures. Permits tissue sampling and stricture dilation. More expensive than barium swallow.
CONTINUOUS AMBULATORY INTRAESOPHAGEAL pH MONITORING
Intraesophageal pH monitoring is used to assess and evaluate GERD-related reflux symptoms such as chest pain, asthma, cough, or hoarseness and to evaluate patient response to drug therapy. Continuous esophageal pH monitoring is usually performed in ambulatory patients with a nasally inserted pH probe fixed at about 5 cm above the LES. A battery-powered computer continuously records esophageal pH over a 24-h period. An event marker can be activated by the patient and correlates reflux episodes with symptoms, body position, or activity. A reflux event is identified when the intraesophageal pH falls below 4. Provides a quantitative evaluation of the amount of time the esophageal pH remains <4. The patient cannot eat acidic foods and must refrain from taking pH-altering medications during the testing period.
ESOPHAGEAL MANOMETRICS
Manometric assessment or the esophagus provides measurements of LES pressure and esophageal musculature contractility. Manometrics are used preoperatively to evaluate peristaltic function because disordered peristalsis may influence the type of antireflux surgery.
PROVOCATIVE TESTS
The Bernstein test is a provocative test used primarily to determine if chest discomfort is secondary to esophageal acidification. Normal saline is infused into the middle of the esophagus for 5 to 15 min followed by an infusion of 0.1 *N* hydrochloric acid. If symptoms occur within 30 min of the infused acid, the saline is reinfused to relieve the symptoms. Complete relief of symptoms by the saline solution is not required. Acid is then infused again to provoke symptoms. The appearance of chest discomfort in a patient blinded to the infusion sequence constitutes a positive test result.

SOURCE: Adapted with permission from PF Kahrilas: *Sleisenger & Fordtran's Gastrointestinal and Liver Disease: Pathophysiology/Diagnosis/Management*, 6th ed. Philadelphia, PA, WB Saunders, 1998; and KR DeVault: Updated guidelines for the diagnosis and treatment of gastro-esophageal reflux disease. *Am J Gastroenterol* 94:1434, 1999.

empirical (potent acid suppression) therapy is often used to confirm the diagnosis. Most patients with mild uncomplicated heartburn do not require additional tests to establish the diagnosis. Whether additional tests should be performed or whether the patient should be referred to a specialist depends on the clinical question that is being asked (e.g., Are the patient's symptoms due to reflux? Is there esophageal damage? Are extraintestinal manifestations esophageal in origin?). Patients in whom empirical therapy is unsuccessful should have further diagnostic tests.[6]

UPPER GASTROINTESTINAL ENDOSCOPY

Upper endoscopy (see Table 18-2) is the procedure of choice to detect the severity of mucosal injury, document esophageal healing, and rule out Barrett's esophagus, esophageal cancer, and other esophageal or GI causes of reflux-type symptoms.[6] Endoscopy (with biopsy) of the esophageal mucosa is indicated for patients who are unresponsive or refractory to potent antisecretory drug therapy or in those with dysphagia, odynophagia, or GI bleeding, to rule out esophageal cancer; in patients with long-standing GERD, to rule out Barrett's esophagus; and in patients with atypical symptoms, when the response to empirical therapy is difficult to evaluate. Esophageal strictures can be detected by endoscopy in most cases, but certain strictures (e.g., esophageal webs) are best evaluated by barium swallow. It is important to recognize that a normal endoscopy does not rule out symptomatic GERD and the presence of esophagitis does not always indicate that esophagitis is the cause of the patient's symptoms. Additional tests, such as 24-h esophageal pH monitoring, may be necessary to correlate symptoms with the presence of acid in the esophagus, aid in the diagnosis, and help guide therapy.

Barrett's esophagus is a histologic diagnosis that, at the time of endoscopy, is recognized by the displacement of the squamocolumnar junction or Z line (the boundary between the pale pink squamous esophageal mucosa and the deep red columnar gastric mucosa) into the lumen of the esophagus. Barrett's esophagus is also suspected when deep-red patches of columnar epithelium exist within the lighter squamous mucosa. Most cases of dysplasia, however, occur in the absence of an endoscopically visible lesion.[8] If Barrett's esophagus is confirmed, periodic endoscopic surveillance with biopsy is indicated to monitor for the development of dysplasia. The optimal frequency of endoscopic surveillance in patients without dysplasia has yet to be determined but recommendations range from every 18 to 24 months to every 5 years.[2,8,9] If dysplasia is present more intense monitoring (e.g., every 6 to 12 months) or esophageal resection is needed, depending on a number of factors including the age of the patient and the grade (low versus high) of dysplasia.[2,8,9]

RADIOGRAPHIC STUDIES

Barium radiography (see Table 18-2) rarely shows free GER of the contrast agent and thus is less useful for the diagnosis of GERD. Although a double-contrast barium esophagogram may be used to rule out esophageal ulcers, with certain types of esophageal strictures (e.g., esophageal webs), hiatal hernia, or extrinsic compression, radiography fails to detect most cases of esophagitis or Barrett's esophagus so endoscopy is preferred.[2,6] A normal radiograph rarely precludes the need for subsequent endoscopy, whereas an initial endoscopic examination rarely requires additional testing before proceeding with treatment.

AMBULATORY ESOPHAGEAL pH MONITORING

Continuous ambulatory intraesophageal 24-h pH monitoring (see Table 18-2) provides quantitative information on the temporal relationship between esophageal acid exposure and reflux events.[2,6] Esophageal pH monitoring is unnecessary in most patients with GERD, but it may be used to document persistent and excessive acid reflux in these patients despite drug or surgical treatment and to correlate atypical symptoms such as chest pain with acid reflux.

ESOPHAGEAL MANOMETRY

Esophageal manometry is most useful in facilitating the placement of ambulatory pH probes and in managing patients with GERD being considered for surgery. Documentation of ineffective peristalsis may require that the patient either avoid surgery or influence the selection of the antireflux surgical procedure.[6]

PROVOCATIVE TESTS

Provocative tests, such as the Bernstein test (see Table 18-2), are sometimes part of the manometric examination and are used to help clarify the diagnosis of GERD. Provocative tests have limited usefulness in the diagnosis of GERD.[6]

PREGNANCY

A compatible history given by a pregnant woman is usually sufficient to diagnose GERD, and further diagnostic testing is not indicated. Although upper GI endoscopy appears to be safe during pregnancy, its use should be limited to those women suspected of having strictures or ulceration. Radiography should be avoided during pregnancy.

Clinical Course

The clinical course of patients with GERD is highly variable. Most symptomatic patients with mild heartburn will respond to lifestyle changes and nonprescription medications. Acid suppression effectively relieves symptoms and heals esophagitis, but the efficacy of various regimens depends on the drug dose, duration of therapy, and the severity of the esophagitis. Unfortunately, GERD symptoms return in a substantial number of patients if treatment is discontinued. The majority of patients can be managed medically, but some will develop esophageal stricture, bleeding, or Barrett's esophagus. New antireflux surgical techniques, such as laparoscopic fundoplication, are alternatives for high-risk patents with medically intractable symptoms or complications and in younger patients who are either unwilling or unable to take medications chronically. In most cases, however, the long-term results of these new surgical procedures are not known.

Therapeutic Goals

The management of GERD should be individualized and directed at relieving symptoms and healing esophagitis with the most cost-effective treatment regimens.[2,6,11,12] Preventing symptomatic recurrence and maintaining esophageal healing increases quality of life and decreases costs associated with diagnostic testing, physician visits, and lost productivity. Sustained acid suppression may prevent complications.

Nonpharmacologic Therapy

Lifestyle modifications (Table 18-3), aimed at decreasing reflux events or enhancing esophageal clearance, are recommended for both nonpregnant or pregnant women with symptomatic GERD.[1,5,11,12] However, the effectiveness of these modifications depends on a number of factors including patient compliance, the frequency and severity of GERD symptoms, and individual differences in patient response. Lifestyle modifications that are most likely to be effective include refraining from lying down after a meal, avoiding eating at least 2 h before bedtime, and elevating the head of the bed or using a foam wedge. Elevating the head of the bed and use of the wedge allow gravity to increase esophageal acid clearance during sleep, especially if nocturnal symptoms are present. The patient should be advised to stop or decrease smoking, especially during pregnancy, because smoking increases reflux symptoms and exposes the fetus to harmful agents. The risk of noncompliance with overly restrictive dietary measures is high because diet is widely variable and only a few foods (e.g., high-fat, mints, chocolate) and beverages (e.g., alcohol, caffeine) tend to be problematic in most patients. Thus, it is best to initially suggest that the patient avoid those foods and beverages that are most troublesome. Medications listed in Table 18-1 also decrease LES pressure and may precipitate or worsen GERD symptoms.

Table 18-3

Lifestyle Modifications Recommended for Patients with GERD*

GENERAL MODIFICATIONS
• Avoid wearing tight-fitting clothing • Avoid medications that promote reflux (if possible) • Discontinue/decrease smoking • Sleep on a 10-inch foam wedge in place of pillows or elevate head of bed 6–8 inches • Reduce weight (if overweight and not pregnant) • Take nonprescription antacids or H_2-receptor antagonists
DIETARY MODIFICATIONS
• Avoid eating at least 2 h before bedtime • Avoid consumption of chocolate, peppermint, spearmint • Avoid consumption of caffeinated and decaffeinated coffee, tea, cola • Avoid consumption of carbonated beverages • Avoid consumption of tomato and citrus fruits/juices • Avoid consumption of spicy foods • Avoid overindulging on fatty foods • Discontinue/decrease alcohol consumption • Reduce meal size and eat more frequent smaller meals

*General and dietary lifestyle modifications should be individualized for each patient; effectiveness of each modification will vary from patient to patient.

Pharmacotherapy

Therapeutic options for treating GERD include antacids, alginic acid/antacid products, sucralfate, H_2-receptor antagonists (H$_2$RAs), proton pump inhibitors (PPIs), and promotility agents. Medications that inhibit gastric acid secretion are usually most effective because they reduce acidity and decrease the volume of the potential refluxate.

ANTACIDS AND ANTACID/ ALGINIC ACID PREPARATIONS

EFFICACY　Antacids neutralize gastric acid, inactivate pepsin, bind bile acids, and increase LES pressure. They are widely used because they provide rapid (within minutes) and effective relief of intermittent mild to moderate heartburn and dyspepsia. The neutralizing capacities of available antacids vary; regular strength antacids generally have one-half the acid-neutralizing capacity of a high-potency

antacid (Table 18-4). Symptom relief lasts about 30 min in fasting individuals; when given 1 h after meals, food acts as a buffer for about 1 h and the antacid effect is prolonged 2 to 3 h. Aluminum-, magnesium-, and calcium-containing salts, when used alone or in combination, provide similar efficacy when the dosage contains the same acid-neutralizing capacity.

Alginic acid, a highly viscous substance thought to float on the surface of gastric contents and mechanically prevent mucosal contact of the irritant refluxate, is available as a combination product with varying amounts of aluminum hydroxide, magnesium trisilicate, and sodium bicarbonate (Gaviscon). Clinical studies suggest that Gaviscon is as effective as antacids when used to control mild to moderate reflux symptoms; however, individual patients often claim that Gaviscon is superior to antacids. Because Gaviscon is usually more expensive, treatment should be initiated with a less costly antacid.[13]

Table 18-4

Oral Drug Treatment Regimens Used to Relieve GERD Symptoms, Heal Esophagitis, or Maintain Esophageal Healing

Drug (Brand Name)	Nonprescription Regimens	Prescription Regimens			FDA Pregnancy Class	Relative Cost*
		GERD Symptoms	Esophageal Healing	Maintenance of Esophageal Healing		
Antacids						
Regular potency (Mylanta, Maalox)	15–30 mL 1 h after meals or prn		Not indicated	Not indicated	None	$
High-potency (Mylanta II, Maalox TC)	15 mL 1 h after meals or prn		Not indicated	Not indicated	None	$
Alginic Acid-Antacid						
Gaviscon	2–4 tablets after meals or prn		Not indicated	Not indicated	None	$$
H$_2$-Receptor Antagonists						
Cimetidine (Tagamet HP, Tagamet, various)	Up to 200 mg bid	300 mg qid	800 mg bid or 400 mg qid	800 mg bid or 300–400 mg qid	B	$$–$$$
Famotidine (Pepcid AC, Pepcid)	Up to 10 mg bid	20 mg bid	20–40 mg bid	20–40 mg bid	B	$$–$$$$
Nizatidine (Axid AR, Axid)	Up to 75 mg bid	150 mg bid	150 mg bid	150 mg bid	B	$$–$$$$
Ranitidine (Zantac-75, Zantac, various)	Up to 75 mg bid	150 mg bid	150 mg bid–qid	150 mg bid–qid	B	$$–$$$$

Table 18-4

Oral Drug Treatment Regimens Used to Relieve GERD Symptoms, Heal Esophagitis, or Maintain Esophageal Healing (*Continued.*)

DRUG (BRAND NAME)	NONPRESCRIPTION REGIMENS	PRESCRIPTION REGIMENS			FDA PREGNANCY CLASS	RELATIVE COST*
		GERD SYMPTOMS	ESOPHAGEAL HEALING	MAINTENANCE OF ESOPHAGEAL HEALING		
PROTON PUMP INHIBITORS						
Lansoprazole (Prevacid)	None	15 mg qd	30 mg qd	15–30 mg qd	B	$$$$
Omeprazole (Prilosec)	None	20 mg qd	20–40 mg qd	20 mg qd	C	$$$$
Pantoprazole (Protonix)	None	?	40 mg qd	?	?	$$$$
Rabeprazole (Aciphex)	None	?	20 mg qd	?	?	$$$$
PROMOTILITY AGENTS						
Cisapride (Propulsid)	None	10–20 mg qid	10–20 mg qid	Not indicated	C	$$$$
Metoclopramide (Reglan, various)	None	10 mg qid	10 mg qid	Not indicated	B	$$–$$$
MUCOSAL DEFENSE						
Sucralfate (Carafate, various)	None	1 g qid	1 g qid	Not indicated	B	$$–$$$

*Relative cost of drug treatment is expressed as $ = least expensive to $$$$ = most expensive; actual cost varies depending on many factors including the availability of the drug as a nonprescription product, availability as a generic drug, total daily dosage regimen, and price differences among pharmacies and third-party payors.

DOSING REGIMENS   The oral dosage regimens of antacids and Gaviscon used to treat GERD are presented in Table 18-4. Magnesium-containing antacids should be avoided in patients with renal failure (see Side Effects and Drug Interactions).

SIDE EFFECTS AND DRUG INTERACTIONS   The GI adverse effects of antacids are dose dependent; diarrhea predominates with magnesium/aluminum containing antacids (Mylanta, Maalox, various) and constipation occurs with aluminum-containing (Alternagel, various) and calcium-containing (Tums, various) products. Magnesium-containing antacids should not be used in patients with a creatinine clearance less than 30 mL/min because magnesium may accumulate and lead to central nervous system (CNS) toxicity (e.g., lethargy, seizures). Aluminum-containing antacids (except aluminum phosphate) form insoluble salts with dietary phosphorus and impair oral phosphate absorption. Hypophosphatemia may occur with long-term use and in patients with low dietary phosphate intake (e.g., alcoholism, malnutrition) or when aluminum-containing antacids are used in combination with sucralfate (an aluminum-containing salt of a sulfated disaccharide). Hypercalcemia may occur in patients with normal renal function taking more than 20 g/d of calcium carbonate (equivalent to 27 tablets of a product such as TUMS-EX, which contains 300 mg elemental calcium [750 mg calcium carbonate] per tablet) and in renal failure patients taking more than 4 g/d. The milk-alkali syndrome (hypercalcemia, alkalosis, renal stones, increased blood urea nitrogen, increased serum creatinine) is associated with high calcium intake in patients with systemic alkalosis.[13]

Antacids may interact with numerous medications by increasing intragastric pH (e.g., ketoconazole), increasing urinary pH (e.g., salicylates), and decreasing drug absorption (e.g., tetracycline, fluoroquinolones). The fluoroquinolone interaction is most important because coadministration with antacids can dramatically reduce their bioavailability.[14] When possible, it is best to separate antacids from other oral medications by at least 2 h.

USE IN PREGNANCY   Magnesium-, aluminum-, and calcium-containing antacids, when used in low dosages, are considered safe for women to use for relieving reflux symptoms during pregnancy. Antacids containing sodium bicarbonate should be avoided because of the potential to cause fluid retention and metabolic alkalosis in the mother and fetus.[4,5] Electrolyte disturbances, including hypercalcemia and hypermagnesemia, have been reported in neonates and fetuses of mothers taking high antacid dosages (i.e., exceeding the usual therapeutic doses).[4] Although alginic acid, itself, appears safe during pregnancy because it is not absorbed, high dosages of Gaviscon should be avoided because of the sodium bicarbonate. No information is available regarding the use of antacids in nursing mothers.[4]

SUCRALFATE

EFFICACY   Sucralfate (Carafate, various), an aluminum-containing salt of a sulfated disaccharide, is a mucosal protectant that acts topically and has no clinically important effect on gastric acid. Sucralfate is not recommended as a first-line agent in relieving symptoms, healing erosive esophagitis, or maintaining esophageal healing because its therapeutic efficacy is variable and generally inferior to antacids, H_2RAs, and PPIs.[2,11,12]

DOSING REGIMEN   The oral dosage regimen of sucralfate used to treat GERD is presented in Table 18-4.

SIDE EFFECTS AND DRUG INTERACTIONS   Sucralfate is usually well tolerated. Constipation is the most common adverse effect and occurs in about 2 percent of patients. Dry mouth, nausea, and abdominal discomfort occur infrequently. Aluminum accumulation leading to CNS toxicity may occur in patients with chronic renal failure especially if they are taking an aluminum-containing antacid.

Sucralfate may reduce the bioavailability and effectiveness of orally administered medications, specifically, fluoroquinolones, tetracycline, digoxin, quinidine, warfarin, L-thyroxine, phenytoin, and ketoconazole, when taken at the same time.[14] Drug interactions may be avoided or minimized by giving the potentially interacting drug either 2 h before or 4 h after the sucralfate dose. Alternative therapy may be warranted in patients taking oral fluoroquinolones.

USE IN PREGNANCY Because sucralfate has limited systemic absorption and few adverse effects, it is sometimes recommended to treat heartburn during pregnancy; however, its less-than-optimal efficacy must be considered.[5] No data are available regarding transfer of sucralfate into breast milk.

H$_2$-Receptor Antagonists

EFFICACY The four available H$_2$RAs, cimetidine (Tagamet, various), ranitidine (Zantac, various), famotidine (Pepcid), and nizatidine (Axid), provide similar efficacy in relieving symptoms of GERD.[6,11,12] In contrast to antacids, the onset of symptom relief following an oral H$_2$RA dose is about 30 to 45 min.[15] Low H$_2$RA doses (see Table 18-4), recommended for nonprescription use, can prevent and relieve heartburn. Patients unresponsive to 2 weeks of treatment with a nonprescription H$_2$RA or 1 month with conventional prescription dosage regimens should be reevaluated. A 4- to 6-week H$_2$RA treatment regimen with conventional prescription dosages (see Table 18-4) may also heal mild esophagitis, but results are disappointing in patients with moderate to severe esophagitis.[11,16] Higher doses (see Table 18-4) and a longer duration of therapy (e.g., 8 to 12 weeks) are generally required, although healing rates will vary depending on disease severity.[11,16] Low H$_2$RA maintenance doses (e.g., ranitidine 150 mg at bedtime), used in peptic ulcer disease (PUD), are not effective in patients with esophagitis.[17] Typically, the maintenance dose of the H$_2$RA is similar to the higher dosage regimen needed for esophageal healing. Symptomatic recurrence may develop when maintenance therapy is instituted with a less potent antisecretory regimen.

DOSING REGIMENS The oral dosage regimens of cimetidine, ranitidine, famotidine, and nizatidine used to treat GERD are presented in Table 18-4. A reduction in the H$_2$RA daily dose is recommended in patients with moderate to severe renal impairment.

SIDE EFFECTS AND DRUG INTERACTIONS The short-term (<12 weeks) and long-term (>12 weeks) safety of the H$_2$RAs are similar and have been well documented.[12,13,17] The most frequently occurring adverse effects include GI (diarrhea, abdominal pain, constipation, nausea, flatulence) and CNS (headache, fatigue, dizziness) symptoms, which occur in 1 to 8 percent and 1 to 5 percent of patients, respectively; confusion has been reported with oral dosages of all four H$_2$RAs, primarily in the elderly and patients with renal impairment. Transient skin rashes (maculopapular, acneiform, and urticaria) have been occasionally reported in less than 1 percent of patients taking H$_2$RAs. Thrombocytopenia and neutropenia occur in less than 0.001 percent of patients and are usually reversible; agranulocytosis and aplastic anemia are rare. Recurrence may develop with rechallange with the same drug or with any of the other H$_2$RAs. Cimetidine is associated with a small increase in serum creatinine presumably secondary to competitive inhibition of renal tubular secretion of creatinine.

All four H$_2$RAs increase gastric pH and significantly decrease the absorption of drugs such as ketoconazole (see antacids). Cimetidine interacts with hepatic cytochrome P450 (CYP450) isoforms to inhibit the metabolism of numerous drugs, including theophylline, warfarin, phenytoin, imipramine, amitriptyline, nortriptyline, chlordiazepoxide, and diazepam.[14] Ranitidine interacts less extensively with CYP450 isoforms and thus the potential for hepatic drug interactions is less than with cimetidine. Famotidine and nizatidine do not interact with drugs metabolized by hepatic CYP450 isoforms and are usually preferred when there is a potential hepatic drug interaction with either cimetidine or ranitidine. A comprehensive review of H$_2$RA drug interactions can be found elsewhere.[14]

USE IN PREGNANCY Data, especially controlled trials, evaluating the safety of H$_2$RAs during pregnancy are limited. One prospective cohort study (N = 230) evaluated H$_2$RAs during pregnancy and compared them with controls matched for age, tobacco, and alcohol use.[5] Most women (88 percent) took an H_2RA during their first trimester; of the available H_2RAs, ranitidine was the most widely used. The investigators concluded that there was no increased risk of teratogenicity or premature births, but information regarding H_2RA dose, frequency, and duration of use were not included. All four H_2RAs cross the placenta and are secreted into human breast milk.[4,5] Although cimetidine is reported to cause antiandrogen-related impaired sexual development in male animals, adverse effects on the human fetus have not been documented.[4] The adverse effects of nizatidine on animal fetuses is concerning; however, the Food and Drug Administration (FDA) recently upgraded the drug from Pregnancy Category C to B. There are fewer human data on the use of famotidine use during pregnancy (see Table 18-4).

PROTON PUMP INHIBITORS

EFFICACY The PPIs, omeprazole (Prilosec), lansoprazole (Prevacid), rabeprazole (Aciphex), and pantoprazole (Protonix), provide rapid relief of symptoms and esophageal healing because of their profound antisecretory effect.[6,18–22] Numerous clinical trials have established the superiority of the PPIs over conventional and high-dose H_2RAs in patients with moderate to severe symptoms and esophagitis.[11,12,18–22] Lansoprazole 30 mg/d provides more prolonged gastric acid suppression than omeprazole 20 mg/d, but the difference in the duration of the antisecretory effect is variable between patients and does not necessarily lead to improved efficacy.[16]

The comparative efficacy of all four PPIs is an important issue especially as it relates to relief of GERD symptoms, esophageal healing, and maintenance of healing. In most comparative trials, symptomatic relief and esophageal healing rates at 4 and 8 weeks were similar when omeprazole 20 mg/d was compared to lansoprazole 30 mg/d.[18–20,23,24] However, several studies suggest that lansoprazole 30 mg/d provides more rapid relief of heartburn than omeprazole 20 mg/d in the first few days of treatment.[23] This may be related to lanso-

prazole's higher initial bioavailability. In one European trial, lansoprazole 30 mg/d provided similar rates of esophageal healing and symptom relief as omeprazole 40 mg/d.[25] Higher daily dosages, more frequent administration, and a longer duration of treatment may be necessary for patients with severe esophagitis. Patients aged 60 or older with symptomatic GERD may require more aggressive antisecretory therapy than their younger counterparts.[26]

The PPIs are also highly effective in maintaining esophageal healing and when used in recommended maintenance doses (see Table 18-4) provide similar efficacy.[17–22] When omeprazole 20 mg/d was compared to ranitidine 150 mg tid, cisapride 10 mg tid, and ranitidine plus cisapride for maintenance therapy in patients with reflux esophagitis, omeprazole was more effective than ranitidine or cisapride alone.[27] A combination of omeprazole plus cisapride was more effective than ranitidine plus cisapride. When used in recommended dosages (see Table 18-4), the newer PPIs (pantoprazole and rabeprazole) provide rates of esophageal healing, maintenance of esophageal healing, and heartburn resolution similar to those of omeprazole and lansoprazole.[18–21]

DOSING REGIMEN The oral dosage regimens of PPIs used to treat GERD are presented in Table 18-4. A dosage reduction does not appear necessary in patients with renal impairment. However, a dosage reduction should be considered in patients with severe hepatic dysfunction.

SIDE EFFECTS AND DRUG INTERACTIONS The short-term adverse effects of all four PPIs are similar and resemble the type and frequency reported with the short-term use of the H_2RAs.[28,29] GI effects (diarrhea, abdominal pain, nausea, flatulence, and constipation) and CNS effects (headache, dizziness) are most common and occur in 1 to 5 percent and 1.5 to 7 percent, respectively. Despite the theoretical concern about potent gastric acid suppression, the long-term adverse effects of the PPIs appear similar to their short-term effects. To date, no cases of gastric carcinoid or gastric cancer in humans have been attributed to the long-term use of either omeprazole or lansoprazole.[28,29]

Although pantoprazole and rabeprazole appear to have a similar safety profile, their long-term effects are not as well established.

The PPIs may potentially interact with other medications by altering the hepatic metabolism of drugs taken concurrently or by increasing gastric pH. Omeprazole interacts selectively with specific hepatic CYP450 isoenzymes and may inhibit the metabolism of phenytoin, diazepam, or warfarin; however, there have been very few documented hepatic drug interactions with omeprazole.[14,19,30] Lansoprazole may slightly increase theophylline clearance; however, the lansoprazole-theophylline interaction does not appear to be clinically important.[14,19,30] Although pantoprazole (and possibly rabeprazole) may theoretically have a lower potential for metabolic drug interactions, clinically important interactions with omeprazole and lansoprazole rarely occur given their widespread use.[21,22,30] Because the PPIs have such a potent effect on gastric acid, the bioavailability of drugs such as ketoconazole may be altered when taken concomitantly (see section on antacids).[30]

USE IN PREGNANCY   There are no prospective clinical trials of PPI use during pregnancy. Although women taking omeprazole have apparently given birth to healthy infants, there are several reports of congenital malformations.[5] Less is known about the safety of lansoprazole, pantoprazole, and rabeprazole during pregnancy.

PROMOTILITY AGENTS

EFFICACY   The promotility agents in the United States include cisapride, metoclopramide, and bethanechol; however, metoclopramide and bethanechol are no longer used because of troublesome adverse effects. Cisapride increases LES pressure, enhances gastric emptying, and improves esophageal clearance. Its efficacy in relieving heartburn is similar to standard H$_2$RA dosage regimens.[6,12,31] In most studies, cisapride is superior to placebo in healing mild esophagitis, but its effectiveness in healing moderate to severe esophagitis is variable.[11,32] The optimal maintenance dose of cisa-

pride has yet to be determined.[11,33] For the majority of patients with GERD, cisapride, when used as a single agent, offers no important therapeutic advantage over standard doses of the H$_2$RAs, has a greater potential for serious adverse effects and drug interactions, and is more expensive.

DOSING REGIMEN   The oral dosage regimens of promotility agents used to treat GERD are presented in Table 18-4. A dosage reduction should be considered in patients with severe hepatic dysfunction. Cisapride is contraindicated in patients with renal failure.

SIDE EFFECTS AND DRUG INTERACTIONS   Cisapride has relatively few CNS adverse effects when compared with metoclopramide and bethanechol. Headache (20 percent) is the most common side effect. Diarrhea (15 percent), abdominal cramping (10 percent), nausea (8 percent), and flatulence (3 percent) occur frequently but tend to resolve with continued use. In a small number of patients, headache, diarrhea, and abdominal pain may be intolerable and require discontinuing the drug. Numerous cases of serious cardiac arrhythmias (e.g., ventricular tachycardia, ventricular fibrillation, torsades de pointes, prolongation of QT interval) have been reported in patients taking cisapride, a number of which have led to fatalities.[34] Many of these patients were receiving concomitant treatment with other drugs that increased plasma cisapride concentration or had other disorders predisposing them to arrhythmias.

Cisapride is contraindicated (black box warning) in patients receiving drugs that inhibit hepatic CYP450 3A4 (e.g., ketoconazole, itraconazole [Sporanox], fluconazole [Diflucan], erythromycin, clarithromycin [Biaxin], nefazodone [Serzone], ritonavir [Norvir], indinavir [Crixivan]) and with grapefruit juice as these agents may markedly increase the serum cisapride concentration and lead to prolongation of the QT interval resulting in ventricular arrhythmias and death.[34–36] In addition, cisapride is contraindicated when taken with medications that prolong the QT interval and increase the risk of arrhythmias, including Class IA (e.g., quinidine, procainamide) and Class III (e.g., sotalol) antiarrhythmics, tricyclic antidepressants (e.g., amitriptyline), tetracyclic antidepressants (e.g., maprotiline), certain antipsychotic medications (e.g., certain phenothiazines, sertindole), astemizole (Hismanal), bepridil (Vascor), and sparfloxacin (Zagam).

Cardiac arrhythmias (sometimes with syncope), cardiac arrest, and sudden death have also been reported in patients not taking the above-mentioned contraindicated drugs. Most of these patients had a history of cardiac disorders (e.g., prolonged QT interval, ventricular arrhythmias, ischemic heart disease, congestive heart failure), renal failure, uncorrected fluid and electrolyte disorders (e.g., hypokalemia, hypomagnesemia), or respiratory failure that predisposed them to arrhythmias with cisapride.[34] Because cisapride is also contraindicated in women with these conditions, the potential benefits of using the drug should be weighed against the risks. An electrocardiogram should be considered before therapy with cisapride is initiated.[34]

USE IN PREGNANCY   In animal studies, cisapride has been associated with lower birth weights and has adversely affected survival. However, a multicenter prospective observational cohort study (N = 129) evaluating the safety of cisapride during pregnancy concluded that cisapride use during pregnancy was not associated with increased risk of congenital malformations, decreased birth weight, or spontaneous abortions.[5] This study was unable to detect minor increases in fetal malformation due to the small number of evaluable patients. Until more information is available, cisapride should not be used routinely for the treatment of GERD during pregnancy.

COMBINING MEDICATIONS

Antacids may be used when needed as an adjunct to antisecretory or promotility drug therapy; however, frequent dosing may indicate the need to reevaluate the primary therapy. Optimizing the dose of a PPI is usually more effective than combining an H_2RA with cisapride, except in patients with delayed gastric emptying (e.g., diabetes mellitus). The concurrent use of two differ-

ent PPIs or two different H_2RAs is not rational. Although the concurrent use of an H_2RA and a PPI should not be routinely advocated, a study in healthy subjects suggests that a bedtime dose of an H_2RA (ranitidine 150 or 300 mg) in addition to a PPI (omeprazole 20 mg at breakfast and dinner) was superior to an additional bedtime dose of a PPI (omeprazole 20 mg) in maintaining intragastric pH above 4 and preventing nocturnal acid breakthrough.[37] Why the H_2RA provided better control of nocturnal acid is unclear, but it may be related to the fact that PPIs are not activated in the fasting state and that H_2RA inhibition of gastric acid is independent of food intake. Additional studies in patients with GERD are required to support the combined use of these medications. Treatment with an antisecretory drug and sucralfate should be reserved for patients with severe esophageal mucosal injury who do not respond to combined treatment with antisecretory drugs and a promotility agent.

ERADICATING *H. PYLORI* INFECTION

The relationship between *H. pylori* and GERD is complicated and eradication of the infection in GERD patients remains controversial. There are three important issues regarding *H. pylori* and GERD: (1) GERD may develop de novo following the eradication of *H. pylori* in patients with PUD; (2) the development of atrophic corpus gastritis (a potentially precancerous condition) may be accelerated in *H. pylori*-positive patients receiving long-term treatment with PPIs; and (3) *H. pylori* might be linked to the pathogenesis of Barrett's esophagus.[38,39] Although questions regarding the relationship between *H. pylori* and GERD remain unanswered at this time, an argument can be made for documenting *H. pylori* and eradicating the infection in young patients receiving PPI maintenance therapy and in patients with long-standing GERD.

Tests used to detect *H. pylori* include those that require endoscopy and biopsy of the gastric mucosa (rapid urease test, histology, culture) and those that do not (serology, urea breath tests). Office-based serologic testing is the nonendoscopic method of choice because results are immediate and the test is inexpensive.[40] Because serology detects antibodies to *H. pylori*, the test should not be used to confirm eradication posttreatment. Eradication of *H. pylori* is not recommended in women who are pregnant or nursing because the regimens contain drugs that should not be used in these conditions (e.g., clarithromycin, metronidazole, tetracycline). Several excellent reviews provide additional information on *H. pylori* testing and treatment.[40,41]

Pharmacoeconomic Considerations

The H$_2$RAs are the most economical when used intermittently to relieve mild, infrequent GERD symptoms.[42] The PPIs are the drugs of choice for healing moderate to severe esophagitis because they are more cost-effective than H$_2$RAs.[43,44] PPIs are reported to improve health-related quality of life in patients with symptomatic erosive esophagitis.[45] A cost-utility analysis suggests that for most patients with moderate to severe esophagitis, medical management may be less costly than laparoscopic fundoplication.[46]

Management Strategies

RELIEVING SYMPTOMS AND HEALING THE ESOPHAGUS

An algorithm for managing GERD is presented in Fig. 18-1.[1,6,47] Self-medication with antacids or nonprescription H$_2$RAs and lifestyle modifications are reasonable for patients with mild episodic typical GERD symptoms. When nonprescription therapy fails, empirical therapy should be initiated with a 4- to 6-week course of a standard H$_2$RA prescription dosage regimen (see Table 18-4). If the patient has had a previous unsuccessful response to an H$_2$RA, treatment should be initiated with a PPI.

The choice of a specific drug within a class should be based on cost and the potential for clinically important drug interactions. If symptoms recur, the patient should be retreated and placed

on maintenance therapy or referred to a gastroenterologist, depending on the frequency and severity of the recurrence.

Patients with initial moderate to severe symptoms or esophagitis should be treated with a PPI and monitored for relief of symptoms. Lifestyle modifications should be reaffirmed. An upper endoscopy should be performed in patients with dysphagia, odynophagia, GI bleeding, chronic symptoms (>5 years), chest pain, and extraintestinal or refractory symptoms. Once the diagnosis of esophagitis has been established, the patient should be switched to a PPI (see Table 18-4). If symptoms persist, the PPI dose may be increased or the duration of treatment extended beyond 4 to 8 weeks. Patients unresponsive to PPIs or those with delayed gastric emptying may require the addition of a promotility agent (cisapride).

MAINTAINING REMISSION

Patients most likely to require long-term medical management include those with initial moderate to severe esophagitis, esophagitis resistant to H$_2$RAs, need for prolonged treatment, symptomatic recurrence within months of healing, and a long duration of symptoms before initial therapy. Although an H$_2$RA or cisapride may be used to maintain remission in patients with nonerosive GERD or mild initial esophagitis, the PPIs are superior to conventional and high-dose H$_2$RAs and cisapride in patients with moderate to severe reflux esophagitis, esophageal stricture, or Barrett's esophagus.[11,47,48] Once an effective therapeutic regimen is obtained, it should be maintained for 2 to 3 months.[47] After this time, an effort should be made to lower the PPI dosage or switch to an H$_2$RA in an attempt to sustain remission with the lowest effective antisecretory therapy.

If symptoms recur, the full therapeutic dose should be reinstituted. Antireflux surgery may be a viable and cost-effective option in a young, otherwise healthy patient.[47,49] Because *H. pylori*-positive patients receiving long-term PPI therapy may have a propensity to develop atrophic gastritis, consideration should be given to detecting and eradicating

Figure 18-1

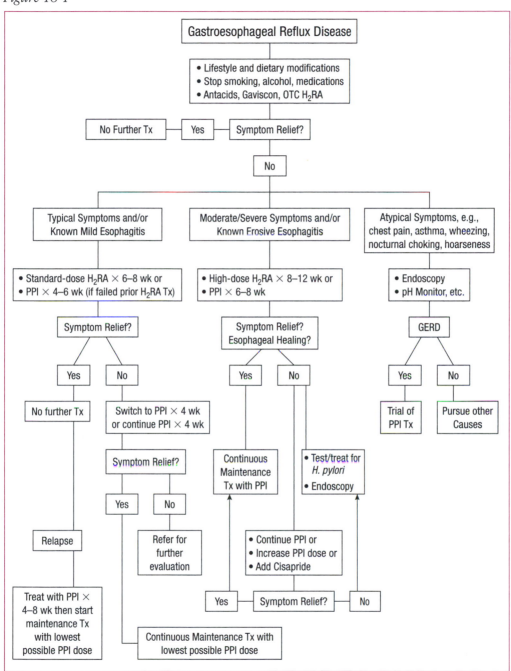

Algorithm for managing patients with gastroesophageal reflux disease.
ABBREVIATIONS: GERD, gastroesophageal reflux disease; H₂RA, H₂-receptor antagonist; OTC, over the counter; PPI, proton pump inhibitor; Tx, treatment.

H. pylori in young GERD patients or those receiving long-term PPI maintenance therapy (see previous section on eradicating *H. pylori* infection).[38]

MANAGING GERD DURING PREGNANCY

Pregnant women should be reassured that GERD is a common occurrence during a normal pregnancy. In most women, adherence to lifestyle modifications is all that is needed. In women with moderate to severe GERD symptoms, the risk of using medications must be discussed with the patient because most safety information is based on animal data. First-line therapy should consist of drugs that are minimally absorbed (antacids, sucralfate). Treatment should be initiated with low-dose antacids. If high or frequent antacid dosing is required, consideration should be given to switching to sucralfate. Although it appears that H_2RAs (preferably ranitidine or cimetidine) are well tolerated by the fetus when used to treat the heartburn of pregnancy, their use should be limited to those women who do not respond to lifestyle modifications, antacids, or sucralfate. PPIs and cisapride are not recommended during pregnancy and should be reserved for pregnant women with severe symptoms or are unresponsive to other treatments. The risks and benefits of systemic medications must be discussed with the mother and her consent should be obtained prior to use.

Nonsteroidal Anti-Inflammatory Drug-Induced Ulcers

Peptic ulcers occur most often when either *H. pylori* or NSAIDs (including aspirin) disrupt the GI mucosa.[50,51] NSAID-induced injury to the GI tract occurs primarily in the stomach, but ulcers can occur in the duodenum, small intestine, and colon.[50,52] Complications, including ulcer bleeding and perforation, occur with use of both prescription and nonprescription NSAIDs.[50,53,54] NSAID risk is complicated by undocumented nonprescription NSAID consumption because patients and physicians are often unaware that such medications are being taken. When NSAID use was assessed by history in patients who presented to the hospital with an upper GI bleed, 42 percent of the NSAIDs consumed were not prescribed.[50]

Table 18-5 identifies factors associated with an increased risk for NSAID-related GI complications. Patients with a history of PUD or ulcer-related complications and those taking concurrent corticosteroids or anticoagulants are at high risk for serious GI complications.[50,53,55] The risk for NSAID-related complications increases in patients over 60 years of age, with those over 75 years of age at highest risk.[53] Although the risk of ulcer complications increases with NSAID dose and duration of therapy, low-dose aspirin (e.g., 75 to 100 mg/d) and nonaspirin NSAIDs (e.g., ibuprofen, naproxen, diclofenac) may cause complications after a few days of treatment.[50,53] The combination of advanced age and other risk factors increase the probability of life-threatening GI complications. Smoking (more

Table 18-5

Factors That Increase the Risk of Nonsteroidal Anti-Inflammatory Drug (NSAID)-Induced Gastrointestinal (GI) Complications

Prior history of peptic ulcer disease
Prior history of ulcer-related complications, e.g., perforation, bleeding
Concurrent use with glucocorticoids
Coagulopathy or concurrent use with anticoagulants
Patient age (greater than 60 years)
High NSAID dose, multiple NSAIDs, increased duration of therapy
Prior history of cardiovascular disease
Poor general health/arthritis-related disability
Smoking or alcohol use
Helicobacter pylori?
Gender (female > male)?

than 10 cigarettes a day) and alcohol use also increase the risk for NSAID-induced ulcers, but may not be independent risk factors. Whether *H. pylori* is an independent risk factor for NSAID-induced ulcers remains controversial.[56] Although the risk of NSAID-induced GI complications is higher in women, data are conflicting as to whether being female is an independent risk factor. The increased risk of ulcers in older women is most likely related to an increased consumption of NSAIDs.[53]

Epidemiology

The NSAIDs are the most widely prescribed medications in the world.[50] About 1 percent of Americans use NSAIDs daily and more than 25 million prescriptions are written for NSAIDs annually. The availability of nonprescription NSAIDs has further expanded the use of these medications. The lifetime prevalence of PUD in the United States is 5 to 10 percent and is comparable in men and women.[51] Although hospitalizations and mortality for PUD have decreased during the last 40 years, mortality rates from this disease have increased in patients over 75 years of age and in women.[53] This rise has been attributed to an increase in NSAID consumption and the fact that gastric ulcer (GU), which is more common with NSAIDs, is associated with a higher mortality than duodenal ulcer (DU). Chronic NSAID use leads to ulceration in 4 to 12 percent of patients; life-threatening complications (bleeding, perforation, obstruction) occur in 2 to 4 percent of patients who take NSAIDs for a year.[50] About 200,000 to 400,000 of the 20 million regular NSAID users in the United States require hospitalization each year for NSAID-related GI complications.[53]

Pathophysiology

Use of NSAIDs is associated with a wide range of alterations in the GI tract. The pathophysiology of NSAID-induced injury is linked to both direct irritation of the gastric mucosa and systemic prostaglan-

din inhibition.[50] The initial injury occurs because of local toxicity, but GU formation correlates directly with the ability of the NSAID to inhibit endogenous prostaglandin synthesis and impair mucosal defense mechanisms. Cyclooxygenase (COX) is the rate-limiting enzyme responsible for the production of mucosal prostaglandins from arachidonic acid. Two COX isoforms have been identified: cyclooxygenase-1 (COX-1), which is found in the stomach, kidney, intestine, and platelets and plays an important role in the maintenance of normal organ integrity; and cyclooxygenase-2 (COX-2), which is induced and upregulated in areas of inflammation.[50,52] Inhibition of COX-1 is linked to GI damage, whereas inhibition of COX-2 is associated with the anti-inflammatory effects of NSAIDs. All NSAIDs inhibit COX-1 and COX-2 to varying degrees, resulting in a beneficial anti-inflammatory response and a potential to cause GI toxicity.

The difference in the relative risk of specific NSAIDs to cause an ulcer appears to correlate directly with their ability to inhibit COX-1.[52,57] Drugs such as aspirin and indomethacin are potent COX-1 inhibitors, whereas etodolac (Lodine) and nabumetone (Relafen) have greater COX-2 selectivity that closely parallels a decrease in ulcer risk.[52] Enteric-coated aspirin, parenteral or rectal aspirin, or NSAIDs and NSAID prodrugs decrease local gastric irritation, but all act systemically to inhibit prostaglandins and are potentially ulcerogenic. The highly selective COX-2 inhibitors (e.g., celecoxib [Celebrex] and rofecoxib [Vioxx]), although similar in efficacy to the nonselective COX NSAIDs, significantly lower the risk for GI toxicity when compared to naproxen, ibuprofen, and diclofenac.[57,58]

Clinical Presentation

The most frequent GI symptoms of patients taking NSAIDs include dyspepsia and epigastric pain often accompanied by heartburn, bloating, and belching.[50,51] In about two-thirds of ulcer patients the pain is epigastric; in others it presents as a vague abdominal discomfort or cramping. Patients with DU frequently complain of hunger and nocturnal epigastric pain that awakens them from sleep. Vomiting, anorexia, and weight loss are more common in patients with GU. Epigastric pain usually diminishes or disappears with treatment, but relief of pain does not directly correlate with ulcer healing. Recurrence of ulcer pain usually suggests a recurrent ulcer. Changes in the character of the pain may indicate ulcer-related complications.

Serious life-threatening GI complications such as bleeding, perforation, and obstruction can occur with NSAID-induced ulcers. Bleeding, perforation, and obstruction are reported to occur at 1, 0.3, and 0.1 percent, respectively, per patient-year of NSAID use.[51] Bleeding may be insidious but often presents as melena or hematemesis. In up to 80 percent of patients with NSAID-related GI bleeding or perforation, the event is silent and not preceded by symptoms.[55] Death occurs primarily in patients who rebleed or continue to bleed after hospitalization. The use of NSAIDs in the elderly is associated with one-third to one-half of all perforated ulcers. Gastric outlet obstruction occurs primarily in patients with long-standing PUD. Surreptitious use of NSAIDs occurs even after surgery for complications of NSAID-induced ulcers.

Diagnosis

Acute ingestion of NSAIDs causes frequent GI symptoms that resolve with continued use, concomitant H$_2$RA, PPI, or misoprostol therapy, or discontinuation of the drug. Symptoms associated with acute ingestion do not correlate with endoscopic damage and do not predict chronic ulceration or complications. Acute injury rarely requires diagnostic evaluation and is of little clinical consequence in most patients. Chronic use, however, is more likely to be associated with GI ulceration, hemorrhage, perforation, and death. Because up to 80 percent of complications may be silent, evaluation with upper GI radiography or upper endoscopy is indicated for patients with upper GI symptoms despite antacid or antisecretory therapy and for those patients with suspected complications (e.g., bleeding, perforation). Colonoscopy may be indicated for patients with lower GI symptoms or bleeding.

Epigastric pain and dyspepsia are common ulcer symptoms. Therefore, it is not possible to confirm PUD or to differentiate a GU from a DU based on symptoms alone. A definitive diagnosis should be established in symptomatic patients taking NSAIDs who are older than 45 years of age (to rule out malignancy), have a history of PUD or related complications, have a long duration of symptoms, and when there is the possibility of another disease or malignancy.[51,59] In these patients, the diagnostic procedure of choice often depends on several factors including the availability and cost of the procedure. Fiberoptic endoscopy is considered the gold standard for diagnosing an ulcer because it permits a direct view of the ulcer crater and tissue biopsies. In most cases, radiography, using double-contrast barium and optimal radiologic techniques, provides comparable results and is less costly than endoscopy. Acid secretory studies and fasting serum gastrin levels are not helpful in establishing the diagnosis of uncomplicated PUD.

Clinical Course

The clinical course of a patient with an NSAID-induced ulcer will vary depending on the presence of established risk factors, whether the NSAID can be discontinued, and whether GI-related complications occur. If the NSAID cannot be discontinued, prophylactic cotherapy with misoprostol or an antisecretory drug or switching to a selective COX-2 NSAID may decrease NSAID-induced complications. Mortality from NSAID-related GI complications is highest in elderly patients with GU.

Therapeutic Goals

Treatment goals depend on the etiology of the ulcer (H. pylori or NSAID-induced), whether the ulcer is initial or recurrent, whether the NSAID is continued or stopped, and whether GI complications have occurred. The aim of drug therapy in a patient with an active ulcer is to relieve ulcer symptoms, accelerate ulcer healing, and prevent ulcer recurrence and complications. If H. pylori is present, it should be eradicated and the ulcer healed. The goal of therapy in high-risk patients who take NSAIDs is to prevent NSAID-induced ulcers and related GI complications.

Nonpharmacologic Therapy

Patients with an NSAID-induced ulcer and those at high risk of developing NSAID-related GI complications should eliminate or reduce cigarette smoking and alcohol usage and, if possible, discontinue the NSAID. The patient should determine which foods and beverages exacerbate their ulcer symptoms and should modify their diet accordingly. Coffee, tea, and cola beverages (even if decaffeinated) tend to be troublesome in patients with PUD.[51]

Pharmacotherapy

SELF-MEDICATION

Nonprescription NSAIDs are widely used for self-medication for the temporary relief of minor aches and pains. Patients who self-medicate with an NSAID should be counseled not to exceed the maximally recommended nonprescription dosage and not to exceed 10 days of treatment unless otherwise directed by a clinician. In addition, patients often self-medicate with antacids or nonprescription H_2RAs to relieve NSAID-induced dyspepsia. Although this is an acceptable practice when used intermittently, the patient should be advised not to exceed the maximally recommended nonprescription H_2RA dosage and duration of therapy and that these agents may mask ulcer symptoms when taken concurrently with an NSAID. All patients who take NSAIDs (nonprescription and prescription) should be alerted to the alarm symptoms associated with ulcer-related complications (e.g., vomiting of blood, blood in stool, lightheadedness, severe abdominal pain).

ANTACIDS

Antacids provide the most rapid relief (within minutes) of ulcer pain and dyspepsia. They may be used as single agents or in combination with other antiulcer medications to relieve ulcer symptoms. Calcium-containing antacids are often avoided in patients with PUD because of the potential to cause acid rebound, but this is most likely a theoretical concern because it appears to be of questionable clinical importance.[60] Although antacids are often used to relieve NSAID dyspepsia, they should not be used as single agents to heal or prevent NSAID-induced ulcers because ulcer healing requires high and frequent dosages and antacids are not effective in preventing NSAID injury to the GI tract.[53,60] (See GERD section for information on antacid adverse effects, drug interactions, and use in pregnancy.)

SUCRALFATE

Standard dosages of sucralfate provide DU and GU healing rates comparable to those observed with the H_2RAs when the NSAID is stopped (Table 18-6).[60] Sucralfate, however, is usually not as effective as antisecretory medications in relieving ulcer pain. If the NSAID is continued or if the ulcer is large or complicated, prolonged treatment (beyond 8 weeks) may be required. Combined therapy with sucralfate and either an H_2RA or a PPI offers no therapeutic advantage for most ulcer patients. The effectiveness of sucralfate in preventing NSAID-induced ulcers is disappointing so the drug should not be used for this indication.[53] (See GERD section for information on sucralfate adverse effects, drug interactions, and use in pregnancy.)

H_2-RECEPTOR ANTAGONISTS

Standard H_2RA dosages of cimetidine, ranitidine, famotidine, and nizatidine provide comparable rates of symptom relief and ulcer healing at 4, 6, and 8 weeks when the NSAID is stopped (see Table 18-6).[60] If the NSAID is continued or if the ulcer is large or complicated, prolonged treatment (beyond 8 weeks) or a higher H_2RA dosage (e.g., famotidine 40 mg bid) appears to be necessary for ulcer healing.[53,61] Although a number of studies have documented a beneficial effect of standard H_2RA dosages (e.g., famotidine 20 mg

Table 18-6

Oral Single-Drug Treatment Regimens Used to Heal Ulcers or Maintain Ulcer Healing

Drug (Brand Name)	Ulcer Healing		Maintenance of Ulcer Healing		Relative Cost*
	Duodenal Ulcer	Gastric Ulcer	Duodenal Ulcer	Gastric Ulcer	
H₂-Receptor Antagonists					
Cimetidine (Tagamet, various)	300 mg qid 400 mg bid 800 mg hs	300 mg qid 800 mg hs	400 mg hs	400–800 mg hs	$–$$
Famotidine (Pepcid)	20 mg bid 40 mg hs	20 mg bid 40 mg hs	20 mg hs	20 mg hs	$$
Nizatidine (Axid)	150 mg bid 300 mg hs	150 mg bid 300 mg hs	150 mg hs	150–300 mg hs	$$
Ranitidine (Zantac, various)	150 mg bid 300 mg hs	150 mg bid 300 mg hs	150 mg hs	150–300 mg hs	$–$$
Proton Pump Inhibitors					
Omeprazole (Prilosec)	20 mg qd	40 mg qd	20 mg qd	20–40 mg qd	$$$$
Lansoprazole (Prevacid)	15 mg qd	30 mg qd	15 mg qd	15–30 mg qd	$$$$
Pantoprazole (Protonix)	30 mg qd	?	?	?	$$$$
Rabeprazole (Aciphex)	20 mg qd	?	?	?	$$$$
Mucosal Defense					
Sucralfate (Carafate, various)	1 g qid 2 g bid	1 g qid 2 g bid	1 g bid	1 g bid	$$–$$$

*Relative cost of drug treatment is expressed as $ = least expensive to $$$$ = most expensive; actual cost varies depending on many factors including the availability of the drug as a nonprescription product, availability as a generic drug, total daily dosage regimen, and price differences among pharmacies and third-party payors.

bid) in preventing NSAID-induced DU, protection against NSAID-induced GU requires higher H_2RA dosages (e.g., famotidine 40 mg bid).[53,61–63] Nonprescription H_2RAs are widely used to relieve NSAID-related dyspeptic symptoms (see section on Self-Medication). (Also see GERD section for information on H_2RA adverse effects, drug interactions, and use in pregnancy.)

PROTON PUMP INHIBITORS

The PPIs are the drugs of choice for the treatment of patients with NSAID-induced ulcers. When taken in recommended dosages (Table 18-6), omeprazole, lansoprazole, pantoprazole, and rabeprazole provide similar rates of ulcer healing and symptom relief.[18,19] It is possible that in some patients, lansoprazole, pantoprazole, and rabeprazole may provide more rapid relief of ulcer symptoms during the first week of therapy.[19] When compared to standard H_2RA ulcer-healing regimens, the PPIs provide more rapid relief of symptoms and ulcer healing.[19] The more rapid response observed with the PPIs results from their potent acid suppression. PPI-based three-drug regimens should be used to eradicate *H. pylori* in *H. pylori*-positive patients, including those taking NSAIDs.[19]

Two large international multicenter trials suggest that omeprazole 20 mg/d is at least as effective as misoprostol 200 μg qid and superior to ranitidine 150 mg bid when used to heal ulcers in patients with arthritis who continued taking NSAIDs.[63,64] In both clinical trials, omeprazole 20 mg/d provided similar ulcer-healing efficacy as omeprazole 40 mg/d. In addition, prophylactic cotherapy with omeprazole 20 mg/d was superior to misoprostol 200 μg bid or ranitidine 150 mg bid in preventing NSAID-induced ulcer recurrence.[63,64] (See GERD section for information on PPI adverse effects, drug interactions, and use in pregnancy.)

PROSTAGLANDINS

EFFICACY Misoprostol (Cytotec) is the drug of choice for preventing NSAID-induced ulcers in high-risk patients taking NSAIDs. Misoprostol, a synthetic prostaglandin E_1 analogue, replenishes mucosal prostaglandins that have been depleted by the NSAID.[53,60] A dosage of 200 μg qid was initially recommended, but frequent GI adverse effects, including diarrhea and abdominal cramping, limited its use. The results from recent clinical studies using a lower misoprostol dose of 200 μg two or three times daily indicate that adequate protection against GU and DU is achieved and that the drug is better tolerated.[53,65,66] Fixed combinations of misoprostol and diclofenac (Arthrotec) may increase compliance, but dosage flexibility is reduced.

SIDE EFFECTS Diarrhea is the most frequent and troublesome adverse effect associated with the use of misoprostol. In controlled trials, diarrhea is reported to develop in 14 to 40 percent of patients taking 800 μg/d.[66] In studies using 400 to 800 μg/d, the incidence of diarrhea averaged 13 percent.[66] The diarrhea, which appears to be dose dependent, usually develops within several weeks of initiating therapy and in most patients subsides within a week after onset or a reduction in the daily dosage. Abdominal cramping (13 to 20 percent) and other GI effects (nausea, flatulence, dyspepsia, vomiting, and constipation) occur in 1 to 4 percent of patients receiving misoprostol, but the incidence of these effects is similar to those receiving placebo.

USE IN PREGNANCY Misoprostol is contraindicated in pregnancy because it is uterotrophic and may endanger the fetus. If misoprostol is inadvertently taken during pregnancy, the drug should be discontinued and the patient warned of the potential hazard (i.e., miscarriage) to the fetus. Misoprostol should be used in women of childbearing age only after determining that they are reliable and able to comply with effective contraceptive measures and after giving both oral and written warnings regarding the hazards associated with the risk of contraceptive failure. In addition, the manufacturer recommends a reliable blood serum pregnancy test be performed within 2 weeks before initiating therapy; the drug should not be provided until the result of the test is reported as negative. If negative, therapy should be initiated on the second or third day of the next normal menstrual cycle.

CYCLOOXYGENASE-2 INHIBITORS

Highly selective COX-2 inhibitors inhibit prostaglandin synthesis at sites of inflammation but spare constitutive prostaglandin synthesis in the GI tract.[58,67] When compared to available NSAIDs, the selective COX-2 inhibitors provide similar anti-inflammatory effects with a marked reduction in the risk for peptic ulcers and ulcer-related GI complications.[68,69] Celecoxib (Celebrex) is the first drug in this class to be approved for the relief of the signs and symptoms associated with osteoarthritis and rheumatoid arthritis. In clinical studies of 12 and 24 weeks' duration, celecoxib (50 to 400 mg bid) was as effective as naproxen 500 mg bid or ibuprofen 800 mg tid and was associated with a significantly lower incidence of endoscopic ulcers.[68] Two studies have compared celecoxib with diclofenac 75 mg bid.[68] One study revealed a statistically significant higher prevalence of endoscopic ulcers in the diclofenac group following 6 months of treatment; the second study revealed no statistically significant difference between cumulative endoscopic ulcer incidence rates after 1, 2, and 3 months of treatment. Although infrequent, serious upper GI bleeding has been observed in patients receiving celecoxib. To date, prospective long-term studies required to compare the incidence of serious upper GI adverse effects in patients taking celecoxib versus other comparable NSAIDs have not been performed.

Studies with rofecoxib (Vioxx), the second available COX-2 NSAID, demonstrate that rofecoxib provides symptomatic relief of osteoarthritis, rheumatoid arthritis, and analgesic relief of acute pain associated with dental extractions, postoperative orthopedic surgery, and dysmenorrhea that is indistinguishable from that observed with ibuprofen.[69] Rofecoxib also has a significantly improved GI safety profile when compared to nonselective COX NSAIDs.

Other highly selective COX-2 NSAIDs are currently at various stages of investigation in the United States. If the results of postmarketing surveillance studies confirm the results of clinical trials, then the selective inhibitors of COX-2 will represent a significant therapeutic advance in the management of inflammation and pain.

OTHER NEW APPROACHES TO SPARE THE GI TRACT

Other new approaches to improving the GI safety of NSAIDs include nitric oxide–releasing NSAIDs, pure enantiomers of chiral NSAIDs, and NSAIDs preassociated with Zwitterionic phospholipids.[52] Nitric oxide derivatives of diclofenac, naproxen, and flurbiprofen have been shown to spare the GI tract in experimental models. Most chiral NSAIDs are racemic mixtures of R- and S-enantiomers. Because the S-enantiomer has a greater effect on inhibiting prostaglandin synthesis, some have suggested the use of the pure R-enantiomer. The results of preliminary studies, however, indicate that the R-enantiomer may have a weaker anti-inflammatory action. In addition, there is concern about in vivo conversion from the R- to the S-enantiomer. The preassociation of an NSAID with a Zwitterionic phospholipid should reduce the ability of the NSAID to associate with phospholipids within the mucous gel layer, thereby reducing NSAID toxicity to the gastric mucosa.

Pharmacoeconomic Considerations

The results of a recent study suggest that misoprostol cotherapy is only cost-effective when used in high-risk patients (see Table 18-6).[70] To date, outcome studies evaluating the cost-effectiveness of prophylactic cotherapy with a PPI or high-dose H_2RA or use of a selective COX-2 inhibitor has not been evaluated.

Management Strategies

HEALING THE ULCER

An algorithm for the treatment of NSAID-induced ulcers is presented in Fig. 18-2. NSAIDs should be discontinued, if possible, when an ulcer

Figure 18-2

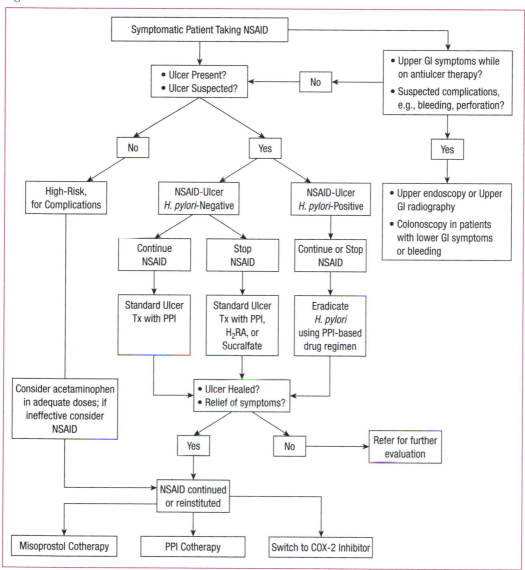

Algorithm for managing patients with nonsteroidal anti-inflammatory drug (NSAID)-induced ulcer.
ABBREVIATIONS: COX-2, cyclooxygenase-2; H_2RA, H_2-receptor antagonist; NSAID, nonsteroidal anti-inflammatory drug; PPI, proton pump inhibitor; Tx, treatment.

is either suspected or confirmed. Acetaminophen should be used for relief of pain. If the NSAID is discontinued, most uncomplicated ulcers will heal within 8 weeks with standard regimens of either an H_2RA or sucralfate. A PPI, however, is generally preferred because of its ability to heal most uncomplicated ulcers in 4 weeks.[53] The PPIs are also the drugs of choice for patients with large or complicated ulcers. If the NSAID must be continued, treatment should be initiated with a PPI.[53] Although H_2RAs will eventually heal most ulcers in the presence of continued NSAID use, higher daily dosages (e.g., famotidine 40 mg bid) or a longer treatment period (e.g., 8 to 12 weeks) will be needed.[53]

ERADICATING *H. PYLORI* INFECTION

If *H. pylori* is present, a PPI-based three-drug regimen should be used to eradicate *H. pylori* and heal the ulcer.[40,41] The PPI should be continued at least 2 to 4 weeks beyond antibiotic treatment to ensure ulcer healing. Eradication of *H. pylori*, however, is not recommended in women who are pregnant or nursing mothers (see GERD section on eradicating *H. pylori* infection).

RELIEVING SYMPTOMS

Patients with ulcers should be monitored for the relief of epigastric pain; pain usually resolves within several days to 1 week of beginning treatment. The presence of symptoms or the return of symptoms after 1 to 2 weeks posttreatment suggests treatment failure or the presence of another disorder. All patients with ulcer, but particularly those at high risk of NSAID-induced ulcers, should be monitored for signs or symptoms of bleeding, obstruction, or perforation (e.g., vomiting of blood, blood in the stool, lightheadedness, nausea/vomiting, severe abdominal pain). Older patients, patients who remain symptomatic or who have recurrent symptoms, or patients who appear to have ulcer-related complications should be referred to a gastroenterologist for a follow-up evaluation.

PREVENTING ULCERS AND ULCER-RELATED COMPLICATIONS

If possible, acetaminophen should be considered as first-line therapy for the treatment of osteoarthritis in elderly women. Acetaminophen in adequate doses (3 to 4 g/d) is as effective, for both acute and long-term therapy, as the NSAIDs in relieving the symptoms of osteoarthritis and improving function. For patients who do not obtain benefits from acetaminophen, NSAID therapy can be considered. Patients at high risk of developing NSAID-induced GI complications should receive prophylactic cotherapy if the NSAID is continued or should be switched to a selective COX-2 NSAID. Misoprostol cotherapy (400 to 600 μg/d) should be instituted in patients at high risk of developing NSAID-induced ulcer complications (see Fig. 18-2). The patient should be advised to report troublesome abdominal cramping and diarrhea, and women of childbearing age should be counseled about the need for adequate contraception. A PPI may be considered for patients unable to tolerate misoprostol. Sucralfate is not effective in preventing NSAID-induced ulcers and therefore should not be used for this purpose. Consideration should be given to switching the patient from a nonselective COX NSAID to a highly selective COX-2 inhibitor. Patients should be advised to report signs or symptoms of a possible ulcer, bleeding, obstruction, or perforation.

Constipation

Constipation is a common symptom encountered in clinical practice.[71,72] It is not, in itself, a disease state, but rather represents the subjective description by the patient of a disturbance of bowel function. The patient usually describes infrequent bowel movements or difficulty passing stool and is frequently concerned about the caliber or consistency of the stool. There is a wide range of normal for bowel movement frequency. Normal bowel frequency can range from two bowel movements per day to two bowel movements per week. There are many myths and misconceptions about normal bowel function, including the fact that some people believe that daily bowel movements are required for heath and that the lack of a daily bowel movement contributes to the accumulation of toxic substances and disease. These and other misconceptions have led to the inappropriate use of laxatives by the public.

Epidemiology

Constipation and its associated symptoms account for one of the most common reasons for patients to consult primary care practitioners. In one study, 1.2 percent of physician visits in the United States were for constipation, twice as many visits were made by women as by men; and the prevalence was between 3 and 5 percent in patients over 65 years of age compared to 1 percent among those less than 60 years old.[71] In addition, studies indicate that the prevalence of self-diagnosed constipation is higher in women and that prevalence increases with increasing age.[71] Thus, constipation is a greater problem for women and for the elderly. Constipation also occurs during pregnancy with a prevalence of 11 to 31 percent, depending on the population studied.[4]

Pathophysiology

Constipation is frequently associated with inadequate ingestion of dietary fiber and fluid and with inactivity.[71,72] Constipation may also be a manifestation of withholding or postponing the urge to defecate as it may blunt the colonic/rectal response and lead to prolonged stool retention. In addition, slowing of colonic transit may result from a primary motor disorder in association with many diseases or from the pharmacologic effects of certain medications (Table 18-7).[71,73]

GI-RELATED CONSTIPATION

The most frequent cause of GI-related constipation is IBS.[71,73] Constipation-predominant IBS occurs most frequently in women and is often associated with other GI symptoms including abdominal pain, bloating, nausea, and genitourinary symptoms. Patients with IBS have a high incidence of prior physical or sexual abuse or psychosocial stress (see section on constipation-predominant IBS). Constipation may also be an indication of obstruction from a colonic tumor or stricture of the colonic lumen.

CONSTIPATION RELATED TO OTHER DISORDERS

Women can have inappropriate contraction of the puborectalis during defecation that inhibits defecation. This finding can be recognized on defecography and responds to biofeedback training. In addition to peripheral neuromuscular disorders, CNS disorders (e.g., brain or spinal cord trauma, cerebrovascular accidents, and Parkinson's disease) can inhibit bowel function. Numerous metabolic and endocrine disorders (e.g., hypothyroidism, hypercalcemia, pheochromocytoma) may also cause constipation (see Table 18-7).[71,73]

CONSTIPATION ASSOCIATED WITH PSYCHOLOGICAL DISORDERS

Constipation may be a symptom of a psychological disorder or a side effect of drug treatment (see Table 18-7). For some patients, constipation may be a manifestation of an affective disorder.[71] Patients with eating disorders, particularly young underweight women, often complain of constipation; prolonged whole-gut transit time has been demonstrated.[71] Depressed patients can become constipated even without anorexia or physical inactivity. Many patients have no obvious cause for constipation but have delayed colonic transit. Transit studies in these patients are often confounded by prolonged cathartic use, which can also delay intestinal transit (colonic inertia).

PREGNANCY

The pathophysiology of constipation in pregnancy is not well understood but is linked to progesterone, which decreases gastric motility, inhibits the smooth muscle of the GI tract, and decreases colonic contractility.[4,74] The lowest progesterone production occurs during the first trimester and the highest production occurs during the third trimester.[75] During pregnancy, motilin (which normally stimulates motility of the small and large intestine) concentration decreases and returns to normal postpartum.[75] It is theorized that motilin may be inhibited by plasma progesterone. Pressure of the gravid uterus on the rectosigmoid colon, increased colonic absorption of sodium and water, and prenatal vitamin supplements that contain iron may also contribute to pregnancy-related constipation.[4]

Table 18-7

Causes of Constipation

FUNCTIONAL	NEUROMUSCULAR
Inadequate dietary fiber Decreased fluid intake Inadequate food intake Immobility Withholding or ignoring the urge to defecate	Parkinson's disease Autonomic neuropathy Multiple sclerosis Spinal cord injury, disease, lesions Scleroderma Intestinal pseudoobstruction (myopathy, neuropathy)
METABOLIC AND ENDOCRINE	**PSYCHOLOGICAL**
Hypothyroidism Diabetes mellitus Electrolyte abnormalities (e.g., hypercalcemia) Pheochromocytoma Porphyria Cushing's syndrome Addison's disease Panhypopituitarism Pregnancy	Anorexia nervosa or bulimia Depression Dementia Obsession about "inner cleanliness" Laxative abuse
	GASTROINTESTINAL
	Obstruction Irritable bowel syndrome Diverticulosis Rectosphincteric dyssynergy, rectocele Prolonged cathartic use, colonic inertia
MEDICATION	
Analgesics (e.g., NSAIDs, opiates) Anticholinergic effects (e.g., antidepressants, antiparkinson, antipsychotics, antihistamine) Antacids (e.g., aluminum- or calcium-containing) Anticonvulsants (e.g., phenytoin) β-blockers (e.g., acebutolol, labetalol) Calcium channel blockers (e.g., nifedipine, verapamil, diltiazem) Chemotherapy (e.g., vinblastin, vincristine) Diuretics (nonpotassium-sparing, e.g., furosemide) H_2-receptor antagonists (e.g., famotidine, ranitidine, cimetidine) Lipid-lowering agents (e.g., pravastatin, simvastatin) Sucralfate (contains aluminum) Iron and iron-containing products (e.g., vitamins)	

SOURCE: Adapted from JE Lennard-Jones[71]; A Wald[72]; RL Longe and JT DiPiro[73]; and LR Schiller.[80]

ELDERLY PATIENTS

Many elderly women develop constipation because of GI or systemic disorders or as a side effect of medications (see Table 18-7). Difficulty in defecation often results from decreased food intake, reduced mobility, and weaker abdominal and pelvic muscles.[71] Limited data suggest that increasing age affects colonic motor function in healthy ambulatory individuals. However, physician visits and laxative use is more pronounced in women over 65 years of age.[72] It is possible that, because older people often describe constipation as the need to strain to defecate, surveys that rely on bowel frequency alone may underestimate the prevalence of constipation in this population. Constipation may present as incontinence or even diarrhea, particularly in institutionalized elderly and children. Incontinence or diarrhea is usually due to liquid stool passing a fecal impaction.

MEDICATION-INDUCED CONSTIPATION

Medications that inhibit the neuromuscular function of the GI tract frequently produce constipation (see Table 18-7).[73,76] In most cases, the effects are dose dependent with higher daily dosages generally more troublesome. Opiates affect all segments of the intestine, but effects are more pronounced on the colon. Medications with anticholinergic effects are commonly used and inhibit bowel function through a parasympatholytic effect.

Clinical Presentation

Patients describe constipation in many ways, either as bowel movement frequency or as having difficulty in defecation, which relates to excessive straining or hard stools or both. It is important to find out what patients mean when they say they are "constipated."

Diagnosis

HISTORY

The patient should be questioned with regard to associated symptoms such as abdominal pain, bloating, nausea, weight loss, and blood in the stool. A life-long problem usually indicates a congenital condition, whereas recent onset suggests an acquired abnormality. Patients should be questioned about frequency and character of bowel movements, typical diet, fluid intake, activity, other diseases or conditions, and prior surgeries. Patients should be asked what medications they have used

to relieve the constipation (recently and in the past) and what medications they are currently taking, with an interest toward medications that might cause constipation. A family history may indicate an inherited neuropathy or familial colon cancer. The social history may reveal past physical or sexual abuse or social stressors.

PHYSICAL EXAMINATION

The physical examination may reveal evidence of non-GI diseases such as hypothyroidism or neurologic diseases that can contribute to constipation (see Table 18-7). The abdominal examination may reveal abdominal masses consistent with the presence of stool or abdominal distention. Bowel sounds are less helpful unless frank obstruction is present. The rectal examination may reveal hard stool in the rectal vault. A careful examination for perianal disease, including fissures and fistulae, should be performed. Anal tone can be assessed by digital examination. On pelvic examination, rectocele may be visualized by bulging into the vagina on bearing down. In cases where a thorough history and physical examination do not isolate an etiology, further diagnostic tests are usually required.

DIAGNOSTIC PROCEDURES

Several diagnostic procedures may be helpful in evaluating the etiology of constipation (Table 18-8). An abdominal flatplate radiograph may demonstrate stool throughout the colon and dilated loops of bowel suggestive of an obstruction or pseudoobstruction. A barium enema or colonoscopy best demonstrates colonic anatomy and the presence of colorectal obstruction or pathology.[71,72] Colonic transit studies are useful in patients who complain of severe constipation and infrequent defecation. These studies are performed by monitoring the passage of radioactive or radiopaque markers through the colon. Standards are based on the specific protocol and results can vary with time in the same patient or with changes in diet or laxative use. Anorectal manometry is most widely used for evaluation of incontinence, but it may

Table 18-8

Diagnostic Procedures Used to Evaluate Patients with Constipation

FLEXIBLE SIGMOIDOSCOPY AND COLONOSCOPY
Flexible sigmoidoscopy and colonoscopy are used to identify lesions that may narrow or occlude the bowel. Colonoscopy is usually recommended because it permits visualization of the entire colon and biopsy (if necessary).
RADIOGRAPHY/BARIUM ENEMA
Abdominal flatplate radiography of the abdomen may detect stool retention in the colon. A barium enema best demonstrates colonic anatomy and the presence of colorectal obstruction or pathology. Radiographic studies provide limited information regarding colonic transit and motor function.
COLONIC TRANSIT STUDIES
Colonic transit studies are useful for patients whose major complaint is infrequent defecation. The patient consumes a high-fiber diet (usually 20–30 g/d) during the study period and is asked to abstain from any medications, laxatives, or enemas that might alter bowel function. Radioactive or radiopaque markers are swallowed, and passage is monitored at different time points. The amount of marker in each region (right, left, and rectosigmoid regions of the colon) is quantitated over time. Standards are set and results vary depending on the specific protocol. Patterns of marker movement may identify colonic inertia or outlet delay.
ANORECTAL MANOMETRY
Manometry uses pressure transducers to measure rectal and anal sphincter function. Pressure recordings of the anal sphincter transducers indicate relaxation or inappropriate contractions of the internal and external anal sphincter; pressure, recorded by a rectal balloon, provides information regarding expulsion effort.
DEFECOGRAPHY
Defecography is a procedure in which thickened barium (approximating stool consistency) is introduced into the rectum. Fluoroscopy is used to monitor the patient while sitting on a specially constructed commode. Defecography is used to assess anorectal structures during expulsion of the barium mixture.

SOURCE: Adapted from JE Lennard-Jones[71]; A Wald[72]; and AL Halverson and BA Orkin.[77]

also provide useful information in patients with severe constipation. Defecography evaluates anorectal structures during expulsion of the barium. In a study of patients with chronic constipation, colonic transit and defecography were found to be most useful in diagnosis.[77]

Therapeutic Goals

Management should be individualized and aimed at education, relieving constipation and its associated symptoms, maintaining adequate nutrition, and preventing further episodes. The goal for patients with acute constipation is to provide symptom relief, whereas the goal for patients with chronic constipation includes proper diet and a decreased reliance on laxatives. For patients with constipation secondary to a definable disease or condition, treatment should be directed at controlling the underlying cause, if possible. Patient education, dietary modifications, and the judicious use of laxatives or enemas are important therapeutic goals.

Nonpharmacologic Management and Dietary Fiber

Patient education should include reassurance and an explanation as to what constitutes "normal bowel habits." Activity and exercise may be recommended for inactive patients. However, studies do not support the beneficial effects of physical activity in relieving constipation.[78] Patients with small, hard stools and those with fever or who live in hot climates should be advised to consume plenty of water.

In patients without significant intestinal or colonic stricture, the initial and most important nonpharmacologic modification used to treat or prevent constipation is to increase the amount of dietary fiber consumed (Table 18-9). Although the specific physiologic effect of fiber is not well understood, it increases stool bulk by retaining water. The resulting increase in fecal mass stimulates colonic motility leading to expulsion of stool; the increased water content softens the consistency of stool, making it easier to pass. Patients may add wheat bran or one of the other high-fiber cereals to their diet followed by a glass of water (see Table 18-9). In the lower bowel, the fiber is acted on by intestinal bacteria producing gas.

Some patients, particularly women and the elderly, find that bran aggravates abdominal bloating and increases flatulence. Patients naive to large amounts of dietary fiber are advised to begin slowly so that their system becomes gradually accustomed to the adverse effects of fiber.[79] Mildly constipated patients should aim for a dietary fiber intake of about 20 to 40 g/d.[72] Dietary fiber should be increased based on the patient's response and tolerance. Most patients begin to notice initial effects in 3 to 5 days, but optimal effects may take as long as 1 month.[73] Patients often are encouraged by the beneficial effects of fiber on the body, including lowing cholesterol and lowering the incidence of certain cancers.

Pharmacotherapy

Therapeutic options for treating or preventing constipation can be divided into three general classes depending on their onset of action: agents that cause softening of the feces in 1 to 3 days; agents that result in soft or semifluid stool in 6 to 12 h; and agents that cause water evacuation in 1 to 6 h

Table 18-9

Fiber Content of High-Fiber and Commonly Ingested Foods

Food	Fiber (g) per 100 g	Approximate Serving Size
CEREALS		
All-Bran	29.9	1/3 cup
100% Bran	29.6	1/2 cup
Bran Buds	27.7	1/3 cup
Wheat germ	14.3	1/4 cup
Raisin Bran	11.3	3/4 cup
Shredded Wheat	9.3	2/3 cup
Wheat Chex	7.4	2/3 cup
Wheaties	7.0	1 cup
Total	7.2	1 cup
Grape Nuts	4.8	1/4 cup
Cheerios	3.8	1 1/4 cup
Special K	0.8	1 1/3 cup
Rice Krispies	0.2	1 cup
FRUITS		
Prunes	11.9	3
Raisins	8.7	1/4 cup
Apricots (dried)	8.1	5 halves
Dates	7.6	3
Apple (with skin)	2.5	1 medium
Banana	2.1	1 medium
Orange	2.0	1
Cantaloupe	1.0	1/4 melon
VEGETABLES (COOKED) AND LEGUMES (COOKED)		
Kidney beans	7.9	1/2 cup
Navy beans	6.3	1/2 cup
Peas	4.7	1/2 cup
Carrots	3.0	1/2 cup
Brussels sprouts	3.0	1/2 cup
Broccoli	2.8	1/2 cup
Corn	2.8	1/2 cup
Spinach	2.3	1/2 cup
Potato (with skin)	1.7	1 medium
BREADS, PASTA (COOKED), AND RICE (COOKED)		
Whole wheat bread	5.7	1 slice
Mixed grain bread	3.7	1 slice
Pumpernickel bread	3.2	1 slice
White bread	1.6	1 slice
Rice (brown)	1.2	1/2 cup
Bagel	1.1	1
Macaroni or spaghetti	0.8	1 cup
Rice (polished)	0.3	1/2 cup
NUTS		
Peanuts	8.1	10 nuts
Almonds	7.2	10 nuts

(Table 18-10).[71–73,80] They can also be categorized based on their mechanisms of action.

BULKING OR HYDROPHILIC AGENTS

Medicinal bulk-forming laxatives are available for patients who cannot consume adequate amounts of dietary fiber (see Table 18-10). The fiber can be of natural origin (psyllium, malt soup extract) or synthetic (polycarbophil, methylcellulose, carboxymethylcellulose). Psyllium is hygroscopic and forms a gel when mixed with water. Polycarbophil is hydrophilic, nonabsorbable, inert, and does not form a gel when mixed with water. Methylcellulose and carboxymethylcellulose are altered forms of cellulose that are resistant to bacterial

Table 18-10

Laxatives Used to Manage Constipation in Adults*

LAXATIVE	BRAND NAME	DAILY DOSAGE RANGE
AGENTS THAT CAUSE SOFTENING OF FECES IN 1–3 D:		
Bulking or hydrophilic agents		
Methylcellulose	Citrucel, various	4–6 g
Carboxymethylcellulose	Disoplex	4–6 g
Malt soup extract	Maltsupex	12–64 g
Polycarbophil	Fibercon, various	1–6 g
Psyllium	Metamucil, various	10–20 g
Emollients		
Docusate calcium	Surfak, various	50–500 mg
Docusate potassium	Diocto-K, various	100–500 mg
Docusate sodium	Colace, various	50–500 mg
Poorly absorbed sugars and polyhydric alcohols		
Lactulose 10 g/5 mL	Cephulac, various	15–60 mL
Sorbitol (10.5 g/15 mL)	Various	15–60 mL
Mineral oil	Various	15–30 mL
Polyethylene glycol 3350	MiraLax	17 g in 8 oz water
AGENTS THAT RESULT IN SOFT OR SEMIFLUID STOOL IN 6–12 H:		
Senna (standardized concentrate)	Senokot, various	15–60 mg
Bisacodyl (oral tablet)	Dulcolax, various	5–15 mg
Magnesium sulfate	Epsom Salt	<10 g (low dose)
AGENTS THAT CAUSE WATERY EVACUATION IN 1–6 H:		
Magnesium hydroxide	Milk of Magnesia	2.4–4.8 g
Magnesium citrate	Citrate of Magnesia	240–300 mL
Magnesium sulfate	Epsom Salt	10–30 g (high dose)
Sodium biphosphate	Fleet enema	9.6–19.2 g
Bisacodyl (rectal suppository)	Dulcolax	10 mg
Polyethylene glycol-electrolyte	GoLightly, various	4 L over 3–4 hr

*All laxative dosages are oral unless otherwise indicated.
SOURCE: Adapted from JE Lennard-Jones[71]; A Wald[72]; RL Longe and JT DiPiro[73]; and LR Schiller.[80]

fermentation and can hold water within the intestine. Fiber supplements should be taken with a full glass of water to prevent esophageal or intestinal obstruction. This is especially important in the elderly or patients who restrict their fluid intake.

SIDE EFFECTS In general, fiber supplements are limited in their use by the same adverse effects that are observed with dietary fiber. Psyllium should not be taken immediately before a meal because it can delay gastric emptying and reduce appetite. Although infrequent, psyllium powder has been reported to cause a hypersensitivity reaction leading to bronchospasm and anaphylaxis.[80–83] Bulk-forming and hydrophilic agents should be used primarily for the long-term treatment of mild constipation (e.g., during pregnancy) and not for the rapid relief of acute, temporary constipation.

EMOLLIENTS

Emollients, also known as surfactants or stool softeners (e.g., Colace, Surfak), are available in various salts (see Table 18-10). These agents are anionic detergents that permit water to interact more effectively with stool solids, thus facilitating mixing of the stool with water and allowing them to soften. They may also inhibit fluid absorption or stimulate secretion in the jejunum.[80] Emollients are not effective in treating constipation, but are sometimes used to prevent constipation in patients where straining at stool should be avoided (e.g., after myocardial infarction or after acute perianal disease or rectal surgery), in patients receiving drugs that decrease bowel motility, and in women with perineal tears after obstetric delivery. Clinical studies, however, indicate that these agents are of little use for prophylactic treatment of constipation in the elderly and bedridden patients.[80] In general, the emollients are nontoxic and relatively safe.

POORLY ABSORBABLE SUGARS AND POLYHYDRIC ALCOHOLS

Lactulose (e.g., Cephulac), a disaccharide, and sorbitol, a monosaccharide, are poorly absorbed sugars that are hydrolyzed, in part, to lactic, acetic, and formic acids by coliform bacteria.[72] When administered orally or rectally, the osmotic action of the metabolites produces fluid accumulation in the colon leading to the formation of soft-formed stools. When used to treat chronic constipation, sorbitol appears to be as effective as lactulose and as well tolerated.[72] Because of its lower cost, consideration should be given to using sorbitol.

Patients should be advised that lactulose and sorbitol can cause flatulence, abdominal bloating, and diarrhea. Lactulose and sorbitol are not used as first-line agents to treat chronic constipation, but may be used in patients, particularly the elderly, who do not respond to dietary fiber or bulk-forming laxatives.

LUBRICANTS

Mineral oil softens and coats the stool to facilitate movement of stool through the GI tract. Adverse effects are rare, but if they occur, they can be serious. Aspiration of the oil can lead to lipoid pneumonia. Long-term use can cause malabsorption of fat-soluble vitamins and foreign body reactions in the intestinal mucosa and regional lymph nodes.[72] In addition, anal seepage may be a problem for some patients.

DIPHENYLMETHANE DERIVATIVES

Diphenylmethane derivatives include bisacodyl (Dulcolax), phenolphthalein, and sodium picosulfate (see Table 18-10).[71–73,80] Bisacodyl and phenolphthalein stimulate the small intestine and colon, whereas sodium picosulfate acts primarily on the colon. Use of these three agents results in fluid accumulation in the bowel and an osmotic action.

The most widely used diphenylmethane derivative is bisacodyl, which is available as an oral tablet and suppository (see Table 18-10). Bisacodyl tablets are enteric coated to prevent gastric irritation and dissolve in the intestine rather than the stomach. Patients should be advised to not chew or crush the tablet. Because its effects are predictable and have a relatively short onset, bisacodyl is often used for the treatment of temporary constipation or as a bowel preparation before diagnostic procedures. Although not usually recommended for daily administration, intermittent doses (every few weeks) of bisacodyl may be used in chronic constipation. The long-term use of bisacodyl, however, is sometimes warranted for the treatment of severe chronic constipation.[71] Adverse effects vary from patient to patient with cramping and liquid stools occurring most often.[71,73]

Phenolphthalein, once the most common nonprescription laxative, was withdrawn by manufacturers from most nonprescription products because animal studies suggested that it might be carcinogenic.[71,80] Laxatives that once contained phenolphthalein (e.g., Modane, Ex-Lax, Evac-U-Gen, Agoral) have been reformulated to contain various alternative laxatives (e.g., bisacodyl, mineral oil, or docusate sodium).[80]

ANTHRAQUINONE DERIVATIVES

Anthraquinone laxatives are derived from plants that produce different anthraquinones; senna leaf and senna pod contain rheindianthrone glucosides, whereas aloe, cascara, and rhubarb produce different families of anthraquinones. Once ingested, the anthraquinones pass into the colon unchanged where colonic bacteria metabolize them and convert them to their active forms.[80] Anthraquinones usually induce defecation within 6 to 8 h after oral administration.[80] Senna, the most widely used anthraquinone, is available for clinical use as a crude vegetable preparation or as a purified and standardized extract. In most cases, intermittent use to treat temporary constipation is acceptable, but chronic use is not recommended.

SIDE EFFECTS Possible adverse effects with the anthraquinones include allergic reactions, electrolyte depletion, and melanosis coli (deposition of dark pigment in the colonic lining).[84,85] Anthraquinones have also been implicated in colonic cancer, but epidemiologic studies do not support this concern.[80] The long-term use of anthraqui-

nones is associated with the development of cathartic colon (colonic inertia).[71,80] Anthraquinones are a common component in "natural" products. The patient should be advised to read the label carefully and discuss all ingredients with the pharmacist or physician.

SALINE LAXATIVES

Saline laxatives are poorly absorbed salts of magnesium, sulfate, phosphate, and citrate that exert an osmotic effect leading to retention of fluid in the GI tract (see Table 18-10). These salts, which may be given orally or rectally, are primarily indicated for acute bowel evacuation before a diagnostic procedure or to treat temporary constipation. Magnesium hydroxide (Milk of Magnesia) may, however, be used regularly in mildly constipated patients because it is generally safe and effective. Magnesium citrate (citrate of magnesia) is available as a carbonated liquid and may be preferred by some patients. Magnesium sulfate (Epsom Salt) has a dose-dependent laxative effect. At higher dosages, its potent cathartic effect produces a large volume of liquid stool.

SIDE EFFECTS Magnesium-containing laxatives, when given orally, may lead to hypermagnesemia in patients with renal impairment and in children.[71,80] Although observed most often in patients with renal failure, hypermagnesemia has been reported in patients with normal renal function.[86]

Phosphate salts may be given orally or as an enema. Phosphate is absorbed by the small intestine, and therefore, larger doses must be given orally to have a laxative effect. One oral phosphate preparation (Fleet) must be diluted before ingestion and followed with three 250-mL glasses of water to prevent vomiting and dehydration.[80] Hyperphosphatemia may occur in patients with renal impairment, and sodium accumulation can result in patients with congestive heart failure.[73] Life-threatening hyperphosphatemia, hypocalcemia, and acidosis have been reported with both the oral and rectal administration of phosphate salts.[87–89]

GLYCERIN

Glycerin is administered as a 3-g suppository and is usually effective. It exerts an osmotic action in the rectum. The onset of action is usually less than 30 min.[73] Although glycerin may cause occasional rectal irritation, it is considered very safe if used on an intermittent basis for constipation, especially in children.

CASTOR OIL

Castor oil is metabolized in the GI tract to ricinoleic acid, which stimulates secretory processes, decreases glucose absorption, and promotes intestinal motility primarily in the small intestine. Its onset of action usually occurs within 1 to 3 h, which makes it suitable as a bowel preparation before a diagnostic or surgical procedure.[73] Castor oil should not be used routinely for the treatment of chronic constipation because of its strong purgative effects. Castor oil may initiate premature uterine contractions in pregnant women and should be avoided.[80]

POLYETHYLENE GLYCOL-ELECTROLYTE LAVAGE/POLYETHYLENE GLYCOL LAXATIVE

A polyethylene glycol (PEG)-electrolyte solution is primarily indicated for the evacuation of the bowel before diagnostic procedures (e.g., colonoscopy) and before colorectal surgery (see Table 18-10). The original preparation (GoLightly) contains sodium sulfate and PEG as its principal osmotic agents. A sulfate-free formulation (NuLightly) contains a high concentration of PEG in place of the sodium sulfate.[80] Both preparations are given as 4 L over several hours and provide similar effects. When given in lower dosages (240 to 300 mL/d) to treat severe chronic constipation, the sulfate-free solution is preferred because the PEG is much less absorbed than the sulfate.[80] The most common adverse effects are nausea, vomiting, abdominal bloating, cramps, and anal irritation.[84] Polyethylene glycol 3350 (MiraLax), a related PEG preparation, is now available for use in treating occasional constipation.

OTHER AGENTS

Gastrointestinal promotility agents such as cisapride (Propulsid, 5 mg tid to 20 mg bid) and erythromycin have been used to treat acute and chronic refractory constipation, but results have been variable.[73,80] There is no place for promotility agents in the routine management of constipation.

Two agents that may be useful for refractory constipation are misoprostol and colchicine. Misoprostol (600 μg qd to tid) has been successfully used to treat refractory constipation, but abdominal cramps and its abortifacient properties limit its use especially in young women.[72] Misoprostol is contraindicated in pregnant women (see misoprostol in NSAID-induced ulcer section). Colchicine (0.6 mg tid) has been used to treat severe constipation. Its mechanism of action is thought to be related to the stimulation of endogenous prostaglandins.[72,80]

Tap-water enemas (about 200 mL water may be instilled rectally) may be used every 3 to 4 days in adults to treat simple constipation, but may result in weakness, shock, convulsions, and coma from water intoxication and dilutional hyponatremia, especially when administered to the elderly, children, or patients with megacolon.[72] Bowel movements usually result within 1 h.[73] Soapsuds enemas are no longer recommended because they cause proctitis and colitis.

NATURAL PRODUCTS

A number of natural products have been used to treat constipation, including aloe, rhubarb, senna, flaxseed, psyllium, buckthorn, cascara, and manna.[72,85] Natural products stimulate propulsive contractions in the colon, decreasing fluid absorption and accelerating intestinal passage of the stool. Psyllium and flaxseed are both effective natural fibers that, when hydrated, form a hydrophilic mucilage that causes intestinal dilation and subsequent defecation (see anthraquinone section for discussion of psyllium). Senna induces a stool of normal (soft) consistency without undue pain or discomfort. Both the leaf and the pod of the senna plant may be used. Aloe- and rhubarb-containing preparations are the most potent; they are best avoided because they produce colic.[72] Cascara and manna produce a mild action with little or no colic.

Management Strategies

PREVENTING CONSTIPATION OR MANAGING MILD COMPLAINTS OF INFREQUENCY OR HARD STOOLS

The approach to preventing and treating constipation begins with an attempt to determine its cause and, when possible, instituting corrective measures (e.g., increase dietary fiber, treat diseases such as hypothyroidism, or discontinue constipating medication). Patients should be assured that, although it is not essential to have daily bowel movements, they should be advised to set aside time daily for an unhurried and, if possible, regular time for defecation. If the patient is inactive, activity should be encouraged. Behavioral treatment aimed at teaching patients to relax muscles of the pelvic floor and to feel smaller volumes of rectal distention may be of assistance to some patients; decreasing psychological stress may be helpful to others.

For patients with mild complaints or infrequency or hard stools, an increase in fluid intake, dietary fiber, or the supplementation of medicinal fiber may be all that is required. An algorithm for preventing and treating constipation is presented in Fig. 18-3.

TREATING TEMPORARY ACUTE CONSTIPATION

Most laxatives with a rapid (within 1 day) onset (see Table 18-10) are acceptable for treating temporary acute constipation, but the most simple and safest measures should be tried before more potent cathartics are used. For most patients, the infrequent (no more than every 2 weeks) use of magnesium hydroxide, senna, bisacodyl, a tapwater enema, or a glycerin suppository usually provides adequate relief. Patients with more severe constipation will usually require more potent laxatives, larger doses of osmotic agents, or smaller daily doses of the gastrointestinal lavage solution.

MANAGING CHRONIC CONSTIPATION

When constipation is chronic, stimulants such as bisacodyl and senna should be avoided because of the potential for cathartic colon. Osmotic agents such as lactulose, sorbitol, and magnesium hydroxide may be effective in these patients. When daily laxative self-treatment is needed for more than 1 week, the patient should be advised to contact the health care provider. If excess straining is a problem, then fiber should be avoided because it only increases the amount of stool that needs to be evacuated.

MANAGING CONSTIPATION IN ELDERLY WOMEN

Managing constipation in the elderly is similar to that of younger patients, although fecal impaction is often a complication, as the anal sphincter tends to become weaker, and inactivity is a problem in bedridden patients. In addition, older patients are more likely to use analgesics and other constipating medications. When fecal incontinence is caused by fecal accumulation, the aim of treatment is to empty the rectum, usually using an enema, and then to keep the rectum empty without causing incontinence. The use of bran tends to cause semisolid stools that may lead to fecal incontinence in the elderly.[71] Alternatively, fiber can increase stool bulk and improve control of stool, particularly in elderly patients with intermittent diarrhea. Laxatives (e.g., senna, lactulose, or sorbitol) may be used to treat constipation in the elderly. However, they must be used carefully and treatment should be individualized; follow-up is key.

MANAGING CONSTIPATION DURING PREGNANCY

Constipation is a frequent occurrence during pregnancy, with most expectant mothers complaining of hard stools rather than a decrease in the frequency of bowel movements. The aim of treatment is to achieve softer stools without the use of medications. Although increasing dietary fiber and taking in adequate fluid may be effective during the early months of pregnancy, most women find it uncomfortable to eat bulky meals during the later

Figure 18-3

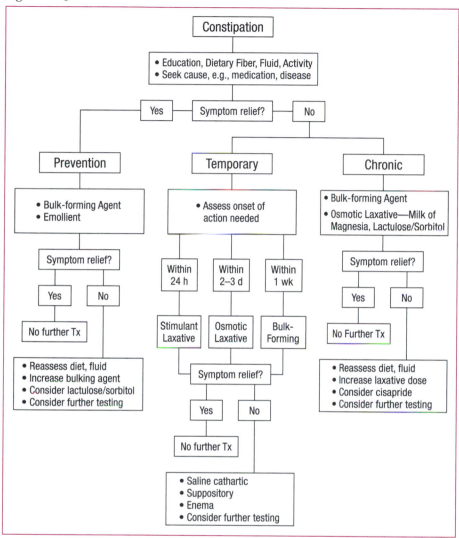

Algorithm for managing patients with constipation.

months. Eating smaller and more frequent meals may be effective, but adding a medicinal bulking agent (see Table 18-10) is also appropriate because these agents are not absorbed.[71] A weekly dose of standardized senna is sometimes recommended when dietary and fiber supplementation fail to relieve symptoms.[71] However, emollients, bisacodyl, and lactulose have been used and appear safe.[71,80] Saline osmotic laxatives may promote fluid retention in the mother and alter fluid and electrolytes in the fetus, although magnesium hydroxide is widely used.[71] Mineral oil should be avoided because it may prevent the absorption of fat-soluble vitamins (A, D, E, K). Castor oil should not be used because it may initiate premature uterine contractions. Misoprostol is contraindicated in pregnant women because it may induce premature labor.

Laxative Abuse

Laxative abuse is most often reported in middle-aged women who use laxatives for weight reduction or control.[73] Laxative abuse is also common among young women with anorexia nervosa and bulimia. These patients often develop cathartic colon, which is usually characterized by a non-functional ileum and colon. Other manifestations of laxative abuse include diarrhea, electrolyte disturbances (particularly hypokalemia), steatorrhea, osteomalacia, and liver disease. Surreptitious use of laxatives can be difficult to diagnose. The treatment of patients who abuse laxatives can be difficult and frequently requires sympathetic medical and psychological support.

Irritable Bowel Syndrome

Irritable bowel syndrome (IBS) is a functional disorder of GI tract characterized by alterations in bowel habits with or without abdominal pain.[90,91] Patients have been grouped based on their dominant symptom (pain-predominant, constipation-predominant, diarrhea-predominant), and the disorder is diagnosed only after the exclusion of organic causes. The belief that IBS is a psychosomatic condition is no longer accurate, although psychological factors play an important role in the exacerbation and perpetuation of symptoms. IBS does not predispose patients to serious conditions such as inflammatory bowel disease (IBD) or cancer and does not alter life expectancy, but it may have a significant impact on the patient's quality of life.[90,91]

Epidemiology

With a prevalence of approximately 20 percent, IBS is recognized as one of the most common GI disorders in primary care.[90] Alternatively, about 20 to 50 percent of patients with IBS are referred to a gastroenterologist. In one U.S. study, the health care costs associated with IBS were estimated at $8 billion annually.[90] In the Western world, women outnumber men by a factor of 2:1, but a higher prevalence in women may reflect patterns of seeking health care rather than actual incidence.[90] Patients with IBS appear to have a much higher prevalence (32 to 44 percent) of previous physical or sexual abuse than patients with organic GI disorders, although how sexual abuse relates to GI dysfunction is unknown.[90]

Pathophysiology

The pathophysiology of IBS is not well understood, but it appears to be multifactorial in origin. The disruption of daily activity (e.g., changes in dietary intake, new medications, increased psychological stress, sleep deprivation, GI infection) usually triggers abdominal pain and its associated symptoms. Three important hypotheses have been proposed to explain the cause of symptoms in IBS.[90,91] First, there exists an underlying disorder of GI motility (altered intestinal motor function); second, patients have a low tolerance for pain or an excessive response to normal signals from the GI tract (visceral hypersensitivity); and third, emotional and psychological factors lead to GI symptoms (psychopathology).

A variety of motor abnormalities in both the small and large bowel have been described in patients with IBS.[90–92] Unfortunately, motor abnormalities often do not correlate with symptoms. High-amplitude contractions have been observed in patients during episodes of crampy abdominal pain.[91,92] An imbalance in autonomic activity has been related to diarrhea-predominant (sympathetic dysfunction) and constipation-predominant (parasympathetic dysfunction) IBS.[90] One investigator studied heart rate variability in women with and without IBS and found that women with IBS had a lower vagal tone compared to women without the syndrome.[93] The fact that not all patients have altered motility yet respond to antispasmodics suggests that the perception of motor activity may be abnormal in some patients rather than the motor activity itself; this finding supports the concept of visceral hypersensitivity. Visceral hypersensitivity, leading to a lower threshold of discomfort, could explain symptoms such as rectal fullness, urgency, incomplete evacuation, and bloating.[90,91] The third hypothesis is derived from studies that report a high rate of psychiatric disorders (e.g., depression, anxiety, panic disorder) in patients with IBS.[90,91,94,95] Psychological distress appears to be an important component of IBS in women and there appears to be a higher prevalence of psychopathology among IBS patients who seek medical advice than among the general population.[94,95] Additionally, IBS patients treated at tertiary hospitals were more likely to report previous physical, sexual, and verbal abuse than those patients with diagnosed organic diseases.[91] Lactose intolerance has been associated with IBS, but its prevalence does not appear to be higher than in the general population.[96]

Clinical Presentation

Most patients with IBS complain of abdominal pain, abdominal distention, and disturbed defecation.[90,91] The Rome diagnostic criteria (Table 18-11) identify specific symptoms that may assist in the evaluation of a patient with suspected IBS. Abdominal pain, the classic symptom of IBS, may be described as aching, burning, crampy, knifelike, or sharp and may be predominant in some patients.[90,91] The pain may be localized or diffuse arising from the small or large bowel or any abdominal region. In most patients, the pain originates from the lower abdomen. Patients frequently complain of bloating and gas with or without abdominal distention.[90,91] However, when the volume of gas was quantitatively measured in patients with IBS and compared to healthy individuals, there was no difference in gas production.[97]

Bloating is least troublesome on awaking but worsens as the day progresses. A number of factors have been proposed to explain bloating including

Table 18-11

Diagnostic Criteria (Rome I) for Irritable Bowel Syndrome*

At least 3 months of continuous or recurrent symptoms of the following:

Abdominal pain or discomfort that is:
- Relieved with defecation, or
- Associated with a change in frequency of stool, or
- Associated with a change in consistency of stool, and

Two or more of the following on at least one-fourth of occasions or days:
- Altered stool frequency (more than three bowel movements per day or less than three per week)
- Altered stool form (lumpy and hard or loose and watery stool)
- Altered stool passage (straining, urgency)
- Feeling of incomplete evacuation
- Passage of mucus
- Bloating or feeling of abdominal distention

*Criteria established for irritable bowel syndrome which were developed by an international working team (Rome). The criteria have not been validated but are recommended for clinical practice and investigative use.

aerophagia (ingestion of air) and the effect of intraluminal bacteria on ingested foods in the diet.[90] Exaggeration of the normal gastrocolonic reflex is common. There also appears to be a correlation between IBS symptoms and the menstrual cycle; abdominal bloating is reported to be higher in the midluteal phase, premenstrual, and menstrual phases of women with IBS.[98]

Patients with IBS experience altered defecation and may present with either diarrhea-predominant, constipation-predominant, or the classic presentation of alternating diarrhea and constipation.[90] It is best not to strictly define diarrhea or constipation (because it may consist of altered stool frequency or consistency), but to relate altered defecation to what is usually normal for the specific patient. In general, diarrhea-predominant IBS is associated with small volumes of loose stool. The first bowel movement of the day is usually of normal consistency followed by softer and increasingly looser stools. Although diarrhea occurs most often in the early part of the day, it is not uncommon to have loose stools after meals. Mucus in the stool is common in IBS. However, the presence of blood in the stool, weight loss, anemia, or nocturnal bowel movements suggest the possibility of IBD and requires further evaluation.

Patients may first experience episodic constipation, which may eventually become chronic and in some cases, resistant to laxatives. Usually the intensity of the abdominal pain is related to the duration of constipation. Pain usually subsides after the bowel movement, but the patient may feel that the evacuation of stool was inadequate.[90] Patients with IBS may also complain of a wide variety of extraintestinal symptoms including urologic disorders, sexual dysfunction, dyspepsia, and GERD.[90,91,99]

Diagnosis

The diagnosis of IBS is based on the identification of a symptom complex compatible with IBS, association of symptoms with factors that produce gut hyperactivity, and exclusion of an organic cause of the symptoms.[90,91,99] Organic diseases that result in abdominal pain and changes in bowel habits (e.g., malignancies, IBD, infections) must be excluded. Lactase deficiency, malabsorption, hyperthyroidism, IBD, parasites, and laxative abuse should be considered in patients with diarrhea. Hypothyroidism, hypercalcemia, colorectal malignancy, and constipating medications should be considered if constipation is present. A history and physical examination should be performed on all patients looking for evidence of other underlying diseases.

HISTORY

The patient should be questioned about abdominal pain, bloating, constipation, diarrhea, nausea, vomiting, weight loss, and blood in the stool. Historical features of IBS-related symptoms should be obtained. A detailed dietary history is especially important if diarrhea and gas bloat are present. Weight loss, anemia, blood in the stool, symptoms suggesting intermittent obstruction, nocturnal diarrhea, vomiting, and dehydration all warrant early evaluation possibly including colonoscopy or barium study. In the absence of these findings, empirical therapy is indicated with vigilant follow-up for the development of signs or symptoms suggesting other diseases (e.g., malignancy, Crohn's disease, ulcerative colitis, celiac sprue, infection).

PHYSICAL EXAMINATION

The physical examination of the patient is generally unimpressive, except that abdominal compression often elicits poorly localized tenderness.

DIAGNOSTIC PROCEDURES

Because the symptoms of IBS are nonspecific and secondary to other less common, but potentially more serious diseases, specific diagnostic tests should be considered, particularly if warning signs are present or develop during follow-up. Diseases such as celiac sprue and Crohn's disease can mimic IBS and require specific diagnostic tests and therapy. Sigmoidoscopy or colonoscopy is useful in excluding IBD and structural lesions, and it assures the patient that there is no underlying organic disease. Mucosal biopsy is only indicated if diarrhea is a predominant symptom. Other tests that may be performed include a complete blood count, examination of stools for ova and parasites (e.g., history of being out of the country), stool for occult blood, fecal leukocytes, radiographic examination of the small bowel, and tests necessary to rule out other organic diseases.

Therapeutic Goals

There is no ideal management strategy for IBS. Nonpharmacologic treatment should be aimed at providing education and reassurance to the patient and modifying the diet to avoid foods or beverages that may contribute to their symptoms. Pharmacotherapy should be aimed at specific symptoms, including abdominal pain and bloating, constipation, diarrhea, and associated psychological disorders, and increasing dietary fiber. The overall approach to treating the IBS patient should be largely nonpharmacologic, with medications targeted to treat specific and resistant symptoms.

Nonpharmacologic Therapy

The treatment of IBS involves a collaborative effort between the patient and the clinician. The value of a positive and supportive relationship with the patient cannot be overestimated because education, reassurance, and emotional support play a central role in the treatment of IBS. The patient should be educated about IBS and its treatment as well as the need to manage stressful life events. Reassurance and psychological support play an important role when dealing with the patient's anxiety and stress and may, in itself, be inherently therapeutic.[90]

STRESS MANAGEMENT

When IBS symptoms are moderate to severe and are either associated with psychological distress or impaired quality of life, psychological or behavior therapy (e.g., hypnosis, psychotherapy, biofeedback, relaxation/stress management, cognitive-behavior treatment, or interpersonal psychotherapy) may reduce anxiety and other psychological symptoms and, in some cases, decrease the severity of GI symptoms.[91] Because there are no comparative data to ascertain which treatments are superior or better for certain patient types, the selection of a specific psychological treatment depends on several factors including patient or clinician preference, cost, and availability.

DIETARY APPROACHES

Many patients believe that their symptoms are caused by specific foods, but such relationships are difficult to establish and patients, unfortunately, often restrict their diet unnecessarily. A prudent approach to dietary modification is to recommend avoiding caffeinated beverages because caffeine may cause diarrhea and produce anxiety, avoiding foods that produce intestinal gas (Table 18-12) because they can contribute to abdominal pain and discomfort, and eliminating lactose (or using lactose-reduced products or lactase) in patients who appear intolerant of lactose-containing foods and beverages. If lactose intolerance cannot be determined by history or dietary restriction, specific tests are available. Maintaining a dietary history is often helpful in identifying foods that may exacerbate specific IBS symptoms.

Although the literature on the effectiveness of high-fiber diets is controversial and patients with IBS who follow such diets often complain of aggravated symptoms (particularly abdominal bloating and distention), they are widely recommended, es-

Table 18-12

Gas-Producing Foods

MAJOR GAS PRODUCERS
Beans
Vegetables (onions, brussels sprouts, celery, carrots)
Fruit (prunes, raisins, apricots, bananas)
Carbohydrates (wheat germ, bagels, pretzels)

MODERATE GAS PRODUCERS
Vegetables (potatoes, eggplant)
Fruit (citrus, apples)
Carbohydrates (pastries, bread)

NORMAL GAS PRODUCERS
Meat, fowl, fish, eggs
Vegetables (lettuce, cucumber, broccoli, peppers, avocado, cauliflower, tomato, asparagus, zucchini, okra, olives)
Fruit (cantaloupe, grapes, berries)
Carbohydrates (rice, popcorn, potato chips)
Nuts (all types)

pecially if the patient has constipation-predominant IBS. Dietary fiber (see Table 18-9) may improve constipation, but is often associated with increased bloating and cramps.

Pharmacotherapy

BULKING AND HYDROPHILIC AGENTS

The use of medicinal fiber supplements (Table 18-13) in patients with IBS is controversial because their effectiveness remains unproven and they may aggravate symptoms of bloating and distention.[90,100–102] Synthetic fiber (e.g., polycarbophil) supplements tend to produce less gas than natural fiber (e.g., psyllium, methycellulose) supplements and are generally preferred when treating IBS.[90] Fiber supplements, because of their hydrophilic properties, bind water in the GI tract, thus preventing excessive dehydration and excessive liquidity of the stool. Therefore, a trial of medicinal fiber may be considered to treat either constipation or diarrhea.[90] Patients with IBS should take fiber supplements with meals, beginning with a low dosage and then cautiously increasing the dose as needed to control constipation or diarrhea.

ANTIDIARRHEAL AGENTS

The antidiarrheal agents, loperamide and diphenoxylate, prolong intestinal transit time, enhance intestinal water and ion absorption, and strengthen rectal sphincter tone (see Table 18-13).[102] These agents are widely used in patients with IBS to decrease diarrhea, urgency, and fecal soiling. Loperamide is preferred over diphenoxylate because it does not cross the blood-brain barrier and is devoid of central opioid-like effects.[90,102] Most clinical trials suggest that, although loperamide is effective in decreasing urgency and bowel movement frequency, global improvement (including abdominal pain) is not usually achieved in patients with abdominal pain and diarrhea-predominant IBS.[102,103] There are no well-controlled studies of diphenoxylate in patients with IBS. The antidiarrheal dosage of these agents will vary from patient to patient and should be titrated based on individual patient

response (see Table 18-13). Patients are often advised to take 1 to 2 tables of loperamide (4 mg) after each loose bowel movement (up to 8 tablets per day). Because the diarrhea seen in IBS is often postprandial, antidiarrheals are generally given before meals. Although opiates such as codeine and morphine have potent effects on colonic motility, they are not routinely used because of their adverse effects and dependence potential. Other agents that have been used experimentally for the treatment of diarrhea-predominant patients include cholestyramine, an agent that binds bile salts, and ondansetron, a 5-hydroxytryptamine ($5-HT_3$) serotonin receptor antagonist, and calcium channel blockers.[90,102]

ANTISPASMODIC AGENTS

Antispasmodic agents are commonly prescribed for IBS patients despite limited data to support their effectiveness (see Table 18-13).[90,102] The rationale for their use is based on the premise that IBS patients have exaggerated patterns of gut motility and that inhibition of this activity provides relief of associated symptoms. Although anticholinergics are most widely used, agents such as calcium channel blockers (e.g., nifedipine, diltiazem, verapamil) and a number of other antispasmodics (not available in the United States) have been proposed because of their relaxant effect on smooth muscle and inhibitory effect on the gastrocolonic response.[102] The anticholinergic antispasmodics are used most often in patients with diarrhea-predominant IBS as they are most helpful in relieving abdominal cramps.[90,100,102] The results of a meta-analysis concluded that anticholinergics were likely to improve the patient's global assessment of well-being and to reduce abdominal pain but that they were no better than placebo in relieving abdominal bloating.[90] Anticholinergics are most effective when used at the onset of acute abdominal pain or before meals. Treatment is often initiated with dicyclomine 10 mg because it tends to have fewer adverse effects (see Table 18-13). Hyoscyamine is available orally and sublingually for acute attacks and is also available in a time-release formulation.

Table 18-13

Medications Used to Treat the Specific Symptoms of Irritable Bowel Syndrome

MEDICATION	BRAND NAME	DOSAGE REGIMEN	SIDE EFFECTS AND DRUG INTERACTIONS
BULKING OR HYDROPHILIC AGENTS			
Psyllium Methylcellulose Polycarbophil	Metamucil, various Citrucel, various Fibercon, various	7–30 g/d 4–6 g/d 1–6 g/d	May cause abdominal distention, bloating, and cramping
ANTIDIARRHEAL AGENTS			
Loperamide Diphenoxylate Cholestyramine	Imodium, various Lomotil, various Various	2–4 mg bid–qid 2.5–5 mg qid 0.5–1 packet qd–bid	May cause constipation
ANTICHOLINERGIC ANTISPASMODIC AGENTS			
Belladonna Dicyclomine Hyoscyamine Propantheline	Various Bentyl, various Various Probanthine, various	5–10 drops tid 10–20 mg tid–qid 0.125–0.25 mg qid 7.5–15 mg tid	May cause dry mouth, blurred vision, sedation, and urinary retention
HETEROCYCLIC ANTIDEPRESSANTS			
Amitriptyline Nortriptyline Imipramine Desipramine Trazodone Nefazodone	Elavil, Endep Aventyl, Pamelor Tofranil, various Norpramin, various Desyrel Serzone	10–75 mg hs 10–100 mg/d 10–100 mg hs 50 mg hs 50–100 mg hs 100 mg bid	May cause dry mouth, blurred vision, sedation, orthostatic hypotension, and weight gain; nortriptyline is less likely to cause orthostatic hypotension in patients with cardiac disease and the elderly but may cause sinus tachycardia and prolong conduction time; use with caution in urinary retention; interacts with SSRIs, alcohol, and inhibitors of CYP450 2D6
SELECTIVE SEROTONIN REUPTAKE INHIBITORS (SSRIs)			
Fluoxetine Sertraline Paroxetine	Prozac Zoloft Paxil	10–60 mg qd 50–200 mg qd 20–50 mg qd	May cause nausea, sedation, insomnia, diarrhea, sexual dysfunction; contraindicated within 2 wk of treatment with monoamine oxidase inhibitors or tryptophan
PROMOTILITY AGENTS			
Cisapride	Propulsid	5–10 mg tid	May cause abdominal cramping, diarrhea; contraindicated with drugs that inhibit CYP450 3A4; prolong the QT interval; and in patients with fluid/electrolyte disorders, underlying cardiac, renal, or pulmonary conditions
5-HT₃ SEROTONIN RECEPTOR ANTAGONISTS			
Alosetron	Lotronex	1 mg bid	Constipation reported in 27–31% of patients; constipation does not appear to increase with increased Tx duration (12 mo); case reports of ischemic colitis/rectal bleeding

SOURCE: Adapted from TG Morales and RE Sampliner[8]; B Kirschbaum[87]; TH Vesa et al[96]; MD Levitt et al[97]; and MM Heitkemper et al.[98]

PROMOTILITY AGENTS

Promotility agents, including 5-HT$_4$ agonists and 5-HT$_3$ antagonists, cisapride, dopamine antagonists (metoclopramide and domperidone), and macrolide antibiotics (erythromycin) have been used to treat patients with IBS. Clinical trials of metoclopramide and domperidone are disappointing, probably because of their lack of action on colonic motility.[90,101,102] Preliminary data from clinical trials suggest that, in patients with severe constipation-predominant IBS, cisapride may increase stool frequency, improve stool consistency, and decrease abdominal pain and distention.[90,102,104] Other reports indicate that cisapride is not helpful for refractory constipation and may, in fact, increase symptoms in diarrhea-predominant patients.[90,91] Although results from studies are conflicting, cisapride should be considered as an alternative for IBS constipation-predominant patients unresponsive to other treatments (see cisapride adverse effects and drug interactions in section on GERD). There are insufficient data to support the role of erythromycin in the treatment of constipation in IBS patients.

ANTIDEPRESSANTS AND ANXIOLYTIC AGENTS

Antidepressants and anxiolytic medications (tranquilizers) have been evaluated for use in the treatment of IBS because many of these agents alter GI motility in addition to their effects on the CNS (see Table 18-13). Of the antidepressants, the tricyclics (e.g., amitriptyline, nortriptyline, imipramine, trimipramine, desipramine) have been studied most extensively for IBS and chronic pain in general. Many of the published studies, however, contain methodological and statistical problems that make it difficult to draw firm conclusions about their effectiveness in treating IBS.[90,100–102]

In addition to their antidepressant effects, tricyclics may offer patients with diarrhea-predominant IBS (with or without abdominal pain) some benefit.[90,91,100–102] The tricyclics also possess analgesic and neuromodulatory properties that appear to be independent of psychotropic effects. The analgesic effects occur sooner (within days) and with a lower dosage than when these agents are used to treat depression (see Table 18-13).[90,91,100–102] Anticholinergic properties are responsible for their antidiarrheal action and may contribute to their analgesic effects. The decision to use an antidepressant depends, in part, on the chronicity of the disorder (because these agents must be used on a continuing basis rather than as needed) and whether the patient has diarrhea or constipation.[91]

SIDE EFFECTS AND DRUG INTERACTIONS Tricyclic antidepressants are likely to cause constipation, whereas nefazodone and trazodone (as well as the selective serotonin reuptake inhibitors [SSRIs]) may cause diarrhea. For more information on the adverse effects and potential drug interactions of these agents see Chap. 9.

Anecdotal reports and uncontrolled studies suggest that the newer SSRIs may be as effective as the tricyclics in controlling chronic pain independent of depression.[91,100,101] They may also benefit patients with depression, phobias, or obsessive-compulsive disorders.[100] Although there is little available information regarding their efficacy in the treatment of IBS, the SSRIs are often preferred over the tricyclic antidepressants because they are associated with fewer adverse effects and potentially fewer drug interactions (see Table 18-13). Tranquilizers and sedatives have been used for years to treat IBS. However, their marginal efficacy and potential for abuse does not support their use in most patients.[91,102]

5-HT$_3$ SEROTONIN RECEPTOR ANTAGONISTS

Alosetron is similar to other 5-HT$_3$ antagonists (e.g., ondansetron). These agents compete with systemic serotonin on 5-HT$_3$ serotonin receptor sites, which are widely distributed within the sensory and enteric neurons of the GI tract (as well as the spinal cord and brain), to delay colonic transit time; alosetron selectively delays left colonic transit time. Alosetron is indicated for the relief of abdominal pain and discomfort in diarrhea-predominant IBS in females; these beneficial effects of alosetron on abdominal pain and bowel function are more consistently demonstrated in females compared with males. Alosetron also improves bowel function (e.g., decreases days with urgency, decreases stool frequency, and produces firmer stools). Relief of pain and discomfort is achieved between 2 and 4 weeks, but benefits often diminish after 1 week of stopping treatment. Improvement in bowel function typically occurs by the end of 1 week. Constipation is the most frequent adverse effect and is reported to occur in 27 to 31 percent of treated patients. Several case reports indicate ischemic colitis or rectal bleeding. Alosetron is the first drug that offers a significant advance in the treatment of IBS in females by improving multiple IBS symptoms.

Figure 18-4

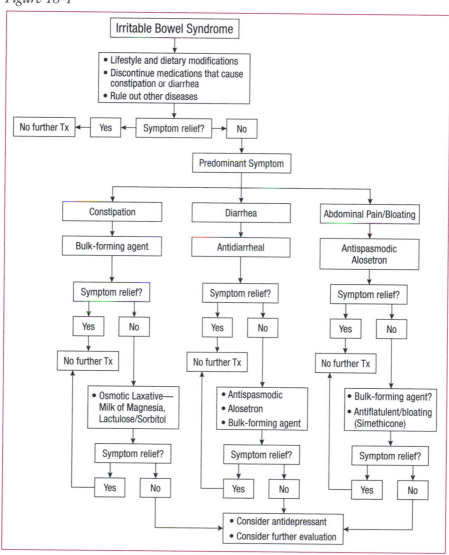

Algorithm for managing the symptoms of irritable bowel syndrome.

Management Strategies

GENERAL APPROACH TO TREATMENT

The clinician should establish an effective and supportive relationship with the patient and provide patient education and reassurance about IBS and its treatment including dietary measures, lifestyle modification, and medications. Most patients with mild symptoms respond to dietary alterations, stress reduction, and occasional nonprescription medications to control abdominal discomfort, bloating, diarrhea, or constipation. Patients with moderate symptoms and more severe disability require pharmacologic treatment. A very small subset of patients have refractory or severe symptoms and a psychosocial disorder. An algorithm for managing patients with IBS is presented in Fig. 18-4.

MANAGING THE CONSTIPATION-PREDOMINANT PATIENT

Patients with constipation-predominant IBS should increase stool bulk and fluid in an attempt to reduce the effort required for defecation. A bulking agent should be added to a high-fiber diet when dietary modifications are inadequate. If possible, constipating medications should be discontinued. Patients should be advised that a high-fiber diet and bulk-forming agents take several weeks to produce a satisfactory result. Fiber should be introduced gradually to minimize distention and gas.

Patients with an inadequate response should take an osmotic laxative such as Milk of Magnesia or lactulose in addition to fiber. Stimulant laxatives should be avoided because of their potential to damage colonic motor function. A trial of cisapride may be indicated in patients with severe or refractory constipation. In general, patients with refractory constipation should be referred to a gastroenterologist for further evaluation.

MANAGING THE DIARRHEA-PREDOMINANT PATIENT

Patients with diarrhea-predominant IBS should be evaluated for an infectious cause of their diarrhea, recent antibiotic use predisposing to colitis induced by *Clostridium difficile*, lactose intolerance, or the ingestion of medications with a laxative effect. Screening for laxative abuse should be considered in patients with refractory diarrhea.

Loperamide or diphenoxylate may be used to reduce defecation frequency or urgency and improve stool consistency. Loperamide, however, is usually the drug of choice for treating diarrhea because it does not cross the blood-brain barrier. Because diarrhea in the IBS patient is often postprandial, the antidiarrheal should be taken before meals. Additional benefit may be achieved by the addition of an anticholinergic antispasmodic agent. Alternatively, a trial of alosetron may be indicated in patients with frequent and recurrent diarrhea. Although many clinicians recommend fiber supplements, their efficacy in diarrhea-predominant IBS is not supported by controlled clinical trials. If the diarrhea is unresponsive to drug therapy, the patient should be referred to a gastroenterologist for further evaluation.

MANAGING ABDOMINAL PAIN AND BLOATING

Anticholinergic antispasmodics are usually recommended for patients with abdominal pain and bloating, especially when symptoms are exacerbated by meals. Alosetron is indicated in patients with abdominal pain and bloating, but onset of relief may take several weeks. A bulk-forming agent may be used for painful IBS, but data for this indication are not convincing. An antiflatulent (e.g., simethicone) may be used when bloating is problematic. Antidepressants are usually reserved for severe, frequent, and refractory abdominal pain. Although the literature supports the use of tricyclic antidepressants, an SSRI may be preferred (because of fewer cardiac side effects and less potential for serious drug interactions) in patients when adverse effects or drug interactions associated with the tricyclics may be a problem.

MANAGING THE PATIENT WITH PSYCHOLOGICAL DISTURBANCES

Biofeedback, hypnosis, and stress-reduction techniques may not relieve abdominal pain or improve bowel habits, but may decrease anxiety. Antidepressants should not be used as a first-line treatment for IBS, but may be considered in patients refractory to other measures. Anxiolytics are not recommended because of their lack of therapeutic superiority over placebo and the possibility of physical dependence.

Summary

Common GI disorders seen in primary care include GERD, NSAID-induced ulcers, constipation, and IBS; they are either more prevalent in women or exacerbated during pregnancy. A better understanding of the pathophysiology, clinical presentation, diagnosis, and management of these disorders should improve the overall heath care of patients and will enable the clinician to better address the special health needs of women.

References

1. Castell DO, Brunton SA, Earnest DL, et al: GERD: management algorithms for the primary care physician and the specialist. *Practical Gastroenterology* April:18, 1998.
2. Kahrilas PF: Gastroesophageal reflux disease and its complications. In: Feldman M, Scharschmidt BF, Sleisenger MH (eds): *Sleisenger & Fordtran's Gastrointestinal and Liver Disease: Pathophysiology/Diagnosis/Management*, 6th ed. Philadelphia: Saunders; 1998:498.
3. Vicari JJ, Peek RM, Falk GW, et al: The seroprevalence of cagA-positive *Helicobacter pylori* strains in the spectrum of gastroesophageal reflux disease. *Gastroenterology* 115:50, 1998.
4. Zimmermann EM, Christman GM: Approach to gastrointestinal disease in the female patient. In: Yamada T, Alpers DH, Laine L, et al (eds): *Textbook of Gastroenterology*, 3rd ed. Philadelphia: Lippincott, Williams & Wilkins, 1999:1059.
5. Broussard CN, Richter CN: Treating gastrooesophageal reflux disease during pregnancy and lactation: what are the safest therapy options? *Drug Safety* 19:325, 1998.
6. DeVault KR, Castell DO: Updated guidelines for the diagnosis and treatment of gastroesophageal reflux disease. *Am J Gastroenterol* 94;1434, 1999.
7. Lagergren J, Bergstrom R, Lindgren A, et al: Symptomatic gastroesophageal reflux as a risk factor for esophageal adenocarcinoma. *N Engl J Med* 340:825, 1999.
8. Morales TG, Sampliner RE: Barrett's esophagus: update on screening, surveillance, and treatment. *Arch Intern Med* 159:1411, 1999.
9. Sampliner RE: Practice guidelines on the diagnosis, surveillance, and therapy of Barrett's esophagus. *Am J Gastroenterol* 93:1028, 1998.
10. Sharma P, Sampliner RE, Camargo E: Normalization of esophageal pH with high-dose proton pump inhibitors therapy does not result in regression of Barrett's esophagus. *Am J Gastroenterol* 92:582, 1997.
11. Boyce HW: Therapeutic approaches to healing esophagitis. *Am J Gastroenterol* 92(suppl):22S, 1997.
12. Klinkenberg-Knol EC, Festen HPM, Meuwissen SGM: Pharmacological management of gastrooesophageal reflux disease. *Drugs* 49:695, 1995.
13. Pinson JB, Weart CW: Acid-peptic products. In: Covington TR, Berardi RR, Young LY, et al (eds): *Handbook of Nonprescription Drugs*, 9th ed. Washington, DC: American Pharmaceutical Association; 1996:193.
14. Welage LS, Berardi RR: Drug interactions with antiulcer agents: considerations in the treatment of acid-peptic disease. *J Pharm Prac* 7:177, 1994.
15. Abramowicz A (ed): Over-the-counter H_2-receptor antagonists for heartburn. *Med Drugs Lett Ther* 37:95, 1995.
16. Howden CW: Optimizing the pharmacology of acid control in acid-related disorders. *Am J Gastroenterol* 92(suppl):17S, 1997.
17. Richter JE: Long-term management of gastroesophageal reflux disease and its complications. *Am J Gastroenterol* 92(suppl):30S, 1997.
18. Richardson P, Hawkey CJ, Stack WA: Proton pump inhibitors: pharmacology and rationale for use in gastrointestinal disorders. *Drugs* 56:307, 1998.
19. Berardi RR, Welage LS: Proton pump inhibitors in acid-related disease. *Am J Health Syst Pharm* 55:2289, 1998.

20. Langtry HD, Wilde MI: Omeprazole: a review of its use in *Helicobacter pylori* infection, gastro-oesophageal reflux disease and peptic ulcers induced by non-steroidal anti-inflammatory drugs. *Drugs* 56:447, 1998.

21. Fitton A, Wiseman L: Pantoprazole: a review of its pharmacological properties and therapeutic use in acid-related disorders. *Drugs* 51:460, 1996.

22. Prakash A, Faulds D: Rabeprazole. *Drugs* 55:261, 1998.

23. Castell DO, Richter JE, Robinson MJ, et al: Efficacy and safety of lansoprazole in the treatment of erosive reflux esophagitis. *Am J Gastroenterol* 91:1749, 1996.

24. Mee AS, Rowley JL, and the Lansoprazole Clinical Research Group: Rapid symptom relief in reflux oesophagitis: a comparison of lansoprazole and omeprazole. *Aliment Pharmacol Ther* 10:757, 1996.

25. Mulder CJ, Dekker W, Gerretsen M, et al: Lansoprazole 30 mg versus omeprazole 40 mg in the treatment of reflux oesophagitis grades II, III and IVa (a Dutch multicentre trial). *Eur J Gastroenterol Hepatology* 8:1101, 1996.

26. Collen MJ, Abdulian JD, Chen YK: Gastroesophageal reflux disease in the elderly: more severe disease that requires aggressive therapy. *Am J Gastroenterol* 90:1053, 1995.

27. Vigneri S, Termini R, Leandro G, et al: A comparison of five maintenance therapies for reflux esophagitis. *N Engl J Med* 333:1106, 1995.

28. Freston JW: Long-term acid control and proton pump inhibitors: interactions and safety issues in perspective. *Am J Gastroenterol* 92:51S, 1997.

29. Garnett WR: Considerations for long-term use of proton-pump inhibitors. *Am J Health Syst Pharm* 55:2268, 1998.

30. Unge P, Andersson A: Drug interactions with proton pump inhibitors. *Drug Safety* 16:171. 1997.

31. Barone JA, Jessen LM, Colaizzi JL, et al: Cisapride: a gastrointestinal prokinetic drug. *Ann Pharmacother* 28:488, 1994.

32. Schutze K, Bigard MA, Van Waes L, et al: Comparison of two dosing regimens of cisapride in the treatment of reflux oesophagitis. *Aliment Pharmacol Ther* 11:497, 1997.

33. McDougall NI, Watson RGP, Collins JSA, et al: Maintenance therapy with cisapride after healing of erosive oesophagitis: a double-blind placebo-controlled trial. *Aliment Pharmacol Ther* 11:487, 1997.

34. Propulsid (cisapride) package insert. Janssen, Titusville, NJ. June, 1998.

35. Bedford TA, Rowbotham DJ: Cisapride: drug interactions of clinical significance. *Drug Safety* 15:167, 1996.

36. Wysowski DK: Cisapride and fatal arrhythmias. *N Engl J Med* 335:290, 1996.

37. Peghini PL, Katz PO, Castell DO: Ranitidine controls nocturnal gastric acid breakthrough on omeprazole: a controlled study in normal subjects. *Gastroenterology* 115:1335, 1998.

38. O'Connor HJ: Review article: *Helicobacter pylori* and gastro-oesophageal reflux disease—clinical implications and management. *Aliment Pharmacol Ther* 13:117, 1999.

39. Kuipers EJ, Lundell L, Klinkenberg-Knol EC, et al: Atrophic gastritis and *Helicobacter pylori* infection in patients with reflux esophagitis treatment with omeprazole or fundoplication. *N Engl J Med* 334:1018, 1996.

40. Howden CW, Hunt RH: Guidelines for the management of *Helicobacter pylori* infection. *Am J Gastroenterol* 93:2330, 1998.

41. Salcedo JA, Al-Kawas F: Treatment of *Helicobacter pylori* infection. *Arch Intern Med* 158:842, 1998.

42. Kunz K, Arundell E, Cisternas M, et al: Economic implications of self-treatment of heartburn/nonulcer dyspepsia with nonprescription famotidine in a managed care setting. *J Managed Care Pharm* 2:263, 1996.

43. Zagari M, Villa KF, Freston JW: Proton pump inhibitors versus H_2-receptor antagonists for the treatment of erosive gastroesophageal disease: a cost-comparative study. *Am J Managed Care* 1:247, 1995.

44. Bloom BS: Cost and quality effects of treating erosive oesophagitis: a re-evaluation. *Pharmaco-Economics* 8:139:1995.

45. Mathias SD, Castell DO, Elkin EP, et al: Health-related quality of life of patients with acute erosive reflux esophagitis. *Dig Dis Sci* 41:2123, 1996.

46. Heudebert GR, Marks R, Wilsox M, et al: Choice of long-term strategy for the management of patients with severe esophagitis: a cost-utility analysis. *Gastroenterology* 112:1078, 1997.

47. Moss SF, Arnold R, Tytgat GNJ, et al: Consensus statement for management of gastroesophageal reflux disease. *J Clin Gastroenterol* 27:6, 1998.

48. Howden CW, Castell DO, Cohen S, et al: The rationale for continuous maintenance treatment of reflux esophagitis. *Arch Intern Med* 155:1465, 1995.

49. Walker SJ, Baxter ST, Morris AI, et al: Review article: controversy in the therapy of gastro-oesophageal reflux disease: long-term proton pump inhibition

or laparoscopic anti-reflux surgery? *Aliment Pharmacol Ther* 11:249, 1997.

50. Cryer B: Nonsteroidal anti-inflammatory drugs and gastrointestinal disease. In: Feldman M, Scharschmidt BF, Sleisenger MH (eds): *Sleisinger and Fordtran's Gastrointestinal and Liver Disease: Pathophysiology/Diagnosis/Management*, 6th ed. Philadelphia: Saunders; 1998:343.

51. Soll AH: Peptic ulcer and its complications. In: Feldman M, Scharschmidt BF, Sleisenger MH, (eds): *Sleisinger and Fordtran's Gastrointestinal and Liver Disease: Pathophysiology/Diagnosis/Management*, 6th ed. Philadelphia: Saunders; 1998:620.

52. Wallace JL: Nonsteroidal anti-inflammatory drugs and gastroenteropathy: the second hundred years. *Gastroenterology* 112:1000, 1997.

53. Lanza FL: A guideline for the treatment and prevention of NSAID-induced ulcers. *Am J Gastroenterol* 93:2037, 1998.

54. Lanza FL, Codisponti JR, Nelson EB: An endoscopic comparison of gastroduodenal injury with over-the-counter doses of ketoprofen and acetaminophen. *Am J Gastroenterol* 93:1051, 1998.

55. Singh G, Rosen DR, Morfield D, et al: Gastrointestinal tract complications of nonsteroidal anti-inflammatory drug treatment in rheumatoid arthritis. *Arch Intern Med* 156:1530, 1996.

56. Wilcox CM: Relationship between nonsteroidal anti-inflammatory drug use, *Helicobacter pylori*, and gastroduodenal mucosal injury. *Gastroenterology* 113(suppl):S85, 1997.

57. Cryer B, Feldman M: Cyclooxygenase-1 and cyclooxygenase-2 selectivity of widely used nonsteroidal anti-inflammatory drugs. *Am J Med* 104:413, 1998.

58. Hawkey CJ: COX-2 inhibitors. *Lancet* 353:307, 1999.

59. Soll AH: Medical treatment of peptic ulcer disease: practice guidelines. *JAMA* 275:622, 1996.

60. Berardi RR: Peptic ulcer disease. In: DiPiro JT, Talbert RL, Yee GC, et al (eds): *Pharmacotherapy: A Pathophysiologic Approach*, 4th ed. Stamford, CT: Appleton & Lange; 1999:548.

61. Hudson N, Taha AS, Russell RI, et al: Famotidine for healing and maintenance in nonsteroidal anti-inflammatory drug-associated gastroduodenal ulceration. *Gastroenterology* 112:1817, 1997.

62. Taha AS, Hudson N, Hawkey CJ: Famotidine for the prevention of gastric and duodenal ulcers caused by nonsteroidal antiinflammatory drugs. *N Engl J Med* 334:1435, 1996;.

63. Yeomans ND, Tulassy Z, Juhasz L, et al: A comparison of omeprazole with ranitidine for ulcers associated with nonsteroidal antiinflammatory drugs. *N Engl J Med* 338:719, 1998.

64. Hawkey CJ, Karrasch JA, Szczepanski L, et al: Omeprazole compared with misoprostol for ulcers associated with nonsteroidal antiinflammatory drugs. *N Engl J Med* 338:727, 1998.

65. Raskin JB, White RH, Jackson JE, et al: Misoprostol dosage in the prevention of nonsteroidal anti-inflammatory drug-induced gastric and duodenal ulcers: a comparison of three regimens. *Ann Intern Med* 123:344, 1995.

66. Silverstein FE: Improving the gastrointestinal safety of NSAIDs: the development of misoprostol—from hypothesis to clinical practice. *Dig Dis Sci* 43:447, 1998.

67. Donnelly MT, Hawkey CJ: Review article: COX-II inhibitors—a new generation of safer NSAIDs? *Aliment Pharmacol Ther* 11:227, 1997.

68. Celebrex (celecoxib) package insert. Searle & Co., Skokie, IL, June, 1999.

69. Vioxx (rofecoxib) package insert. Merck & Co., Inc., West Point, PA, June, 1999.

70. Maetzel A, Ferraz MB, Bombardier C: The cost-effectiveness of misoprostol in preventing serious gastrointestinal events associated with the use of nonsteroidal anti-inflammatory drugs. *Arthritis Rheum* 41:16, 1998.

71. Lennard-Jones JE: Constipation. In: Feldman M, Scharschmidt BF, Sleisenger MH (eds): *Sleisinger and Fordtran's Gastrointestinal and Liver Disease: Pathophysiology/Diagnosis/Management*, 6th ed. Philadelphia: Saunders; 1998:174.

72. Wald A: Evaluation and management of constipation. *Clinical Perspectives in Gastroenterology* 1:106, 1998.

73. Longe RL, DiPiro JT: Diarrhea and constipation. In: DiPiro JT, Talbert RL, Yee GC, et al (eds): *Pharmacotherapy: A Pathophysiologic Approach*, 4th ed. Stamford, CT: Appleton & Lange; 1999:599.

74. Bonapace ES, Fisher RS: Constipation and diarrhea in pregnancy. *Gastroenterol Clin North Am* 27:197, 1998.

75. Baron TH, Ramiriz B, Richter JE: Gastrointestinal motility disorders during pregnancy. *Ann Intern Med* 118:266, 1993.

76. Lisi DM: Drug-induced constipation. *Arch Intern Med* 154:461, 1994.

77. Halverson AL, Orkin BA: Which physiologic tests are useful in patients with constipation? *Dis Colon Rectum* 41:735, 1998.

78. Robertson G, Meshkinpour H, Vandenberg K, et al: Effects of exercise on total and segmental colon transit. *J Clin Gastroenterol* 16:300, 1993.

79. Schaefer DC, Cheskin LJ: Constipation in the elderly. *Am Fam Physician* 58:907, 1998.

80. Schiller LR: Clinical pharmacology and use of laxatives and lavage solutions. *J Clin Gastroenterol* 28:11, 1999.

81. Sussman GL, Dorian W: Psyllium anaphylaxis. *Allergy Proc* 11:241, 1990.

82. Freeman GL: Psyllium hypersensitivity. *Ann Allergy* 73:490, 1994.

83. Vaswani SK, Hamilton RG, Valentine MD, et al: Psyllium laxative-induced anaphylaxis, asthma, and rhinitis. *Allergy* 51:266, 1996.

84. Guttuso JM, Kamm MA: Adverse effects of drugs used in the management of constipation and diarrhoea. *Drug Safety* 10:47, 1994.

85. Blumenthal M: *The Complete German Commission E Monographs: Therapeutic Guide to Herbal Medicines.* Boston: Integrative Medicine Communications; 1998.

86. Qureshi T, Melonakos TK: Acute hypermagnesemia after laxative use. *Ann Emerg Med* 28:552, 1996.

87. Kirschbaum B: The acidosis of exogenous phosphate intoxication. *Arch Intern Med* 158:405, 1998.

88. Filho AF, Lassman MN: Severe hyperphosphatemia induced by a phosphate-containing oral laxative. *Ann Pharmacother* 30:141, 1996.

89. Pitcher DE, Ford RS, Nelson MT, et al: Fatal hypocalcemic, hyperphosphatemic, metabolic acidosis following sequential sodium phosphate-based enema administration. *Gastrointest Endosc* 46:266, 1997.

90. Olden KW, Schuster MM: Irritable bowel syndrome. In: Feldman M, Scharschmidt BF, Sleisenger MH (eds): *Sleisinger and Fordtran's Gastrointestinal and Liver Disease: Pathophysiology/Diagnosis/Management*, 6th ed. Philadelphia: Saunders; 1998:1536.

91. Drossman GA, Whitehead WE, Camilleri M, et al: Irritable bowel syndrome: a technical review for practical guideline development. *Gastroenterology* 112:2120, 1997.

92. Muller-Lissner S, Coremans G, Dapoigny M, et al: Motility in irritable-bowel syndrome. *Digestion* 58:196, 1997.

93. Heitkemper M, Burr RL, Jarrett M, et al: Evidence for autonomic nervous system imbalance in women with irritable bowel syndrome. *Dig Dis Sci* 43:2093, 1998.

94. Jarrett M, Heitkemper M, Cain KC, et al: The relationship between psychological distress and gastrointestinal symptoms in women with irritable bowel syndrome. *Nurs Res* 47:154, 1998.

95. Lydiard RB: Anxiety and the irritable bowel syndrome: psychiatric, medical, or both? *J Clin Psychiatry* 58(suppl):51, 1997.

96. Vesa TH, Seppo LM, Marteau PR, et al: Role of irritable bowel syndrome in subjective lactose intolerance. *Am J Clin Nutr* 67:7, 1998.

97. Levitt MD, Furne J, Olsson S: The relation of passage of gas and abdominal bloating to colonic gas production. *Ann Intern Med* 124:422, 1996.

98. Heitkemper MM, Jarrett M, Cain KC, et al: Daily gastrointestinal symptoms in women with and without a diagnosis of IBS. *Dig Dis Sci* 40:1511, 1995.

99. Fass R, Fullerton S, Naliboff B, et al: Sexual dysfunction in patients with irritable bowel syndrome and non-ulcer dyspepsia. *Digestion* 59:79, 1998.

100. Wald A: Irritable bowel syndrome. *Curr Treat Options Gastrenterol* 2:13, 1999.

101. Farthing MJG: New drugs in the management of irritable bowel syndrome. *Drugs* 56:11, 1998.

102. Pace F, Coremans G, Dapoigny M, et al: Therapy of irritable bowel syndrome—an overview. *Digestion* 56:433, 1995.

103. Efskind PS, Bernklev T, Vatn MH: A double-blind placebo-controlled trial with loperamide in irritable bowel syndrome. *Scand J Gastroenterol* 31:463, 1996.

104. Farup PG, Hovdenak N, Wetterhus S, et al: The symptomatic effect of cisapride in patients with irritable bowel syndrome and constipation. *Scand J Gastroenterol* 33:128, 1998.

Diana Curran

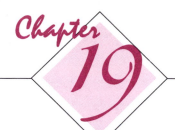

Gallbladder Disease

Overview

Doctors teach medical students the motto, "female, fat, fertile, and forty," to remember who is at risk for gallbladder disease. Although trite, it largely holds true. Women more often than men have gallstones, and obesity and multiparity are additional risk factors. Diseases of the gallbladder include gallstones, cholecystitis, and rarely cancer.

Gallstones

The overall prevalence of gallstones among those over age 40, based on autopsy series, is 20 percent for women and 8 percent for men. The disease affects 16 to 20 million people in the United States with an estimated 1 million new cases per year.[1] Women outnumber men at least 2:1 in prevalence. Prevalence varies by ethnic background and increases with advancing age and in association with several disease states and conditions such as diabetes and pregnancy.

Less than one-third of people with asymptomatic gallstones will ever develop symptoms.[1,2] Demographic characteristics such as age, sex, and number or size of stones do not predict who will develop symptoms or require surgery. In a study of asymptomatic gallstones in adults, the cumulative risk for the development of symptoms requiring surgery was 10 percent at 5 years, 15 percent at 10 years, and 18 percent at 15 years and 20 years.[3]

Cholecystitis

Cholecystitis, or inflammation of the gallbladder wall, occurs in over 90 percent of patients with symptomatic gallstones.

ACUTE CHOLECYSTITIS

Acute cholecystitis, associated with pain lasting 6 h or more, occurs in about 10 percent of patients with symptomatic gallstones. Bacteria can be cultured from bile in 20 to 30 percent of patients with acute cholecystitis during the first few days of the attack, but by day 7 to 10, almost 80 percent of cultures are positive.[4] Conservative treatment with intravenous antibiotics and hospitalization will relieve symptoms for about 75 percent of patients. Another 25 percent will develop complications requiring urgent or emergent cholecystectomy. Among the patients who achieve remission, 25 percent will have recurrence within 1 year and 60 percent within 6 years.[1]

Complications of acute cholecystitis include emphysematous gallbladder, chronic cholecystitis, gangrene, perforation, and hydrops or edema in the gallbladder wall. Both ischemia and gangrene, a gas-producing bacterial infection, can result in emphysematous gallbladder. These complications are more prevalent among elderly men and patients with diabetes, as is perforation. Nearly 10 percent of patients with acute cholecystitis develop gangrene and perforate their gallbladder; 20 percent develop jaundice.[5]

CHRONIC CHOLECYSTITIS

Chronic inflammation, from recurrent bouts of infection and mechanical obstruction, may be asymptomatic for years or may be mildly symptomatic. Complications from chronic cholecystitis are rare and include porcelain gallbladder, empyema, and hydrops. Porcelain gallbladder, discussed later, is associated with a high likelihood of progression to gallbladder cancer. Empyema usually results from superinfection of the underlying inflamed gallbladder. Hydrops or mucocele result from prolonged obstruction, usually by a solitary stone. Over time, a distended lumen progresses to form an epithelized mucocele that may be palpable on examination. Emergency surgery is indicated for both conditions because of the high risk for gangrene, perforation, and death.[1]

Gangrene of the gallbladder is rare and associated with bacterial infections and with underlying conditions such as diabetes, vasculitis, arterial occlusion, or torsion. Local perforation can occur, resulting, most commonly, in an abscess forming under the omentum that requires drainage. Free perforation is rare but is associated with about a 30 percent mortality rate.

Gallbladder Cancer

Carcinoma of the gallbladder is rare and occurs in fewer than 6000 individuals in the United States per year. Biliary tract cancer incidence and mortality vary widely around the world and are roughly 30 times more common in high-risk compared to low-risk populations. The highest incidence occurs in Chile and Japan and among Native American women in New Mexico.[6] For Chilean women, cancer of the gallbladder is the number one cause of cancer mortality with a rate of 13.3/100,000.[7] Great Britain and Greece have the lowest incidence. In the United States, African Americans have a gallbladder cancer incidence of 2.3 to 3.0/100,000 per year, whereas whites have an incidence of 4.5/100,000 for men and 11.5/100,000 for women; in Southwestern Native Americans, the incidence is 16.2/100,000 for men and 46.4/100,000 for women.[8] These differences in prevalence suggest an environmental or genetic influence or both.

Gallbladder cancer is more common among patients with gallstones, but the lifetime risk overall is low, 0.3 to 1 percent, about the same as operative mortality.[4] Native Americans with cholelithiasis, however, have a higher gallbladder cancer incidence, 3 to 5 percent. Based on data from a large case-control study of three races, the estimated percentage of patients with gallstones who would develop gallbladder cancer is 0.13 to 0.15 percent for blacks, 0.26 to 0.5 percent for whites, and 0.94 to 1.5 percent for Native Americans.[8] The number of cholecystectomies required to prevent one case of gallbladder cancer ranged from 769 (95 percent CI 370 to 1428) for black men to 67 (95 percent CI 57 to 76) for Native American women.

The role of bacterial infection as a causative agent for gallbladder disease and cancer is currently under investigation. In a 1994 European study, no bacteria were found in bile aspirates from patients without gallbladder disease. In contrast, 32 percent of patients with symptomatic gallstones, 41 percent with acute cholecystitis, 58 percent with a common bile duct stone, and 81 percent with a carcinoma of the gallbladder had bacteria present in the bile.[9] Both *Salmonella typhi* and *Helicobacter* spp. isolates have been cultured from the gallbladders of patients with chronic cholecystitis.[7] Although compelling evidence is mounting in support of a causal relationship between bacterial infection and cancer, it remains unproven.

Two other conditions, adenomatous polyps of the gallbladder and porcelain gallbladder, are strongly associated with gallbladder cancer. Adenomatous polyps, especially when they are larger than 1.0 cm in diameter or when they exhibit rapid growth, are an absolute indication for cholecystectomy because of the increased risk of carcinoma.[10] Porcelain gallbladder, caused by chronic cholecystitis resulting in calcium salt deposits in the gallbladder wall, appears as a halo-type outline on plain films of the abdomen. Porcelain gallbladder has a nearly 50 percent likelihood of progression to carcinoma *and should be considered a precancerous condition.*

Pathophysiology

The gallbladder is a storage organ for bile produced by the liver. Bile is comprised of salts, phospholipids, and cholesterol. A balance in the concentrations of these constituents is necessary to keep them soluble. Mechanisms that alter the balance will lead to precipitation of cholesterol or pigment forming sludge or stones. At least three factors are necessary for the formation of stones: (1) cholesterol or pigment supersaturation of bile (index >1), (2) a kinetic defect that accelerates crystal nucleation, and (3) gallbladder hypomotility or stasis.

Cholesterol supersaturation of bile is lithogenic and many factors may contribute. Enteric neuropathy slows intestinal transit, resulting in increased anaerobic bacterial enzymatic formation of deoxycholate, a substrate for cholesterol. This leads to hepatic cholesterol hypersecretion. Estrogen causes hypersecretion of cholesterol in bile, and progesterone causes delayed conversion of cholesterol to cholesterol esters.

During pregnancy, the composition of the bile acid pool changes, resulting in a marked increase in cholesterol concentration by the third trimester. This is the physiologic explanation for the increased risk of gallstones in women and during pregnancy. Among obese individuals, excess hepatic cholesterol secretion appears to be the primary mechanism for gallstone formation.[11]

Gallbladder motility defects lead to stasis of bile creating the opportunity for stone formation. Motility is controlled by hormonal and neural factors.[12] Among patients with diabetes mellitus, neuropathy may cause delayed gallbladder emptying. During pregnancy, the gallbladder is slower to respond to a meal.

Risk Factors

Independent risk factors for gallbladder disease are listed in Table 19-1. Patients with multiple risk factors are at much higher risk.

Demographic Factors

The incidence of gallbladder disease varies worldwide. In the United States, it is more common among Mexican Americans but less common among African Americans. A researcher in Texas who conducted ultrasound evaluations on over a thousand randomly selected Mexican Americans found a prevalence of gallstones of 40.2 percent for women and 19.2 percent for men over age 45, double the U.S. average.[13] In contrast, African Americans have a prevalence rate of about 5 percent.[2]

Gallstone disease increases with age and runs in families. The U.S. Asymptomatic Gallstone Study performed ultrasound on 2041 patients (297 men and 1744 women) who had no history of gallstones or biliary disease.[14] The prevalence of asymptomatic gallstones in women was 5 percent for age 20 to 29, 9 percent for age 30 to 39, and 11 percent for age 40 and over. Family history of a first-degree relative with gallstones increases the risk by about 10 percent.[15]

Pregnancy and increased parity are both risk factors for gallstones. During pregnancy, cholesterol gallstones develop more readily because of hormone-mediated effects on cholesterol saturation of bile and gallbladder contractility.[16] A 1993 study found a prevalence of gallstones of 12.2 percent in almost 1000 women evaluated by ultrasound immediately after giving birth. Only large stones (>1 cm diameter) were likely to be symptomatic, and 29 percent of small stones (<6 mm diameter) dissolved spontaneously during the postpartum period.[17] The number of pregnancies also increases risk as demonstrated in the U.S. Asymptomatic Gallstone Study. Among women with zero, three, and six or more prior pregnancies, the prevalence of gallstones was 3.7 percent, 7.6 percent, and 16.7 percent, respectively, for all age groups.[14] Even when controlling for age, the risk associated with pregnancy persisted and increased by 2 percent per additional pregnancy. Other studies report that parity of three or more is the threshold for increased associated risk.[15]

Health Habits

DIET

Certain diets are associated with the formation of gallstones. Low-cholesterol diets increase the risk of gallstone formation,[18] as do high-fat and high-calorie diets.[19] Rapid weight loss diets such as the very-low-calorie diets (500 to 800 kcal/d) with 1 to 3 g fat per day increase the risk of developing gallstones by 11 to 25 percent.[20] The mechanism of gallstone formation was thought to be due

Table 19-1

Predisposing Factors Associated with Gallbladder Disease in Women

DEMOGRAPHICS	HEALTH HABITS	DISEASE STATES	DRUGS
Female Gender	Diets	Obesity	Clofibrate
Ethnic background	Very-low-calorie	NIDDM	Thiazide diuretics
Native American	Low-cholesterol	Cystic fibrosis	Ceftriaxone
Mexican American	High-fat	Dehydration due to:	Hypersensitivity to:
Chilean	High-calorie	Surgery	Erythromycin
Asian	Rapid weight loss	Trauma	Ampicillin
Advancing age	Smoking	ICU patients	Chemotherapy via
Family history	Sedentary lifestyle	Cirrhosis	hepatic artery
Pregnancy		Biliary tract infections	infusion pumps
Parity >3		Chronic hemolytic states	Octreotide
			Cyclosporine

ABBREVIATIONS: ICU, intensive care unit; NIDDM, non-insulin-dependent diabetes mellitus.

to gallbladder stasis resulting from insufficient fat in the gut to stimulate contraction. However, a prospective study evaluating a 900-kcal/d liquid diet with 30 g fat, equally divided and given three times a day, enough to maximally stimulate gallbladder emptying, did not reduce risk.[21] The mechanism by which very-low-calorie diets increase gallstone formation continues to be investigated.

SMOKING

Smokers have an increased risk of gallstones. Although a recent case-control study on smoking and gallstones failed to find a significantly increased risk of gallstones among current or past smokers, subgroup analyses revealed a higher risk of gallstones among women smokers under age 35 (OR = 3.5, 95 percent CI 1.2 to 9.8), and during the first 1 to 8 years of smoking (OR = 2.8, 95 percent CI 1.1 to 7.1).[22]

ALCOHOL USE

Moderate alcohol usage does not appear to add to the risk of gallstones and may be protective, but data are limited. In a large California study,

investigators found that women over age 50 who drank an average of 5.1 mL alcohol per week had no increased risk of gallstones.[23] In another study, a lower alcohol intake (11.7 g weekly versus 20.3 g weekly) was independently predictive of gallstones among women with diabetes mellitus.[15]

Alcohol abuse and cirrhosis of the liver are associated with increased incidence of cholelithiasis. Among these patients, pigment stones (caused by unconjugated, insoluble bilirubin in the bile) are more common than cholesterol stones. In a study of 356 patients with cirrhosis, the risk of stones was higher in those with a greater severity and duration of disease ($P < 0.001$) as well as in those with previous alcohol abuse (41.5 versus 28.3 percent). Prospective follow-up of the patients with cirrhosis without gallstones (N = 182) who later developed cholelithiasis (11.5 percent) demonstrated the same relationship to severity and duration of disease.[24]

EXERCISE

A sedentary lifestyle is associated with increased gallstones and may be related to obesity. In women, low levels of leisure time physical activity in the

Second National Health and Nutrition Examination Survey (NHANES II) population independently predicted gallbladder disease.[25] Exercise, at least in men, is proven to reduce the risk of symptomatic gallstones.[26]

Comorbid Medical Conditions

OBESITY

Obesity is a risk factor for gallstones, more so for women than men. Overweight women with a body mass index (BMI) of 30 or greater have at least double the risk compared to women with a BMI of 25 or less.[27] Risk increases with increasing BMI. In the Nurses Health Study, symptomatic gallstone disease was 3.7 to 7.4 times greater for women with a BMI of 30 or above compared to those with a BMI of 24 or less.[28] Central obesity or increased waist/hip ratio is also associated with a higher prevalence even if the BMI does not meet criteria for obesity.[27] Although a reduced weight may decrease the risk of gallstones, there is an increased risk of gallstone development during or immediately following weight loss (10 to 25 percent), and roughly one-third of these become symptomatic.[23]

DIABETES MELLITUS

The association between diabetes mellitus and increased risk of gallstones is debated. In the San Antonio Heart Study, individuals with diabetes self-reported a gallbladder disease prevalence of 34.2 percent in women and 7.2 percent in men.[29] In this study, duration of diabetes was positively associated with gallbladder disease, but hyperglycemia was not, suggesting a trend consistent with advancing age rather than severity of disease. Additionally, women with diabetes were almost twice as likely as controls to have gallstones (41.8 versus 23.1 percent), and the risk was highest in the younger age group (30 to 59). This correlates with the hormonal effect expected during the childbearing years. No increase in the prevalence of gallstones was reported in a study of patients who primarily had type 1 diabetes.[30]

The largest study to date, including both patients with insulin-dependent and non-insulin-dependent diabetes mellitus (NIDDM), found a higher incidence of gallstones among all groups of patients with diabetes, but only women with NIDDM were at increased risk independent of other risk factors.[15] This suggests that the higher incidence of gallbladder disease reported for patients with diabetes is likely secondary to other risk factors that are common among patients with NIDDM such as obesity. In summary, women with NIDDM appear to be at higher risk of developing gallstones, and the risk may be limited to women with NIDDM who are premenopausal.

HYPERLIPIDEMIA

Data are conflicting about the relationship between plasma lipid levels and gallbladder disease. In an epidemiologic study of women over age 50, an elevated triglyceride level (average 122 mg/dL versus 98 mg/dL) was associated with an increased risk of gallbladder disease.[23] In the New Zealand diabetes study, decreased high-density lipoprotein cholesterol and elevated low-density lipoprotein cholesterol levels were independent risk factors for gallstones.[15]

CYSTIC FIBROSIS

Individuals with cystic fibrosis have a very high prevalence of gallbladder disease including nonfunctioning gallbladders (30 percent), microgallbladders (8 to 30 percent), and gallstones (4 to 30 percent).[31] This may be due to the slow intestinal transport or altered gallbladder motility associated with pancreatic dysfunction among patients with cystic fibrosis. Gastrointestinal symptoms are common among patients with cystic fibrosis, and gallbladder disease should be strongly considered in the differential diagnosis of abdominal pain. Prophylactic cholecystectomy is not recommended because operative morbidity and mortality are high (10 and 5 percent, respectively) for traditional open surgery, even among patients undergoing aggressive treatment. No outcome data have been reported, however, for laparoscopic surgery in this population.

CHRONIC HEMOLYTIC STATES

Chronic hemolytic states such as sickle cell anemia are associated with pigment stones.[1] Hemolysis releases bilirubin, a substrate in bile, and supersaturation with bilirubin leads to pigment stones. Other disease states associated with pigment stones are alcoholic cirrhosis (as noted above) and biliary tract infections such as cholangitis or parasitic infestation.

DEHYDRATION

Dehydration, following surgery or trauma, predisposes patients to acalculous cholecystitis (ACC). Patients in the intensive care unit (ICU) also have an increased risk of ACC because of gallbladder stasis associated with fasting, total parenteral nutrition (TPN), sedation, ventilation, infection, and shock. In a study of 30 consecutive ICU patients, ultrasound evidence of gallbladder abnormalities was found in 18 patients within 2 days of admission.[32] Clinical significance is unlikely because the findings were early in the ICU course and no patients required surgery.

Hormone Therapy

ORAL CONTRACEPTIVES

An association between oral contraceptives (OCs) and gallstones was found in the early 1970s by several researchers. It is unlikely, however, that this is currently an important risk factor for gallbladder disease because of the lower estrogen content of modern OCs. In 1993, the results of a meta-analysis of all controlled epidemiologic studies published through March of 1992 showed only a slight increase in the incidence of benign gallbladder disease (OR = 1.36, 95 percent CI 1.15 to

1.62) for ever-versus never-use of oral contraceptives.[33] The authors postulated that the use of low-dose OCs would likely further weaken the association because of the dose-effect relationship demonstrated in several studies.

So far this is proving to be true. In 1994, a follow-up to a large multicenter prospective epidemiologic study in Great Britain reported no significant association between OC use and gallbladder disease. From 1968 to 1974, the Oxford Family Planning Association contraceptive study recruited women aged 25 to 39 who were using some form of birth control. After reaching age 45, the women who either had never used OCs or had 8 or more years of use were followed. Seventy percent of the OC users were taking a product containing 50 μg estrogen. Of the 482 women with gallbladder disease, the relative risk of gallstones was 1.1 (95 percent CI 0.9 to 1.3) for ever- versus never-use, and the relative risk for use 8 or more years was 1.1 (95 percent CI 0.8 to 1.3).[34] It appears that OCs pose little or no threat for symptomatic gallstone disease, and the presence of gallstones should no longer be considered a contraindication to their use.

ESTROGEN REPLACEMENT THERAPY

Concern about the relationship between estrogen replacement therapy and gallstones stemmed from a reported increased risk of gallstones in men with prostate cancer who were treated with exogenous estrogen. Additionally, a study in 1974 reported a relative risk of 2.5 for gallbladder disease in postmenopausal women taking replacement estrogen.

Since then, there is little evidence of an increased risk of gallstones among women on hormone replacement therapy.[35] A large epidemiologic study of women age 50 found no association between current estrogen use and benign gallbladder disease.[23] A case-control study of 235 Italian women under age 75 years with gallstones and 538 control subjects found a relative risk (RR) for ever-use of estrogen replacement of 1.9, not significant (95 percent CI 1.0 to 3.6) by multiple logistic regression analysis. No evidence supported an increased risk with increased duration of use.[36] A randomized prospective trial of postmenopausal women with coronary disease (average age 66.7 years) given estrogen and progestin versus placebo found a relative hazard of gallbladder disease of 1.38 (95 percent CI 1.00 to 1.92).[37] In this study, women were followed for 4 to 5 years and 25 to 30 percent discontinued the hormones within 3 years of study enrollment. In summary, current data are insufficient to conclude whether estrogen replacement therapy has a significant influence on gallbladder disease.

Other Medications

Several medications have a negative effect on the gallbladder. A summary of drug-induced gallbladder disease published in 1992 is available for those interested in a more comprehensive review.[35] The following information is adapted from this summary (see Table 19-1).

LIPID-LOWERING AGENTS

Of the lipid-lowering agents, clofibrate, at doses of 1g bid, is the only drug proven to increase gallstone formation and may do so up to eightfold. Clofibrate increases the output of cholesterol in the bile and feces, causing supersaturation of biliary cholesterol. Gemfibrozil has similar properties, and a few studies suggest an increased risk, but long-term effects on gallstone formation are not yet determined. Nicotinic acid increases cholesterol saturation of bile and may increase the risk of gallstones, but data are inconclusive. Cholestyramine at a dose of 16 g/d does not increase gallstones or cholecystectomy. The 3-hydroxy-3-methylglutaryl coenzyme A (HMG-coA) reductase inhibitors do not increase risk and, with the reduction in biliary cholesterol saturation, may even be protective.

DIURETICS

Thiazide diuretics increase the risk of acute cholecystitis in several reports, but prospective studies are lacking. In a case-control drug surveil-lance study, the relative risk of acute cholecystitis was 2.0 (95 percent CI 1.4 to 2.7) for those who used thiazide diuretics within a month of admission compared with those who never used the drug.[38] A significant trend of increasing relative risk with duration of use more than 5 years was also found. Whether this effect is on gallstone formation or on the development of acute cholecystitis in the setting of preexisting gallstones is yet to be investigated.

ANTIBIOTICS

Parenteral ceftriaxone causes precipitation of its calcium salt in the gallbladder and induces sludge in those on high doses (>2 g/d), but this effect is reversed when the drug is discontinued.[39] Ultrasound evidence of sludge occurred in 43 percent of children in a small prospective study and caused symptoms in 19 percent of those.[40] In adults, about one in four develop pseudolithiasis.[35] The sludge clears within several days to 2 months after ceftriaxone is discontinued. Symptoms appear to be rare, but if they develop, the drug should be discontinued and the patients followed closely.

Acute ACC associated with the initiation of intravenous ampicillin or erythromycin was reported in 12 cases from 1982 to 1987.[41] The mechanism appears to be a hypersensitivity reaction because histologic examination of the gallbladders revealed a massive eosinophilic infiltrate. The author recommends that these drugs be discontinued if symptoms of acute ACC occur.

CANCER CHEMOTHERAPIES

Chemotherapy, given through implanted hepatic artery infusion pumps, increases the risk of chemical cholecystitis; prophylactic cholecystectomy at the time of implantation is advocated by several authors.[42,43] Percutaneous pumps generally are not associated with chemical cholecystitis.[35]

Octreotide, a somatostatin analogue used in the management of acromegaly, metastatic carcinoid tumors, vasoactive intestinal polypeptide-secreting tumors, and gastrointestinal or pancreatic fistulas, is another agent associated with gallstones. Long-term use of octreotide causes gallstone formation in up to 50 percent of patients in the first year of use.[35] A controlled trial of 18 patients also found that 50 percent developed gallstones while taking octreotide in varying therapeutic dosages.[44] The likely mechanism is through inhibition of gall-bladder contraction as well as changes in the bile composition that promote cholesterol precipitation.

Cyclosporine immunosuppressive therapy is associated with cholelithiasis. In a prospective study of 27 gallstone-free heart transplant recipients, 9 of 26 male patients developed gallstones during therapy, and 7 of these during the first year of treatment.[45] Risk factors for the development of cyclosporine-induced gallstones during the immediate postoperative period included high blood concentrations of the drug, diabetes mellitus, and obesity. In a series of renal transplant recipients, the incidence of cholelithiasis was only 2.4 percent of patients taking cyclosporine and prednisone.[46] Additionally, these patients usually develop moderate or severe hepatotoxic events. The mechanism may be direct hepatocyte injury or altered bile composition, but is not yet clearly defined.

Principal Diagnoses

The diagnostic differential of gallbladder diseases includes pancreatitis, peptic ulcer disease, acute hepatitis, and other inflammatory conditions of the abdomen and pelvis such as appendicitis, diverticulitis, and pelvic infections. Table 19-2 displays the history, physical examination, and laboratory findings that assist in distinguishing gallbladder disease from other illnesses.

Symptomatic Gallstones

Most patients with gallstones are asymptomatic. Symptoms can begin, however, when a stone ob-structs the cystic duct or common bile duct. This obstruction creates pressure and distention that cannot be relieved by biliary contractions.

HISTORY AND PHYSICAL EXAMINATION

Patients often present with a history of recurrent bouts of abdominal pain known as biliary colic. They typically complain of right upper quadrant, epigastric, or back pain, described as a severe steady ache or pressure, which can be associated with radiation to the right scapula or shoulder. This "gallbladder attack" usually begins suddenly and lasts 1 to 4 h, is associated with nausea and vomiting, and may cause a residual dull ache for about 24 h. The pain is often nocturnal and may peak around midnight. Although biliary colic is frequently preceded by a fatty meal, it may also occur with a normal meal or after a prolonged fast. Patients with gallstones often complain of epigastric fullness, dyspepsia, or flatulence, but these symptoms are not specific to cholelithiasis.[1]

The physical examination is usually normal, although some patients may have mild to moderate right upper quadrant pain to palpation.

LABORATORY AND DIAGNOSTIC TESTING

No laboratory testing is indicated for the diagnosis of biliary colic because tests, including complete blood counts and liver function tests, are usually normal or nonspecific.

The potential role, advantages, and disadvantages of available diagnostic tests to assess the gallbladder are noted in Table 19-3. Gallbladder ultrasound (GBUS) is the diagnostic test of choice in the evaluation of biliary colic. For diagnosing gallstones as small as 1 to 2 mm, GBUS has a sensitivity of 84 to 97 percent and specificity of 95 to 100 percent; for diagnosing acute cholecystitis, sensitivity is 88 to 94 percent and specificity is 78 to 80 percent.[6] Ultrasound findings of gallstones, sludge, a dilated common bile duct, or a thickened gallbladder wall are indicative of gallbladder disease. The role of other tests will be discussed below.

Table 19-2

Differentiating Features Between Gallbladder Disease, Pancreatitis, Peptic Ulcer Disease, and Hepatitis

	SYMPTOMATIC GALLSTONES	ACUTE CHOLECYSTITIS	PANCREATITIS	PEPTIC ULCER DISEASE	HEPATITIS
HISTORY	1–4 h of RUQ pain preceded by fatty meal Recurrent, nocturnal Nausea ± vomiting Vague gastrointestinal c/o	> 6 h RUQ pain, radiates to back Nausea ± vomiting	Severe, persistent mid-epigastric LUQ pain, radiates to RUQ or back Associated with alcohol use Nausea and vomiting	Aching or burning episodic epigastric pain, may radiate Onset 1–3 h after meals or NSAID usage Relieved with antacids, vomiting, or eating	± RUQ pain Malaise/fatigue Anorexia Dark urine Pruritus
PHYSICAL EXAM	RUQ tenderness	Fever + Murphy's sign RUQ rigidity, guarding ± Palpable gallbladder ± Jaundice	Low-grade fever Abdominal distention Epigastric tenderness Diminished bowel sounds	Epigastric tenderness	Low-grade fever Tender, palpable liver ± Splenomegaly Jaundice
LABORATORY FINDINGS	Normal	↑WBC, 12–15,000 ↑Amylase ↑AST, ALT ±Mildly ↑bilirubin, < 4	↑Amylase ↑Lipase ↑WBC, < 20,000 Mild hypocalcemia	± Guaiac positive stool	Bilirubinuria ↑AST, ALT
RADIOLOGY FINDINGS	Gallstones on U/S	+ HIDA scan or OCG Gallstones, ± dilated bile ducts on U/S	Pleural effusions and/or calcified pancreas on KUB Pseudocysts and/or abscess on U/S or CT ± contrast	Duodenal or stomach ulcer on UGI or endoscopy	None

ABBREVIATIONS: ALT, alanine transaminase; AST, aspartate transaminase; c/o, complaints; CT, computed tomography; HIDA, hepatoiminodiacetic acid; KUB, abdominal series x-rays; LUQ, left upper quadrant; NSAID, nonsteroidal anti-inflammatory drug; OCG, oral cholecystography; RUQ, right upper quadrant; UGI, upper gastrointestinal barium swallow; U/S, ultrasound; WBC, white blood cell count.

Table 19-3

Diagnostic Tests for Gallbladder (GB) Disease

DIAGNOSTIC TEST	POTENTIAL ROLE	ADVANTAGE	DISADVANTAGE
Gallbladder ultrasound (GBUS)	Gallstones Acute cholecystitis Chronic cholecystitis	Noninvasive No preparation No radiation	Not always able to visualize GB
Oral Cholecystogram (OCG)	Gallstones Acute cholecystitis Chronic cholecystitis Acalculous cholecystitis	Gold standard Visualizes GB functioning Useful when unable to visualize GB on ultrasound	Radiation esposure Preparation Fasting state Dye exposure
Plain x-ray	Pigment stones Gangrene and/or perforation Porcelain GB	Visualizes complications of acute cholecystitis	Misses most gallstones
HIDA scan with or w/o cholecystokinin	Acalculous cholecystitis Acute cholecystitis Evaluation of GB empyting	Useful when unable to visualize GB on ultrasound	Radiation exposure IV administration
CT scan	Gallstones Monitoring dissolution therapy	Useful if GBUS and OCG equivocal	Cost Radiation exposure
Endoscopic retrograde cholangio-pancreatogram (ERCP)	Common bile duct stones Other causes of obstruction such as tumors	Visualizes common bile duct stones in absence of dilated ducts Relieve obstruction by sphincterotomy with ERCP Biopsy of tumors	Invasive
Intraoperative transhepatic cholangio-pancreatogram	Common bile duct stones	When ERCP fails	Intraoperative

ABBREVIATION: HIDA, hepatoiminodiacetic acid.

Acute Cholecystitis

HISTORY AND PHYSICAL EXAMINATION

Fever or chills associated with biliary colic is often an indication of acute cholecystitis. Patients may complain of increasing and spreading tenderness across the abdomen over 6 h duration. Anorexia, nausea, and vomiting are common.

Among patients who are in the ICU, especially those who are receiving TPN or mechanical ventilation, these symptoms may represent ACC. This condition occurs in 5 to 10 percent of patients with acute cholecystitis.[4] Half of the cases of ACC can be explained by an underlying condition that will resolve with time.

Physical examination findings of acute cholecystitis classically include tenderness of the right upper quadrant that worsens with deep inspiration (Murphy's sign). An enlarged gallbladder may be palpable in up to 20 percent of patients with acute cholecystitis.[5] Patients may also appear jaundiced.

Empyema and gangrene of the gallbladder are infrequent but serious complications of acute cholecystitis. Patients with empyema present with severe signs of infection including high fever, marked abdominal pain, and a very elevated white blood count. Patients with gangrene of the gallbladder also have more severe symptoms; however, if perforation occurs, the symptoms may suddenly abate only to be followed by signs of generalized peritonitis. These signs include diffuse abdominal pain, rebound tenderness (increasing pain on release of pressure from abdominal palpation), and abdominal muscle rigidity. Bowel sounds will disappear, and signs of shock including hypotension, tachycardia, and oliguria commonly occur.

LABORATORY AND DIAGNOSTIC TESTING

Laboratory tests that may be helpful in differentiating uncomplicated cholecystitis from other diagnoses include white blood cell count, liver enzymes (aspartate transaminase, alanine transaminase), serum amylase, and bilirubin level. The patient with acute cholecystitis usually has a mild leukocytosis (10,000 to 15,000 white cells/mL) with a left shift on differential. Roughly 25 percent of patients have modest elevations in serum transaminases and about 45 percent will have a mild elevation in bilirubin (<5 mg/dL).[1]

Plain abdominal x-ray and abdominal computed tomography (CT) scans have limited usefulness in the diagnosis of gallstones or acute cholecystitis. Roughly 85 percent of gallstones will be missed on plain films.[4] CT scans visualize gallstones over 80 percent of the time but cost twice as much as GBUS.[5] The diagnosis of gangrene, however, can be made on plain films; air-fluid levels (from gas-forming bacterial organisms) are seen in the biliary tree or gallbladder. In addition, when peritonitis is suspected, plain films may reveal dilated large and small loops of bowel with edema of the small-bowel wall.

In the patient with acute cholecystitis, GBUS is the diagnostic test of choice, and gallstones are usually visualized (90 to 95 percent of cases) (Fig. 19-1). An additional advantage of GBUS is that scanning of the liver, bile ducts, and pancreas can be accomplished simultaneously.[1]

The oral cholecystogram has been largely replaced by GBUS. However, it is the preferred test when ultrasound is limited or when acalculous disease is suspected. For this test, the patient receives 3 g iopanoic acid after dinner and fasts overnight; films are taken the next morning. If necessary, this is repeated. A single dose of contrast will visualize the gallbladder in up to 75 percent of patients, and a second dose will visualize an additional 15 percent.[5] Liver and gastrointestinal diseases that interfere with the absorption of the iopanoic acid

Figure 19-1

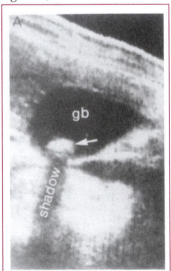

Ultrasound of gallbladder with solitary stone visualized. *(Reproduced with permission from AS Fauci et al, eds: Harrison's Principles of Internal Medicine, 14th ed. New York, McGraw-Hill, 1998.)*

will cause false-positive tests. The reported false-positive rate is 4 percent and the false-negative rate is 10 percent.[6]

Patients with gallbladder symptoms who do not have gallstones on ultrasound or cholecystography may benefit from scintiscanning with hepatic 2,6-dimethyliminodiacetic acid (HIDA) or other similar agents. Cholescintigraphy evaluates gallbladder function in response to a meal or cholecystokinin (CCK), the hormone that stimulates gallbladder contraction, after injection with radioactive organic anions that are taken up by hepatocytes and selectively secreted into the biliary system. Abnormal cholescintigraphy may predict which patients with biliary symptoms without gallstones will benefit from surgery.[47] HIDA scanning with CCK has a sensitivity of 97 percent and specificity of 90 percent.[5] Obstruction of the common bile duct results in nonvisualization.

Acalculous cholecystitis is diagnosed by finding a tense gallbladder without stones, with or without sludge, and poor emptying and motility on either oral cholecystogram or HIDA scanning.

Endoscopic retrograde cholangiopancreatography (ERCP) is useful in finding common bile duct stones in the absence of a dilated duct. It is often used as an adjunct to laparoscopic cholecystectomy. Intraoperative transhepatic cholangiopancreatogram is useful when ERCP fails.[48]

Figure 19-2 presents an algorithm for the work-up and management of patients with biliary colic who present in the primary care setting. Initial decision-making is often based on the presence of fever to differentiate between symptomatic gallstones and acute cholecystitis.

Gallbladder Cancer

HISTORY AND PHYSICAL EXAMINATION

Most patients ultimately diagnosed with gallbladder cancer present with a clinical picture similar to those with benign gallbladder disease. In an epidemiologic study in Chile of all cases of gallbladder cancer diagnosed between January 1987 and December 1990, investigators found that more

than 95 percent of the cases were diagnosed preoperatively as having either symptomatic gallstones or cholecystitis.[49] The majority of patients with gallbladder cancer report right upper quadrant pain that may be intermittent or continuous.[50] Some patients report a change in the character of the pain from intermittent to constant. Common symptoms and signs of gallbladder cancer are listed in Table 19-4. The most common reported symptoms are pain or tenderness, weight loss, anorexia, nausea, and vomiting. The most common signs are hepatomegaly and jaundice. A palpable mass is present in 24 to 40 percent of patients.

LABORATORY AND DIAGNOSTIC TESTING

The results of laboratory tests are nonspecific and may reveal anemia, elevation of liver function tests, and leukocytosis. Plain abdominal film may be used to diagnose a porcelain gallbladder; the gallbladder will appear as a halo-type outline. Findings on GBUS depend on the stage of the disease;

Table 19-4

Common Signs and Symptoms in Cancer of the Biliary System

	PERCENTAGE OF PATIENTS WITH GALLBLADDER CANCER
Pain and/or tenderness	52–97
Weight loss	44–77
Hepatomegaly	34–65
Anorexia	33–52
Jaundice	40–54
Nausea and vomiting	8–64
Palpable gallbladder or right upper quadrant mass	24–40
Fatty food intolerance	20–33
Chills and/or fever	12–20
Ascites	10–13
Diarrhea	<10
Other	<10

SOURCE: Adapted with permission from J Ahlgren: Neoplasms of the hepatobiliary tract: *Medical Oncology*, 2nd ed. New York, McGraw-Hill, 1993.

Figure 19-2

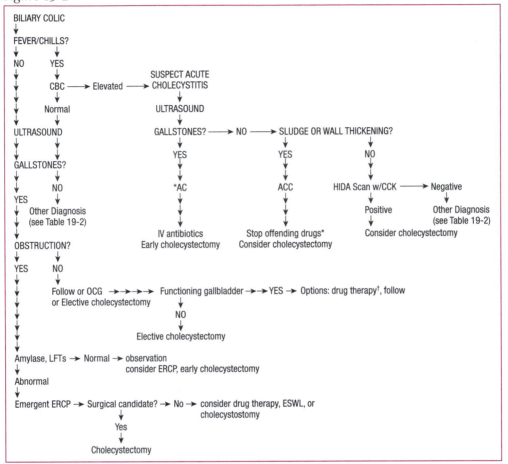

Decision-tree for the work-up of biliary colic.

Abbreviations: *AC, acute calculous cholecystitis; ACC, acalculous cholecystitis; CBC, complete blood count; CCK, cholecytokinin (stimulates gallbladder contraction); Dx, diagnosis; HIDA, hepatic dimethyliminodiacetic acid; ERCP, endoscopic retrograde cholagiopancreatography; ESWL, extracorporeal shock wave lithotripsy; LFTs, liver function tests; OCG, oral cholecystogram.

†Best results in nonobese women with small, floating, radiolucent stones.

early disease may present as focal asymmetric gallbladder wall thickening, whereas more advanced disease may be associated with invasion of the biliary tree, with associated dilation of the cystic or common bile duct. CT scanning is often used to further investigate direct local extension of the tumor or to detect the presence of liver metastases. Gallbladder cancer is not usually suspected preoperatively and is only identified following histologic evaluation of the surgical specimen.

Treatment

Prevention

Primary prevention may be possible for patients at high risk, but to date, no studies have proven a reduced incidence of gallbladder disease by modifying risk factors.

DIET

Dietary changes for primary prevention of gallstone disease are still theoretical. Unfortunately, no dietary recommendations are known to prevent either the formation of gallstones or the conversion of asymptomatic gallstones to symptomatic disease. High-fiber diets could theoretically prevent gallstone formation by increasing intestinal motility, which decreases the deoxycholate substrate available to the liver for conversion to cholesterol. However, according to a Scandinavian review, among patients who had successful gallstone dissolution therapy, placement on fiber-rich diets did not reduce the recurrence rate.[51] Smaller but more frequent meal intervals could reduce bile storage in the gallbladder.

Everhart reviewed obesity and weight loss with regard to gallstone disease and reported three interesting findings: (1) gallstone disease risk is reduced during dieting for those who avoid prolonged fasting, (2) animal studies show reduced nucleation of supersaturated bile in low saturated fatty acid diets, and (3) in humans, restricting dietary fat and cholesterol is of no benefit in asymptomatic patients.[52] In the Ulm (Germany) Gallstone Study of 1116 blood donors who underwent GBUS, however, no vegetarians in the study were found to have gallstone disease (N = 48).[53]

VITAMIN C

Vitamin C supplementation has theoretical benefits in the prevention of gallstone disease because it is required for cholesterol catabolism. Data on women from the Heart and Estrogen-Progestin Replacement Study (HERS) research group showed vitamin C supplementation was associated with a reduced prevalence of gallstones (OR = 0.5, 95 percent CI 0.31 to 0.81) and cholecystectomy (OR = 0.38, 95 percent CI 0.21 to 0.67), but only in association with any alcohol consumption.[54] Nondrinkers did not appear to benefit from vitamin C. Data reported from NHANES II (1976–1980) of 20,000 Americans, showed that a high serum ascorbic acid level correlated with an approximately 50 percent lower prevalence of gallbladder disease in women, although the quantity used by the subjects is not reported.[25] Other antioxidants may play a role, but the data are insufficient to support general recommendations for supplementation with antioxidants other than vitamin C.

EXERCISE

Exercise, at least in men, is proven to reduce the risk of symptomatic gallstones. A large prospective cohort study of American male health professionals, followed from 1986 to 1994, found increased physical activity was inversely related to the risk of symptomatic gallstones. Physically active men under age 65 had a relative risk of 0.58 (CI = 0.44 to 0.78), and physically active men over age 65 had a relative risk of 0.75 (CI = 0.52 to 1.09).[26] These investigators estimate that 34 percent of cases of symptomatic gallstones in men could be prevented by endurance-type exercise of just 30 min, five times per week. Although encouraging, these data may not extrapolate to women.

PREVENTING GALLBLADDER CANCER

Gallbladder cancer may be a preventable disease. Among patients who are at high risk of gallbladder cancer (Chilean or Native American women), early diagnosis of the precursors to cancer such as gallstones, gallbladder polyps, and chronic gallbladder inflammation, combined with cholecystectomy, could greatly reduce cancer risk. Gallbladder dysplasia takes an estimated 15 years to develop into neoplasia,[49] and screening these patients with GBUS may be indicated. Cholecystectomy for patients with adenomatous polyps or porcelain gallbladder to prevent gallbladder cancer is clearly warranted.

Asymptomatic Gallstones

Less than 33 percent of individuals with asymptomatic gallstones will ever develop symptoms,[1,2] and only about 3 percent (most following warning signs) develop complications such as acute cholecystitis, pancreatitis, or obstructive jaundice.[3] Based on these data, prophylactic cholecystectomy for asymptomatic gallstones is not generally recommended.

Prophylactic cholecystectomy is recommended in certain high-risk patients with gallstones, including Chilean women, Native Americans, and those with polyps, porcelain gallbladder, and implanted hepatic artery infusion pumps. In addition, gallstones in children are more likely to be symptomatic, and the gallbladder should be removed.[55]

Symptomatic Gallstones

Although avoiding fat-rich meals may reduce the recurrence of symptoms for patients with gallstones and biliary colic, most authors recommend more definitive treatment for these patients. The preferred treatment for patients with recurrent episodes of symptomatic gallstones, in the absence of complications, is elective surgery. Expectant management is reasonable for those who are at high risk for a surgical procedure. Without surgery, however, 50 percent will experience recurrence of symptoms within 5 years.[5]

SURGERY

Cholecystectomy reduces the morbidity and mortality risk from complications of untreated symptomatic gallstone disease such as acute cholecystitis, pancreatitis, and cancer. Evidence from mortality trends reported from 1955 to 1990 supports this conclusion; mortality from gallbladder disease in North America dropped by 70 percent for men and 80 percent for women in conjunction with increased use of surgery.[56]

Open cholecystectomy has been replaced by laparoscopic cholecystectomy as the surgical procedure of choice because of reduced mortality, morbidity, hospital length of stay, and readmission rates associated with the laparoscopic approach. This is true even among patients over age 60.[57]

Following the rise in the use of the laparoscopic technique, the perioperative mortality rate dropped from 1.4 percent (1989) to 0.3 to 0.6 percent (1991–1992). The mortality rate is significantly reduced in the elderly as well.[58] In Maryland, between 1989 and 1992, risk of mortality dropped 33 percent per procedure.[59]

Laparoscopic cholecystectomy also offers the most definitive relief of symptoms.[5] Data collated from multiple studies involving over 4000 patients revealed several key points: complications from laparoscopic cholecystectomy occur in about 4 percent, conversion to open cholecystectomy occurs in about 5 percent, mortality is low (<0.1 percent), and bile duct injuries and retained stones occur in less than 5 percent.[1] Early postoperative complications include atelectasis, bleeding, infection, and thromboembolism.

Beyond the immediate postoperative period, cholecystectomy appears to be very successful with near total or complete resolution of symptoms in 75 to 90 percent.[1] However, postoperative symptoms can persist. A prospective analysis of 92 patients followed for over 2 years found abdominal pain continued in 30 percent of patients.[60] Most symptoms (e.g., abdominal bloating, dyspepsia, heartburn, fat intolerance, nausea, and vomiting) significantly improved after cholecystectomy. Diarrhea, constipation, and excessive flatus did not significantly improve. A multicenter questionnaire study asked about symptoms 5 to 10 years after cholecystectomy and found that more women had abdominal pain or dyspepsia than men (42 versus 29 percent, $P = 0.01$), but 93 percent had improved overall or were cured.[61] Persistent gastrointestinal symptoms may indicate another underlying condition such as peptic ulcer disease or gastroesophageal reflux.

MEDICATIONS

Drug therapy should be reserved for patients who refuse surgery or who cannot undergo cholecystectomy for medical reasons. This is due to the low efficacy of treatment, both immediately and in the long term. Dissolution therapy can be accomplished with either ursodeoxycholic acid (UDCA) or methyl *tert*-butyl ether (MTBE) (Table 19-5). Following treatment with either agent, gallstones recur in 50 percent of patients within 5 years of completed dissolution therapy.[62] Recurrence rates are higher with multiple stones and for patients over age 50.

URSODEOXYCHOLIC ACID   UDCA is an oral medication taken for months to years. It has few side effects, results in about 50 percent dissolution in 2 years, and is useful in patients with small (<2 cm diameter), radiolucent stones.[62] Ideal candidates for UDCA treatment are women who refuse therapy and who are thin, have stones smaller than 1.5 cm in diameter, floating stones as visualized by oral cholecystography, or stones of low density on CT scan and a functioning gallbladder. Among obese patients on weight loss plans that include very-low-calorie diets, UDCA has been shown to prevent the formation of gallstones.[55] It should also be considered in the treatment of patients with recurrent stones in the common bile duct after cholecystectomy.

METHYL *TERT*-BUTYL ETHER   Contact dissolution with MTBE works rapidly and has greater effectiveness than UDCA, at least in the short-term. MTBE dissolves any size cholesterol gallstone that is not CT dense and leaves behind innocuous debris.[63] The goal of MTBE therapy is complete dissolution of all fragments to prevent recurrence. It is a safe treatment but requires an interventional radiologist to insert a percutaneous transhepatic catheter to deliver the medication directly into the gall-

Table 19-5

Dissolution Therapy for Gallstones

	URSODEOXYCHOLIC ACID (UDCA)	**METHYL *TERT*-BUTYL ETHER (MTBE)**
DESCRIPTION	Bile Acid	Cholesterol solvent
INDICATION	Radiolucent, noncalcified gallstones < 2 cm diameter, mild-moderate symptoms	Any size and number of low-density cholesterol gallstones on computed tomography
DOSE	8–10 mg/kg/d divided 2–3 doses/d, available as 300-mg tablet	Continuous infusion and aspiration at 4–6 cycles/min
DURATION	Months to years	4–30 h
COST	$200–250/100 tablets*	Approximately $70 for 4 L*
SIDE EFFECTS	Diarrhea	Perforation
		Pain, fever, nausea/vomiting
PREGNANCY CATEGORY	B	Safety not known
COMMENTS	Useful in poor surgical candidates and obese patients who are on weight loss regimens	Not available at most hospitals
		Invasive
EFFICACY	50% dissolution within 2 y	70% dissolution within 6–7 h
RECURRENCE	50% recurrence within 5 y	50% recurrence within 5 y
FOLLOW-UP	Ultrasound q 6 mo until dissolved	Unknown
	Continue 1–3 mo, repeat ultrasound, and stop if no recurrence	

*Cost to pharmacy; for MTBE does not include cost of preparation for use or physician costs.

bladder. The medication is continuously infused and aspirated four to six cycles per minute to achieve dissolution. Treatment lasts an average of 6 h for a solitary stone (range, 4 to 23 h) and 7 h for multiple stones (range, 4 to 30 h). This procedure risks perforation; of 25 patients in one consecutive series, 1 patient required urgent cholecystectomy due to bile peritonitis and 1 patient required surgery later for symptomatic recurrence.[62] Complete dissolution was achieved in 18 of 25 (72 percent), but 4 (22 percent) had recurrence within a year and a half.

Regular follow-up ultrasound examinations should be undertaken after gallstone dissolution, but data are lacking on the optimal interval. Continuous postdissolution treatment is not justified due to cost.[64]

PROSTAGLANDIN INHIBITORS   Prostaglandin inhibitors such as indomethacin and other nonsteroidal anti-inflammatory drugs (NSAIDs) may play a role in prevention of gallstone formation and relief of biliary colic.[65] Limited evidence for the efficacy of this treatment, however, precludes recommendations.

OTHER MEDICATIONS   Other medications have been investigated, but none appear to offer significant advantages. In patients with diabetes, abnormal gallbladder motility may be treatable with the D_2-dopamine receptor antagonist levosulpiride.[66] However, because asymptomatic disease does not require treatment, this should be considered experimental and of questionable usefulness. Cisapride showed promise, in animal studies, on gallbladder motility, but in humans it did not alleviate dyspeptic symptoms despite improved gallbladder kinetics.[67]

Cholecystitis

Options in the management of patients with cholecystitis primarily include stabilization and surgery. Elective surgery is preferable to emergency surgery because of the reduced risk of complications.

STABILIZATION

Acutely ill patients benefit from hospitalization and symptomatic treatment until stabilization; treatment includes intravenous rehydration, repair of electrolyte abnormalities, elimination of oral intake, and nasogastric suction for patients who are experiencing vomiting. Intravenous antibiotics are usually initiated to cover Enterobacteriaceae (68 percent), Enterococci (14 percent), Bacteroides (10 percent), and *Clostridium* spp. (7 percent).[68] Suggested agents include an antipseudomonal β-lactamase-susceptible penicillin with or without metronidazole, or ampicillin and gentamicin with or without metronidazole, or imipenem cilistatin (Primaxin®), or meropenem, or ticarcillin/clavulanate (Timentin®), or piperacillin-tazobactam, or ampicillin/subactam (Unasyn®).[68]

Pain control can usually be achieved with meperidine (Demerol®) or pentazocine (Talwin®). These agents are preferred over morphine because morphine may be more likely to produce spasm of the sphincter of Oddi.[1]

Some patients require ERCP for stone removal of an obstructing stone and/or cholecystostomy with drainage; the latter is often necessary for patients with empyema of the gallbladder who may not respond to antibiotics alone and for debilitated patients for whom surgery may pose an unacceptable risk.

Remission of acute symptoms within 2 to 7 days can be expected in approximately 75 percent of patients treated medically.[1] Complications of cholecystitis including empyema, gangrene, or perforation may require emergency surgical intervention with appropriate antibiotic coverage.

SURGERY

Early surgical intervention, often within days of the acute attack, is recommended. The timing of cholecystectomy in acute cholecystitis was evaluated prospectively in a randomized study of 99 patients, conducted in China. The investigators found that initial conservative treatment followed by delayed interval surgery did not reduce morbidity or the conversion rate to open chole-cystectomy.[69] In fact, delayed surgery led to a longer hospital stay (11 versus 6 days, $P < 0.001$) and a longer recovery period (19 versus 12 days, $P < 0.001$).

Delayed surgery may be indicated, however, for patients who have comorbid illnesses that impose an unacceptable risk for surgery and for those in whom the diagnosis of acute cholecystitis is in doubt.[1]

MEDICATION

Prostaglandin inhibitors such as indomethacin and other NSAIDs may play a role in patients with acute cholecystitis as well. Indomethacin given to patients twice daily rectally for acute cholecystitis significantly reduced gallbladder volume and pain after 48 h in one small study in Venezuela.[70] Because of limited evidence for the efficacy of this treatment, recommendations cannot be offered.

Gallbladder Cancer

The prognosis for gallbladder cancer when diagnosed as an incidental finding at the time of cholecystectomy is excellent, with over 95 percent survival. Unfortunately for patients presenting with symptoms more typical of cancer (e.g., weight loss, anorexia), over 75 percent of gallbladder carcinomas are unresectable at the time of diagnosis.[1] Ninety-five percent of these patients will die within the first year. None of the current treatments including radical surgery, radiation, and chemotherapy appear to improve survival.

Gallbladder Disease During Pregnancy

Cholecystectomy appears to be safe in pregnancy, but data are limited. In a retrospective study of five pregnant women in Puerto Rico, laparoscopic cholecystectomy performed in the setting of complicated gallbladder disease did not result in complications for the mother or fetus in any of the cases.[71] These results are supported by a retrospective case series, from 1986 to 1993 in North Carolina, of 19 pregnant women (4 in the first trimester, 10 in the second, and 5 in the third) in whom conservative treatment for symptomatic gallstones failed and who required surgical resection with either open or laparoscopic technique. All of the women did well in the immediate postoperative period, only 4 required tocolysis, and the 2 patients who delivered prematurely did so 10 and 15 weeks following surgery.[72] These authors conclude that cholecystectomy should be considered primary management of symptomatic gallstones in pregnancy. However, this conclusion is based on retrospective studies of a small number of women who had complicated cholecystitis. Conservative treatment and delayed surgery is the standard of care in women with uncomplicated symptomatic gallstones and will likely remain so until stronger evidence is reported.

Alternative Approaches

Little information has been published on alternative therapies for the management of gallbladder disease. Percutaneous techniques for acute cholecystitis or common bile duct obstruction previously had a role in the management of high-risk patients, but have largely been replaced by laparoscopic cholecystectomy.[73] In one study, diagnostic percutaneous gallbladder puncture and cholecystostomy was successful in 125 of 127 patients. Major complications such as peritonitis, bleeding, hypotension, and adult respiratory distress occurred in 8.7 percent, minor complications occurred in 3.9 percent, and 3.1 percent (N = 4) died as a result of an underlying condition.[74]

Biliary extracorporeal shockwave lithotripsy (ESWL) is an alternative approach to standard treatment. A Japanese study comparing 15 patients with CT-lucent stones and 18 patients with dense calcified stones found all 5 patients with stones under 1 cm diameter cleared with ESWL regardless of density.[75] Larger stones that are CT-lucent completely cleared 93 percent of the time, but denser stones only cleared 64 percent of the time. A prospective 4-year study of 280 patients with symptomatic gallstones achieved fragmentation in 81 percent; of these, 66.4 percent achieved stone clearance within 12 months.[76] An average of 2.1 ESWL sessions were required per patient, 68 percent required analgesia during therapy, and 31.4 percent experienced side effects (such as colic) after treatment. Severe complications (e.g., impacted fragments in the ampulla of Vater followed by pancreatitis) occurred in 7 patients (2.5 percent); all required urgent endoscopic sphincterotomy. Four patients (1.4 percent) required emergency cholecystectomy within 4 weeks of ESWL, and another 16 (5.7 percent) had elective cholecystectomy; no patient died. These authors conclude that biliary ESWL is not recommended for patients with stones larger than 3 cm or volume of 14 cm^3 size because of the high rate of complications associated with large fragment volume. ESWL is not currently approved by the U.S. Food and Drug Administration (FDA) for the treatment of gallstones.

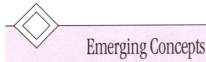

Emerging Concepts

Improved Surgical Techniques

Laparoscopic cholecystectomy is the current preferred surgical technique, but it requires air to be pumped into the peritoneal cavity to create the operating field. This pneumoperitoneum is associated with cardiopulmonary side effects such as reduced lung volume and abnormal heart rhythms. An electric-powered abdominal wall lifter that raises the abdominal wall to create the operating field may prove useful in the future as an alternative to pneumoperitoneum during laparoscopic cholecystectomy. A small study found the technique successful in 16 of 20 patients (80 percent).[77] This technique has the advantage of allowing the

surgeon to directly palpate the abdominal organs rather than to rely solely on visualization, as with the current technique.

Diagnostic Strategies

Diagnostic fine-needle puncture of the gallbladder for biliary lipid analysis and nucleation time may be an adjunct to ultrasonography in the future. In a study of 207 patients with gallstones, ultrasound-guided bile aspiration performed under local anesthesia with a 22-gauge needle was safe, quick, and without major side effects such as bleeding, bile leakage, or acute inflammation.[78] Infection was identified in 10.1 percent. Minor side effects were experienced; 11.6 percent of patients reported mild abdominal symptoms, 3.4 percent required analgesia, and 1.0 percent had biliary colic. One patient went on to elective cholecystectomy. With this technique, the authors found that patients with a solitary stone had significantly longer nucleation times than those with multiple stones but that lipid indices and the presence of infection did not correlate with the number of stones. The predictive accuracy of this procedure in identifying those who will develop symptoms has yet to be determined.

New Treatments

Thermal ablation by means of injection of hot contrast media into the gallbladder has been studied in dogs. This procedure resulted in 11 of 13 animals undergoing successful ablation.[79] Two of the dogs were killed prematurely at 8 and 17 days due to bile leakage and gallbladder rupture, respectively. Future directions for this technique are speculative, but this appears to be a potential option for those unable or unwilling to undergo cholecystectomy. Human research using this technique has not yet been reported.

The role of NSAIDs in the treatment of acute gallbladder pain has yet to be adequately researched but has potential for short-term relief. The role of infection in gallbladder cancer is currently being actively researched because this may be a treatable environmental condition causing high cancer rates in areas such as Chile.

References

1. Greenberger NS, Isselbacher KJ: Diseases of the gallbladder and bile ducts. In: Fauci AS, Braunwald E, Isselbacher KJ, et al (eds): *Harrison's Principles of Internal Medicine*, 14th ed. New York: McGraw-Hill; 1998; 1725.

2. Zubler J, Markowski G, Yale S, et al: Natural history of asymptomatic gallstones in family practice office practice. *Arch Family Med* 7:230, 1998.

3. Gracie WA, Ransohoff DF: The natural history of silent gallstones: the innocent gallstone is not a myth. *N Engl J Med* 307:798, 1982.

4. Mezey E, Bender JS: Diseases of the biliary tract. In: Barker LR, Burton JR, Zieve PD (eds): *Principles of Ambulatory Medicine*, 4th ed. Baltimore: Williams & Wilkins; 1995:1333.

5. Moscati, RM: Cholelithiasis, cholecystitis and pancreatitis. *Emerg Med Clin N Am* 14:719, 1996.

6. Tavani A, Megri E, La Vecchia C: Biliary tract tumors. *Annali dell Instituto Superiore di Sanita* 32:615, 1996.

7. Fox, JG, Dewhirst FE, Shen Z, et al: Hepatic *Helicobacter* species identified in bile and gallbladder tissue from Chileans with chronic cholecystitis. *Gastroenterology* 114:755, 1998.

8. Lowenfels AB, Lindstrom CG, Conway MJ, Hastings PR: Gallstones and the risk of gallbladder cancer. *J Natl Cancer Inst* 75:77, 1985.

9. Csendes A, Becerra M, Burdiles P, et al: Bacteriological studies of bile from the gallbladder in patients with carcinoma of the gallbladder, cholelithiasis, common bile duct stones and no gallstones disease. *Eur J Surg* 160:363, 1994.

10. Farinon AM, Pacella A, Cetta F, Sianesi M: Adenomatous polyps of the gallbladder. *Hepatobiliary Surgery* 3:251, 1991.

11. Andersen T: Liver and gallbladder disease before and after very-low-calorie diets. *Am J Clin Nutr* 56:235S, 1992.

12. Tierney S, Pitt HA, Lillemoe KD: Physiology and pathophysiology of gallbladder motility. *Surg Clin N Am* 73:1267, 1993.

13. Hanis CL, Hewett-Emmett D, Kubrusly LF, et al: An ultrasound survey of gallbladder disease among Mexican Americans in Starr County, Texas: frequencies and risk factors. *Ethnic Diseases* 3:32, 1993.

14. Hopper KD, Landis R, Meilstrup J, et al: The prevalence of asymptomatic gallstones in the general population. *Invest Radiol* 26:939, 1991.

15. Chapman BA, Wilson IR, Frampton CM, et al: Prevalence of gallbladder disease in diabetes mellitus. *Dig DisSci* 41:2222, 1996.

16. Everson GT: Pregnancy and gallstones. *Hepatology* 17:159, 1993.

17. Valdivieso V, Covarrubias C, Siegel F, et al: Pregnancy and cholelithiasis: pathogenesis and natural course of gallstones diagnosed in early puerperium. *Hepatology* 17:1, 1993.

18. Dickerman JL: Gallbladder disease and coronary artery disease: is there a link? *J Am Osteopath Assoc* 91:359, 1991.

19. Kuller LH: Dietary fat and chronic diseases: epidemiologic overview. *J Am Dietary Assoc* 97:S9, 1997.

20. Yang H, Petersen GM, Roth MP, et al: Risk factors for gallstone formation during rapid weight loss. *Dig Dis Sci* 37:912, 1992.

21. Vezina WC, Grace DM, Hutton LC, et al: Similarity in gallstone formation from 900-kcal/day diets containing 16 g vs 30 g of daily fat. *Dig Dis Sci* 43:554, 1998.

22. McMichael AJ, Baghurst PA, Scragg RK: A case-control study of smoking and gallbladder disease: importance of examining time relations. *Epidemiology* 3:519, 1992.

23. Mohr GC, Kritz-Silverstein D, Barrettt-Conner E: Plasma lipids and gallbladder disease. *Am J Epidemiol* 134:78, 1991.

24. Benvegnu L, Noventa F, Chemello L, et al: Prevalence and incidence of cholecystolithiasis in cirrhosis and relation to the etiology of liver disease. *Digestion* 58:293, 1997.

25. Simon JA, Hudes ES: Serum ascorbic acid and other correlates of gallbladder disease among U.S. adults. *Am J Public Health* 88:1208, 1998.

26. Leitzmann MF, Giovannucci EL, Rimm EB, et al: The relation of physical activity to risk for symptomatic gallstone disease in men. *Ann Intern Med* 128:417, 1998.

27. Jung RT: Obesity as a disease. *Br Med Bull* 53:307, 1997.

28. Stampfer MJ, Maclure KM, Colditz GA, et al: Risk of symptomatic gallstones in women with severe obesity. *Am J Clin Nutr* 55:652, 1992.

29. Haffner SM, Diehl AK, Valdez R, et al: Clinical gallbladder disease in NIDDM subjects. Relationship to duration of diabetes and severity of glycemia. *Diabetes Care* 16:1276, 1993.

30. Persson GE, Thulin AJG: Prevalence of gallstone disease in patients with diabetes mellitus. *Eur J Surg* 157:579, 1991.

31. Jebbink MC, Heijerman HG, Masclee AA, et al: Gallbladder disease in cystic fibrosis. *Neth J Med* 41:123, 1992.

32. Molenat F, Boussuges A, Valantin V, et al: Gallbladder abnormalities in medical ICU patients: an ultrasonographic study. *Intensive Care Med* 22:356, 1996.

33. Thijs C, Knipschild P: Oral contraceptives and the risk of gallbladder disease: a meta-analysis. *Am J Public Health* 83:1113, 1993.

34. Vessey M, Painter R: Oral contraceptive use and benign gallbladder disease; revisited. *Contraception* 50:167, 1994.

35. Michielsen PP, Fierens H, Van Maercke YM: Drug-induced gallbladder disease: incidence, etiology and management. *Drug Safety* 7:32, 1992.

36. La Vecchia C, Negri E, D'Avanzo B, et al: Oral contraceptives and non-contraceptive oestrogens in the risk of gallstone disease requiring surgery. *J Epidemiol Community Health* 46:234, 1992.

37. Hulley S, Grady D, Bush T, et al: Randomized trial of estrogen plus progestin for secondary prevention of coronary heart disease in postmenopausal women. *JAMA* 280:605, 1998.

38. Rosenberg L, Shapiro S, Slone D, et al: Thiazides and acute cholecystitis. *N Engl J Med* 303:546, 1980.

39. Shiffman ML, Keith FB, Moore EW: Pathogenesis of ceftriaxone-associated biliary sludge. In vitro studies of calcium-ceftriaxone binding and solubility. *Gastroenterology* 99:1772, 1990.

40. Schaad UB, Wedgewood-Krucko J, Tschaeppeler H: Reversible ceftriaxone-associated biliary pseudolithiasis in children. *Lancet* 2:1411, 1989.

41. Parry SW, Pelias ME, Browder W: Acalculous hypersensitivity cholecystitis: hypothesis of a new clinicopathologic entity. *Surgery* 104:911, 1988.

42. Pietrafitta JJ, Anderson BG, O'Brien MJ, et al: Cholecystitis secondary to infusion chemotherapy. *J Surg Oncol* 31:287, 1986.

43. Ottery FD, Scupham RK, Weese JL: Chemical cholecystitis after intrahepatic chemotherapy. The case for prophylactic cholecystectomy during pump placement. *Dis Colon Rectum* 29:187, 1986.

44. Ho KY, Weissberger AJ, Marbach P, et al: Therapeutic efficacy of the somatostatin analog SMS 201-995 (octreotide) in acromegaly. Effects of dose and frequency and long-term safety. *Ann Intern Med* 112:173, 1990.

45. Spes CH, Angermann CE, Beyer RW, et al: Increased incidence of cholelithiasis in heart transplant recipients receiving cyclosporin therapy. *J Heart Transplant* 9:404, 1990.

46. Lorber MI, Van Buren CT, Flechner SM, et al: Hepatobiliary and pancreatic complications of cyclosporin therapy in 466 renal transplant recipients. *Transplantation* 43:35, 1987.

47. Kloiber R, Molnar CP, Shaffer EA: Chronic biliary-type pain in the absence of gallstones: the value of cholecystokinin cholescintigraphy. *AJR Am J Roentgenol* 159:509, 1992.

48. Goldbert HI: Imaging of the biliary tract. *Curr Opin Radiol* 4:62, 1992.

49. Roa I, Araya JC, Villaseca M, et al: Preneoplastic lesions and gallbladder cancer: an estimate of the period required for progression. *Gastroenterology* 111:232, 1996.

50. Ahlgren J: Neoplasms of the hepatobiliary tract. *Medical Oncology*, 2nd ed. New York: McGraw-Hill, 1993:710.

51. VanBerge HGP, Portincasa P, vanErpecum KJ: Effect of lactulose and fiber-rich diets in relation to gallstone disease. *Scand J Gastroenterol* 222:68, 1997.

52. Everhart JE: Contributions of obesity and weight loss to gallstone disease. *Ann Intern Med* 119:1029, 1993.

53. Kratzer W, Kachele V, Mason RA, et al: Gallstone prevalence in relation to smoking, alcohol, coffee consumption, and nutrition. The Ulm gallstone study. *Scand J Gastroenterol* 32:953, 1997.

54. Simon JA, Grady D, Snabes MC, et al: Ascorbic acid supplement use and the prevalence of gallbladder disease. Heart and Estrogen-Progestin Replacement Study (HERS) Research Group. *J Clin Epidemiol* 51:257, 1998.

55. Pokorny WJ, Saleem M, O'Gorman RB, et al: Cholelithiasis and cholecystitis in childhood. *Am J Surg* 148:742, 1984.

56. La Vecchia C, Levi F, Lucchini F, et al: Trends in mortality from non-neoplastic gallbladder disease. *Ann Epidemiol* 5:215, 1994.

57. Mayol J, Martinez-Sarmiento J, Tamayo FJ, et al: Complications of laparoscopic cholecystectomy in the aging patient. *Age Aging* 26:77, 1997.

58. Feldman MG, Russell JC, Lynch JT, et al: Comparison of mortality rates for open and closed cholecystectomy in the elderly: Connecticut statewide survey. *J Laparoendosc Surg* 4:165, 1994.

59. Steiner CA, Bass EB, Talamini MA, et al: Surgical rates and operative mortality for open and laparoscopic cholecystectomy in Maryland. *N Engl J Med* 330:403, 1994.

60. Gui GP, Cheruvu CV, West N, et al: Is cholecystectomy effective treatment for symptomatic gallstones? Clinical outcomes after long-term follow-up. *Ann R Coll Surg* 80:25, 1998.

61. Middlefart HV, Kristensen JU, Laursen CN, et al: Pain and dyspepsia after elective and acute cholecystectomy. *Scand J Gastroenterol* 33:10, 1998.

62. Schoenfield LJ, Marks JW: Oral and contact dissolution of gallstones. *Am J Surg* 165:427, 1993.

63. McNulty J, et al: Dissolution of cholesterol gallstones using methyl *tert*butyl ether: a safe effective treatment. *Gut* 32:1550, 1991.

64. Fachbereich G, Deutsche KD, Wiesbaden BD: Prevention of recurrence after successful gallstone dissolution. *Z Gastroenterol* 29:301, 1991.

65. Babb RR: Managing gallbladder disease with prostaglandin inhibitors. *Postgrad Med* 94:127, 1993.

66. Mansi C, Savrino V, Vigneri S, et al: Effect of D2-dopamine receptor antagonist levosulpiride on diabetic cholecystoparesis: a double-blind crossover study. *Aliment Pharmacol Ther* 9:185, 1995.

67. Marzio L, DiFelice F, Laico MG, et al: Gallbladder hypokinesia and normal gastric emptying of liquids in patients with dyspeptic symptoms. A double-blind placebo-controlled clinical trial with cisapride. *Dig Dis Sci* 37:262, 1992.

68. Gilbert DN, Moellering RC, Sande MA: *The Sanford Guide to Antimicrobial Therapy 1998*, 28th ed. Hyde Park, VA: Antimicrobial Therapy; 1998.

69. Lo CM, Liu CL, Fan ST, et al: Prospective randomized study of early versus delayed laparoscopic cholecystectomy for acute cholecystitis. *Ann Surg* 227:461, 1998.

70. Anez MS, Martinez D, Pacheco JL, et al: Indomethacin in the treatment of acute cholecystitis and biliary colic. *GEN* 45:32, 1991.

71. Reyes TR: Laparoscopic cholecystectomy in pregnancy. *Bol Asoc Med P R* 89:9, 1997.

72. Davis A, Katz VL, Cox R: Gallbladder disease in pregnancy. *J Reprod Med* 40:759, 1995.

73. Cheslyn-Curtis S, Lees WR, Hatfield AR, et al: Percutaneous techniques for the management of symptomatic gallbladder stones. *Dig Dis* 10:208, 1992.

74. vanSonnenberg E, D'Agnostine HB, Goodacre BW, et al: Percutaneous gallbladder puncture and cholecystostomy: results, complications and caveats for safety. *Radiology* 183:167, 1992.

75. Mori T, Shimono K, Moriyama S, et al: The efficacy of extracorporeal shock wave lithotripsy on single dense calcified gallstones according to computed tomography. *Surg Today* 23:387, 1993.

76. Schreiber F, Steindorfer P, Pristautz H, et al: Complications and surgical interventions during 4 years of biliary extracorporeal shockwave lithotripsy. *Hepatogastroenterology* 43:1124, 1996.

77. Tsoi EK, Smith RS, Fry WR, et al: Laparoscopic surgery without pneumoperitoneum. A preliminary report. *Surg Endosc* 8:382, 1994.

78. Tudyka J, Kratzer W, Kuhn K, et al: Diagnostic value of fine-needle puncture of the gallbladder: side effects, safety, and prognostic value. *Hepatology* 21:1303, 1995.

79. Coleman CC, Vennes JA, Posalaky IP, et al: Thermal ablation of the gallbladder. *Radiology* 180:363, 1991.

Barbara Kaplan-Machlis
Kathleen P. Bors

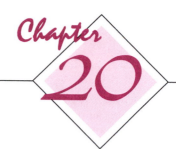

Osteoporosis

Overview: Women's Concerns

More than 28 million women in the United States are affected by osteoporosis or have low bone mass.[1] Four out of five people with osteoporosis are women; for women over age 50 years this results in a 40 percent lifetime risk for fractures. A high percentage of these women will become temporarily or permanently disabled, particularly after hip fracture, and up to 20 percent will die within a year of a hip fracture.

Women may not appreciate the true risk of this disease and therefore may fail to take appropriate preventive or treatment actions. A 1995 Gallup survey, supported by the American Heart Association and the American Medical Women's Association, asked 505 American women ages 45 to 75 nationwide about their views on the leading causes of death among women. Women identified breast cancer as the leading cause of death, suggesting that it accounted for 40 percent of female mortality; heart disease came second, accounting for 19 percent. Actual mortality statistics show a clear discrepancy between real and perceived health threats. Cardiovascular diseases are the leading causes of death among women (accounting for 45 percent of mortality) and breast cancer ranks eighth out of nine categories, accounting for only 4 percent of deaths. A woman's lifetime risk of hip fracture is equal to her combined risk of developing breast, uterine, and ovarian cancer.[1]

Prevalence and Health Risks

Definition

Osteoporosis is defined as a universal, gradual reduction in bone mass to a point where the skeleton is compromised, resulting in fractures from minimal trauma.[2] The 1993 Consensus Development Conference sponsored by the National Osteoporosis Foundation (NOF), the European Foundation for Osteoporosis and Bone Disease, and the National Institute of Arthritis and Musculoskeletal and Skin Diseases further defined osteoporosis as a "systemic skeletal disease characterized by low bone mass and microarchitectural deterioration of bone tissue, with consequent increase in bone fragility and susceptibility to fracture."[2] In 1994, the World Health Organization (WHO) used clinical criteria to establish diagnostic categories for osteoporosis that focus on preventing fragility fractures. Using bone mineral density (BMD) testing, the WHO defined "normal" as BMD or bone mineral content (BMC) within 1.0 standard deviation (SD) of the young adult mean.[3] WHO defines osteopenia as BMD or BMC measurement 1.0 to 2.5 SD below the gender-matched young adult mean. Osteopenia is often referred to as the first stage of osteoporosis and carries a twofold increase risk of fracture. Osteoporosis is defined as BMD or BMC measurement 2.5 SD or more below the gender-matched, young adult mean, because most fragility fractures occur below this bone density. (Table 20-1). Osteoporosis is advanced osteopenia to the point where a reduction of total bone (protein and minerals) occurs and carries a four- to five-fold increased risk of fracture.

Prevalence

In 1996, the NOF estimated that approximately 29 million people aged 50 and over in the United States had osteoporosis or were at risk of developing this disease; this number is expected to rise to over 41 million by the year 2015.[4] Even among young women, 16 percent were found by the third National Health and Nutrition Examination Survey (NHANES III) to have a BMD below normal (T score < −1).[5]

Osteoporosis is often considered the "silent disease" because its progression is insidious and most individuals are unaware of the disease until a bone fracture occurs. About 1.2 million osteoporosis-related fractures are reported each year in the United States. One in every two women and one of every eight men will suffer an osteoporosis-related fracture at some time during their lives.[6]

VERTEBRAL FRACTURES

About 40 percent of women will have at least one vertebral fracture by the time they are 80 years of age. Vertebral compression fractures are often the first osteoporosis-related fracture to occur. (Fig. 20-1). Vertebral fractures can be painless and go undetected until a noticeable loss of height results (> 1 inch). The consequences of these fractures are severe for many individuals. Multiple thoracic fractures may result in restrictive lung disease (manifested by exertional dyspnea, decreased exercise tolerance, and altered spirometry findings), and lumbar fractures may lead to a reduced abdominal cavity, limiting stomach capacity and leading to early satiety and impaired gastric emptying. Limited bladder capacity may also occur, causing or exacerbating problems already common among elderly and postmenopausal women (e.g., urinary incontinence, nocturia, and other bladder dysfunction). Abdominal distortion may also contribute to dyspareunia and sexual dysfunction in osteoporotic women. Postural disfigurement and height changes can further result in reduced mobility (including bending and reaching) and chronic pain.

HIP FRACTURES

The annual hip fracture incidence alone is estimated to range from 147,000 to 250,000, with approximately 80 percent resulting from minor trauma. Sufferers of hip fractures have a 5 to 20 percent greater risk of dying within the first year

Table 20-1

Diagnostic Categories for Osteoporosis

NORMAL	A value for BMD or BMC within 1 standard deviation of the young adult reference mean.	T-score between +1.0 and −1.0
OSTEOPENIA (**LOW BONE MASS**)	A value for BMD or BMC > 1 SD below the young adult mean but < 2.5 SD below this value.	T-score between −1.0 and −2.5
OSTEOPOROSIS	A value of BMD or BMC 2.5 SD or more below the young adult mean.	T-score of < −2.5
SEVERE OSTEOPOROSIS (**ESTABLISHED OSTEOPOROSIS**)	A value of BMD or BMC of 2.5 SD or more below the young adult mean in the presence of one or more fragility fractures.	T-score of < −2.5 and the presence of one or more fragility fractures.

ABBREVIATIONS: BMD, bone mineral density; BMC, bone mineral content; SD, standard deviation.
SOURCE: National Institute of Arthritis and Musculoskeletal and Skin Diseases.[6]

Figure 20-1

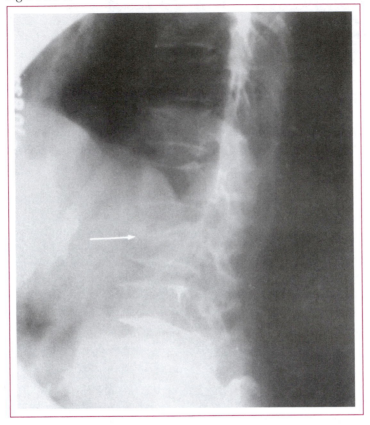

X-ray of a vertebral compression fracture. (*Reproduced with permission from Krane SM, Holick MF: Metabolic bone disease. In: Fauci AS, Braunwald E, Isselbacher KJ, et al, eds: Harrison's Principles of Internal Medicine, 14th ed. New York, McGraw-Hill, copyright 1998.*)

of their injury compared to others in the same age group; an additional 13 percent mortality is expected within the next year. Fifty percent of people with hip fracture will be unable to walk without assistance during their remaining lifetime. Fifty percent of women and men 60 years or older hospitalized for hip fractures will be discharged to a nursing home and about 25 percent will still reside in the nursing home 1 year later.[6] Both hip and vertebral fractures can also cause psychological symptoms including depression, anxiety, fear, and anger, which can impede recovery and profoundly reduce quality of life.[7]

Economic Costs

The estimated economic burden of osteoporosis ranges from $6 to $18 billion and by the year 2040, projected treatment costs will reach $240 billion.[8] The escalating economic cost of osteoporosis appears due to the aging population and increasing life span.

Pathophysiology

Normal Bone Growth, Development, and Maintenance

Bone mineral density is highly correlated with bone strength and with fracture risk.[9] Skeletal weakness, which develops in osteoporosis, results in part from structural and quantitative abnormal connections or alterations in bone quality. These include changes in bone turnover and in rate of repair, as well as loss of connectivity of the trabecular elements that comprise cancellous bone. (Figs. 20-2 and 20-3). Such changes contribute to skeletal weakness; however, some of these changes in bone quality are the direct result of bone loss.

Bone is a living tissue in a constant state of turnover and renewal. Bone remodeling maintains healthy bone with an ability to store calcium essential for bone density, bone strength, and other vital body functions. Bone responds to physiologic demands and repairs microstructural defects. Two major multinucleated, monocyte/macrophage lineage cell types, osteoclasts and osteoblasts, are involved with bone remodeling. Osteoclasts resorb bone and osteoblasts synthesize new bone matrix. Osteoid (the organic matrix of bone) subsequently calcifies to fill in defects resulting from osteoclast activity. Overall bone turnover is determined by the skeletal summation of metabolic activity generated by osteoclastic/osteoblastic coupling.[8,10]

Figure 20-2

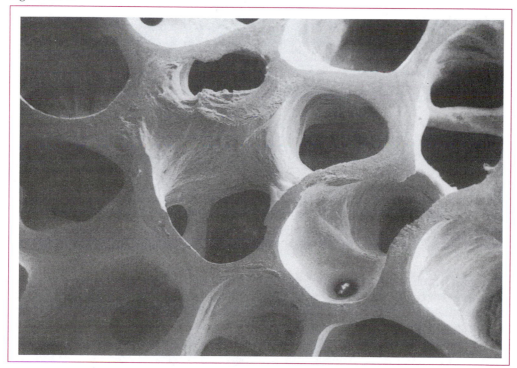

Trabecular/cancellous bone—normal bone. (*Reproduced with permission from Lindsay R, Kelly P: Osteoporosis in postmenopausal women. In: Wren BG, Nachtigall LE, eds: Clinical Management of the Menopause. New York, McGraw-Hill, copyright 1996.*)

Figure 20-3

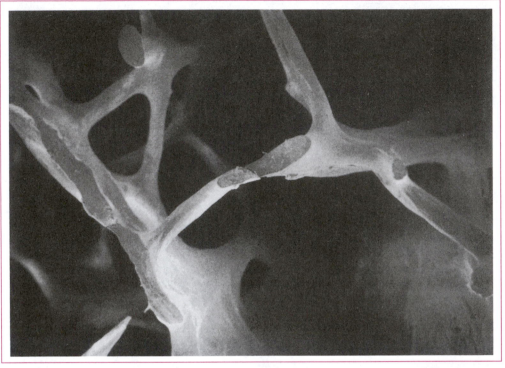

Trabecular/cancellous bone—osteoporotic bone. (*Reproduced with permission from Lindsay R, Kelly P: Osteoporosis in postmenopausal women. In: Wren BG, Nachtigall LE, eds: Clinical Management of the Menopause. New York, McGraw-Hill, copyright 1996.*)

During growth and development, net bone formation exceeds resorption. The critical years for building bone mass begin in preadolescence. Peak bone mass occurs at about age 20 for the hip and during the early thirties for the spine. During the fourth decade in both genders, skeletal bone loss begins. At menopause, the rate of bone loss accelerates sharply. Estrogen receptors, present in bone, directly affect bone cell function by inhibiting osteoclastic bone resorption. With the decline in estrogen levels, osteoclastic and osteoblastic activity increase, but excess osteoclastic resorption occurs, causing a net bone loss of up to 2 to 3 percent per year for approximately 5 years.[11] Total lifetime losses may equal 30 to 40 percent of peak mass for women and 20 to 30 percent for men.

Bone loss may occur in either trabecular or cortical bone from an imbalance of skeletal remodeling that favors bone resorption. Trabecular bone is spongy or cancellous and comprises 80 percent of the adult skeleton while cortical bone is compact or tubular and comprises 20 percent of the adult skeleton. Cortical bone predominates in the shafts of long bones, whereas trabecular bone is concentrated in the vertebrae, ends of long bones, pelvis, and other flat bones. Trabecular bone has a greater surface area than cortical bone and is therefore metabolically more active. Bone remodeling is a dynamic process necessary to provide calcium for extracellular function, for repair and removal of old bone, and to maintain skeletal elasticity. Bone remodeling occurs at about one million bone sites at any given time and within a given year, remodeling occurs in 25 percent of trabecular and 3 percent of cortical bone. The complete bone remodeling cycle (bone resorption followed by formation of bone matrix and then mineralization of the matrix) takes up to 8 months to occur.[12]

AGING CHANGES

Maximal BMD of cortical bone occurs in men and women in the second to fourth decade of life, followed by a slow decline.[13] Women have less bone mass at skeletal maturity, requiring less bone to be lost before the threshold for fractures is reached. Initial skeletal bone loss begins during the fourth decade of life and occurs at a rate of 0.3 to 0.5 percent per year for both genders. At the time of menopause, the rate of bone loss accelerates sharply for approximately 5 years and then occurs more slowly until about age 70. At age 70, the rate of bone loss increases again in one-third of women and doesn't change in one-third of women; one-third of women experience a decrease in the rate of bone loss.

Types of Osteoporosis

At least three types of osteoporosis exist. Postmenopausal osteoporosis or type I, will be the focus of this chapter. It occurs within the first 15 to 20 years following menopause and results from a disproportionate loss of trabecular bone that leads to an increase in painful crush-type vertebral fractures, fractures of the distal part of the forearm, ankle fractures, and occasionally, loss of teeth.

Type II or senile osteoporosis affects both men and women older than age 70. In type II osteoporosis cortical and trabecular bone density values show a proportionate loss. The clinical manifestations of type II osteoporosis are multiple vertebral, hip, and radius fractures.

Type III osteoporosis or osteoporosis secondary to other diseases or medications occurs in either gender at any age.[10] A listing of the diseases and medications is shown in Table 20-2.

Risk Factors

The goal of osteoporosis prevention and treatment is to decrease the risk of fracture. Table 20-2 lists multiple genetic, environmental, medical, and social conditions that can influence an individual's likelihood of developing osteoporosis.[8,12,13] Four risk factors that have been demonstrated in a large, ongoing, prospective U.S. study to be key factors in determining the risk of hip fracture (independent of BMD) include personal history of fracture as an adult, history of fracture in a first-degree relative, current cigarette smoking, and low body weight (< 127 lb).[14,15] To assess a patient's risk for bone fragility, the provider should review the patient's clinical history with special attention to risk factor assessment and potential interventions to decrease risk.[11] Bone loss can be slowed or reversed if risk factors (e.g., physical inactivity, low dietary calcium intake, tobacco use or hyperthyroidism) are identified and treated.[12]

BONE MASS

Low bone mass, as measured by BMD testing, is the single best predictor of increased fracture risk.[2,12] BMD testing can be used to establish a diagnosis of osteoporosis, estimate future fracture risk, and monitor medical conditions that contribute to the progression of osteoporosis or offer follow-up on therapeutic intervention. Most fragility fractures occur with a BMD more than 2.5 SD below the young adult mean. Yet, bone mass alone does not determine fracture risk. Age also contributes to a woman's risk of sustaining a fracture in her lifetime.[16] In addition to bone loss associated with aging, age-related extraskeletal factors that influence fracture risk include an increased likelihood of falling and a decreased ability to adequately respond to a fall to lessen the force of impact.[11]

Table 20-2

Factors Commonly Associated with Osteoporosis

GENETICS
White or Asian ethnicity
Positive family history
Small body frame (< 58 kg or 127 lb.)
Vitamin D receptor allele anomaly
Early natural menopause
Later menarche

LIFESTYLE
Smoking
Sedentary lifestyle
Nulliparity
Excessive exercise

NUTRITIONAL FACTORS
Milk intolerance
Lifelong low dietary calcium intake
Alcoholism
Consistently high animal protein intake
Vegetarian diet*
Vitamin D deficiency

DRUG THERAPY
Glucocorticoid drugs
Chronic lithium therapy
Chemotherapy
Gonadotropin-releasing hormone agonist or antagonist therapy
Anticonvulsant drugs
Extended tetracycline use[†]

(continued)
Diuretics producing calciuria[†]
Phenothiazine derivatives[†]
Cyclosporin[†]
Aluminum-containing antacids[†]
Methotrexate
Heparin

MEDICAL DISORDERS
Endocrine Diseases
Cushing's syndrome
Diabetes mellitus type 1
Primary hyperparathyroidism
Addison's disease
Hematologic Diseases
Multiple myeloma
Hemolytic anemia
Pernicious anemia
Systemic mastocytosis
Lymphoma, leukemia
Rheumatologic Diseases
Rheumatoid arthritis
Ankylosing spondylitis
Gastrointestinal Diseases
Malabsorption syndromes (e.g., Crohn's disease)
Chronic liver disease (e.g., primary biliary cirrhosis)
Other Diseases
Anorexia nervosa
Osteogenesis imperfecta
Low testosterone levels (men)

*Vegetarian diets vary in the quantity and types of calcium containing foods. Vegan-type vegetarian diets are more likely to be associated with low calcium intake and an increased risk for osteoporosis.

[†] Not yet associated with decreased bone mass although identified as either toxic to bone in animals or inducing calciuria and/or calcium malabsorption in human beings.

SOURCE: Modified with permission from Scheiber TB, Torregrosa L: Evaluation and treatment of postmenopausal osteoporosis. *Semin Arthritis Rheum* 27:245, 1988; Eastell R: Treatment of postmenopausal osteoporosis. *N Engl J Med* 338:736, 1998.

MEDICATIONS

Several medications contribute to a woman's risk of developing osteoporosis (see Table 20-2). Corticosteroids are the most common drug class implicated in causing osteoporosis. Corticosteroid-induced osteoporosis-related fractures occur in 30 to 50 percent of patients receiving chronic therapy (i.e., > 7.5 mg/d of prednisone for > 6 months). Chronic corticosteroid therapy blocks the maturation of osteoblasts resulting in decreased bone formation, decreased gastrointestinal absorption of calcium, and increased renal calcium excretion. Excessive levothyroxine therapy (> 200 μg/d or > 1.6 μg/kg) can result in increased osteoclast activity and decreased serum calcium concentrations. High-dose and chronic heparin administration (> 15,000 U/d for > 3 to 6 months), often used for thromboprophylaxis during pregnancy, can cause increased bone resorption and decreased formation. This complicates the physiologic bone demineralization that occurs during pregnancy and lactation. As a result, symptomatic osteoporosis can occur in 2 percent of women due to long-term heparin use during pregnancy. Chronic anticonvulsant therapy with phenytoin or a barbiturate (bone loss may begin as early as 6 months into therapy), especially with combined use of these agents, can result in decreased intestinal calcium absorption, hypocalcemia, and decreased serum vitamin D.[17]

Principal Diagnosis

Clinical Presentation

The common clinical presentation of a woman with osteoporosis is shortened stature (> 1 inch), kyphosis and cervical lordosis (frequently referred to as dowager's or widow's hump), or a fracture, most commonly of the vertebra, hip, or forearm. Because the development of osteoporosis is insidious, the clinical manifestation of acute pain associated with fracture is often the first symptom and is noted long after significant bone loss has occurred.[7] The fractures frequently occur after minor trauma, such as bending, lifting, jumping, and falling from the standing position.[10] Recurrent fractures are common and the time frame is unpredictable. Vertebral body collapse is the most frequently seen fracture, especially in early postmenopausal women. As a result, back pain of variable intensity and spine deformities occur.

Some patients have a fracture discovered on routine x-ray or in relationship to a reduction in height. Collapsed vertebra rarely lead to spinal cord compression.[10] Acute fracture-related pain usually completely resolves in 2 to 3 months. However, the acute phase of vertebral fracture may be followed by chronic back pain, characterized as a nagging, deep, dull pain localized to the general area of the fracture.

History

Osteoporosis is a disease that does not affect everyone, can be prevented, and should be appropriately treated when recognized. Osteoporosis results from failure to reach appropriate peak bone mass, significant and rapid postmenopausal loss of bone mass, ongoing age-related bone loss, and secondary risk factors (see Table 20-2).[10]

The patient's history is probably the most critical part of the evaluation and should include family history of osteoporosis and other bone disease, loss of height, presence of chronic or acute back pain, assessment of risk factors (see Table 20-2), history of fractures, and personal or family history of nephrolithiasis. A thorough menstrual history documenting the length of exposure to endogenous estrogen should also be taken, including when the patient experienced menarche and menopause, type of menopause (surgical or natural), and periods of amenorrhea not associated with pregnancy. In patients with established osteoporosis or with suspected spine fracture, a thorough history that details pain, its character, where it radiates, and what exacerbates and improves it should also be solicited.

Physical Examination

The physical examination is performed to identify and evaluate clinical signs and symptoms of osteoporosis. Height should be measured accurately. The spine should be examined for symmetry, kyphosis, and cervical lordosis. Tenderness to light or firm palpation over the spinous processes and paraspinous muscle spasm should be noted. Range of motion (e.g., extension, side bending, and flexion) should also be determined. Particular attention should be paid to dentition and the presence of oral bone loss; manifestations of osteoporosis in the mouth may include tooth loss and edentualism. The neck should be examined to look for an enlarged thyroid gland and pulse should be taken to assess signs of hyperthyroidism. An abdominal examination will reveal whether the abdomen is protuberant (associated with gastrointestinal or bladder symptoms or sexual dysfunction). Women should have breast and pelvic examinations to detect evidence for lowered estrogen levels and to assess the safety of postmenopausal estrogen as a treatment option. Gait (steadiness and pain) and posture (e.g., kyphosis) should be assessed and the patient should be observed ascending and descending stairs. Finally, mobility should be observed to assess if the patient is using good body mechanics during sit to stand, transfers, bed mobility, and lifting objects from low surfaces.[18]

Aspects of the physical examination that suggest increased risks of osteoporosis are those reflective of known risk factors for osteoporotic fracture. (see Table 20-2). Specific attention should also be given to race and family history, body weight (< 127 lb), unexplained bony tenderness of spine or hip, evidence of tobacco use or alcohol abuse not uncovered by the history, evidence of recurrent falls, and a general assessment for poor health and frailty.[14]

Diagnostic Procedures

BMD MEASUREMENT

Although risk factors often precede fractures, using only clinical features to identify individuals most likely to suffer a fracture will miss approximately 30 percent of those with osteoporosis. BMD is the strongest known predictor of fracture risk.[9,19,20] Fracture risk increases as BMD decreases. BMD measures the amount of calcium present in the region of bone being evaluated. BMD measurements do not predict absolute fracture probability for an individual, but estimate a relative risk of fracture compared with a control group (i.e., reference normal population—T-score or average BMD for age and gender—Z-score).[21]

CLINICAL UTILITY OF BMD MEASUREMENT Conventionally, osteoporosis is defined as 2.5 SD below the T-score value that indicates mean peak bone mass in a reference population of 30-year-old individuals. Alternatively, a Z-score of -1.0 places a patient in the 25th percentile for BMD for that age and gender group and a score of -2 identifies those in the 2.5 percent or lower BMD. Defining an absolute cutoff point of BMD below which fractures will occur and above which they will not is impossible. However, risk of fracture increases with the number of skeletal sites having low bone mass. A BMD value does not discriminate between patients with and without fractures nor does it diagnose fractures, but this measure can be used to determine fracture risk.

GUIDELINES FOR USE OF BMD MEASUREMENT Most recently, the NOF in collaboration with a multispecialty council of medical experts in the field of bone health, provided guidelines for when, where, and in whom to measure BMD (Table 20-3).[14] Calculation of a cost/benefit ratio for osteoporosis screening is complex because costs include screening, treatment, effectiveness of treatment, potential changes in quality of life and independent living, and fracture cost.21 BMD measurement should be used to identify individuals at risk (see Table 20-3) so that timely interventions can be initiated to prevent osteoporosis-related fractures, thus reducing the morbidity, mortality, and cost of the disease.[22] Perhaps the most optimal time to obtain BMD testing in women is during perimenopause, when the decision to begin estrogen replacement therapy (ERT) is often made. BMD measurement can be used to diagnose osteoporosis, influence a clinical decision, and monitor changes in risk over time.[9]

Table 20-3

Indications for Bone Mineral Density (BMD) Studies

*All postmenopausal women under age 65 who have one or more additional risk factors for osteoporosis (other than menopause)
All women aged 65 and older regardless of additional risk factors
Postmenopausal women who present with fractures (to confirm diagnosis and determine disease severity)
Women who are considering therapy for osteoporosis, if BMD testing would facilitate the decision
Women who have been on hormone replacement therapy for prolonged periods
*Individuals receiving, or planning to receive, long-term glucocorticoid (steroid) therapy
*Individuals with primary hyperparathyroidism
*Individuals with vertebral abnormalities
*Individuals being monitored to assess the response or efficacy or an approved osteoporosis drug therapy

NOTES: The decision to test for BMD should be based on an individual's risk profile, and testing is never indicated unless the results could influence a treatment decision.
*Medicare covers all FDA-approved bone density technologies for the respective indications as of July 1, 1998; frequency of testing is once every 2 years; benefit applies to individuals in all Medicare plans, including managed care; Medicare will only reimburse for bone densitometry tests when ordered by the treating health care provider.
SOURCE: Modified with permission from Kanis JA: Diagnosis of osteoporosis. *Osteoporosis Int*. 7(Suppl 3): S108, 1997.

TECHNOLOGY FOR MEASUREMENT OF BMD　Table 20-4 compares several technologies for bone mass measurement.[23] Dual x-ray absorptiometry (DEXA) is the most widely used technology for obtaining bone mass measurement. This procedure is highly reproducible, is accurate, uses a low radiation dose, and is capable of measuring bone density at axial and appendicular skeletal sites.[24]

However, there is debate about which bones should be used for BMD estimation and measurement. At this time, DEXA measurement at the proximal femur is thought to be the most useful for predicting fracture and measurement at the lumbar spine is most accurate for monitoring response to therapy.[12]

FOLLOW-UP BMD MEASUREMENT　BMD measurement should not be obtained more frequently than the time required to detect a change in bone mass. For example, the average amount of postmenopausal bone loss is about 2 percent per year, slightly higher than the precision of many available instruments.[25] In clinical practice, a precision of 1 percent is rarely achieved; only changes of more than 3 percent in the spine and 6 percent in

the hip are considered clinically significant.[21] Therefore, postmenopausal women should not undergo scanning more often than every 1.4 years. However, for patients on chronic glucocorticoid therapy, more frequent BMD measurements are recommended (e.g., every 6 months) due to the potential rapid rate of bone loss (as much as 17 percent of the skeleton within the first 6 to 12 months of prednisone therapy at a dose of 30 mg/d).[23]

LIMITATIONS OF DEXA TECHNOLOGY　Several limitations of DEXA scanning should be noted. Criteria used to define "normal population" for the reference databases differ among instruments so the same measured value may lie within different parts of the reference range and may be assigned a different fracture risk depending on the system used.[21] However, differences in normative data between manufacturers (with variations of as much as an entire standard deviation) are being corrected by the information collected in the NHANES III. As a result, experts recommend that longitudinal follow-up be performed using the same instrument, whenever possible.[21]

Table 20-4

Noninvasive Measurements of Bone Mineral Density*

MODALITY	ADVANTAGES	DISADVANTAGES	RELATIVE COST*
DEXA	Considered gold standard Total body measurements Hip/spine/wrist measurements Low radiation exposure May perform serial tests	Area measurement study Limited mobility of equipment	$$
Peripheral DEXA	Low radiation exposure Equipment mobile	Limited to study of wrist or heel Area measurement study Limited correlation to spine/hip	$
QCT	Volumetric measurement May perform serial tests	High radiation exposure Recalibration between tests Limited mobility of equipment Difficulty measuring the hip	$$$
RA	Requires only a x-ray unit and phantom Equipment mobile	Limited to study of phalanges Limited as screening test Limited correlation to hip/spine	$
SXA	Equipment mobile	Limited to forearm/heel study Limited as screening test Limited correlation to spine/hip	$
Ultrasound	Equipment mobile Radiation free	Limited to calcaneous study Limited as screening test Limited correlation to spine/hip	$

*$, low cost per test/equipment; $$, moderate cost of equipment, moderate to low cost per test; $$$, moderate cost per test.
ABBREVIATIONS: DEXA, dual x-ray absorptiometry; QCT, quantitative computed tomography; RA, radioabsorptiometry; SXA, single x-ray absorptiometry.
SOURCE: Modified with permission from Eastell R: Treatment of postmenopausal osteoporosis. *N Engl J Med* 338:736, 1998.

Quality control is also important to maintain high precision in BMD measurements. Spinal BMD can be affected by the presence of scoliosis and vertebral compression fractures. Single vertebrae are difficult to define technically when compression fractures have occurred. Also, the distribution of osteoporosis could vary within the spine, with differential involvement of the dorsal spine and lumbar spine. As a result, BMD values do not discriminate between patients with and those without fractures.[21] Frequency of densitometry testing is limited, because clinically meaningful changes depend on adequate time periods between measurements. In such cases, treatment responses may be monitored with measurements of biochemical markers (see below).

ACCESS TO BMD MEASUREMENT   Lack of access to BMD testing may limit its usefulness in areas where the equipment is not yet available, such as in smaller rural communities and for women who have transportation difficulties (e.g., frail elderly women). On July 1, 1998, Medicare announced coverage for all Food and Drug Administration (FDA)-approved bone density technologies (see Table 20-4).[14] As a result, access to DEXA testing should improve and more patients should be able to undergo BMD assessment for determination of fracture risk.

LABORATORY TESTING

Serologic and urine markers of bone turnover may reflect bone formation or bone resorption. Biochemical markers for bone resorption (urine pyridinoline, deoxypyridinoline, *N*- and *C*-telopeptides of the cross-links of collagen) and bone formation (serum osteocalcin, bone-specific alkaline phosphatase, and carboxyl-terminal extension peptide of type I procollagen) have been identified.[12] Studies suggest that increased levels of biochemical markers of resorption indicate bone turnover and that these "markers" may predict increased risk of fracture independent of BMD level.[7]

However, biochemical markers cannot measure bone quality or quantity of skeletal mineralization. As a result, biochemical markers cannot replace BMD measurement when diagnosing osteoporosis, but may be used as a means of monitoring the adequacy of osteoporosis treatment. For example, biochemical markers can determine if a patient is a rapid bone loser and changes in bone turnover can be detected within 1 to 3 months of initiating antiresorptive therapy. In contrast, at least 1 year is required to determine if a change in bone mass has occurred using BMD testing. Specifically, biochemical markers are useful in the following clinical situations: patients with borderline BMD test results or when the patient or physician is not convinced by the BMD results, patients already committed to a treatment program in whom a baseline BMD study was not obtained, and patients who are doubtful about whether to continue a treatment program.[8]

Recently, two clinically available tests (urinary deoxypyridinoline and the cross-linked *N*-telopeptide) that are very sensitive and accurate indicators of bone turnover have been approved by the FDA. These urine tests measure collagen cross-links and can be of value in identifying rapid bone loss in selected patients. However, biochemical test results may have assay and diurnal variability; diurnal variation may be eliminated by using a second morning void. Also, for individual patients, a drop in biochemical markers is not always predictive of an increase in bone mass, although this has been shown to be highly correlated in groups of patients. As a result, biochemical marker determinations do not obviate the need for repeat BMD measurements.[18] Currently, urinary collagen cross-link testing is expensive (approximately $50/test) but much less expensive than DEXA.

Treatment

Prevention

Osteoporosis prevention is pertinent to the health of women across their life span. The development and progression of osteoporosis depends on two separate processes: the formation of bone mass during childhood and young adulthood and rate of bone loss in later life.[26] Young women should meet or exceed their body's calcium needs to build bone mass crucial to protect against osteoporosis. In 1997, the National Academy of Sciences (NAS) issued substantively increased recommendations for dietary allowances of calcium (Table 20-5).[10] Educating women regarding the importance of adequate calcium intake and calcium sources should be a part of the health maintenance examination. Ideally, calcium intake should be derived from natural food sources and dietary supplements should be viewed as an adjunct for achieving recommended intake.

Primary and secondary prevention activities should be promoted among middle-aged and older adults who are at risk for osteopenia and osteoporosis. Modalities include lifestyle modification such as weight-bearing exercise, dietary advice,

Table 20-5

Recommended Intake and Sources of Calcium and Vitamin D

AGE GROUP	ELEMENTAL CALCIUM (MG/DAY)	DIET[†] (SERVINGS PER DAY)	SUPPLEMENTS[‡] (NUMBER PER DAY)	VITAMIN[*] D (IU/DAY)	DIET[§] (SERVINGS PER DAY)	SUPPLEMENTS[#] (NUMBER PER DAY)
Adolescents/young adults (both genders) 9–18 y	1300	4–5	4–5	200	2	1
Pregnant and lactating women						
14–18 y	1300	4–5	4–5	200	2	1
19–50 y	1000	3–4	3–4	200	2	1
Adults (nonpregnant)						
19–50 y	1000	3–4	3–4	200	2	1
50–65 y on ERT or males	1000	3–4	3–4	400	4	2
50–65 years not on ERT	1500	5	5	400	4	2
> 65 y (both genders)	1500	5	5	600	6	3

* One microgram (m) cholecalciferol = 40 IU vitamin D

† 1 serving of dairy approximately 300 mg obtained with 1 cup of milk, 1 cup calcium-fortified orange juice

‡ Calcium carbonate available as Tums Ex = 1 tablet = approximately 300 mg elemental calcium

§ Recommended 10–15 min in sun, 2–3 times per week; dietary sources may contain significant amounts of saturated fat and cholesterol except for low fat milks; 1 cup milk contains approximately 100 IU vitamin D

#Vitamin D_3 (cholecalciferol) is sold over the counter as vitamin supplements; 1 capsule equals approximately 200 IU vitamin D (see individual label for description of contents)

calcium supplementation, pharmacologic therapies (e.g., hormone replacement therapy [HRT], raloxifene, alendronate), and bone densitometry for high-risk individuals. Also, reassessment of BMD should be conducted in patients at high risk for osteoporosis due to drug therapy (e.g., long-term treatment with corticosteroids, anticonvulsants, heparin, or excessive levothyroxine therapy) or in those patients on osteoporosis treatment to determine adequacy of drug therapy. Tertiary prevention is recommended for middle-aged and elderly individuals who have been diagnosed with osteoporosis or who have already suffered an osteoporotic fracture. The goal of tertiary prevention is to limit future disability and provide rehabilitation.[8] Measures include exercise, calcium supplementation, pharmacologic therapies, and fall prevention.

NONPHARMACOLOGIC APPROACHES

Maximizing peak bone mass involves development of healthy dietary habits and nonsedentary lifestyles beginning during the teenage years. Several dietary and lifestyle behavior changes have been recommended to preserve bone.

CAFFEINE Excessive caffeine reduces mineralization of the skeleton and increases renal excretion of calcium.[27] Caffeine ingestion should be decreased to the equivalent of less than 2 to 5 cups of coffee per day.

SMOKING CESSATION Smoking cessation is important because smoking has been associated with lower bone mass and increased fracture rates. Cigarette smoking also causes earlier menopause and increases metabolism of endogenous and exogenous sex hormones.[28]

ALCOHOL INGESTION   An association between alcohol use and low bone density and fractures has been found in some, but not all studies. Alcohol may induce nutritional deficiencies in calcium, vitamin D, and magnesium,[29] and reducing alcohol intake may improve the overall health of individual patients.[13] Evidence also indicates that alcohol may cause dysfunction of osteoblasts and thereby impair bone formation and mineralization.[30] Frequent consumption of even moderate quantities of alcohol (e.g., 1 to 2 drinks daily) can lead to reduced bone mass.[31]

EXERCISE   The specific type, duration, and style of exercise needed to maintain a strong musculoskeletal structure has not been determined. However, two types of exercise have been shown to significantly increase bone density in randomized clinical trials. These are weight-bearing exercise (walking, jogging, basketball, soccer, hiking, dancing, skiing, aerobic dancing, gymnastics, and stair climbing) and resistive exercise (weight training and vigorous water exercises).[18] The magnitude of BMD change in the spine and hip over several months to 1 year following two to four times per week, regular, progressive exercise is between 0.5 to 3 percent in both young and postmenopausal women. Therefore, women can gain two benefits from increased aerobic and strengthening exercises: prevention of bone loss and fewer falls (because muscle tone is improved).[32] Studies suggest that bones that are most directly stressed by exercise have the greatest increase in BMD. Exercise programs designed to improve body mechanics and general conditioning do not directly increase BMD, but may prevent falls and traumatic injuries and reduce the rate of fractures.

Amenorrhea associated with vigorous exercise programs (e.g., elite athletes who have functional hypogonadism or women with anorexia nervosa) has caused decreased vertebral BMD.[18] Amenorrhea occurs in 35 to 40 percent of highly trained endurance women athletes as a result of low gonadotropin concentrations and is associated with accelerated bone resorption, resulting in an increased risk of osteoporosis. In some cases, oral contraceptives have been administered to amenorrheic athletes to overcome this estrogen-deficiency state.[10]

FALL PREVENTION   Prevention of falls is critical for decreasing a patient's risk of sustaining fractures (Table 20-6).[18] Elderly patients with known gait instability should be encouraged to use a cane or walker when ambulating, even when moving about their own homes. Activities that cause compressive forces on the spine or deep flexion of the spine (e.g., lying supine instead of laterally in bed, erect standing for long periods of time, isometric abdominal contraction, slouched sitting, standing flexed forward from the waist, sitting flexed forward) should be avoided because these activities can encourage occurrence of vertebral compression fractures.[18]

Pharmacologic Prevention and Treatment Modalities

AVOIDING MEDICATION-INDUCED OSTEOPOROSIS AND FRACTURES

Pharmacists and prescribers should review patient medication profiles for potential therapies that are associated with increased falls (e.g., psychotropic, antihypertensive, and diuretic medications) and those associated with an increased risk of osteoporosis (see Table 20-2).

MEDICATIONS ADVERSELY AFFECTING BMD   Corticosteroid use should be limited to the lowest effective dose and duration or inhaled steroids should be used. Levothyroxine dosing should be monitored so that the thyroid-stimulating hormone is within the normal range (0.4 to 10 mIU/L). Heparin use should be limited to the lowest effective dose and shortest duration possible and low molecular weight heparins may be substituted; however, data are conflicting with regard to overall

Table 20-6

Safety Tips for Fall Prevention

Remove throw rugs and make certain that carpet edges are securely fastened to the floor.

Reduce clutter, especially in traffic areas.

Install or maintain sturdy handrails at stairs.

Increase wattage of lighting in hallways, bathrooms, kitchens, stairwells, and entrances to home.

Use night lights near bed, in hallways, and in bathrooms to improve night safety.

Install safety handrails in shower, tub, and around toilet; bathtubs and shower stalls should have nonskid surfaces.

When you must reach for something high, use a safety step-stool (one with wide steps and a friction surface to stand on); a type equipped with a high handrail is preferred.

If a cane or walker has been recommended, use it to help increase your stability.

Wear supportive, cushioned, low-heeled shoes; avoid scuffs (backless bedroom slippers) and high heels.

Avoid rushing to answer the phone or doorbell; a portable phone that you can take from room to room with you is a good idea for security and safety.

Have sand or salt available to spread on porches, stairs, and sidewalks during snowy, icy weather.

SOURCE: From Duke University Medical Center Bone and Metabolic Clinic. Modified with permission from Tresolini CP, Gold DT, Lee LS, eds: *Working with Patients to Prevent, Treat, and Manage Osteoporosis: A Curriculum Guide for the Health Professions,* 2nd ed. San Francisco: National Fund for Medical Education; 1998.

osteoporosis risk of low molecular weight heparin. Anticonvulsant therapy should be administered with concomitant vitamin D supplementation of 4000 to 10,000 IU/week and baseline vitamin D deficiencies should be corrected.

MEDICATIONS THAT INCREASE RISK FOR FALLS Psychotropic medications should be minimized or discontinued if altered balance or confusion result. In general, sedative use should be avoided in the treatment of elderly women. If adverse cognitive side effects occur, sedatives should be discontinued or switched to short-acting agents (e.g., lorazepam, zolpidem). Diuretics should be given during the day to prevent the need for nocturnal voiding. Falls are associated with poor vision (lighting, lack of use of corrective lenses) and impaired balance during the night when individuals arise to urinate. Orthostatic blood pressure problems should be resolved through dosage modifications as necessary and slow rising from lying and sitting positions should be encouraged (see Chap. 17).

PHARMACOLOGIC TREATMENT OF OSTEOPOROSIS

Most medications used to prevent or treat osteoporosis act by decreasing bone resorption (estrogen, bisphosphonates, raloxifene, calcitonin).[7,8] Remodeling space occurs when bone has been resorbed but not yet replaced; this often occurs in postmenopausal osteoporosis. The antiresorptive agents decrease the rate of initiation of new remodeling cycles, thus decreasing remodeling space. Filling of the remodeling space accounts for the 5 to 10 percent gain in BMD seen with antiresorptive therapy. This process usually takes 2 to 3 years after which there is little change in BMD. A 5 to 10 percent increase in BMD is associated with a 50 percent decrease in fracture rates. Other drugs (fluoride, parathyroid hormone [PTH]) increase bone formation, but none are currently approved for osteoporosis treatment. Newly formed bone either overfills cavities or is added to sites that were not previously resorbed. Drugs that stimulate bone formation result in annual rates of increase in BMD similar to antiresorptive therapies, but the increase continues beyond two years.[13] Table 20-7 lists pharmacologic treatment strategies for osteoporosis.

CALCIUM

Physiologic Effects. Almost all of the body's calcium content is stored in bone. Equilibrium exists between the body's calcium requirements and bone resorption. Serum calcium concentration, PTH, and vitamin D interact to control the resorption of bone to meet the body's calcium needs. On average, regardless of age, the American diet contains insufficient calcium.[33] The NOF recommends daily intake of calcium through a healthy diet with incremental supplementation as needed. Dietary calcium should be increased with dairy products, calcium-fortified juices, green leafy vegetables (e.g., collard and turnip greens and broccoli), and lactose-modified foods, when appropriate (Table 20-8).

Therapeutic Effects. Only a few studies of calcium supplementation (usually with concurrent vitamin D administration) have been conducted that have sufficient sample sizes, adequate duration of follow-up, and a scientifically sound study design to evaluate fracture incidence. These studies generally find fracture rates lower with calcium supplementation when compared to placebo.[34,35] Comparison studies find calcium to be less beneficial with respect to both increased BMD and decreased fracture rates than HRT. Because most studies of HRT included calcium supplementation, adequate dietary or supplemental calcium should be advocated in estrogen users.[36] Synergy between calcium and other osteoporosis prevention and treatment modalities is the key to promoting bone health for women of all ages.

Dosing Regimens. Pharmacists should assist patients in selecting the appropriate calcium supplement and regimen. Calcium may be ingested either in food or through oral supplementation (see Tables 20-7 and 20-8).

Calcium carbonate contains the most elemental calcium by weight (40 percent). Calcium carbonate has acid-dependent absorption and should be taken with meals or vitamin C to increase absorption. Although calcium citrate has acid-independent absorption, the salt contains less elemental calcium and is more costly. Elderly patients, however, may have difficulty absorbing calcium due to decreased acid secretion, so calcium carbonate should be taken with meals or calcium citrate can be substituted. Calcium citrate is also recommended for patients taking daily H_2-receptor blockers or proton pump inhibitors. Calcium is an actively transported substance and the absorption process becomes saturated at about 500 mg. Therefore, divided doses of 500 mg or less should be ingested to enhance the amount absorbed. Calcium products with dolomite or bone meal have been reported to contain lead and should be avoided as calcium supplements.

Side Effects and Contraindications. Few side effects are associated with calcium therapy. The most common side effect is constipation, often occurring at a higher incidence in elderly patients; bloating and abdominal pain may also occur. A sudden increase in calcium intake may promote bloating and constipation, so a gradual increase in consumption is advised. Caution should be exercised in patients with a history of kidney stones, although doses up to 2000 mg/d are generally considered safe.

Drug Interactions Calcium can decrease iron, tetracycline, ciprofloxacin, etidronate, phenytoin, and fluoride absorption when given concomitantly; however, these interactions can be avoided by spacing doses (e.g., administering calcium 1 h before or 2 to 3 h after the other agent).

VITAMIN D AND ITS METABOLITES Vitamin D is a hormone synthesized when skin is exposed to adequate amounts of sunlight. Vitamin D can also be obtained from dietary intake; it is metabolized in the liver to 1-hydroxyvitamin D. Further metabolism

Table 20-7

Pharmacologic Treatment Strategies for Osteoporosis*

DRUG	BRAND NAME	DAILY DOSE	COST/ MONTH#	COMMON SIDE EFFECTS	NOTES
CALCIUM					
Calcium carbonate (OTC)	Tums, Oscal, Oyst-cal	500 mg qd–tid to achieve goal	$4.75–12.80	Bloating, abdominal pain, constipation	Take with food and vitamin C; increase dose slowly; consider citrate for elderly
Calcium citrate (OTC)	Citracal	400 mg qd–qid			
Tricalcium phosphate (OTC)	Posture	600 mg qd–tid			
VITAMIN D					
Calcitrol	Rocaltrol	0.25 µg	$35.91	Hypercalcemia	
Ergocalciferol/ Cholecalciferol (D_2/D_3) (OTC)	Delta-D	200–600 IU qd	$1.00		
HORMONE-REPLACEMENT THERAPY†					
ERT					
Conjugated equine estrogen	Premarin	0.625 mg qd	$14.13	Breast tenderness, menstrual bleeding, migraine headaches	Consider natural estrogen to reduce side effects or continuous dosing regimens
Ethinyl estradiol	Estrace	1 mg qd	$11.69		
HRT (estrogen & progesterone)					
Medroxyprogesterone	Provera	5 mg cyclic 2.5 mg continuous	$7.60 $12.59	Weight gain; pedal edema	Evaluate if irregular bleeding continues after 6 mo; irregular bleeding usually declines with continuance
Micronized progesterone	Prometrium	200 mg cyclic 100 mg continuous	$11.34 $14.18		
Combined‡	Prempro	0.625 mg E/2.5 mg P continuous	$20.05		
	Premphase	0.625 mg E/5 mg P cyclic	$18.38		

Table 20-7

Pharmacologic Treatment Strategies for Osteoporosis* (*Continued.*)

DRUG	BRAND NAME	DAILY DOSE	COST/ MONTH#	COMMON SIDE EFFECTS	NOTES
			SELECTIVE ESTROGEN RECEPTOR MODULATORS		
Raloxifene	Evista	60 mg qd	$59.40	Hot flashes; leg cramps	
			BISPHOSPHONATES		
Alendronate	Fosamax	10 mg qd	$53.54	Dyspepsia, nausea, muscle pain, esophagitis	Take 30 min prior to breakfast after an overnight fast with 8 oz of water; maintain upright position
			CALCITONIN		
Salmon calcitonin	Miacalcin	1 spray (200 IU) into one nostril qd	$81.65§	Rhinitis, epistaxis	Perform nasal exam prior to start of treatment and any time nasal complaints occur
	Calcimar	50–100 IU SC 3 times per week	$62.70//	Nausea, anorexia, diarrhea, abdominal pain, flushing	Consider night-time dosing

*All medications available per prescription only unless otherwise specified.

†Doses of hormones may vary; details on ERT/HRT can be found in Chap. 4.

‡Daily dosage equals one tablet for both combined therapies.

§Price calculated based on 22 doses per bottle, therefore 1.5 bottles per month required; 1 bottle (2 ml) = $54.43.

//Price calculated based on generic equivalent using 50 IU three times weekly; 1 vial = 8 doses, therefore 2 vials per month required; 1 vial = $31.35.

#Prices determined using average wholesale price from 1998 Drug Topics® Red Book. Montvale, NJ: Medical Economics Company, Inc.

Table 20-8

Calcium Content of Selected Foods (adapted from National Osteoporosis Foundation, 1991)

DAIRY FOODS	CONTENT CALCIUM (MG)	NONDAIRY FOODS	CONTENT CALCIUM (MG)
Skim milk, 1 cup	300	Calcium-fortified orange juice, 1 cup	300
Lowfat milk, 1 cup	295	Salmon, canned, with bones, 3 oz	167
Whole milk, 1 cup	290	Oysters, raw, 13–19 medium	226
Yogurt (plain, lowfat), 1 cup	415	Sardines, canned with bones, 3 oz	372
Frozen yogurt (fruit), 1 cup	240	Shrimp, canned, 3 oz	98
Swiss cheese, 1 oz	270	Collard greens, cooked, 1 cup	357
Cheddar, mozzarella, or Muenster cheese, 1 oz	205	Turnip greens, cooked, 1 cup	252
Cottage cheese (lowfat), 4 oz	78	Broccoli, cooked, 1 cup	100
Part-skim ricotta cheese, 4 oz	335	Soybeans, cooked, 1 cup	131
Vanilla ice cream, 1 cup	176	Tofu, 4 oz	108*
Soft-serve vanilla ice cream, 1 cup	236	Almonds, 1 oz	75

*Calcium content of tofu varies depending on processing method; check nutritional label on package for precise calcium content.

to the active metabolite, 1, 25-dihydroxyvitamin D (calcitriol), occurs in the kidney. Calcitriol (Rocaltrol) increases calcium absorption and may have direct effects on bone cells. However, in a study of 622 postmenopausal women with a history of vertebral fractures treated with either calcitriol or calcium for 3 years, calcitriol resulted in no change in the rate of vertebral fractures, whereas the calcium group exhibited an increased rate of vertebral fractures; BMD was not measured.[37]

Vitamin D supplementation (Table 20-7 and 20-9) may be needed for the elderly, patients lacking exposure to sunlight (e.g., residents in long-term care facilities), or individuals with renal disease because a decrease in calcitriol synthesis can occur. Seasonal variations exist for serum vitamin D concentrations; thus seasonal differences in dosage requirements may also exist. Current Recommended Dietary Allowances, especially for the elderly, may be too low (see Table 20-5).[26] The National Institutes of Health Consensus Development Conference recommends intakes of 600 to 800 IU/d for the homebound or institutionalized elderly.

Side Effects and Contraindications. Vitamin D products can cause hypercalcemia and hypercalciuria if doses greater than 800 IU are ingested. Patients receiving higher than 800 IU of vitamin D daily should be under the care of a physician and serum calcium levels should be monitored annually. Patients who are active kidney stone formers and the elderly with elevated blood calcium levels should be evaluated on an individual basis. A decrease in dose or dietary calcium restriction may be required. High serum calcium concentrations could decrease verapamil activity. Concomitant thiazides may increase the serum calcium concentrations. Cholestyramine, mineral oil, phenytoin, and barbiturates can decrease vitamin D concentration.

HORMONE REPLACEMENT THERAPY

Bone Effects. Estrogen has multiple actions that influence bone health and overall women's health. Actions that influence bone density include regulation of calcium absorption and excretion by directly or indirectly modulating PTH, calcitonin, activated vitamin D, and intestinal calcium receptors, and regulation of metabolic bone activity by exerting effects on estrogen receptors located on osteoclasts and osteoblasts.[38] Estrogen produces a transient uncoupling of bone remodeling, slowing resorption and allowing formation to continue until a new equilibrium is established.

Other Effects. Consensus regarding potential extraskeletal benefits such as cardiovascular protection, improvement of vasomotor symptoms, and reduction in overall mortality is available elsewhere,[39] and discussed in Chap. 4. Controversy regarding breast cancer risk and other side effects often dissuades women from beginning HRT.[40] Both potential benefits and risks of HRT need to be discussed prior to initiation of therapy in postmenopausal women.

Therapeutic Effects. ERT or HRT (estrogen with progestin for women with an intact uterus) is one of two first-line therapies for the prevention and treatment of osteoporosis. The U.S. Preventive Services Task Force recommends that all postmenopausal women receive counseling about HRT, regardless of age.[41] The estrogen effect on bone remodeling appears to operate at all ages and is independent of the course or time since onset of menopause. Recent data suggest that ERT be continued into late life for the maintenance of high bone density.[42] Past estrogen use does not provide long-term benefit for preservation of bone density. However, the optimal age for initiating ERT is controversial because similar bone density benefit was observed in women who began ERT after age 60.

Studies have shown that ERT consistently preserves both cortical and trabecular bone. Data suggest that the greatest positive effect is seen during the period of accelerated bone loss, immediately following menopause. A significant increase of 5 to 10 percent in bone mass may occur over several years if estrogen therapy has been initiated within the first 3 to 6 years following menopause. This increase in BMD is associated with a decrease in

fracture rates. Pharmacoeconomic studies support ERT use for fracture prevention. In one cohort study of nearly 9000 women with 15 or more years of estrogen use, a 40 percent reduction in all cause mortality was observed.[43]

More recently, the postmenopausal estrogen/ progestin interventions trial (PEPI), a large, 3-year, prospective trial of 4 different HRT regimens versus placebo, demonstrated significant gains in BMD from baseline at the spine and hip in treatment arms versus placebo.[36] From this study and others, the following conclusions regarding ERT can be made: (1) earlier initiation of estrogen in the postmenopausal phase of accelerated bone turnover will result in better maintenance of bone mass; (2) estrogen exerts its primary beneficial effects on bone only so long as it is taken; (3) benefit will accrue even if estrogen is started many years after menopause; and (4) benefit is lost when ERT is discontinued. Ettinger and Grady recommend that based on estimates of the effect of estrogen treatment on BMD and the effect of changes in BMD on osteoporosis fracture risk, estrogen therapy should start at menopause and continue to the end of life to be most effective. They estimate that this would reduce osteoporotic fracture risk by over 70 percent.[44]

Dosing Regimens. The suggested doses for ERT for osteoporosis prevention are presented in Table 20-7. The majority of epidemiologic data about the safety and efficacy of estrogens relate to oral use; conjugated equine estrogens (Premarin) 0.625 mg is the most common dose studied. However, estrogens reduce bone turnover when administered transdermally, percutaneously, subcutaneously, and intravaginally, provided doses are sufficient.[45]

Vaginal estrogen creams are not routinely used for systemic purposes due to very short half-lives and minimal effects in the systemic circulation or on the endometrium unless given frequently and for a long period of time. Vaginal estradiol tablets and vaginal rings are also available, but use is limited to treatment of genitourinary symptoms because these dosage forms do not provide protection against osteoporosis or ischemic heart disease.[46]

Continuous HRT (estrogens and progesterones dosed daily) appears to be similar to cyclic HRT in preserving bone mass at cortical and trabecular bone sites.[47] In addition, continuous therapy resulted in 93 percent compliance after 1 year of treatment compared with 66 percent compliance in women on traditional cyclic therapy.[48] Cyclic therapy is preferred during the first 5 years of menopause because a more physiologic hormone delivery is provided and less breakthrough bleeding occurs.

Side Effects and Contraindications.   Common adverse effects for HRT include vaginal spotting and bleeding; breast tenderness and breast enlargement, especially in older women; and pedal edema.

Compliance with ERT/HRT is an important issue to address. The two most common reasons women discontinue usage are vaginal bleeding and breast tenderness. Women need to be educated about vaginal bleeding and its expected onset, frequency, and duration. Dosage manipulations may be required to control and eliminate vaginal bleeding. If continuous therapy is used and amenorrhea does not develop after 6–12 months, following a workup to rule out abnormal causes of bleeding is suggested; predictable bleeding patterns with cyclic therapy may be preferred for these women. Breast tenderness may decrease with time. Other management options are described in Chap. 4. The benefits versus risks, including adverse reactions, must be continually assessed.

BISPHOSPHONATES

Bone Effects.   Bisphosphonates are analogues of pyrophosphate that adsorb onto the surface of hydroxyapatite crystals, especially at sites of active bone remodeling. Bisphosphonates inhibit bone resorption by decreasing osteoclastic activity and reducing the rate at which bone remodeling occurs. Specifically, bisphosphonates adsorb to bone hydroxyapatite, become a permanent part of bone structure, and are resistant to enzymatic hydrolysis. The estimated half-life of bisphosphonates is similar to the half-life of bone (1 to 10 years). When osteoclasts bind to the bisphosphonate bone surface, its structure and function are altered, preventing adherence. When osteoclasts phagocytize bone crystals containing these agents, their metabolic activity is inhibited and their ability to resorb additional bone is reduced.

Bisphosphonates are poorly absorbed orally and cause gastroesophageal irritation.[49] The prototype bisphosphonate, etidronate, although not approved for treatment of osteoporosis, has been studied in two prospective randomized controlled trials.[50,51] Results demonstrated increases in lumbar spine BMD and significant reductions in rates of new vertebral fractures. Because etidronate also inhibits bone mineralization and osteomalacia may result, studies of etidronate used a cyclic dosage regimen of daily treatment for 14 days followed by calcium supplementation alone for 3 months. In 1995, a significant advancement in osteoporosis treatment with bisphosphonates occurred when alendronate (Fosamax) was approved for the treatment of osteoporosis (see Table 20-7 for dosing and cost information). The dose of alendronate that inhibits bone resorption is much lower than the dose that inhibits mineralization; therefore, use of alendronate does not lead to bone mineralization problems.

Therapeutic Effects.   Alendronate is approved for both the prevention and treatment of osteoporosis in postmenopausal women. Two large controlled trials confirmed its efficacy for treatment of postmenopausal osteoporosis. The first study followed 994 women with osteoporosis (T-scores < -2.5 SD, with or without baseline vertebral fractures) who were aged 45 to 80 years and at least 5 years postmenopausal.[52] After 3 years, alendronate treatment resulted in significant gains in BMD versus placebo at the lumbar spine (+8.8 percent), femoral neck (+5.9 percent), and trochanter (+7.8 percent). The Vertebral Deformity Study of the Fracture Intervention Trial subsequently reported results from 2027 women aged 55 to 81 years with low femoral neck BMD and at least one vertebral fracture.[53] Women were randomly assigned to 3 years of alendronate treatment or placebo. A significant increase ($P < 0.001$) in posteroanterior spine (6.2 percent) and lateral spine BMD (6.8 percent) were observed in the alendronate-treated women versus placebo.

A recent, double-blinded, placebo-controlled, 6-year study of oral alendronate versus HRT in 1609 healthy postmenopausal women aged 45 to 59 years, prompted the FDA to approve the 5-mg alendronate dose (half the 10-mg treatment dose) for prevention of osteoporosis. This study, the Early Postmenopausal Interventional Cohort trial, enrolled women who were more than 6 months menopausal (average 6.1 years) recruited from four study centers in the United States and Europe.[54] Women receiving placebo lost BMD at all measured sites, but patients treated with alendronate 5 mg demonstrated statistically significant increases in BMD at lumbar spine, hip, and total body ($P < 0.001$). Responses to estrogen-progestin were 1 to 2 percentage points greater than the 5-mg dose of alendronate. Both therapies were well tolerated with safety profiles similar to placebo.

Side Effects and Contraindications. Alendronate appears to be a safe and effective nonhormonal option for prevention of postmenopausal bone loss.[55] The most common adverse effects are abdominal pain, nausea, constipation, diarrhea, flatulence, esophageal ulcer, and acid reflux (3 to 7 percent); headache, and musculoskeletal pain (2 to 3 percent); and taste perversion or dysphagia (1 percent). In a study of 475,000 patients taking alendronate, 51 patients (0.01 percent) had esophageal abnormalities that were considered medication related and serious. On closer examination, each case of esophageal abnormality could be traced to inappropriate administration, that is ingesting less than 8 oz of water when administering the drug or assuming a supine position before 30 min after taking the medication. Esophageal stricture is an absolute contraindication to treatment with alendronate and gastroesophageal reflux disease is a relative contraindication to treatment.

Prevention with 5 mg of alendronate daily should be considered for women who are at high risk for osteoporosis (see Table 20-2) or if BMD testing results indicate low bone mass or osteopenia (T-score between -1 and -2.5). Less than 1 percent of a dose is absorbed, so alendronate must be taken after an overnight fast and 30 min before breakfast with at least 8 oz water (no juice or coffee, tea, mineral water, or other medications); patients should remain upright for at least 30 min and until food is consumed after ingestion to prevent esophagitis and esophageal ulcers. Alendronate is well tolerated; a discontinuance rate of 4 percent versus 6 percent for placebo was demonstrated in a 3-year multicentered trial.

SELECTIVE ESTROGEN RECEPTOR MODULATORS

Bone Effects. Selective estrogen receptor modulators (SERMs) are a structurally diverse group of compounds that interact with the estrogen receptor to elicit either an estrogen agonist or an estrogen antagonist response, depending on the target tissue and physiologic context. SERMs are compounds that can bind to and activate the estrogen receptor, but have tissue-specific effects distinct from estradiol.

Raloxifene, the only SERM approved by the FDA for the prevention or treatment of osteoporosis, has a 1.5 to 2.9 times higher affinity for the estrogen receptor than estradiol. Raloxifene specifically mimics the desirable actions of estrogen on lipids and the skeleton while acting as an antiestrogen in breast and uterine tissue.[56] Raloxifene is absorbed rapidly after oral administration. Dosing and cost information can be found in Table 20-7.

Therapeutic Effects. An interim 2-year analysis of placebo-controlled osteoporosis prevention trials (N = 3300 women) showed that raloxifene is safe and well tolerated. Raloxifene increased bone density by 2 to 3 percent compared to placebo and reduced low-density lipoprotein (LDL) and total cholesterol by 10 to 12 percent. No increased risk of myocardial infarction or stroke has been observed.[57] These changes are similar to the beneficial changes that occur in women on ERT. In contrast to ERT, raloxifene does not appear to cause adverse changes in levels of serum triglycerides; the beneficial effects of ERT on high-density lipoprotein (HDL) cholesterol, however, are not seen with raloxifene.

In a recent, double-blinded, randomized, parallel trial of 390 healthy postmenopausal women, raloxifene in doses of 60 or 120 mg/d was compared to HRT (conjugated estrogens 0.625 mg and medroxyprogesterone 2.5 mg/d) or placebo to determine early lipid and coagulation parameter changes. Raloxifene was found to favorably alter biochemical markers of cardiovascular risk by decreasing LDL cholesterol, fibrinogen, and lipoprotein (a), without raising trigylcerides. When compared to HRT, raloxifene had no effect on HDL cholesterol and plasminogen activator inhibitor-1, and less effect on lipoprotein (a).[59]

Long-term clinical trials are necessary to determine if the favorable biochemical effects are associated with cardiovascular disease protection. Raloxifene is administered without progestins because no endometrial or breast stimulation occurs. In fact, women treated with raloxifene experienced lower rates of endometrial and breast stimulation compared to placebo.[60]

At this time, raloxifene appears to be an alternative to ERT as first-line treatment for prevention or treatment of osteoporosis. Raloxifene also offers an alternative to ERT in postmenopausal women intolerant to or who have contraindications to estrogen treatment. Information regarding cardiovascular benefits compared to ERT is not yet available. (See Addendum on p. 663.)

Side Effects and Contraindications. The majority of adverse effects that occur during raloxifene therapy are mild and do not require discontinuation of treatment. The most common adverse effects reported were hot flashes and leg cramps (1 percent). Raloxifene does not prevent menopausal hot flashes. In fact, hot flashes are observed more commonly during the first 6 months of therapy.

Analysis of raloxifene-treated women showed an increased risk of venous thrombolic events defined as deep vein thrombosis, pulmonary embolism, and retinal vein thrombosis. Risk is greatest during the first 4 months of therapy. Similar to estrogen, raloxifene should be discontinued at least 72 h before and during prolonged immobilization (surgery recovery, prolonged bed rest). Women taking raloxifene should also be advised to avoid prolonged restriction of movement during travel.

Raloxifene should be used with caution in patients with hepatic disease or impairment; however, specific dosing adjustment guidelines have not been established.

Raloxifene is classified as Pregnancy Category X. It should not be administered to patients who are or may become pregnant due to risk for teratogenicity.

Drug Interactions   Drug-drug interactions have been identified between raloxifene and cholestyramine (60% reduction in the absorption and enterohepatic cycling of raloxifene); therefore, administration should be separated 1 hour before or 2 to 3 h after cholestyramine. In addition, coadministration of raloxifene and warfarin results in a 10 percent decrease in prothrombin time. Monitoring of International Normalized Ratio/prothrombin time is advised when using these drugs concomitantly. Because raloxifene is 95 percent bound to plasma proteins, caution is advised when administering with other highly bound drugs like clofibrate, indomethacin, ibuprofen, diazepam, and diazoxide because increased free drug concentrations of these agents may occur, resulting in greater pharmacologic effect or toxicity. Finally, concomitant administration of raloxifene and systemic estrogens is not recommended.

CALCITONIN

Bone Effects.   Calcitonin, a polypeptide hormone that acts as an antiresorptive agent, has been widely used to reverse bone loss observed in Paget's disease of bone, malignant and hyperparathyroid hypercalcemia, and osteoporosis. Calcitonin decreases osteoclast bone attachment, motility, life span, and numbers, along with altering the cellular structure. Bone density is preserved because the mineral, matrix, and collagen material is not broken down. Calcitonin may also preserve BMD by positively effecting osteoblasts.[12] In 1995, intranasal salmon calcitonin (Miacalcin) was approved by the FDA for the treatment of postmenopausal osteoporosis for women at least 5 years postmenopause who cannot or will not take estrogen (see Table 20-7).

Therapeutic Effects.   Studies using nasal salmon calcitonin are of relatively small size and shorter duration than HRT and bisphosphonate trials. Clinical trials have shown a stabilization or increase in bone mass, especially lumbar bone density (3 percent over a 2-year period) when compared to placebo. Cortical bone either remains constant or has a slight increase. Patients with high bone turnover, such as corticosteroid-induced osteoporosis, respond better to calcitonin than those with normal or low bone turnover rates. However, elderly women who often have a low bone turnover rate have demonstrated decreased bone resorption with calcitonin.[12]

Overgaard et al. studied 208 women aged 68 to 72 years with established osteoporosis for 2 years using 200 IU calcitonin intranasally daily in a placebo-controlled, blinded study.[62] Women treated with intranasal calcitonin demonstrated a 3 percent gain in lumbar BMD. Although not powered to detect reduction in fracture rates, the investigators reported an approximately one-third reduction in the rate of new vertebral compression fractures.

Some trials of continuous administration of calcitonin for 2 years have found that increases in bone density plateau or decrease after 12 to 18 months. Potentially, neutralizing antibodies, which develop in 40 to 70 percent of patients treated with subcutaneous calcitonin, appear to reduce

calcitonin's effect and may be partly responsible for the resistance sometimes observed with continuous long-term treatment.[10] Interestingly, resistance to both the subcutaneous and intranasal formulations may occur (usually after 18 to 24 months of therapy); however, intermittent therapy may prevent resistance. Overall, calcitonin has been effective in decreasing biochemical markers of bone turnover and preventing bone loss in osteoporosis. However, nasal calcitonin appears to be less effective than estrogen or alendronate at preventing bone loss at the hip.[7]

Analgesic Effect   In addition to its antiresorptive bone properties, calcitonin exerts a primary analgesic effect for some patients following acute vertebral crush fracture. Treatment may lead to early recovery and avoids the complications of prolonged bed rest. Calcitonin has gained additional interest for osteoporosis pain control.[63] Both subcutaneous and intranasal administration bring pain relief within 1 to 12 weeks to patients with osteoporotic or metastatic bone pain. Analgesic effects can be seen within 3 days when used for acute bone fractures; chronic osteoporosis-related bone pain improvement may be slower, taking several months for maximal effect to be observed.[18] Daily administration is initially used and then decreased to 50 to 100 IU two or three times a week. Potential mechanisms of action include decreased prostaglandin synthesis, altered intracellular calcium concentrations, or increased β-endorphin synthesis.

Side Effects and Contraindications.   Side effects of parenteral administration include anorexia, metallic/salty taste, nausea, vomiting and diarrhea (10 to 20 percent); flushing of face, ears, and occasionally upper body (10 percent); and rash that is generalized or at an injection site (5 percent). Less common side effects are increased urination, pruritus, and puffiness of the hands and feet. Most side effects decrease over time and may also decrease with nighttime administration. Due to the chronicity of osteoporosis and disadvantages inherent to injectable formulations, the nasal formulation is recommended for treatment of established osteoporosis. Approximately 10–25 percent of nasal calcitonin is absorbed and this product produces fewer side effects. The nasal spray is administered one spray (200 IU) per day, alternating nostrils to minimize local side effects. The most commonly reported adverse effects include rhinitis (12 percent); epistaxis (4 percent); and sinusitis (2 percent); normal saline "rinse" is suggested as a measure to reduce local irritation. Baseline nasal examinations with visualization of the nasal mucosa, turbinates, septum, and mucosal blood vessel status are recommended with repeat examinations at any time nasal complaints occur; approximately 4 percent of patients discontinue treatment due to local effects.[64] Drug holidays may be considered for excessive irritation. As with other

treatments for osteoporosis, concurrent calcium (1500 mg elemental per day) and vitamin D (400 IU/d) are recommended for optimal effects.

PHYTOESTROGENS Phytoestrogens are naturally occurring plant sterols that exert effects similar to estrogen.[65] One type of phytoestrogen is the isoflavones, which are found in soy beans, garbanzo beans, and other legumes. The isoflavones genestein and daidzein have a molecular structure similar to that of estradiol.[66] These phytoestrogens have a low binding affinity for estrogen receptor (ER)-α and a high affinity for ER-β; the key beneficial effects on bone and heart may be mediated through ER-β. Each gram of soy protein contains 4 to 5 mg phytoestrogen and for positive effects, a woman would require approximately 60 mg/d.[67] Asian women typically ingest 40 to 80 mg/d, where-

Table 20-9

Vitamin D Content of Selected Foods

FOOD CATEGORY	FOOD	SERVING SIZE	VITAMIN D CONTENT
Dairy foods	Milk—fortified with vitamin D	1 cup	100 IU
	Swiss cheese	3½ oz (100 g)	100 IU
	Edam cheese	3½ oz (100 g)	84 IU
	Pudding—mix, made with vitamin D-fortified milk	½ cup	50 IU
Eggs	Egg, medium, boiled	1	23 IU
Fats and candy	Margarine	3½ oz (100 g)	320 IU
		1 tablespoon	46 IU
	Milk chocolate with almonds	1 oz	10 IU
	Milk chocolate	1 oz	25 IU
	Chocolate with crisped rice	1 oz	20 IU
Fish and meats	Salmon, canned	3½ oz (100 g)	500 IU
	Sardines, canned in oil	3½ oz (100 g)	300 IU
	Chicken liver, simmered	3½ oz (100 g)	67 IU
	Pork bacon, cooked	1 slice	3 IU
	Hotdog, beef	1	11 IU
Cereals	Corn flakes, Kellogg's	1¼ oz	50 IU
	Frosted mini-wheats	4 biscuits	50 IU
	Product 19	¾ cup	50 IU
	Raisin Bran, Kellogg's	¾ cup	50 IU

SOURCE: Abstracted from Pennington JAT, Church HN: *Food Values of Portions Commonly Used,* 14th ed. New York: Harper & Row; 1985.

as American women ingest only about 3 mg/d.[63] One trial found that administration of 45 g soy grits daily increased BMD by 5.4 percent after three months of treatment.[68] The isoflavone content of common soy foods is shown in Table 20-10.[65]

Ipriflavone, an isoflavone synthesized from the soy isoflavone daidzein, is being investigated in clinical trials. Ipriflavone inhibits osteoclast production, inhibits PTH responsiveness, and increases osteoblast maturation. Clinical trials with ipriflavone have found an increase in radial bone density, no change in lumbar bone density, and a decrease in bone pain.[12] Tentative evidence suggests that phytoestrogens may have similar effects in maintaining bone density to those of ipriflavone.

To date, data are insufficient to recommend particular dietary practices or changes, but encouraging findings from laboratory and clinical studies indicate the need for further research to clarify the role of phytoestrogens for osteoporosis treatment.

Algorithms for the Evaluation and Treatment of Osteoporosis

The NOF has published universal recommendations for all patients to maximize and preserve bone mass including an adequate intake of calcium and vitamin D, regular weight-bearing exercise, avoidance of tobacco use and alcohol abuse, and treatment of other fracture risk factors (e.g.,

Table 20-10

Isoflavones in Foodstuffs

FOODSTUFF	SERVING SIZE	ISOFLAVONES
Tofu, tempeh	100 g	62–112 mg
Miso	120 g	40 mg
Soy milk	250 g	40 mg
Texturized soy protein	100 g	138 mg
Soy beans, roasted	100 g	162 mg
Green soy	100 g	135 mg

SOURCE: Taylor M: Alternatives to conventional hormone replacement therapy. *Comp Ther* 23:514, 1997.

impaired vision).[14] Figure 20-4 provides an algorithm for the treatment of pre- and perimenopausal women with one or more risk factors for osteoporosis and Fig. 20-5 provides an algorithm for the management of postmenopausal women at risk for osteoporosis. The algorithms incorporate NOF recommendations and data obtained from the literature.[8,14] Treatment for osteoporosis should be based on strong evidence that an intervention will prevent fractures and their consequences, that expected benefits outweigh any potential adverse effects, and that a reasonable use of resources are represented.

Combination Drug Therapy

At present, combination drug therapy for osteoporosis has not been approved by the FDA. However, studies with ERT in combination with bisphosphonates have shown a greater increase in BMD at both the hip and spine sites that with either treatment alone.[69] In fact, alendronate data are currently being reviewed by the FDA for a combination therapy indication with ERT.

Emerging Concepts

Fluoride

Although research is being conducted on slow-release fluoride formulations, fluoride is not approved for osteoporosis treatment in the United States. Fluoride (sodium fluoride or monofluorophosphate) may increase osteoblasts through a mitogenic effect, resulting in increased bone formation. The fluoride ion serves as a hydroxy radical in the hydroxyapatite crystals, forming fluorapatite, which alters the size and structure of crystals and results in increased bone crystallinity and a decrease in solubility. The net effect is a mineral

Figure 20-4

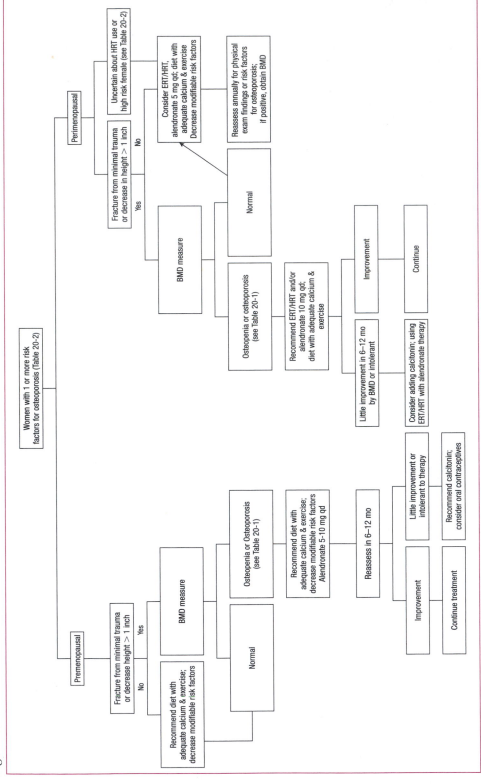

Algorithm for the evaluation and treatment of osteoporosis in pre- and peri-menopausal women with one or more risk factors for osteoporosis.

Figure 20-5

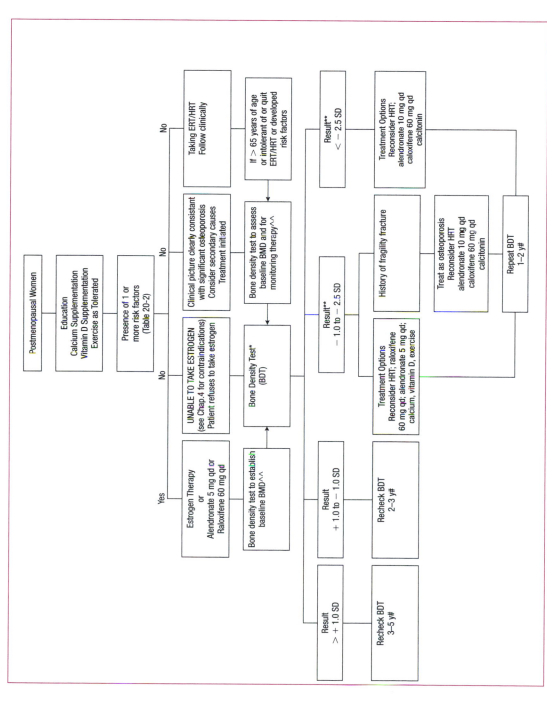

Algorithm for the evaluation and treatment of osteoporosis in postmenopausal women. (*Modified with permission from PD Miller et al, for the Society of Clinical Densitometry. Semin Arthritis Rheum 25:361, Copyright 1996.*)[9]

^^Based on National Osteoporosis Foundation, Washington, DC, Copyright 1998.[14]

*Using T-score   **Consider secondary causes (Table 20–2)

#Reassess annually for physical findings and risk factors of osteoporosis

ABBREVIATIONS: BDT, bone density testing; BMD, bone mineral density; ERT, estrogen replacement therapy; HRT, hormone replacement therapy; qd, once daily; SD, standard deviation.

system more resistant to resorption. Fluoride also uncouples the normal bone remodeling process to favor formation over resorption.

Bone density has been shown to increase with fluoride, but the bone formed may be somewhat disorganized, resulting in immature woven bone rather than lamellar bone. Fluoride-made bone appears to be more resistant to compressive forces, but less to torsional strain, which is believed to be responsible for hip fractures.[70] Some studies report an increase or no change in hip or peripheral fractures in fluoride-treated patients versus placebo. In one study of 202 osteoporotic women, treatment with sodium fluoride resulted in an 8 percent per year increase in lumbar spine BMD over the 4-year study period. However, there was substantial bone loss from the forearm that indicated redistribution of bone mineral from the cortical to trabecular bone.[71] The large amounts of newly formed matrix in trabecular bone require large amounts of calcium absorption, so to compensate, minerals are removed from cortical bone, making it weaker and more susceptible to fractures. Researchers propose the use of lower doses and sustained-release fluoride products with sufficient calcium and vitamin D to decrease the negative effect on cortical bone. Currently lower doses (10 to 20 mg fluoride), sustained-release products, and intermittent therapy are being investigated.[72]

Other Treatments

HORMONAL METHODS

At present, several additional agents are being investigated for the treatment of osteoporosis. PTH stimulates bone turnover, differentiation of new bone and remodeling units, and renal tubular reabsorption of calcium. The few clinical studies using PTH report no clinically significant benefits. In addition, only parenteral formulations are available, precluding use as a first-line agent.[12]

Tibolone is a synthetic hormone being evaluated as an estrogen substitute due to preliminary data that supports its efficacy at decreasing bone loss without causing vaginal bleeding.[73,74] Oral contraceptives have also been explored to maintain bone mass in premenopausal and perimenopausal women, elite anthletes, and anorexia nervosa patients with amenorrhea. In fact, oral contraceptive use during the perimenopausal time frame to avoid periods of estrogen deficiency may be advocated in the future.[10]

ANTIRESORPTIVE AGENTS

Several investigational antiresoptive agents are being studied. Because prostaglandins may have a role in bone remodeling, research with nonsteroidal anti-inflammatory drugs is being conducted to determine if decreased prostaglandin production could influence bone. Other antiresorptive agents under investigation include echistatin and potassium bicarbonate, which are thought to minimize bone destruction by creating a better acid–base balance (i.e., correcting acid imbalances) in the body.

BONE-FORMING AGENTS

Investigational bone formation agents such as recombinant growth hormone and insulin-like growth factors (IGF-I, IGF-II, transforming growth factor-β) have also been investigated for treating osteoporosis. Growth hormone and IGF have been associated with stimulating both bone formation and bone resorption. In growth hormone clinical trials, bone formation and resorption have been stimulated, based on blood and urine indices, but minimal to no changes occur in BMD.[75] Most likely, these agents will not be given as single agents but may have a future role in combination therapy to stimulate or mimic the normal bone remodeling process.

References

1. *Stand up to Osteoporosis: Your Guide to Staying Healthy and Independent through Prevention and Treatment.* Washington, DC: National Osteoporosis Foundation; 1997:10.

2. Concensus Development Conference: Diagnosis, prophylaxis, and treatment of osteoporosis. *Am J Med* 94:646, 1993.

3. The WHO Study Group: *Assessment of Fracture Risk and Its Application to Screening for Postmenopausal Osteoporosis.* Technical Report Series, No. 843. Geneva, Switzerland: World Health Organization; 1994.

4. National Osteoporosis Foundation: *1996 and 2015 Osteoporosis Prevalence Figures: State-by-State Report.* Washington, DC: Author; 1997.

5. Ott SM: Osteoporosis and osteopmalacia. In: Hazzard WR, Blass JP, Ettinger Jr WH, et al (eds): *Principles of Geriatric Medicine and Gerontology,* 4th ed. New York: McGraw-Hill; 1999:Chap. 80.

6. National Institute of Arthritis and Musculoskeletal and Skin Diseases. Washington, DC: National Institutes of Health. National Resource Center for Osteoporosis and Related Bone Diseases, 1997. Internet page at URI: http://www.nrc@nof.org.

7. Hurley DL, Khosla S: Update on primary osteoporosis. *Mayo Clin Proc* 72:943, 1997.

8. Scheiber LB, Torregrosa L: Evaluation and treatment of postmenopausal osteoporosis. *Semin Arthritis Rheum* 27:245, 1998.

9. Miller PD, Bonnick SL, Rosen CJ, for the Society for Clinical Densitometry, et al: Clinical utility of bone mass measurements in adults: consensus of an international panel. *Semin Arthritis Rheum* 25:361, 1996.

10. Oconnell MB, Bauwens SF: Osteoporosis and osteomalacia. In: DiPiro JT, Talbert RL, Yee GC, et al (eds): *Pharmacotherapy: A Pathophysiologic Approach,* 3rd ed. Stamford, CT: Appleton & Lange; 1997; 1689.

11. Golden BD: The prevention and treatment of osteoporosis. *Arthritis Care and Research* 11:124, 1998.

12. Eastell R: Treatment of postmenopausal osteoporosis. *N Engl J Med* 338:736, 1998.

13. Riggs BL, Melton LJ III: Clinical heterogeneity of involutional osteoporosis: implications for preventive therapy. *J Clin Endocrinol Metab* 70:1229, 1990.

14. National Osteoporosis Foundation. *Physician's Guide to Prevention and Treatment of Osteoporosis.* Washington DC: Author, 1998.

15. Black DM: Why elderly women should be screened and treated to prevent osteoporosis. *Am J Med* 98(suppl 2A):67S, 1995.

16. Kanis JA: Diagnosis of osteoporosis. *Osteoporosis Int* 7(suppl 3):S108, 1997.

17. Riggs BL: Osteoporosis. In: Wyngaarden JB, Smith LH Jr (eds): *Cecil Textbook of Medicine,* 18th ed. Philadelphia: Saunders; 1988:1510.

18. Tresolini CP, Gold DT, Lee LS, eds.: *Working with Patients to Prevent, Treat, and Manage Osteoporosis: A Curriculum Guide for the Health Professions,* 2nd ed. San Francisco: National Fund for Medical Education; 1998.

19. Melton LJ, Atkinson EJ, O'Fallon WM, et al: Long-term fracture prediction by bone mineral assessed at different skeletal sites. *J Bone Miner Res* 8:1227, 1993.

20. Cummings SR, Black DM, Nevitt MC, et al: Bone density at various sites for prediction of hip fractures. *Lancet* 341:72, 1993.

21. Levis S, Altman R: Bone densitometry: clinical considerations. *Arthritis Rheum* 41:577, 1998.

22. Jonsson B, Christiansen C, Johnell O, et al: Cost-effectiveness of fracture prevention in established osteoporosis. *Osteoporosis Int* 5:136, 1995.

23. Johnston CC, Slemenda CW, Melton LJ: Current concepts: clinical use of bone densitometry. *N Engl J Med* 324:1105, 1991.

24. Jergas M, Genant HK: Current methods and recent advances in the diagnosis of osteoporosis. *Arthritis Rheum* 36:1649, 1993.

25. Christiansen C: Osteoporosis: diagnosis and management today and tomorrow. *Bone* 17:513S, 1995.

26. Finn SC: The skeleton crew: Is calcium enough? *J Womens Health* 7:31, 1998.

27. Massey LK, Whiting SJ: Caffeine, urinary calcium, calcium metabolism and bone. *J Nutr* 123:1611, 1993.

28. Baron JA, LaVecchia CL, Levi F: The antiestrogenic effect of cigarette smoking in women. *Am J Obstet Gynecol* 162:505, 1990.

29. Moniz C: Alcohol and bone. *Br Med Bull* 50:67, 1994.

30. Diamond T, Stiel D, Lunzer M, et al: Ethanol reduces bone formation and may cause osteoporosis. *Am J Med* 86:282, 1989.

31. Klein RF: Alcohol-induced bone disease: impact of ethanol on osteoblast proliferation. *Alcohol Clin Exp Res* 21:392, 1997.

32. Nelson ME, Fiatarone MA, Morganti CM, et al: Effects of high-intensity strength training on multiple risk factors for osteoporotic fractures. *JAMA* 272:1909, 1994.

33. Reid IR, Ames RW, Evans MC, et al: Long-term effects of calcium supplementation on bone loss

and fractures in postmenopausal women: a randomized controlled trial. *Am J Med* 98:331, 1995.

34. Recker RR, Hinders S, Davies KM, et al: Correcting calcium nutritional deficiency prevents spine fracture in elderly women. *J Bone Miner Res* 11:1961, 1996.

35. Carr CJ, Shamgraw RF: Nutritional and pharmaceutical aspects of calcium supplementation. *Am Pharm* 27:49, 1987.

36. The Writing Group for the PEPI trial: Effects of hormone therapy on bone mineral density: results from the postmenopausal estrogen/progestin interventions (PEPI) trial. *JAMA* 276:1389, 1996.

37. Tilyard MW, Spears GFS, Thomson J, et al: Treatment of postmenopausal osteoporosis with calcitriol or calcium. *N Engl J Med* 326:357, 1992.

38. Notelovitz M: Estrogen therapy and osteoporosis: principles & practice. *Am J Med Sci* 313:2, 1997.

39. Grodstein F, Stampfer MJ, Colditz GA, et al: Postmenopausal hormone therapy and mortality. *N Engl J Med* 330:1062, 1997.

40. Lindsay R, Bush TL, Grady D, et al: Therapeutic controversy: estrogen replacement in menopause. *J Clin Endocrinol Metab* 81:3829, 1996.

41. US Preventive Services Task Force: *Guide to Clinical Preventive Services,* 2nd ed. New York: Williams & Wilkins; 1995.

42. Schneider DL, Barrett-Connor EL, Morton DJ: Timing of postmenopausal estrogen for optimal bone mineral density. *JAMA* 277:543, 1997.

43. Henderson BE, Paganini-Hill A, Ross RK: Decreased mortality in users of estrogen replacement therapy. *Arch Intern Med* 151:75, 1991.

44. Ettinger B, Grade D: Maximizing the benefit of estrogen therapy for prevention of osteoporosis. *Menopause: The Journal of the North American Menopause Society* 1:19, 1994.

45. Lindey R: Therapeutic controversy: estrogen replacement in menopause. *J Clin Endocrinol Metab* 81:3829, 1996.

46. Jacobs S, Hillard TC: Hormone replacement therapy in the aged: a state of the art review. *Drugs Aging* 8:193, 1996.

47. Grey AB, Cundy TF, Reid IR: Continuous combined oestrogen/progestin therapy is well tolerated and increases bone density at the hip and spine in postmenopausal osteoporosis. *Clin Endocrinol* 40:671, 1994.

48. Doren M, Reuther G, Minne HW, et al: Superior compliance and efficacy of continuous combined oral estrogen-progestogen therapy in postmenopausal women. *Am J Obstet Gynecol* 173: 1446, 1995.

49. Francis RM: Bisphosphonates in the treatment of osteoporosis in 1997: a review. *Curr Ther Res* 58: 656, 1997.

50. Miller PD, Watts NB, Licata AA, et al: Cyclical etidronate in the treatment of postmenopausal osteoporosis: efficacy and safety after seven years of treatment. *Am J Med* 103:468, 1997.

51. Masud T, Mulcahy B, Thompson AV, et al: Effects of cyclical etidronate combined with calcitriol versus cyclical etidronate alone on spine and femoral neck bone mineral density in postmenopausal osteoporotic women. *Am Rheum Dis* 57:346, 1998.

52. Liberman UA, Weiss SR, Broll J, et al., for the Alendronate Phase III Osteoporosis Treatment Study Group: Effect of oral alendronate on bone mineral density and the incidence of fractures in postmenopausal osteoporosis. *N Engl J Med* 333:1437, 1995.

53. Black DM, Cummings SR, Karpf DB, et al: Randomized trial of effect of alendronate on risk of fracture in women with existing vertebral fractures. *Lancet* 348:1535, 1996.

54. Hosking D, Chilvers CED, Christiansen C, et al., for the Early Postmenopausal Intervention Cohort Study Group: Prevention of bone loss with alendronate in postmenopausal women under 60 years of age. *N Engl J Med* 228:485, 1998.

55. McClung M, Clemmesen B, Daifotis A, et al., for the Alendronate Osteoporosis Prevention Study Group: Alendronate prevents postmenopausal bone loss in women without osteoporosis: a double-blind, randomized, controlled trial. *Ann Intern Med* 128: 253, 1998.

56. Ashworth LE: Focus on raloxifene: a selective estrogen receptor modulator for prevention of osteoporosis in postmenopausal women. *Formulary* 33:305, 1998.

57. Delmas PD, Bjarnason NH, Mitlak BH, et al: Effects of raloxifene on bone mineral density, serum cholesterol concentrations, and uterine endometrium in postmenopausal women. *N Engl J Med* 337:1641, 1997.

58. Ettinger B, Black DM, Mitlak BH, et al: Reduction of vertebral fracture risk in postmenopausal women with osteoporosis treated with raloxifene: results from a 3-year randomized clinical trial. *JAMA* 282 (7):637,1999.

59. Walsh BW, Kuller LH, Wild RA, et al: Effects of raloxifene on serum lipids and coagulation factors in healthy postmenopausal women. *JAMA* 279: 1445,1998.

60. Boss SM, Huster WJ, Neild JA, et al: Effects of raloxifene hydrochloride on the endometrium of postmenopausal women. *Am J Obstet Gynecol* 177: 1458,1997.

61. Cummings SR, Eckert S, Krueger A, et al: The effect of raloxifene on risk of breast cancer in postmenopausal women: results from the MORE randomized trial. *JAMA* 281(23):2189, 1999.

62. Overgaard K, Hansen MA, Jensen SB, Christiansen C: Effect of salcatonin given intranasally on bone mass and fracture rates in established osteoporosis: a dose-response study. *BMJ* 305:556, 1992.

63. Gennari C, Agnusdei D, Camporeale A: Use of calcitonin in the treatment of bone pain associated with osteoporosis. *Calcif Tissue Int* 49(suppl 2):S9, 1991.

64. Plosker GL, McTavish D: Intranasal salcatonin (salmon calcitonin): a review of its pharmacological properties and role in the management of postmenopausal osteoporosis. *Drugs Aging* 8:378, 1996.

65. Taylor M: Alternatives to conventional hormone replacement therapy. *Comp Ther* 23:514, 1997.

66. Barnes S: Evolution of the health benefits of soy isoflavones. *Proc Soc Exp Biol Med* 217:386, 1998.

67. Tham DM, Gardner CD, Haskell WL: Clinical review 97: potential health benefits of dietary phytoestrogens: a review of the clinical, epidemiological and mechanistic evidence. *J Clin Endocrinol Metab* 83:2223, 1998.

68. Murkies A: Phytoestrogens—what is the current knowledge? *Aust Fam Physician* 27(suppl 1):S47, 1998.

69. Seeman E: Osteoporosis: trials and tribulations. *Am J Med* 103(2A):74S, 1997.

70. Kanis JA: Treatment of symptomatic osteoporosis with fluoride. *Am J Med* 95(suppl 5A):S53, 1993.

71. Riggs BL, Hodgson SF, O'Fallon WM, et al: Effect of fluoride treatment on the fracture rate in postmenopausal women with osteoporosis. *N Engl J Med* 322:802, 1990.

72. Yves Reginster JY, Meurmans L, Zegels B, et al: The effect of sodium monofluorophosphate plus calcium on vertebral fracture rate in postmenopausal women with moderate osteoporosis: a randomized, controlled trial. *Ann Intern Med* 129:1, 1998.

73. Studd J, Arnala I, Kicovic PM, et al: A randomized study of tibolone on bone mineral density in osteoporotic postmenopausal women with previous fractures. *Obstet Gynecol* 92(4 Pt 1):574, 1998.

74. Lippuner K, Haenggi W, Birkhaeuser MH, et al: Prevention of postmenopausal bone loss using tibolone or conventional peroral or transdermal hormone replacement therapy with 17-beta-estradiol and dydrogesterone. *J Bone Miner Res* 12:806, 1997.

75. Rubin CD: Southwestern Internal Medicine Conference: growth hormone—aging and osteoporosis. *Am J Med Sci* 305:120, 1993.

Addendum

Investigators from the Medical Outcomes of Raloxifene Evaluation (MORE) study, a 25-country, 3-year placebo-controlled trial of raloxifene use in almost 7,000 postmenopausal women with osteoporosis, found that 60 mg/d of raloxifene increased BMD in both the spine (2.6 percent) and the femoral neck (2.1 percent).[58] More importantly, raloxifene decreased the risk of vertebral fracture (RR = 0.7, 95 percent, CI = 0.5–0.8); 10 percent of women receiving placebo had at least one new vertebral fracture vs. 6.6 percent of those on raloxifene. Although raloxifene use was associated with an increased risk of venous thromboembolism (1 percent vs. 0.3 percent for placebo; RR = 3.1, 95 percent CI = 1.5–6.2), raloxifene does not causal vaginal bleeding or breast tenderness. The MORE trial also demonstrated that raloxifene decreased the risk of estrogen receptor-positive breast cancer by 90 percent (RR = 0.10, 95 percent CI = 0.04–0.24); it did not decrease the risk for estrogen receptor-negative invasive breast cancer. Raloxifene was also found not to increase the risk for endometrial cancer (RR = 0.8, 95 percent CI = 0.2–2.7).[61]

Index

Page numbers ending in "*f*" refer to illustrations: those ending in "*t*" refer to tables.

ISBN 0-07-069767-1

9 780070 697676

90000